Evidence-Based Chronic Pain Management

Edited by

Catherine F. Stannard MB ChB, FRCA, FFPMRCA

Consultant in Pain Medicine
Pain Clinic, Macmillan Centre
Frenchay Hospital
Bristol, UK

Eija Kalso MD, DMedSci

Professor of Pain Medicine
University of Helsinki and Pain Clinic
Department of Anaesthesia and Intensive Care Medicine
Helsinki University Central Hospital
Finland

Jane Ballantyne MD, FRCA

Professor of Anesthesiology and Critical Care
Penn Pain Medicine Center
Hospital of the University of Pennsylvania
Philadelphia
PA, USA

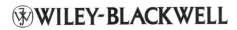
WILEY-BLACKWELL

A John Wiley & Sons, Ltd., Publication

BMJ Books

ISBN: 9781405152914

Library of Congress Cataloging-in-Publication Data

Evidence-based chronic pain management / edited by Catherine F. Stannard, Eija Kalso, Jane Ballantyne.
    p. ; cm.
  Includes bibliographical references and index.
  ISBN 978-1-4051-5291-4
  1. Chronic pain.   I. Stannard, Catherine F.   II. Kalso, Eija, 1955-   III. Ballantyne, Jane, 1948-
  [DNLM: 1. Pain—therapy. 2. Chronic Disease. 3. Evidence-Based Medicine. WL 704 E925 2010]
RB127.E95 2010
616′.0472—dc22
                                                                          2009042743
A catalogue record for this book is available from the British Library.

Set in 9.5/12pt Minion by Macmillan Publishing Solutions, Chennai, India

Printed and bound in Singapore by Fabulous Printers Pte Ltd

1   2010

Contents

Evidence-Based Medicine Series

Updates and additional resources for the books in this series are available from:
www.evidencebasedseries.com

List of contributors

Amy Abernethy MD
Associate Director
Duke Comprehensive Cancer Center
Associate Professor of Medicine
Duke University Medical Center
Durham, NC, USA

Paulin Andréll MD
Pain Centre, Department of Medicine
Sahlgrenska University Hospital/Östra
Göteborg University
Göteborg, Sweden

Andrew P. Baranowski BSc Hons, MBBS, FRCA, MD, FFPMRCA
Consultant and Honorary Senior Lecturer in Pain Medicine
The Pain Management Centre
The National Hospital for Neurology and Neurosurgery
University College London Hospitals
London, UK

Ralf Baron MD
Head, Division of Neurological Pain Research and Therapy
Department of Neurology
Universitaetsklinikum Schleswig-Holstein
Kiel, Germany

Rae Frances Bell MD, PhD
Senior Consultant Anaesthetist
Head of Multidisciplinary Pain Clinic/Research Fellow
Regional Centre of Excellence in Palliative Care
Haukeland University Hospital Bergen, Norway

Andreas Binder MD
Division of Neurological Pain Research and Therapy
Department of Neurology
Universitaetsklinikum Schleswig-Holstein
Kiel, Germany

Allan Binder
Lister Hospital
E & N Hertfordshire NHS Trust
Stevenage, UK

L. Vandy Black MD
Division of Pediatric Hematology
Johns Hopkins University
Baltimore, MD, USA

Mats Börjesson MD, PhD
Associate Professor, Sahgrenska University Hospital/Östra
Department of Medicine and Pain Center
Göteborg, Sweden

Michael Chester MBBS MRCP MD FESC
Consultant Cardiologist & Director
National Refractory Angina Centre
Royal Liverpool and Broadgreen University Hospital
Liverpool, UK

Steven P. Cohen MD
Johns Hopkins Medical Institutions
Baltimore, MD
Walter Reed Army Medical Center
Washington, DC, USA

Beverly Collett MB.BS, FRCA, FFPMRCA
Consultant in Pain Medicine
Pain Management Service
University Hospitals of Leicester
Leicester, UK

Paul Creamer MD, FRCP
Consultant Rheumatologist
Southmead Hospital, Bristol, UK

Christina Daousi MRCP, MD

Senior Lecturer and Honorary Consultant Physician in
Diabetes & Endocrinology
University Hospital Aintree
Clinical Sciences Centre
Liverpool, UK

Sheena Derry MA

Senior Research Officer
Nuffield Department Anaesthetics
University of Oxford
Oxford, UK

Anthony Dickenson PhD

Professor of Neuropharmacology
Department of Pharmacology
University College London
London, UK

Anthony Dragovich MD

Assistant Professor of Anesthesiology
Womack Army Medical Center
Fort Bragg, NC, USA

Robert H. Dworkin PhD

Professor of Anesthesiology, Neurology, Oncology, and
Psychiatry
University of Rochester School of Medicine and
Dentistry
Rochester, NY, USA

Christopher Eccleston PhD

Professor of Psychology & Director
Centre for Pain Research and
Coordinating Editor of Pain Palliative and Supportive Care
Cochrane Review Group
University of Bath, Bath, UK

Edzard Ernst MD, PhD, FMed Sci, FSB, FRCP, FRCP (Edin.)

Laing Chair of Complementary Medicine
Peninsula Medical School
Universities of Exeter and Plymouth
Exeter, UK

Nanna B. Finnerup MD, PhD

Associate Professor, Danish Pain Research Center
and Department of Neurology
Aarhus University Hospital, Aarhus, Denmark

Victoria Harvey PhD

Department of Pharmacology
University College London
London, UK

Winfried Häuser MD

Head, Psychosomatic Medicine
Department Internal Medicine 1
Center of Pain Therapy
Klinikum Saarbrücken
Saarbrücken, Germany

Rita Janes MD

Consultant in Oncology
Department of Oncology
Helsinki University Hospital
Helsinki, Finland

Troels Staehelin Jensen MD, DMSc

Professor of Experimental and Clinical Pain Research
Danish Pain Research Center and Department of Neurology
Aarhus University Hospital
Aarhus, Denmark

Mark I. Johnson PhD, BSc

Professor of Pain and Analgesia
Faculty of Health, Leeds Metropolitan University
and Leeds Pallium Research Group
Leeds, UK

Francis J. Keefe PhD

Professor & Director, Pain Prevention and Treatment
Research Program
Department of Psychiatry and Behavioral Sciences
Duke University Medical Center
Durham, NC, USA

Henriette Klit MD

Danish Pain Research Center and Department of Neurology
Aarhus University Hospital
Aarhus, Denmark

Bart Koes PhD

Professor of General Practice
Erasmus MC-University Medical Center
Rotterdam, The Netherlands

Austin Leach FRCA, FFPMRCA

Consultant in Pain Medicine
National Refractory Angina Centre
Royal Liverpool and Broadgreen University Hospital
Liverpool, UK

Raphael Leo MA, MD

Associate Professor, Department of
Psychiatry
School of Medicine and Biomedical Sciences
State University of New York at Buffalo
Buffalo, NY, USA

Bengt Linderoth MD, PhD

Professor & Head; Functional
Neurosurgery
and Applied Neuroscience Research
Program
Karolinska Institutet
Stockholm, Sweden

Sarah Love-Jones

Frenchay Hospital
Bristol, UK

Clas Mannheimer MD

Professor & Head, Multidisciplinary
Pain Center
Department of Medicine
Sahlgrenska University Hospital/Östra
University of Göteborg
Göteborg, Sweden

Ellen McGough PhD, PT

Biobehavioral Nursing and Health Systems
University of Washington
Washington, DC, USA

Henry McQuay DM, FRCA, FRCP(Edin)

Nuffield Professor of Clinical Anaesthetics
John Radcliffe Hospital
University of Oxford
Oxford, UK

Andrew Moore DSC

Research Director
Nuffield Department of Anaesthetics
University of Oxford
John Radcliffe Hospital
Oxford, UK

David B. Morris PhD

University Professor
University of Virginia
Charlottesville
VA, USA

Timothy J. Ness MD, PHD

Simon Gelman Endowed Professor
Department of Anesthesiology
University of Alabama at Birmingham
Birmingham, AL, USA

Lone Nikolajsen MD, PhD

Consultant, Department of Anaesthesiology
and Danish Pain Research Center
Aarhus University Hospital
Aarhus, Denmark

Turo J. Nurmikko MD, PhD

Professor of Pain Science
Neuroscience Research Unit
School of Clinical Sciences
University of Liverpool
Liverpool, UK

Alec B. O'Connor MD, MPH

Associate Professor of Medicine
University of Rochester School of
Medicine and Dentistry
Rochester, NY, USA

Frederick M. Perkins MD

Chief, Anesthesia
United States Department of Veteran Affairs
White River Junction, VT, USA

Frank Petzke MD

Uniklinik Köln, Department of Anesthesiology
and Postoperative Intensive Care Medicine
University Hospital of Cologne
Köln, Germany

James P. Robinson MD, PhD

Department of Rehabilitation Medicine
University of Washington
Washington, DC, USA

Tiina Saarto MD, PhD

Consultant in Oncology and
Head, Department of Oncology
Helsinki University Hospital
Helsinki, Finland

Michael Schatman PhD, CPE

Research Director, Pain and Addiction Study Foundation
Bellevue, WA, USA

David L. Scott BSc, MD, FRCP

Professor of Clinical Rheumatology
Department of Rheumatology and Weston Education
Centre
Kings College London School of Medicine
London, UK

Tamara J. Somers PhD

Assistant Professor, Department of Psychiatry
and Behavioral Sciences
Duke University Medical Center
Durham, NC USA

Claudia Sommer MD

Professor of Neurology
Universität Würzburg
Würzburg, Germany

William Stones MD

Chair, Department of Obstetrics and Gynaecology
Aga Khan University Hospital
Nairobi, Kenya

Kristina B. Svendsen MD, PhD

Danish Pain Research Center and Department of Neurology
Aarhus University Hospital
Aarhus, Denmark

Peer Tfelt-Hansen MD DMSc

Danish Headache Centre
Department of Neurology
University of Copenhagen
Glostrup Hospital
Glostrup, Denmark

Kati Thieme PhD

Center for Neurosensory Disorders
Thurston Arthritis Research Center
University of North Carolina
Chapel Hill, NC, USA

Maurits van Tulder PhD

Professor, Department of Health Sciences
and EMGO Insitute for Health and Care Research
Faculty of Earth and Life Sciences
VU University
Amsterdam, The Netherlands

Joseph Wallach MD

Department of Psychiatry
School of Medicine and Biomedical Sciences
State University of New York at Buffalo
Buffalo, NY, USA

Joanna M. Zakrzewska MD, FDSRCS, FFDRCS

Division of Diagnostic, Surgical and Medical Sciences
Eastman Dental Hospital
UCLH NHS Foundation Trust
London, UK

Preface

Evidence-based medicine is now firmly established as a basis for clinical decision making. It is also advocated by national and international institutions and policy makers. Systematic reviews are used for the writing of guidelines and consensus documents relating to clinical practice.

Evidence-based pain management had its start around 15 years ago when the doctoral thesis *Meta-Analysis of Randomised Clinical Trials in Pain Relief* by Alejandro Jadad-Bechara was approved at the University of Oxford. The first database that was used for Dr Jadad's thesis was compiled from articles that were hand searched and photocopied. Today's meta-analyses are facilitated considerably by advances in electronic database and search engine technology.

In 1998 Oxford University Press published *An Evidence-Based Resource for Pain Relief* by Henry McQuay and Andrew Moore. This was followed by Bandolier's *Little Book of Pain* and *Making Sense of the Medical Evidence*. These books and many original papers based on meta-analyses and systematic reviews have changed the way in which clinical research papers are assessed. Many early studies addressed methodological issues. One of the most obvious consequences of these seminal papers was the improvement in the design of clinical trials in pain relief in line with the developments in other fields of medicine. Randomization, blinding and the appropriate selection control groups, both active and inactive, were the most important issues. More recently, the CONSORT and QUORUM statements have provided guidance on how these factors should be addressed in clinical trials.

Trial sensitivity and the placebo response are particularly important questions in studies of pain relieving interventions. Trial sensitivity means that there should be enough pain to be relieved. Expectation and conditioning are important in both the placebo effect and in pain relief. Another challenge has been the number of patients needing to be included in a treatment arm in order to provide the study with enough power to produce reliable results. In addition to trial quality, issues of validity have become increasingly important. Validity involves understanding both the clinical condition and the interventions that are studied. This means systematic reviews and meta-analyses need collaboration between contributors who have competence in search and meta-analytical methods and clinicians who are experienced in the clinical field being studied.

Traditional randomized and controlled trials concentrate on the mean effect and what happens to the majority, i.e. the average patient. With increasing understanding of the genetic and environmental effects on individual differences the average response needs to be considered critically. Evidence-based medicine will provide the basis for treatment choices but the patient's individual characteristics also need to be considered. Clinical trial methodology must be developed in order to take patient variability into consideration. Performing meta-analyses based on individual patient data could provide new possibilities for understanding the pathophysiology of chronic pain.

During the production of this book a prolific US researcher in the field of pain was shown to have fabricated data in some 21 studies published in peer-reviewed journals. The fraud is believed to be one of the largest known cases of academic misconduct and was widely reported in the American media.

Academic dishonesty on this scale produces enormous collateral damage. The papers were withdrawn from the journals (and all relevant references have been removed from this book). All authors and publishers in the field have had to re-examine the fraudulent material and mitigate the influence of these studies. Systematic reviews and meta-analyses containing the data have needed to be recalculated. The episode has brought to the fore discussions regarding academic integrity and probity and highlights the vigilance with which journal editors, publishers and readers of scientific material must exclude sources of bias and to identify data that may mislead either deliberately or unintentionally.

We have been fortunate to attract international leaders in the field of pain management, as well as experts in systematic analysis, to contribute to this book on evidence-based chronic pain management. The involvement of such individuals is a testament to a shared recognition that a book that consolidates evidence supporting and refuting the many available approaches to managing chronic pain will be a valuable addition to the literature. We hope this book will guide practitioners in their treatment choices by helping them to identify which treatments offer the greatest hope of improving pain for patients, and those therapies which evidence suggests have low likelihood of success, poor cost-effectiveness, or both.

Cathy Stannard
Eija Kalso
Jane Ballantyne

List of abbreviations

ACC — anterior cingulate cortex/American College of Cardiology
ACE — angiotensin-converting enzyme
ACEI — angiotensin-converting enzyme inhibitor
ACR — American College of Rheumatology
ADR — adverse drug reaction
AE — adverse effects
AIMS — Arthritis Impact Measurement Scale
AL-TENS — acupuncture-like TENS
ANS — autonomic nervous system
APF — antiproliferative factor
ATP — adenosine triphosphate
BOCF — baseline observations carried forward
BPS/IC — bladder pain syndrome/interstitial cystitis
BT — behavior therapy
CABG — coronary artery bypass graft
CAD — coronary artery disease
CAM — complementary and alternative medicine
CBFV — coronary blood flow velocity
CBM — cannabis-based medicine
CBT — cognitive behavioral therapy
CD — Crohn's disease
CDLBP — chronic diskogenic low back pain
CER — control event rate
CGRP — calcitonin gene-related peptide
CI — confidence interval
CNCP — chronic noncancer pain
CNS — central nervous system
COMT — catecholamine-O-methyltransferase
CONSORT — Consolidated Standards of Reporting Trials
COX — cyclo-oxygenase

COXIBs — COX-2 inhibitors
CP — central pain
CPDN — chronic painful diabetic neuropathy
CPSP — central post-stroke pain
CR — controlled release
CRP — C-reactive protein
CRPS — complex regional pain syndrome
CT — computed tomography
CVA — cerebrovascular accident
CVD — cardiovascular disease
CWP — chronic widespread pain
D — double blinded
DAS — Disease Activity Scale
DBS — deep brain stimulation
DH — dorsal horn
DHE — dihydroergotamine
DMARDs — disease-modifying antirheumatic drugs
DMSO — dimethylsulfoxide
DP — directional preference
DRG — dorsal root ganglia
EBM — evidence-based medicine
EDSS — Expanded Disability Status Scale
EECP — external enhanced counterpulsation
EER — experimental event rate
EFNS — European Federation of Neurological Societies
EMDA — electromotive drug administration
EMG — electromyogram
ER — extended release
ERCP — endoscopic retrograde cholangiopancreatography
ES — effect size
ESCS — electrical spinal cord stimulation
ESI — epidural steroid injections
ESR — erythrocyte sedimentation rate

FBSS	failed back surgery syndrome	MRI	magnetic resonance imaging
FBT	fentanyl buccal tablet	MS	multiple sclerosis
FDA	Food and Drug Administration	MTP	metatarsophalangeal
FMS	fibromyalgia syndrome	NA	noradrenaline
FSS	functional somatic syndrome	NAC	N-acetylcysteine
GABA	γ-aminobutyric acid	NGF	nerve growth factor
GI	gastrointestinal	NMDA	N-methyl-D-aspartate
GLA	γ-linolenic acid	NNH	number needed to harm
GM-CSF	granulocyte macrophage-colony stimulating factor	NNT	number needed to treat
		NO	nitric oxide
GnRH	gonadotrophin-releasing hormone	NRAC	National Refractory Angina Centre
GTN	glyceryl trinitrate	NSAIDs	nonsteroidal anti-inflammatory drugs
HLA	human leukocyte antigen	NSE	negative sexual events
HNP	herniated nucleus pulposus	OA	osteo-arthritis
HPA	hypothalamic-pituitary-adrenal axis	ODI	Oswestry Disability Index
HRQOL	health-related quality of life	OMT	optimal medical therapy
HZ	herpes zoster	OR	Odds ratio
IAP	intermittent acute porphyria	OTFC	oral transmucosal fentanyl citrate
IASP	International Association for the Study of Pain	PAF	primary afferent fibers
		PAG	periaqueductal gray
IBD	inflammatory bowel disease	PBS	painful bladder syndrome
IBS	irritable bowel syndrome	PCI	percutaneous coronary intervention
IC	interstitial cystitis	PDN	painful diabetic neuropathy
IDDS	intrathecal drug delivery system	PEMF	pulsed electromagnetic field
IDET	intradiskal electrothermal therapy	PENS	percutaneous electrical nerve stimulation
IL	interleukin		
IMMPACT	Initiative on Methods, Measurement, and Pain Assessment in Clinical Trials	PET	positron emission tomography
		PHN	postherpetic neuralgia
		PIP	proximal interphalangeal
IN	intranasal	PL	placebo
ISDN	isosorbide dinitrate	PMP	pain management program
IT	intrathecal	PMR	percutaneous myocardial laser revascularization
ITT	intention to treat		
IV	intravenous	PPS	pentosanpolysulfate
IVRA	intravenous regional anesthesia	PSN	presacral neurectomy
IVRS	intravenous regional sympatholysis	PT	physical therapist/therapy
LA	locus coeruleus/left anterior	PTS	painful tonic seizures
LBP	low back pain	QALY	quality-adjusted life-year
LOCF	last observation carried forward	QST	quantitative/qualitative sensory testing
LP	long-term potentiation	QUOROM	quality of assessement of systematic reviews
LUNA	laparoscopic uterine nerve ablation		
LV	left ventricle	RA	rheumatoid arthritis
MAOI	monoamine oxidase inhibitor	RCT	randomized clinical/controlled trial
MCP	metacarpophalangeal	RDC	Research Diagnostic Criteria
MEG	magnetoencephalographic	RF	rheumatoid factor/radiofrequency
MHC	major histocompatibility complex	RR	relative risk
MI	myocardial infarction	RVM	rostroventral medulla
MRA	magnetic resonance angiography	SD	standard deviation

SCI	spinal cord injury	TG	therapeutic gain
SCS	spinal cord stimulation	THC	δ-9-tetrahydrocannabinol
SI	sacroiliac	TMD	temporomandibular disorders
SIP	sympathetically independent pain	TMJ	temporomandibular joint
SLR	straight leg raising	TMR	transmyocardial myocardial laser revascularization
SMA	supplementary motor area		
SMD	standard mean difference	TMS	transcranial magnetic stimulation
SMP	sympathetically maintained pain	TN	trigeminal neuralgia
SNRI	serotonin and noradrenaline reuptake inhibitor	TNF-α	tumor necrosis factor α
		TOTPAR	total pain relief
SP	substance P	TRP	transient receptor potential
SPID	sum of pain intensity difference	TSE	transcutaneous spinal electroanalgesia
SP-SAP	substance P-saporin	TTF	time to treatment failure
SRT	self-regulatory treatments	TTX	tetrodotoxin
SSRI	Selective serotonin reuptake inhibitors	UC	ulcerative colitis
SUNA	short-lasting neuralgiform pain with autonomic symptoms	VAS	visual analog scale
		VATS	video-assisted thoracoscopic sugery
SUNCT	short-lasting unilateral neuralgiform headaches with conjunctival tearing	VVS	vulval vestibulitis syndrome
		VZV	varicella zoster virus
TCA	tricyclic antidepressant	WHO	World Health Organization
TENS	transcutaneous electrical nerve stimulation	WMD	weighted mean difference
TFESI	transforaminal epidural steroid injection		

PART 1

Understanding evidence and pain

CHAPTER 1

Why evidence matters

Andrew Moore and Sheena Derry

Pain Research, Nuffield Department of Anaesthetics, John Radcliffe Hospital, Oxford, UK

Introduction

There are two ways of answering a question about what evidence-based medicine (EBM) is good for or even what it is. One is the dry, formal approach, essentially statistical, essentially justifying a proscriptive approach to medicine. We have chosen, instead, a freer approach, emphasizing the utility of knowing when "stuff" is likely to be wrong and being able to spot those places where, as the old maps would tell us, "here be monsters." This is the *Bandolier* approach, the product of the hard knocks of a couple of decades or more of trying to understand evidence.

What both of us (and Henry McQuay and other collaborators over the years), on our different journeys, have brought to the examination of evidence is a healthy dose of skepticism, perhaps epitomized in the birth of *Bandolier*. It came during a lecture on evidence-based medicine by a public health doctor, who proclaimed that only seven things were *known* to work in medicine. By *known*, he meant that they were evidenced by systematic review and meta-analysis. A reasonable point, but there were unreasonable people in the audience. One mentioned thiopentone for induction of anesthesia, explaining that with a syringe and needle anyone, without exception, could be put to sleep given enough of this useful barbiturate; today we would say that it had an NNT of 1. So now we had seven things known to work in medicine, plus

thiopentone. We needed somewhere to put the bullet points of evidence; you put bullets in a bandolier (a shoulder belt with loops for ammunition).

The point of this tale is not to traduce well-meaning public health docs, or meta-analyses, but rather to make the point that evidence comes in different ways and that different types of evidence have different weight in different circumstances. There is no single answer to what is needed, and we have often to think outside what is a very large box. Too often, EBM seems to be corralled into a very small box, with the lid nailed tightly shut and no outside thinking allowed.

If there is a single unifying theory behind EBM, it is that, whatever sort of evidence you are looking at, you need to apply the criteria of quality, validity, and size. These issues have been explored in depth for clinical trials, observational studies, adverse events, diagnosis, and health economics [1], and will not be rehearsed in detail in what follows. Rather, we will try to explore some issues that we think are commonly overlooked in discussions about EBM.

We talk to many people about EBM and those not actively engaged in research in the area are frequently frustrated by what they see as an impossibly complicated discipline. Someone once quoted Ed Murrow at us, who, talking about the Vietnam war, said that "Anyone who isn't confused doesn't really understand the situation" (Walter Bryan, *The Improbable Irish*, 1969). We understand the sense of confusion that can arise, but there are good reasons for continuing to grapple with EBM. The first of these is all about the propensity of research and other papers you read to be wrong. You need to know about that, if you know nothing else.

Evidence-Based Chronic Pain Management. Edited by C. Stannard, E. Kalso and J. Ballantyne. © 2010 Blackwell Publishing.

Most published research false?

It has been said that only 1% of articles in scientific journals are scientifically sound [2]. Whatever the exact percentage, a paper from Greece [3], replete with Greek mathematical symbols and philosophy, makes a number of important points which are useful to think of as a series of little laws (some of which we explore more fully later) to use when considering evidence.

- The smaller the studies conducted in a scientific field, the less likely the research findings are to be true.
- The smaller the effect sizes in a scientific field, the less likely the research findings are to be true.
- The greater the number and the fewer the selection of tested relationships in a scientific field, the less likely the research findings are to be true.
- The greater the flexibility in designs, definitions, outcomes, and analytical modes in a scientific field, the less likely the research findings are to be true.
- The greater the financial and other interests and prejudices in a scientific field, the less likely the research findings are to be true. (These might include research grants or the promise of future research grants.)
- The hotter a scientific field (the more scientific teams involved), the less likely the research findings are to be true.

Ioannidis then performs a pile of calculations and simulations and demonstrates the likelihood of us getting at the truth from different typical study types (Table 1.1). This ranges from odds of 2:1 on (67% likely to be true) from a systematic review of good-quality randomized trials, through 1:3 against (25%

likely to be true) from a systematic review of small inconclusive randomized trials, to even lower levels for other study architectures.

There are many traps and pitfalls to negotiate when assessing evidence, and it is all too easy to be misled by an apparently perfect study that later turns out to be wrong or by a meta-analysis with impeccable credentials that seems to be trying to pull the wool over our eyes. Often, early outstanding results are followed by others that are less impressive. It is almost as if there is a law that states that first results are always spectacular and subsequent ones are mediocre: the law of initial results. It now seems that there may be some truth in this.

Three major general medical journals (*New England Journal of Medicine*, *JAMA*, and *Lancet*) were searched for studies with more than 1000 citations published between 1990 and 2003 [4]. This is an extraordinarily high number of citations when you think that most papers are cited once if at all, and that a citation of more than a few hundred times is almost as rare as hens' teeth.

Of the 115 articles published, 49 were eligible for the study because they were reports of original clinical research (like tamoxifen for breast cancer prevention or stent versus balloon angioplasty). Studies had sample sizes as low as nine and as high as 87,000. There were two case series, four cohort studies, and 43 randomized trials. The randomized trials were very varied in size, though, from 146 to 29,133 subjects (median 1817). Fourteen of the 43 randomized trials (33%) had fewer than 1000 patients and 25 (58%) had fewer than 2500 patients.

Of the 49 studies, seven were contradicted by later research. These seven contradicted studies included

Table 1.1 Likelihood of truth of research findings from various typical study architectures

Example	Ratio of true to not true
Confirmatory meta-analysis of good-quality RCTs	2:1
Adequately powered RCT with little bias and 1:1 prestudy odds	1:1
Meta-analysis of small, inconclusive studies	1:3
Underpowered and poorly performed phase I–II RCT	1:5
Underpowered but well-performed phase I–II RCT	1:5
Adequately powered exploratory epidemiologic study	1:10
Underpowered exploratory epidemiologic study	1:10
Discovery-orientated exploratory research with massive testing	1:1000

one case series with nine patients, three cohort studies with 40,000–80,000 patients, and three randomized trials, with 200, 875 and 2002 patients respectively. So only three of 43 randomized trials were contradicted (7%), compared with half the case series and three-quarters of the cohort studies.

A further seven studies found effects stronger than subsequent research. One of these was a cohort study with 800 patients. The other six were randomized trials, four with fewer than 1000 patients and two with about 1500 patients.

Most of the observational studies had been contradicted, or subsequent research had shown substantially smaller effects, but most randomized studies had results that had not been challenged. Of the nine randomized trials that were challenged, six had fewer than 1000 patients, and all had fewer than 2003 patients. Of 23 randomized trials with 2002 patients or fewer, nine were contradicted or challenged. None of the 20 randomized studies with more than 2003 patients were challenged.

There is much more in these fascinating papers, but it is more detailed and more complex without becoming necessarily much easier to understand. There is nothing that contradicts what we already know, namely that if we accept evidence of poor quality, without validity or where there are few events or numbers of patients, we are likely, often highly likely, to be misled.

If we concentrate on evidence of high quality, which is valid, and with large numbers, that will hardly ever happen. As Ioannidis also comments, if instead of chasing some ephemeral statistical significance we concentrate our efforts where there is good prior evidence, our chances of getting the true result are better. This may be why clinical trials on pharmaceuticals are so often significant statistically, and in the direction of supporting a drug. Yet even in that very special circumstance, where so much treasure is expended, years of work with positive results can come to naught when the big trials are done and do not produce the expected answer.

Limitations

Whatever evidence we look at, there are likely to be limitations to it. After all, there are few circumstances in which one study, of whatever architecture, is likely to be able to answer all the questions we need to know about an intervention. For example, trials capturing information about the benefits of treatment will not be able to speak to the question of rare, but serious, adverse events.

There are many more potential limitations. Studies may not be properly conducted or reported according to recognized standards, like CONSORT for randomized trials (www.consort-statement.org), QUOROM for systematic reviews, and other standards for other studies. They may not measure outcomes that are useful, or be conducted on patients like ours, or present results in ways that we can easily comprehend; trials may have few events, when not much happens, but make much of not much, as it were. Observational studies, diagnostic studies, and health economic studies all have their own particular set of limitations, as well as the more pervasive sins of significance chasing, or finding evidence to support only preconceptions or *idées fixes*.

Perfection in terms of the overall quality and extent of evidence is never going to happen in a single study, if only because the ultimate question – whether this intervention will work in this patient and produce no adverse effects – cannot be answered. The average results we obtain from trials are difficult to extrapolate to individuals, and especially the patients in front of us (of which more later).

Acknowledging limitations

Increasingly we have come to expect authors to make some comment about the limitations of their studies, even if it is only a nod in the direction of acknowledging that there are some. This is not easy, because there is an element of subjectivity about this. Authors may also believe, with some reason, that spending too much time rubbishing their own results will result in rejection by journals, and rejection is not appreciated by pointy-headed academics who live or die by publications.

Even so, the dearth of space given over to discussing the limitations of studies is worrying. A recent survey [5] that examined 400 papers from 2005 in the six most cited research journals and two open-access journals showed that only 17% used at least one word denoting limitations in the context of the scientific work presented. Among the 25 most cited journals, only one (*JAMA*) asks for a comments section on study limitations, and most were silent.

Statistical testing

It is an unspoken belief that to have a paper published, it helps to report some measure with a statistically significant difference. This leads to the phenomenon of significance chasing, in which data are analyzed to death and the aim is to find any test with any data that show significance at the paltry level of 5%. A P value of 0.05, or significance at the 5% level, tells us that there is a 1 in 20 chance that the results occurred by chance. As an aside, you might want to ask yourself how happy you are with 1 in 20; after all, if you throw two dice, double six seems to occur frequently and that is a chance of 1 in 36. If you want to examine evidence with a cold and fishy eye, try recognizing significance only when it is at the 1 in 100 level, or 1%, or a P value of 0.001; it often changes your view of things.

Multiple statistical testing

The perils of multiple statistical testing might have been drummed into us during our education but as researchers, we often forget them in the search for "results," especially when such testing confirms our pre-existing biases. A large and thorough examination of multiple statistical tests underscores the problems this can pose [6].

This was a population-based retrospective cohort study which used linked administrative databases covering 10.7 million residents of Ontario aged 18–100 years who were alive and had a birthday in the year 2000. Before any analyses, the database was split in two to provide both derivation and validation cohorts, each of about 5.3 million persons, so that associations found in one cohort could be confirmed in the other cohort.

The cohort comprised all admissions to Ontario hospitals classified as urgent (but not elective or planned) using DSM criteria, and ranked by frequency. This was used to determine which persons were admitted within the 365 days following their birthday in 2000, and the proportion admitted under each astrological sign. The astrological sign with the highest hospital admission rate was then tested statistically against the rate for all 11 other signs combined, using a significance level of 0.05. This was done until two statistically significant diagnoses were identified for each astrological sign.

In all, 223 diagnoses (accounting for 92% of all urgent admissions) were examined to find two statistically significant results for each astrological sign. Of these, 72 (32%) were statistically significant for at least one sign compared with all the others combined. The extremes were Scorpio, with two significant results, and Taurus, with 10, with significance levels of 0.0003 to 0.048.

The two most frequent diagnoses for each sign were used to select 24 significant associations in the derivation cohort. These included, for instance, intestinal obstructions and anemia for people with the astrological sign of Cancer, and head and neck symptoms and fracture of the humerus for Sagittarius. Levels of statistical significance ranged from 0.0006 to 0.048, and relative risk from 1.1 to 1.8 (Fig. 1.1), with most being modest.

Protection against spurious statistical significance from multiple comparisons was tested in several ways.

When the 24 associations were tested in the validation cohort, only two remained significant: gastrointestinal haemorrhage and Leo (relative risk 1.2), and fractured humerus for Sagittarius (relative risk 1.4).

Using a Bonferoni correction for 24 multiple comparisons would have set the level of significance acceptable as 0.002 rather than 0.05. In this case, nine of 24 comparisons would have been significant in the derivation cohort, but none in the both derivation and validation cohort. Correcting for all 14,718 comparisons used in the derivation cohort would

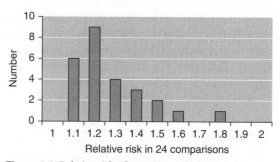

Figure 1.1 Relative risk of associations between astrological sign and illness for the 24 chosen associations, using a statistical significance of 0.05, uncorrected for multiple comparisons.

have meant using a significance level of 0.000003, and no comparison would have been significant in either derivation or validation cohort.

This study is a sobering reminder that statistical significance can mislead when we don't use statistics properly: don't blame statistics or the statisticians, blame our use of them. There is no biologic plausibility for a relationship between astrological sign and illness, yet many could be found in this huge data set when using standard levels of statistical significance without thinking about the problem of multiple comparisons. Even using a derivation and validation set did not offer complete protection against spurious results in enormous data sets.

Multiple subgroup analyses are common in published articles in our journals, usually without any adjustment for multiple testing. The authors examined 131 randomized trials published in top journals in 6 months in 2004. These had an average of five subgroup analyses, and 27 significance tests for efficacy and safety. The danger is that we may react to results that may have spurious statistical significance, especially when the size of the effect is not large.

Size is everything

The more important question, not asked anything like often enough, is whether any statistical testing is appropriate. Put another way, when can we be sure that we have enough information to be sure of the result, using the mathematical perspective of "sure," meaning the probability to a certain degree that we are not being mucked about by the random play of chance? This is not a trivial question, given that many results, especially concerning rare but serious harm, are driven by very few events.

In a clinical trial of drug A against placebo, the size of the trial is set according to how much better drug A is expected to be. For instance, if it is expected to be hugely better, the trial will be small but if the improvement is not expected to be large, the trial will have to be huge. Big effect, small trial; small effect, big trial; statisticians perform power calculations to determine the size of the trial beforehand. But remember that the only thing being tested here is whether the prior estimate of the expected treatment effect is actually met. If it is, great, but when you calculate the effect size from that trial, using number

needed to treat (NNT), say, you probably have insufficient information to do so because the trial was never designed to measure the *size of the effect*. If it were, then many more patients would have been needed.

In practice, what is important is the size of the effect – how many patients benefit. With individual trials we can be misled. Figure 1.2 shows an example of six large trials (213–575 patients, 2000 in all) of a single oral dose of eletriptan 80 mg for acute migraine, using the outcome of headache relief (mild or no pain) at 2 hours. NNTs measured in the individual trials range from 1.6 to 3.1, an almost twofold difference in the estimate of the size of the effect (overall, the NNT was 2.6). Even with these excellent trials, impeccably conducted, variations in response with eletriptan (between 56% and 69% in individual trials) and placebo (between 21% and 40%) mean that there is uncertainty over the size of the effect. For many treatments and dose/drug/condition combinations, we have much less information, fewer events, and much more uncertainty over the size of the effect.

Consider Figure 1.3, which looks at the variation in the response to placebo in over 50 meta-analyses in acute pain. In all the 12,000 or more patients given placebo, the response rate was 18% (meaning not that placebo **caused** 18% of people to have at least 50% pain relief over 6 hours, but that 18% of people in trials like

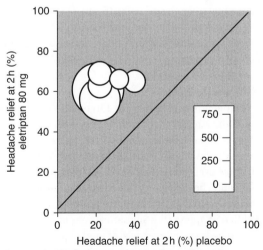

Figure 1.2 Headache response at 2 hours for oral eletriptan 80 mg. Size of symbol is proportional to number of patients in a trial.

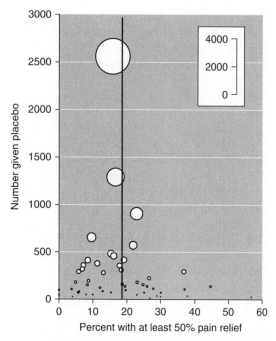

Figure 1.3 Percentage of patients with at least 50% pain relief with placebo in 56 meta-analyses in acute pain. Size of symbol is proportional to number of patients given placebo. Vertical line is the overall average.

these will have at least 50% pain relief over 6 hours if you do nothing at all). With small numbers, the measured effect with placebo varies from 0% to almost 50%. Only when the numbers are large is there greater consistency, and there are many other examples like this of size overcoming variability caused by the random play of chance.

How many events?

A few older papers keep being forgotten. When looking at the strengths and weaknesses of smaller meta-analyses versus larger randomized trials, a group from McMaster suggested that with fewer than 200 outcome events, research (meta-analyses in this case) may only be useful for summarizing information and generating hypotheses for future research [7]. A different approach using simulations of clinical trials and meta-analyses arrived at pretty much the same conclusion, that with fewer than 200 events, the magnitude and direction of an effect become increasingly uncertain [8].

Just how many events are needed to be reasonably sure of a result when event rates are low (as is the case for rare but serious adverse events) was explored some while ago [9]. This looks at a number of examples, varying event rates in experimental and control groups, using probability limits of 5% and 1%, and with lower and higher power to detect any difference. Higher power, greater stringency in probability values, lower event rates, and smaller differences in event rates between groups all suggest the need for more events and larger numbers of patients in trials. Once event rates fall to about 1% or so, and differences between experimental and control to less than 1%, the number of events needed approaches 100 and number of patients rises to tens of thousands.

All of which points to the inescapable conclusion that with few events, our ability to make sense of things is highly impaired. As a rule of thumb, we can probably dismiss studies with fewer than 20 events, be very cautious with 20–50 events, and reasonably confident with more than 200 events – if everything else is OK.

Subgroup analyses

Almost any paper you read, be it analysis of a clinical trial, an observational study or meta-analysis of either, will involve some form of subgroup analysis, such as severity of condition, age or sex. In addition to the problems of multiple testing, subgroup analyses also tend to involve small numbers – because the more you slice and dice the data, the fewer the number of actual events – and, if they are clinical trials, remove the benefits of randomization. They almost always introduce the danger of some unknown confounding.

One of the best examples of the dangers of subgroup analysis, due to unknown confounding, comes from a review article examining the 30-day outcome of death or myocardial infarction from a meta-analysis of platelet glycoprotein inhibitors [10]. Analysis indicated different results for women and men (Fig. 1.4), with benefits in men but not women. Statistically this was highly significant (P<0.0001).

In fact, it was found that men had higher levels of troponins (a marker of myocardial damage) than women and when this was taken into account, the difference between men and women was understandable, with more effect with greater myocardial damage; sex wasn't the source of the difference.

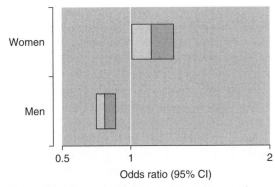

Figure 1.4 Subgroup analysis in women and men of death or MI with platelet glycoprotein inhibitors (95% confidence interval).

Trivial differences

It is worth remembering what relative risks tell us in terms of raw data (Table 1.2). Suppose we have a population in which 100 events occur with our control intervention, whatever that is. If we have 150 events with an experimental, the relative risk is now 1.5. It may be statistically significant, but most events were those occurring anyway. If there were 250 events, the relative risk would be 2.5, and now most events would occur because of the experimental intervention.

Large relative risks may be important, even with more limited data. Small relative risks, probably below 2.0 and certainly below about 1.5, should be treated with caution, especially where the number of

Table 1.2 Rules of causation

Feature	Comment
Consistency and unbiasedness of findings	Confirmation of the association by different investigators, in different populations, using different methods
Strength of association	Two aspects: the frequency with which the factor is found in the disease, and the frequency with which it occurs in the absence of the disease. The larger the relative risk, the more the hypothesis is strengthened
Temporal sequence	Obviously, exposure to the factor must occur before onset of the disease. In addition, if it is possible to show a temporal relationship, as between exposure to the factor in the population and frequency of the disease, the case is strengthened
"Biologic gradient (dose–response relationship)"	Finding a quantitative relationship between the factor and the frequency of the disease. The intensity or duration of exposure may be measured
Specificity	If the determinant being studied can be isolated from others and shown to produce changes in the incidence of the disease, e.g. if thyroid cancer can be shown to have a higher incidence specifically associated with fluoride, this is convincing evidence of causation
Coherence with biologic background and previous knowledge	The evidence must fit the facts that are thought to be related, e.g. the rising incidence of dental fluorosis and the rising consumption of fluoride are coherent
Biologic plausibility	The statistically significant association fits well with previously existing knowledge
Reasoning by analogy	Common sense, especially when you have other similar examples for types of intervention and outcome
Experimental evidence	This aspect focuses on what happens when the suspected offending agent is removed. Is there improvement? The evidence of remission – or even resolution of significant medical symptoms – following explanation obviously would strengthen the case It is unethical to do an experiment that exposes people to the risk of illness, but it is permissible and indeed desirable to conduct an experiment, i.e. a randomized controlled trial on control measures. If fluoride is suspected of causing thyroid dysfunction, for example, the experiment of eliminating or reducing occupational exposure to the toxin and conducting detailed endocrine tests on the workers could help to confirm or refute the suspicion

events is small, and even more especially outside the context of the randomized trial.

The importance of a relative risk of 2.0 has been accepted in US courts [11]. "A relative risk of 2.0 would permit an inference than an individual plaintiff's disease was more likely than not caused by the implicated agent. A substantial number of courts in a variety of toxic substance cases have accepted this reasoning."

Confounding by indication

Bias arises in observational studies when patients with the worst prognosis are allocated preferentially to a particular treatment. These patients are likely to be systematically different from those not treated or treated with something else (paracetamol rather than nonsteroidal anti-inflammatory drugs (NSAID) in asthma, for instance).

Confounding, by factors known or unknown, is potentially a big problem, because we do not know what we do not know and the unknown could have big effects, like troponin above. When relative risks are small, say below about 1.3, potential bias created because of unknown confounding, or confounding by indication improperly adjusted, becomes so great that it makes any conclusion at best unreliable. This is especially important when interpreting observational studies that appear to link a particular intervention with a particular outcome.

Adverse events

Evidence around adverse events is important, complicated, yet often poor. It is impossible to do justice to adverse event evidence in a few paragraphs, so perhaps it is worth sticking to the highlights.

Adverse events are important because the "value" of a particular therapeutic intervention depends on both potential benefit and potential harm in the individual. To assess this trade-off, we need evidence for both, and while evidence about benefit is generally well documented, at least in clinical trials of newer interventions, evidence about harm has been neglected.

Long-term drug therapy is increasingly being used for primary prevention. Asymptomatic patients may be asked to tolerate adverse effects when the likelihood of therapeutic benefit is small. Adverse events are a major influence on compliance and the most common reason for discontinuation in clinical practice. A medicine not taken is one that cannot work. There is an increasing tendency for more openness and accountability in clinical decision making, with patients asking for more information and taking a more active role in their care.

Adverse events occur in the absence of treatment, something to remember when looking at data. Symptoms commonly listed as adverse events in clinical trials happen to all of us at some time. Fortunately most of them are not serious and even if severe, are reversible. Most are not related to any therapeutic intervention. Groups of medical and nonmedical people in the USA in the 1960s [12], and medical students in Germany in the 1990s [13], who were free of disease and not in any kind of trial or taking any medication, were asked about symptoms. Most participants were in their 20s. They were given a list of symptoms and asked to record whether or not they had experienced any in the previous 3 days. Overall, 83% experienced at least one of the symptoms and only 17% reported none. There were no major differences between medical and nonmedical participants, or between studies carried out 30 years apart. The most common symptom reported by at least 40% was fatigue. Having an idea of the background rate of an adverse event in a study population is important as it can affect tolerability, and also how easy it is to establish a causal association with the intervention.

Another example of common adverse events would be constipation, something we worry about a lot when prescribing opioids. Constipation occurs in about 15% of people with chronic pain using weak opioids [14].

The overall average percentage of people with constipation in a systematic review of constipation prevalence in the US was about 15% (1 in 7 adults [15]). The range was 1.9–27%, depending to some extent on how constipation was ascertained. Most reports were in the range of 12–19%, with some self-reported prevalence being higher and two face-to-face questioning reports below 4%. There was a distinctly higher prevalence in women compared with men in almost every study, irrespective of method of ascertainment. Prevalence of constipation in women was on average about twice as high as in men. There was also a consistent finding of higher constipation prevalence in non-Caucasian people, by a factor of about 1.4 to 1, though nonwhite racial groups were not subdivided. Other trends were for decreased prevalence in people with highest income and highest educational attainment or years of education, though these may well be measuring different aspects of the same phenomenon. Older age, especially age over 70 years, was also associated with higher constipation rates.

With any examination of adverse events, it is worth bearing in mind that what we want to establish is causation. The most important *aide-mémoire* is the Bradford-Hill rules, summarized in Table 1.2. They ask about strength of association, timing, dose–response, and other linking evidence. We need more than association to proceed to causation.

Safety

Claims are all too often made about safeties that are unfounded. To some extent, it depends what one means by safety, but members of the public say that they want to know about any adverse event that occurs at a rate more frequently than 1 in 100,000 [16]. To be even remotely confident about an adverse event occurring at a rate 10 times more frequently than that (1 in 10,000), we would need information from about 2 million people.

Clinical trials, even meta-analyses of clinical trials, will not have this amount of information. Nor will most observational studies or even meta-analyses of observational studies. Things may be changing, because large databases are beginning to be interrogated to provide data on safety. Caution is required because of confounding by indication and small numbers of events, so that individual studies can give very different results. For instance, a systematic review looking at NSAIDs and risk of myocardial infarction showed that the risk for naproxen compared to non-use of NSAIDs varied linearly between a relative risk of 0.5 and one of 1.5 (with a mean of 1.0).

Large database studies may also surprise. A good example of the surprising results of database studies (good as in good study, as well as a surprising result) indicated that long-term use of proton pump inhibitors significantly increased risk of hip fracture in older people [17]. It might be that the risk of using a proton pump inhibitor with NSAID incurs a bigger risk to life from hip fracture than did the gastrointestinal bleed the proton pump inhibitor was protecting against.

In any event, claims of absolute safety cannot be made, and we will see more examples of rare but serious adverse events in future than ever we did in the past.

Importance of the individual patient

The two quotations below come from people who argued vehemently over the role and importance of EBM yet agreed on the importance of the individual within the system.

"Evidence-based medicine is the conscientious, explicit and judicious use of current best evidence in making decisions about the care of individual patient." [18].

"Managers and trialists may be happy for treatments to work on average; patients expect their doctors to do better than that." [19].

This underlines the importance of looking at information from the point of view of the individual patient. In acute pain, patients have been shown generally to obtain pain relief that is either very good or poor, but the average of responses to analgesics is at a point where there are few, if any, patients [20]. It is commonly understood that not every patient with a particular condition benefits from treatments known to work (on average). Patients may discontinue therapy because of adverse events as well as lack of efficacy, especially in chronic conditions. A clinical trial may tell us that 50% of patients have pain relief with drug, compared with 20% with placebo, and we applaud a good NNT of 3.3. Yet that obscures the fact that half the patients do not have pain relief but may have adverse effects.

A classic example demonstrating how different we all are is provided by a trial in which depressed patients were randomized to one of three antidepressants which were, on average, the same [21]. Patients initially randomized to one treatment frequently changed to another. By 9 months only 44% were still taking the treatment to which they had been randomized. Some (about 15%) were lost to follow-up after baseline or when on any of the randomized treatments. Others either switched to another antidepressant or stopped treatment because of adverse effects or lack of efficacy, again without any difference between the three antidepressants. Each was taken by about the same proportion, on average, just different patients to those initially randomized. Patients and their doctors found the balance of effect and absence of adverse events that was right for them, and almost 70% had a good outcome over the 9 months of the trial.

The degree of variability between individuals in their physiologic response to drugs is remarkable, and best exemplified by a study of 50 healthy young volunteers who received rofecoxib 25 mg, celecoxib 200 mg or placebo in randomized order, and who underwent a series of tests [22]. There was considerable variability between individuals in cyclo-oxygenase 2 inhibition achieved, and in selectivity, for both of the drugs. Variation between individuals was 50 to several hundred-fold in activity in different *in vitro* tests following a single dose. Differences were associated with genetic polymorphisms and other factors were involved in the variability observed. Similarly, a range of polymorphisms in genes coding for enzymes metabolizing morphine, opioid receptors, and blood–brain barrier transport of morphine by drug receptors all contribute to considerable variability between individuals [23]. A number of mechanisms can influence individual responses to analgesics [24].

There are important practical implications following these findings. They obviously relate particularly to the potential harm of limited formularies, but also challenge how we use average results from trials in making decisions about individual patients.

Outcomes

Where evidence can often let us down is in the outcomes chosen in trials. Outcomes used may not be what we, or patients, want from treatment, but rather what it is possible to measure. Ideally, a satisfactory outcome should involve both benefit and lack of adverse events, because adverse events are often a cause of discontinuation of an otherwise effective therapy.

Things are changing. In migraine, for example, an outcome of mild or no pain 2 hours after therapy changed to no pain at 2 hours, then no pain at 2 hours plus no recurrence or need to use analgesics

over the next 24 hours. The hurdle was getting higher. It was recently raised yet again, when an individual patient meta-analysis identified those patients who were both pain free for 24 hours and had no adverse effects [25]; this amounted to no more than 22% of the total, only 12% more than with placebo. A large randomized comparison of two triptans found about 30% of patients with this outcome [26].

There are other examples where people have sought more relevant outcomes. For instance, a series of different outcomes related to wart clearance and return emerged from a systematic review of genital wart therapy [27], while a longitudinal survey of patients with bipolar disorder suggested that success be judged over longer periods because of the sustained nature of the disorder [28].

There is no reason why we cannot demand more intelligent and comprehensive outcomes to be measured in clinical trials. While it is likely that the combination of benefit plus absence of adverse events will be found only in the minority, this will be a spur for both better use of what therapies we have and determination of better therapies for the future.

Conclusion

Evidence-based medicine is about a number of things. First and foremost, it is about avoiding being misled. That means that we have to have a passing acquaintance with issues of quality, validity, and size, and most of these come down to good old common sense. When a trial is done using two men and a dog and reports a subgroup analysis on the dog as statistically significant, that is not a reason for rushing to change practice.

The second thing that EBM should be about is making things better. This could mean wanting better and more meaningful outcomes or knowing how to assess trial results in terms of an individual patient, or asking the question of knowing which patient will benefit before you treat. It may be slow, but keeping some of these issues in your mind can mean hours of fun asking awkward questions of visiting speakers, a few of which may do some good. Over and above this, of course, is the incorporation of prior evidence in the production of new evidence, especially clinical trials, which are becoming bigger and better, though much more expensive to conduct.

Thirdly, when we collect together all the good evidence on a topic and get rid of the misleading, we often see more clearly. A number of examples exist in pain, especially in acute pain [29], migraine [30], and neuropathic pain [31].

The final message should be about the importance of wisdom. EBM, in its fullest sense, should incorporate evidence from whatever source, your knowledge of the patient, the patient's own preferences, and the circumstances you are in. Evidence should be regarded as a tool, not a rule. Even where there is limited evidence, in combination with clinical experience and wisdom it can produce useful results, perhaps the best example being a treatment algorithm for neuropathic pain [31].

References

1. Moore RA, McQuay HJ. *Bandolier's Little Book of Understanding the Medical Evidence*. Oxford University Press, Oxford, 2006.
2. Smith R. Where is the wisdom: the poverty of medical evidence. *BMJ* 1991; **303**: 798–799.
3. Ioannidis JPA. Why most published research findings are false. *PLoS Med* 2005; **2**: e124. www.plosmedicine.org.
4. Ioannidis JPA. Contradicted and initially stronger effects in highly cited clinical research. *JAMA* 2005; **294**: 218–228.
5. Ioannidis JPA. Limitations are not properly acknowledged in the scientific literature. *J Clin Epidemiol* 2007; **60**: 324–329.
6. Austin PC, Mamdani MM, Juurlink DN, Hux JE. Testing multiple statistical hypotheses resulted in spurious associations: a study of astrological signs and health. *J Clin Epidemiol* 2006; **59**: 964–969.
7. Flather MD, Farkouh ME, Pogue JM, Yusuf S. Strengths and limitations of meta-analysis: larger studies may be more reliable. *Control Clin Trials* 1997; **18**: 568–579.
8. Moore RA, Gavaghan D, Tramer MR, Collins SL, McQuay HJ. Size is everything – large amounts of information are needed to overcome random effects in estimating direction and magnitude of treatment effects. *Pain* 1998; **78**: 209–216.
9. Shuster JJ. Fixing the number of events in large comparative trials with low event rates: a binomial approach. *Control Clin Trials* 1993; **14**: 198–208.
10. Thompson SG, Higgins JPT. Can meta-analysis help target interventions at individuals most likely to benefit? *Lancet* 2005; **365**: 341–346.
11. Federal Judicial Center. *Reference Manual on Scientific Evidence*, 2nd edn. Federal Judicial Center, Washington, DC, 2000, p539.
12. Reidenberg MM, Lowenthal DT. Adverse nondrug reactions. *N Engl J Med* 1968; **279**: 678–679.
13. Meyer FP, Troger U, Rohl FW. Adverse nondrug reactions: an update. *Clin Pharmacol Ther* 1996; **60**: 347–352.
14. Moore RA, McQuay HJ. Prevalence of opioid adverse events in chronic non-malignant pain: systematic review of randomized trials of oral opioids. *Arth Res Ther* 2005; **7**: R1046–R1051.
15. Higgins PD, Johanson JF. Epidemiology of constipation in North America: a systematic review. *Am J Gastroenterol* 2004; **99**: 750–759.
16. Ziegler DK, Mosier MC, Buenaver M, Okuyemi K. How much information about adverse effects of medication do patients want from physicians? *Arch Intern Med* 2001; **161**: 706–713.
17. Yang YX, Lewis JD, Epstein S, Metz DC. Long-term proton pump inhibitor therapy and risk of hip fracture. *JAMA* 2006; **296**: 2947–2953.
18. Sackett DL, Rosenberg WM, Gray JA, Haynes RB, Richardson WS. Evidence based medicine: what it is and what it isn't. *BMJ* 1996; **312**: 71–72.
19. Grimley Evans J. Evidence-based or evidence-biased medicine? *Age Ageing* 1995; **24**: 461–463.
20. Moore RA, Edwards JE, McQuay HJ. Acute pain: individual patient meta-analysis shows the impact of different ways of analysing and presenting results. *Pain* 2005; **116**: 322–331.
21. Kroenke K, West SL, Swindle R, *et al*. Similar effectiveness of paroxetine, fluoxetine and sertraline in primary care. *JAMA* 2001; **286**: 2947–2995.
22. Fries S, Grosser T, Price TS, *et al*. Marked interindividual variability in the response to selective inhibitors of cyclooxygenase-2. *Gastroenterology* 2006; **130**: 55–64.
23. Klepstad P, Dale O, Skorpen F, Borchgrevink PC, Kaasa S. Genetic variability and clinical efficacy of morphine. *Acta Anaesthesiol Scand* 2005; **49**: 902–908.
24. Lötsch J, Geisslinger G. Current evidence for a genetic modulation of the response to analgesics. *Pain* 2006; **121**: 1–5.
25. Dahlof CG, Pascual J, Dodick DW, Dowson AJ. Efficacy, speed of action and tolerability of almotriptan in the acute treatment of migraine: pooled individual patient data from four randomized, double-blind, placebo-controlled clinical trials. *Cephalalgia* 2006; **26**: 400–408.
26. Goadsby PJ, Massiou H, Pascual J, *et al*. Almotriptan and zolmitriptan in the acute treatment of migraine. *Acta Neurol Scand* 2007; **115**: 34–40.
27. Moore RA, Edwards JE, Hopwood J, Hicks D. Imiquimod for the treatment of genital warts: a quantitative systematic review. *BMC Infect Dis* 2001; **1**: 3.
28. Chengappa KN, Hennen J, Baldessarini RJ, *et al*. Recovery and functional outcomes following olanzapine treatment for bipolar I mania. *Bipolar Disord* 2005; **7**: 68–76.
29. Moore A, Edwards J, Barden J, McQuay H. *Bandolier's Little Book of Pain*. Oxford University Press, Oxford, 2003.
30. Oldman AD, Smith LA, McQuay HJ, Moore RA. A systematic review of treatments for acute migraine. *Pain* 2002; **97**: 247–257.
31. Finnerup NB, Otto M, McQuay HJ, Jensen TS, Sindrup SH. Algorithm for neuropathic pain treatment: an evidence based proposal. *Pain* 2005; **118**: 289–305.

CHAPTER 2

Clinical trial design for chronic pain treatments

Alec B. O'Connor[1] and Robert H. Dworkin[2]

[1]Department of Medicine, University of Rochester School of Medicine and Dentistry, Rochester, NY, USA
[2]Departments of Anesthesiology and Neurology, University of Rochester School of Medicine and Dentistry, Rochester, NY, USA

The World Health Organization defines a clinical trial as "any research study that prospectively assigns human participants or groups of humans to one or more health-related interventions to evaluate the effects on health outcomes" [1]. This definition includes the double-blind, randomized clinical trial (RCT), considered the "gold standard" research design for clinical trials, as well as various prospective, uncontrolled, nonblinded cohort designs. In this chapter, we emphasize RCTs because uncontrolled trials produce treatment effect estimates that are substantially less informative than those from RCTs. Even among RCTs, however, study quality varies considerably, and many limitations and sources of bias can exist.

We focus on clinical trials of treatments for chronic pain, conventionally defined as pain that persists beyond 3 months or the normal time of healing [2]. Chronic pain is typically classified based on its presumed etiology, specifically, neuropathic pain versus non-neuropathic inflammatory and musculoskeletal pain. Neuropathic pain is caused by a lesion or disease affecting somatosensory pathways of the peripheral or central nervous system [3], whereas non-neuropathic (i.e. nociceptive) pain reflects stimulation of specialized nociceptors in somatic tissue, with visceral pain often classified separately. We focus on trials of pharmacologic interventions for both of these types of chronic pain in this chapter, although many of the issues we address are also relevant to studies of psychologic therapies, nerve blocks, spinal cord stimulation,

physical therapy, acupuncture or any other procedure that can be used to treat chronic pain. We begin by reviewing the types of clinical trials and research designs that are most commonly used in investigations of chronic pain. Next, we discuss the major components of clinical trials, including the interventions studied, patient selection, and assessment of treatment outcomes. Finally, we discuss the analysis and interpretation of pain and related data in clinical trials, and conclude by summarizing the major sources of bias in clinical trials. Excellent resources are available for investigators undertaking clinical trials of pain treatments and for those who want additional information about the interpretation of clinical trials [4–10].

Clinical trials involve research on human subjects and it is therefore critical that all individuals involved in such studies become familiar with the ethical principles and obligations that apply to such research. This includes the roles and responsibilities of investigators conducting clinical trials, especially the importance of informed consent, and also applicable institutional, local, and national regulations and procedures for study review and approval. It is beyond the scope of this chapter to summarize these issues, particularly given geographic variation in specific considerations, but in-depth reviews are available [11].

Types of clinical trials

When designing a clinical trial or interpreting its results, the first issue that must be considered is the objective of the trial – specifically, what question is the trial is intended to answer? Max [12, 13] emphasized the importance of distinguishing

Evidence-Based Chronic Pain Management. Edited by C. Stannard, E. Kalso and J. Ballantyne. © 2010 Blackwell Publishing.

between pragmatic and explanatory clinical trials [14]. Pragmatic clinical trials have the objective of answering practical questions about patient care; for example, are tricyclic antidepressants (TCA) useful for relieving pain in patients with phantom limb pain? These trials are typically designed to reflect clinical practice to the greatest extent possible, and decisions about various features of the trial are guided by the clinical situation that the results of the trial are intended to inform. The goal of an explanatory clinical trial, however, is to answer a question about the mode of action of a treatment, the etiology of a condition, or both. The methodologic features of an explanatory trial are therefore selected to maximize the likelihood that the trial will answer a specific question about the mechanisms of disease or treatment and without regard to the realities of the clinical situation. In pragmatic trials, the clinical context, tolerability of the treatment, and generalizability of the results are all vitally important, whereas controlling variables and ensuring that a sufficiently large dosage is given become more important considerations in explanatory trials. Of course, answering questions about the likely efficacy of a treatment in clinical practice and about the mechanism of its action are not mutually exclusive. However, these two different objectives generally require different outcome measures, and studies with both goals must be carefully planned to ensure that the objectives and outcomes do not interfere with each other.

In considering clinical trials, a distinction is often made between efficacy and effectiveness trials [15], although some clinical trials combine elements of both. *Efficacy* trials test the hypothesis of whether or not there are beneficial effects of treatment in a group of patients, and the methods and procedures are tightly controlled and standardized. In such studies, threats to the internal validity of the study (e.g. the integrity of the double blind or the inclusion and exclusion criteria) are minimized to the greatest extent possible so that treatment effects or biologic mechanisms can be evaluated accurately. *Effectiveness* trials, on the other hand, are conducted to test the value of a treatment as applied in the "real world" of clinical practice, in which, for example, some patients do not take all the medication they are prescribed. Because of the increased variability, such trials are typically larger than efficacy trials and there

is often less control of methods and procedures. In effectiveness studies, external validity and generalizability are emphasized and the trial is designed so that conclusions can be drawn about the value of the treatment as it is actually used. A simple example of this distinction would be two medications that are found to have equivalent efficacy but differ in effectiveness because one is taken less consistently as a result of its greater side effects.

Prospective cohort trials

In general, cohort studies can demonstrate association but not causation; that is, regardless of the findings of a cohort study, it cannot be concluded that an intervention caused the observed outcomes. Cohort trials lack randomization, which is the most effective method of creating a valid comparison group. As such, cohort trials cannot distinguish the effects of the intervention from other factors that can affect outcomes, such as natural history (e.g. spontaneous remissions), regression to the mean, and placebo effects. Comparisons of outcomes in a treatment cohort with pretreatment values or with historical controls can therefore provide inaccurate or even misleading estimates of treatment benefits. Cohort studies also generally lack blinding, and treatment endpoints can be biased by the expectations of patients and investigators, especially when subjective outcomes such as pain are assessed.

Although the results of cohort trials cannot be used to establish the efficacy of an intervention, they can be useful in providing pilot data showing whether the treatment appears to have a beneficial effect and in demonstrating its safety and tolerability. For example, if no RCTs evaluating an intervention exist but a cohort study demonstrates tolerability, clinicians may feel somewhat reassured that an intervention is likely to be associated with acceptable tolerability. Moreover, large cohort studies are often the best method of detecting rare, serious adverse events [16], and can be used for confirmation of safety in samples much larger and more representative of the general population than those studied in RCTs.

Randomized clinical trials: general considerations

Randomized clinical trials are generally considered the best design for determining whether an intervention is efficacious. Successful randomization of a large group of patients controls for baseline factors, resulting in groups that are essentially identical except for the study treatment. RCTs are therefore the only type of clinical trial for which inferences of causality are appropriate. For example, outcome differences between an active treatment and a placebo group in a large, well-designed placebo-controlled RCT can be inferred to have been caused by the intervention. In general, the results of RCTs should be considered to overrule contradictory findings from other types of studies; an exception to this statement is that most RCTs of treatments for chronic pain are not adequately powered to detect between-group differences in uncommon adverse events.

Investigations of treatments for chronic pain have typically compared the efficacy, tolerability, and safety of a single treatment with placebo. Few RCTs have compared different treatments [17, 18] and even fewer trials have examined whether combinations of treatments are superior to the component treatments examined separately [19, 20]. Studies of combination treatments can use a 2×2 factorial design in which patients are randomized to the combination of two treatments, each of the treatments administered alone (with a placebo matching the other treatment), or double placebo. Such a factorial design not only makes it possible to evaluate the efficacy of the combination, but can also provide a "head-to-head" comparison of the two individual treatments. Given how common combination therapy for patients with chronic pain is in clinical practice, additional combination studies of chronic pain treatments must be conducted to determine which combinations are efficacious and well tolerated and which are not.

Even rarer than RCTs of combinations of different medications are studies examining the benefits of combining different modes of treatments, for example, a medication combined with cognitive-behavioral therapy compared with the medication and cognitive-behavioral therapy each administered alone. Such trials have been a major focus of research on the treatment of various psychiatric disorders for many years, and it is unfortunate that so little effort has been devoted to this type of clinical trial in research on the treatment of patients with chronic pain.

Typically, RCTs examining treatments for chronic pain have been designed to determine if one or more

different treatments (or different dosages of a single treatment) are superior to placebo with respect to pain reduction and other outcomes. One of the reasons that head-to-head trials of chronic pain treatments have rarely been performed is that the sample size required to show that one efficacious intervention is superior to another would typically be much larger than that required to show that an intervention is superior to placebo. RCTs can also be designed to demonstrate that one treatment is either equivalent to or not inferior to another (typically, first-line) treatment [21–23]. However, equivalence and noninferiority trials have generally not been conducted for chronic pain treatments, probably because until recently there have been few treatments for chronic pain that have such well-established efficacy that they could be considered standards with which another treatment can be compared. Such trials typically require fewer subjects than one intended to show that one efficacious treatment provides greater benefit than another, making it possible to demonstrate that two treatments have comparable efficacy but that one offers advantages over another in, for example, cost, convenience or tolerability.

In addition, even chronic pain treatments with well-established efficacy may sometimes fail to be superior to placebo in a given trial. When a standard treatment cannot be considered reliably superior to placebo, then an RCT demonstrating that a new treatment is equivalent or noninferior to the standard treatment may simply reflect that in this particular trial, neither the standard treatment nor the new treatment was efficacious. This lack of assay sensitivity in trials that do not have a placebo group is well recognized [24, 25]. For this reason, equivalence and noninferiority trials of chronic pain treatments would still require a placebo group to demonstrate that the standard treatment was superior to placebo. Only if the standard treatment is shown to be superior to placebo does it become possible to conclude that the new treatment is equivalent or noninferior to a standard efficacious treatment.

Randomization

The critical importance of randomization is demonstrated by the observation that interventions that are shown to be effective in nonrandomized trials have been found to be not effective in randomized trials [6]. There are two primary goals of randomizing subjects. The first is to eliminate both intentional and unintentional bias in the allocation of treatments, which historically has been a significant source of bias in clinical trials. Investigator allocation bias is eliminated by prespecifying a randomization protocol that removes the investigators from the process of selecting which subjects receive which interventions.

The second goal of randomization is to create subject groups that are equivalent in every way except for the intervention. On average, randomization will disperse subject variability evenly between the treatment groups, including both measured variables, such as age and sex, and unmeasured variables, such as pain-relevant genetic polymorphisms that have not yet been identified. The likelihood that randomized groups are truly similar is dependent on the sample size. Smaller groups are more likely to differ in potentially important ways, both among measured and unmeasured variables, whereas between-subject variability is more likely to be dispersed evenly between groups with large sample sizes.

With cross-over designs in which each subject receives more than one intervention, subjects are randomized to different treatment orders, not different treatments. For example, to provide a valid comparison between interventions A and B, an equal number of subjects should be randomized to receive intervention A first and to receive intervention B first. Randomizing by treatment order serves to spread treatment order-related variables evenly between the interventions; these may include differences related to the order of treatment, carry-over effects, or the natural history of the condition.

Two additional aspects of randomization are blocking and stratification. *Blocking* is a method for ensuring that small groups of subjects are randomized evenly. For example, if a block size of four is chosen in a study with two treatment groups, the first four subjects could be randomized in any potential combination that would produce an even number of subjects in the two groups (e.g. ABAB, BABA, or BBAA). After the first block is complete, the next four subjects would be assigned to interventions via a newly randomized sequence. Blocked randomization ensures that randomization does not result in substantially different numbers of subjects being allocated to the different

interventions by chance. *Stratification* refers to dividing subjects into groups according to factors associated with treatment response prior to randomization. For example, if depression is thought to affect treatment response, subjects may be separated into those who are and are not depressed prior to randomization; this reduces the likelihood that a greater number of depressed subjects would be randomized to one intervention than the other due to chance, which might affect estimates of overall treatment response.

Publications reporting the results of clinical trials should include a description of the procedures used for randomization, but many do not [26]. The method of randomization has been included in a scoring system for rating trial quality [27]. In this scoring system, random number generation is considered an appropriate method for randomization, whereas randomization based on patient factors, such as date of birth, hospital number or date of exposure, is considered to potentially introduce bias.

Blinding

A double-blind RCT is one in which the identity of the interventions is concealed from both the subjects and the investigators; typically, the placebo in studies of medications is inert but appears identical to the active medication in color, shape, size, taste, and even odor. This is the best way to reduce potential bias related to knowledge of the intervention. Unblinded or "open-label" studies typically overestimate treatment effects, and interventions that appear highly efficacious in unblinded studies have been shown to be ineffective in blinded studies [6]. The importance of blinding in estimating the magnitude of treatment effects in RCTs should not be underestimated. The average response in the patients receiving placebo, for example, is often greater than the difference between the average response in the placebo and active treatment groups.

Even within double-blind trials, sometimes subjects and investigators can accurately guess which intervention they are receiving, for example, because of the development of characteristic side effects or the effectiveness of the treatment in reducing symptoms. Following completion of participation, subjects and investigators should be asked which intervention they believe was received (or, in the case of cross-over trials, what the treatment sequence was) and what is the basis of their guesses [28]. In a clinical trial of an effective treatment, patients being able to tell which group they were in because of beneficial effects is evidence of treatment efficacy and not an indication of compromised blinding. It is only when patients are able to correctly guess their group based on factors that are unrelated to efficacy, such as side effects, that the adequacy of the blinding and the potential of bias must be considered.

In order to improve the blinding within trials, many chronic pain RCTs have employed "active placebos," which are nonanalgesic medications (rather than inert placebos) with side effects that mimic those of the analgesic medication being studied [19, 29, 30]. The use of active placebos in chronic pain RCTs can be an effective strategy for maintaining the double-blind feature of a clinical trial, particularly in cross-over trials where each subject receives multiple interventions and may therefore be more likely to correctly guess when they are receiving an inert placebo. The use of active placebos, however, remains somewhat controversial. It has recently been argued that "the available evidence does not provide a compelling case for the necessity of an active placebo" in studies of antidepressant medications in patients with depression [31]. Given the difficulty of identifying active placebos for many of the medications used in the treatment of chronic pain, it would be important to determine whether active placebos are necessary in chronic pain trials.

As with randomization, the adequacy of the description of blinding procedures is considered a critical feature when evaluating the quality of published RCTs [27].

Parallel group trials

Parallel group trials are performed by randomizing each eligible subject to only one of two or more treatment groups (also termed treatment "arms"), and differences between groups in treatment outcomes are evaluated. Parallel group designs are considered by many to be the most informative type of clinical trial because they have the fewest limitations, provided that the sample size is large enough to provide an adequate test of the study's primary hypothesis.

Cross-over trials

In situations where the treatment effect has a relatively short and predictable duration and the condition being treated remains constant, a cross-over design can be used in which each subject receives each intervention. For example, in a cross-over trial comparing a new medication with placebo, subjects would be randomized to one of two treatment sequences, either medication first followed by placebo or vice versa. Subjects therefore receive either medication or placebo in the first treatment period, which is typically followed by a "washout" period during which subjects receive no treatment, and then subjects receive in the second treatment period whichever intervention they were not administered in the first period. In this manner, each subject serves as his or her own control. At the end of the trial, the responses of the patients when they were treated with the active medication can be compared to their responses during whichever period they received placebo.

The major advantage of cross-over trials is that they are extremely efficient in terms of sample size. Compared to a two-arm parallel group trial, a two-period cross-over design could require as few as one-quarter the number of subjects to show the same size treatment effect because variability is reduced when subjects serve as their own controls. An additional advantage of cross-over designs when two or more treatments are compared is the ability to evaluate treatment response and other outcomes within the same subjects. For example, are the subjects who have the best responses to one treatment also the ones who respond best to a different treatment [17]?

One of the central assumptions of cross-over trials is that the outcomes in the two (or more) treatment periods are not affected by the order of treatment. This assumption can be violated in different ways. If the natural history of the disease being studied is such that change during the trial is likely, or if a treatment alters the natural course of the disease, then the outcomes during later treatment periods can be expected to differ from outcomes during earlier periods. Another important concern about cross-over trials is the potential for "carry-over effects," that is, the continued effects of an earlier treatment on the outcomes of later periods. The duration of washout periods between treatment periods is often selected not only so that the medication from the first treatment period will have been eliminated before the beginning of the next period but also so that its effects will have disappeared, because such effects can persist longer than the presence of a medication. Carry-over effects can result in different types of error. Overestimation of the pain relief provided by the second treatment can occur if analgesic effects from the first treatment persist and are added to the true effects of the second treatment. On the other hand, overestimation of the side effects of the second treatment can result if side effects from the first treatment persist and are added to the side effects of the second treatment.

Although the relative impact of each of these effects can be mitigated by the random assignment of treatment order (i.e. approximately equal numbers of subjects will get each of the treatments first in the sequence), the assessment of treatment effects and tolerability will be inaccurate in the presence of carry-over or period effects. There are statistical tests that can detect the presence of treatment-by-period interactions and carry-over effects but these tests will generally be underpowered to adequately exclude the presence of such effects.

Nevertheless, the results of cross-over trials have provided a great deal of information about the treatment of chronic pain. For many types of chronic pain, knowledge of natural history supports the assumption of minimal change in pain during the course of the trial. Cross-over trials examining a variety of different medications have found little evidence of carry-over or treatment-by-period effects [17–19, 30]. It is important to recognize, however, that the statistical analysis of cross-over trials is typically a "completer" analysis (i.e. analyzing the responses of subjects who completed the entire trial) rather than the intention-to-treat (ITT) analysis that is typically used in parallel group studies; this can make comparing the results of parallel group and cross-over trials challenging, as will be further discussed below.

Treatment features

Clinical trials typically have a number of different phases. Some trials have a run-in period, which can be used to exclude patients from the trial for various reasons. These include lack of compliance with

protocol requirements (e.g. failure to record daily pain ratings), beneficial response to placebo, poor tolerability of the active medication, and lack of beneficial response to the active medication [32]. RCTs of chronic pain treatments typically have a baseline period that includes pain ratings made on several occasions, typically once daily in a diary. This baseline is of major importance because it makes it possible to analyze the difference between pain during the baseline period and during the treatment phase. Following the baseline period, patients are randomized to two or more treatments. In RCTs of medications for chronic pain, the beginning of treatment may include a period in which dosage is titrated to a designated maximum that is expected to be efficacious and adequately tolerated.

The titration phase is followed by a period of maintenance treatment. Regulatory agencies generally prefer fixed-dosage studies, in which all patients in a treatment arm receive the same dosage of study medication, because this makes it possible to determine the efficacy, safety, and tolerability of specific dosages. However, individual variation in absorption, metabolism, and physiologic distribution of analgesic medications can substantially increase the variability in patients' responses and the number of patients necessary to detect a treatment benefit. Because the dosage a patient receives is adjusted on the basis of both effectiveness and tolerability, flexible dosing not only addresses this variability but also reflects clinical practice more closely than use of a fixed dosage. Some clinical trials have therefore included treatment arms in which the dosage can be increased for additional pain relief or decreased to reduce side effects [33, 34].

Regardless of whether a chronic pain RCT uses a fixed- or flexible-dosage strategy, an important consideration involves the length of the maintenance period. Except for brief proof-of-concept studies designed to demonstrate initial evidence of efficacy, the durations of treatment used in RCTs of chronic pain treatments have typically ranged from 2 to 12 weeks. With chronic pain syndromes, longer durations of treatment are desirable to evaluate whether any beneficial effects of the treatment are maintained over time. Adequate evaluations of the durability of treatment effects are, of course, important in patients who are not likely to spontaneously improve and will therefore require extended treatment.

The treatment phase can be followed by a period during which the treatment is tapered. This is most common in studies of medications that should not be discontinued abruptly, such as opioid analgesics. In medication trials, a follow-up period may also be included to evaluate late adverse events associated with treatment. Follow-up periods are also important in trials of treatments expected to have beneficial effects that persist after treatment has ended.

Comparison groups

Although the use of placebo groups in chronic pain RCTs is generally well accepted, an obvious concern is how to ethically include a placebo group when the hypothesis of the trial is that subjects treated with placebo will experience more pain than those receiving the active treatment. There are at least two approaches that have been used to address this issue. One is to provide rescue analgesics to all subjects who require pain relief. When this is done, use of the rescue analgesic can be examined as an outcome measure, with greater use of rescue treatment being expected in the placebo group than in the active medication group if the treatment being studied is efficacious.

Another strategy is to permit patients in the trial to remain on stable dosages of any analgesic treatments that they were taking before the trial. Because of the availability of efficacious medications for chronic pain, it is likely that patients who are not taking any of these medications or who can be withdrawn from such treatments may be relatively unresponsive to therapy, not only existing therapies but also new treatments. Enrolling such patients in an RCT may therefore make it less likely that a new treatment will demonstrate efficacy. Moreover, prohibiting concurrent use of other analgesics in a chronic pain trial may make it more likely that patients will drop out of the trial, and may also make the results less generalizable to clinical practice, in which combination therapy is very common. Although it has been argued that an evaluating a medication in patients who are already being treated with effective treatments will be less likely to demonstrate efficacy, the limited data available do not support this hypothesis.

A third strategy has been to compare a high dosage of a medication with a low dosage of the same medication rather than with placebo [35]. Although this approach is likely to be more acceptable to patients than the inclusion of a placebo group, the use of a low dosage of an efficacious medication rather than placebo is not without limitations, including: (1) the lack of assay sensitivity if no difference is found between dosages; (2) the need for larger numbers of subjects to show superiority of the higher dosage than would be required with a placebo group if the low dosage is also efficacious; and (3) the same ethical issues raised by use of a placebo group if the low dosage is expected to have no beneficial effects.

Patient selection

Depending on the objectives of the trial and the specific treatment being evaluated, patients with either relatively homogenous conditions (e.g. painful diabetic peripheral neuropathy) or relatively heterogeneous conditions (e.g. peripheral neuropathic pain) can be studied. Careful attention must also be paid to specifying other features of the patients' pain, such as pain intensity and duration. Many studies include a minimum level of baseline pain intensity as one of the inclusion criteria in order to increase the likelihood of demonstrating a benefit of an active treatment versus placebo. Specifying too high a level of baseline pain, however, may augment responses in the placebo group by increasing regression to the mean [33]. Most recent clinical trials of treatments for chronic pain have therefore only included patients who have an average pain intensity of 4 or greater (on a 0–10 numeric rating scale) during the baseline period. The duration of time that pain has been present is also an important consideration. Typically, pain must have been present for at least 3 months to be considered chronic [2], but many studies have required a minimum pain duration of 6 months.

To eliminate patients who may have an increased risk from participating in the study and to increase the likelihood of detecting treatment benefits, clinical trials often restrict enrollment based on characteristics such as age, language, other medical conditions, known allergies, psychiatric disorders, alcohol or drug abuse, and, in women, pregnancy and the ability to conceive. Some studies have also excluded patients who have been refractory to multiple prior treatments for their chronic pain condition. Although some restrictions are necessary in defining a study sample, the use of unnecessary exclusion criteria in clinical trials reduces the generalizability of the results.

Some clinical trials are designed to exclude patients who are less likely to respond favorably to the investigational medication. Such "enriched enrollment" designs have been used to exclude patients who have done poorly with the medication during a run-in period – either because they showed a lack of benefit or because they could not tolerate its side effects – or patients who have a history of poor response to medications thought to share the same mechanism of action as the investigational treatment. Restricting the study sample to patients who are more likely to respond favorably to the study treatment can increase the likelihood that a trial will demonstrate efficacy. However, enriched enrollment designs can have important disadvantages, including limitations in the generalizability of the results because of the representativeness of the randomized sample, as well as the potential for unblinding resulting from prior experience with the medication's side effects during a run-in period. Such trial designs therefore may have greater value in establishing "proof of concept" of a potential analgesic intervention than in evaluating what the effectiveness of a treatment would be in the community.

Assessment of baseline characteristics and co-variates

There are various demographic characteristics of patients enrolled in clinical trials that must be routinely assessed, not only to accurately determine inclusion and exclusion criteria but also for use in data analyses. Depending on the condition being examined, age (e.g. in postherpetic neuralgia), sex (e.g. in fibromyalgia), and other demographic and clinical (e.g. pain duration) characteristics may be important co-variates in analyses of the data. Education, occupation, employment status, workers' compensation and other benefits, and presence of any litigation may also play a role in treatment outcome.

It is very important to record as much detail as possible regarding the patient's medical status in chronic pain clinical trials. This information should include past and present illnesses and injuries, especially any other chronic pain conditions, as well as past and present medical and nonmedical treatments for these conditions. There is a consensus that chronic pain is a complex biopsychosocial phenomenon, and it is especially important in clinical trials to obtain information about past and present psychiatric disorders and treatments, especially mood and anxiety disorders, suicide, and substance and alcohol abuse. Such conditions may be considered exclusion criteria for a trial, and may also serve to moderate the effects of treatment [36].

Treatment outcomes

Analgesic interventions can produce a number of different effects, including pain relief, side effects, improved sleep, psychiatric effects such as reduced depression, medication abuse, inconvenience, and substantial costs. Although the ideal primary outcome measure of a clinical trial assessing a pain intervention might be a single measure that quantified the overall net impact of all these potential effects on, for example, health-related quality of life, there is unfortunately no validated measure that does so.

Recently, the Initiative on Methods, Measurement, and Pain Assessment in Clinical Trials (IMMPACT) has recommended six core outcome domains [37] and specific outcome measures for each of these domains [38] for clinical trials of chronic pain treatments. The six recommended core outcome domains are pain; physical functioning; emotional functioning; participant ratings of improvement and satisfaction with treatment; symptoms and adverse events; and participant disposition (e.g. adherence to the treatment regimen and reasons for premature withdrawal from the trial). Specific outcome measures were selected for four of these domains on the basis of their appropriateness of content, reliability, validity, responsiveness, and participant burden, as follows: (1) pain intensity, assessed by a 0–10 numerical rating scale; (2) physical functioning, assessed by the Multidimensional Pain Inventory or Brief Pain Inventory interference scales; (3) emotional functioning, assessed by the Beck Depression Inventory and/or Profile of Mood States; and (4) participant ratings of overall improvement, assessed by the Patient Global Impression of Change scale. Use of this standard set of outcome domains and recommended measures in chronic pain clinical trials would facilitate the process of developing research protocols, permit pooling of data from different studies, and provide a basis for systematic reviews and meaningful comparisons among treatments.

Except for some very early studies designed to explore the range of potential benefits of a treatment, clinical trials should clearly identify the primary efficacy outcome measure and distinguish it from the secondary endpoints. The distinction between primary and secondary endpoints is necessary for determining the statistical power and required sample size of a clinical trial and requires investigators to identify which endpoint provides the optimal test of the primary study hypothesis. The results of clinical trials that report the results of significance tests for multiple endpoints without indicating which outcome measure was the prespecified primary endpoint are difficult to interpret. The likelihood that the statistical differences between treatments are due to chance can be appreciable when multiple significance tests are performed without a correction for multiple comparisons; identifying one primary endpoint or a limited number of co-primary endpoints minimizes this possibility.

A measure of improvement in pain intensity is typically the primary endpoint in a clinical trial of a treatment for a chronic pain condition [38]. The other outcome domains related to the experience of having chronic pain, including the impact of pain on physical and emotional functioning and other components of health-related quality of life, are then considered secondary endpoints.

Data collection

In designing and interpreting clinical trials, attention must be paid to the specific methods used for administering and collecting outcome data. For example, should a measure of pain intensity be administered by giving patients a questionnaire to complete, reading the questions to patients in face-to-face interviews, reading the questions to patients over the telephone, having patients enter their responses on a device kept in their possession (e.g. a palm-top computer or personal digital assistant), having patients respond by voice or by touch tones to recorded prompts after dialing into a central phone number or after an automatically generated telephone call to them, or having patients enter their responses over the internet (e.g. to an emailed questionnaire or at a designated website)? Deciding among such options is challenging and includes considerations of resources and feasibility as well as reliability and validity.

Unfortunately, there are relatively few studies that have compared the different methods that can be used in the assessment of pain-related outcomes. Moreover, the reliability and validity of these methods probably vary as a result of what is being assessed; it would not be surprising if responses to questions about depression or sexual disability differ depending on whether they are made in a face-to-face interview or on a questionnaire. In addition, the extent to which patients prefer different methods of administration could have a considerable impact on subject retention in clinical trials. Although it is beyond the scope of this chapter to consider these issues further, discussions of these issues with respect to a variety of measures are available [8, 39].

An additional important question regarding the administration of the measures in a clinical trial involves the frequency with which they are administered and what instructions are given regarding the time period to be used by patients when making their responses. Currently, most clinical trials of treatments for chronic pain require patients to make daily ratings of average pain in the past 24 hours and weekly or monthly ratings of the other measures, including secondary pain endpoints and other secondary outcome measures.

The assessment of adverse events is an essential component of clinical trials, and specific protocols differ with respect to the way in which these critical data are collected [38]. Side effects can be assessed using an "active" ascertainment approach, in which subjects are asked directly about the presence of specific side effects (e.g. "have you been dizzy?"). In contrast, a "passive" approach may ask whether subjects have developed "any new symptoms" or "changes in health" or "side effects" since the previous visit. The former approach will be more sensitive for detecting the specific side effects that are assessed, whereas the latter approach may produce more clinically relevant answers; subjects are likely to report particularly troubling side effects with either approach, but relatively insignificant side effects are more likely to be reported by subjects using an active ascertainment approach. An additional consideration is that active ascertainment prioritizes those symptoms that are assessed while relatively de-emphasizing symptoms that are not.

All trial reports should precisely describe how side effects were ascertained, including the wording used, which is particularly important when active ascertainment is used. When comparing different clinical trials, it is important to recognize that side effect frequency can be greatly affected by the approach used. Comparison of the side effect frequencies of placebo groups can be helpful in determining if the side effect ascertainment used in different trials was roughly comparable, although differences among studies in the characteristics of the enrolled patients can complicate such comparisons.

The adequacy of the description of withdrawals and drop-outs in a clinical trial is considered a critical marker of trial quality [27] and has also been emphasized by IMMPACT as one of the core outcome domains for chronic pain clinical trials [38]. The Consolidated Standards of Reporting Trials (CONSORT) were developed to standardize the reporting of clinical trials, and adequate accounting of subject disposition in clinical trials is a critical feature of CONSORT recommendations [23, 40–42]. A checklist and flow diagram of the information regarding research design, methods and procedures, data analysis, and generalizability that should be included in publications are provided; importantly, these guidelines can also be used when designing a clinical trial to ensure that adequate attention will be given to documenting the manner in which the trial is actually conducted, and when interpreting the results of published clinical trials to determine whether the key features of the trial have been described in enough detail to evaluate their quality.

Statistical analysis

It is unfortunate that many clinicians and readers of medical literature are unfamiliar with the often complex statistical analyses required of an RCT because the results and their interpretation depend on the specific statistical analyses performed. Several aspects of the statistical analysis are especially important in the interpretation of RCTs. First, the central hypothesis of the trial should be clearly specified because the hypothesis being tested drives the statistical analysis plan. The most commonly tested hypothesis in an RCT is that one intervention is superior to another (e.g. placebo). Two alternative potential hypotheses

of RCTs are (a) that two interventions are equivalent, and (b) that one intervention is noninferior to another. Both of these statistical analyses require that a margin of equivalence (or noninferiority) be defined, such that if the treatment effect of the new intervention falls within the prespecified margin of the second, then the two are considered equivalent (or one is considered noninferior to the other). The equivalence or noninferiority margin should be small enough that if the treatment effect estimate of the intervention falls anywhere within the margin, it would be considered clinically equivalent to the other intervention.

The plan for the statistical analysis of the data from an RCT (and the published report of its results) should clearly specify the primary outcome measure, the type of statistical test being used to evaluate group differences in the primary outcome, and the way in which the sample size was determined, which is particularly important when interpreting the results of trials that do not find a statistically significant difference between treatments. It is important to recognize that failure to detect between-group differences in a superiority trial does not indicate that the two interventions are clinically equivalent; all that can be concluded from a trial designed to demonstrate superiority that fails to show one group is superior to the other is that neither intervention was superior to the other.

In the course of an RCT, a subject may not finish the trial taking the intervention to which he or she was randomized. The most common type of intervention change is "dropping out," which can occur because of side effects or for reasons unrelated to the intervention, such as death or moving. In some types of trials, "drop-ins" can occur; these refer to switching from one intervention to the other, such as following a surgery versus no surgery randomization. The method by which the analysis considers subjects who do not finish the trial taking the intervention to which they were randomized can have a large impact on treatment estimates. The best method for analyzing parallel group superiority RCTs is generally an ITT analysis, in which all subjects who were randomized to an intervention are included in the final analysis. The most conservative ITT analysis examines all patients randomized, regardless of whether they meet all the inclusion and exclusion criteria and whether they have received even a single dose of the treatment. In many trials a modified ITT analysis is used, for example, only analyzing data from patients who have taken at least one dose of the study medication and who have completed one post-baseline pain diary (the criteria used for defining such modified ITT samples must, of course, be prospectively specified).

An ITT analysis avoids the bias that can occur as a result of selectively excluding subjects from the analysis. Randomized treatment groups from which subjects have been excluded are no longer equivalent to the original randomized groups, and the groups can no longer be assumed to be comparable with respect to measured and unmeasured variables that could be related to treatment outcomes. The results of ITT analyses also more closely reflect the treatment situation outside the clinical trial setting where patients treated in clinical practice, for example, do not have the correct diagnosis or are noncompliant with their treatment. ITT analyses are typically required by regulatory authorities for approval of medications.

Including patients in the analysis who do not have the relevant disorder or who are less likely to derive benefit because of noncompliance, however, makes it difficult to evaluate the true effects of a treatment. In a "per protocol" analysis, only subjects who would be expected to benefit from the treatment are included; that is, those who have the diagnosis for which the treatment is intended and who have received an amount of the treatment that could be expected to have a beneficial effect (as with ITT analyses, the criteria for excluding patients from such analyses should be prospectively defined). Since subjects who cannot tolerate an intervention or who do not respond to an intervention are much more likely to drop out, a per protocol analysis can overestimate the true benefits of the treatment in the population from which the per protocol sample was drawn [43]. However, this type of analysis can be informative when performed in conjunction with an ITT analysis; for example, if a per protocol analysis shows superiority of an intervention over placebo when the ITT analysis does not, then it may be concluded that the treatment can have beneficial effects when it is tolerated and administered as intended, assuming it can also be shown that the two per protocol treatment groups are likely to be comparable with respect to factors associated with treatment outcome [44, 45].

A per protocol analysis is the preferred type of data analysis in certain situations. For example, in equivalence and noninferiority trials, a per protocol analysis is typically preferred because the use of an ITT analysis tends to err towards finding equivalence or noninferiority, although the results of an ITT analysis should also be reported. In cross-over trials, "completer analyses" are usually reported because subjects serve as their own controls. In cross-over trials with more than two periods, subjects providing data for at least two of the periods can be included in analyzing the differences between the treatments administered in those periods [19].

There has been increasing attention to the analysis of missing data in chronic pain RCTs. One of the most commonly used methods is the "last observation carried forward" (LOCF) approach. However, if one assumes that missing data are more likely to occur among non-responders or those who cannot tolerate an intervention, then carrying forward the last observations collected before subjects dropped out can overestimate the beneficial effect of the intervention at the endpoint. In some of its medical reviews for chronic pain indications, the United States Food and Drug Administration has suggested that analysis and presentation of pivotal RCTs for chronic pain conditions should consider patients who have dropped out as non-responders (e.g. with ITT analyses using a "baseline observation carried forward" (BOCF) approach for missing data) [46]. The method of handling missing data can have an impact on treatment effect estimates, and the results of LOCF and BOCF analyses of the same data can differ in important ways. For example, the results of LOCF analyses can overestimate the degree of pain relief when compared to the results of BOCF analyses [46]. Although BOCF analyses can provide a conservative estimate of treatment effects for conditions such as chronic pain, by including baseline data for patients who drop out of the trial for reasons that have little to do with the trial (e.g. change in residence), they can reduce a trial's power to detect treatment benefits."

Regardless of the approach used for missing data in analyzing an RCT, the details must be described in reporting the trial's results. Unfortunately, the manner in which missing data are handled is not always reported, although LOCF analyses seem to be commonly used in industry-sponsored RCTs [47].

Interpretation of results

In analyzing data from clinical trials, establishing the statistical significance and confidence intervals of group differences in treatment outcome is a pivotal first step. It is well known, however, that statistical significance reflects both the magnitude and variability of the treatment effect as well as the sample size. A statistically significant improvement may therefore reflect a benefit that is clinically unimportant. For this reason, determinations of statistical significance must be supplemented by consideration of the clinical importance of changes in outcome measures. Such information provides a basis for evaluating and comparing the impact of chronic pain treatments on pain and health-related quality of life. Because most measures of treatment response in chronic pain trials involve the patient's subjective experience, the patient is the most important judge of whether changes are important or meaningful. For this reason, patient evaluations of overall improvement have been considered a core outcome domain for chronic pain trials [37].

Responder analyses can also assist in interpreting the clinical importance of chronic pain treatment outcomes, for example, analyses of the proportions of patients whose pain decreases from baseline by ≥30% or by ≥50% [48], as well as graphs presenting cumulative proportion of responder analyses [49]. Evaluating the clinical importance of the results of a clinical trial must also consider other factors besides patient assessments of pain reduction and overall improvement, including the characteristics of the disease being treated, the risks of the treatment (i.e. side effects and safety), the convenience of the treatment, and the characteristics of other treatments that are available for the same condition.

Clinical trial quality and sources of bias

There are a large number of potential sources of bias in clinical trials, and many types of bias result in overestimation of treatment effects. In addition, some clinical trial reports draw conclusions that are not justified by the data. For example, publications describing prospective cohort trials sometimes attribute benefits to the treatment when the absence of a control group makes such conclusions unwarranted. RCTs are the optimal clinical trial design for establishing efficacy, yet all RCTs have limitations and some are biased in ways that make the conclusions potentially misleading. Clinical trial reports must therefore be scrutinized carefully to determine if the conclusions are justified given the study design and data analysis, and a systematic method of evaluating RCTs for sources of bias can be employed [7]. In this section we will discuss factors that can decrease the validity of clinical trials, focusing on those that can reduce the internal and external validity of an RCT.

Internal validity

There are a large number of potential sources of bias in clinical trials. Unfortunately, many tend to make treatments appear better than they truly are, and incorporating biased trial results into clinical decision making can result in failure to adequately treat pain, the development of side effects, inconvenience, and unnecessary costs.

The adequacy of randomization is vitally important to the internal validity of an RCT. Some interventions that are consistently effective in nonrandomized trials can be consistently found to be ineffective in randomized trials [6]. Moreover, studies that provide unclear descriptions of the randomization process have also been found to consistently overestimate treatment effects when compared to studies that clearly describe randomization methods [6]. As noted above, treatment allocation methods that are not based on a valid approach to generating random numbers are not considered adequate methods of randomization [27].

Studies with large numbers of subjects who drop out from one or more arms of the trial should be viewed critically because drop-outs can change the composition of the original randomized treatment groups and also make the study sample no longer representative of the intended population. A large number of drop-outs can also indicate that the trial was not carefully designed or conducted. Studies that do not clearly describe the disposition of all study subjects, especially those who drop out, should be viewed critically.

The adequacy of blinding is also very important in the interpretation of clinical trials. Interventions that appear highly efficacious in unblinded studies are sometimes shown to be ineffective in blinded studies [6]. Given the subjective nature of pain measurements and the large placebo effects that are found in pain trials, lack of blinding or unintentional unblinding of either subjects or investigators can lead to substantial bias. Subjects' guesses about their treatment assignment should be assessed when they complete their participation in a study and these results should be described in the published reports of RCTs.

Inappropriate statistical analyses can also compromise internal validity and potentially lead to erroneous conclusions. Failure to state the prespecified primary endpoint raises the possibility that endpoints showing statistically significant effects have been selected for emphasis on the basis of the analyses, which makes interpretation of the trial results hazardous if not impossible. Occasionally, the primary endpoint is specified in the methods section, but the results and conclusions emphasize other endpoints, presumably because analyses of the primary endpoint were not favorable.

Sometimes, it is erroneously concluded that two interventions are equivalent when an RCT designed to test for superiority fails to show it. This is not an appropriate conclusion for a superiority trial showing no group differences; such trials should include a detailed description of the sample size assumptions and statistical power calculations, which will make it possible for readers to determine if assumptions used about the treatment effect size may have accounted for the lack of significant group differences. Equivalence and noninferiority trials require a different statistical analysis plan than superiority trials, including a prespecified equivalence or noninferiority margin for the primary endpoint, which should be based on clinical judgment as well as statistical considerations. Studies that are specifically designed to test for equivalence or noninferiority should state this.

As described above, the sample used in the data analyses should be clearly specified, and, for a superiority trial, the primary analysis should typically be based on an ITT sample. The method of handling missing data should also be specified in advance of the data analyses, and, ideally, alternative methods (e.g. both BOCF and LOCF) would be reported.

External validity

An RCT can have high internal validity yet produce biased estimates of treatment response due to problems of external validity; that is, the results of the trial may not apply to the patients treated in clinical practice. Extrapolation of clinical trial results to patient care can be challenging and potentially lead to patient harm, if, for example, study results from one patient population are inappropriately applied to a different population [50]. There are two aspects of RCTs that commonly reduce external validity: the representativeness of the study sample and the dosing strategies used in the trial.

There are a number of factors that can affect the study sample in ways that limit the generalizability of the subjects' treatment response to other patients. For example, similar RCTs performed in different countries sometimes have very different results [6, 51]. In addition, the mere fact that a subject is willing and able to participate in a clinical trial distinguishes him or her from the broader pool of patients for whom the treatment might be appropriate. Moreover, the recruitment methods investigators employ – for example, identifying patients from clinics or advertising in newspapers – can have a large impact on the types of patients enrolled in an RCT [32, 52].

The inclusion and exclusion criteria are used to define the study sample in an RCT, yet they frequently result in samples that differ substantially from the population for which the treatment is intended [53]. Strictly speaking, the conclusions from a placebo-controlled trial should describe how an intervention compares with placebo *in the sample studied*. The study sample is presumed to represent the population of all patients who meet the inclusion and exclusion criteria; however, the published conclusions in RCTs typically extrapolate the results to the entire population of patients with a particular disorder, not just those who would have been eligible to participate in the trial.

For example, most recent RCTs of treatments for chronic pain have required subjects to have an average pain score of 4 or greater on 0–10 daily diaries rated during a baseline week preceding randomization (a criterion of 5 or greater has also occasionally been used). When efficacy has been demonstrated in such studies, however, it is typically not concluded that the study's results may only apply to patients with moderate or severe pain. Although designing an RCT so that enrollment is limited to patients with moderate or greater pain may increase the likelihood that an active treatment will be superior to placebo, the results of the study may not extrapolate to patients with mild pain.

Another important limitation in interpreting the results of clinical trials involves the dosing strategy, which can have a substantial effect on trial outcome, including evaluations of both efficacy and tolerability. The rate at which the dosage of a medication is titrated, the maximum dosage administered, and whether the dosing strategy involves titration to a fixed dosage or flexible dosing adjusted on the basis of beneficial effects and tolerability can all have a major impact on the generalizability of the trial's results to clinical practice. In RCTs designed to compare the efficacy and tolerability of different medications, the dosing regimens used can be a major determinant of the results [47]. For example, if one medication is titrated more slowly and to a lower dosage than another, it is likely to be better tolerated; similarly, if one medication is titrated to relatively higher dosages than another, it could show greater efficacy when no differences would exist if equianalgesic dosages of the two medications had been used.

Other potential sources of bias

Reports of clinical trials should clearly identify the funding source and any potential conflicts of interest of the investigators. Industry-sponsored trials are typically designed with the objectives of demonstrating the efficacy, superiority, or greater tolerability and safety of the sponsor's product, and it is important to carefully consider potential biases in the study design and data collection, analysis, and interpretation of such trials from this perspective [47, 54, 55]. For example, a recent study found that trials sponsored by for-profit organizations were much more likely to recommend an intervention as the "treatment of choice" than trials sponsored by nonprofit organizations, and that neither the magnitude of the treatment effect nor the occurrence of adverse events explained the association between sponsorship and positive recommendations [56]. Although considerable attention has been paid to various biases associated with industry-sponsored trials, it should be recognized that such trials undergo a high level of scrutiny when they are submitted to

regulatory agencies for product approval. It has been observed that academic investigators are also invested in the outcome of the research they conduct, but it is more difficult to evaluate these "nonfinancial conflicts of interest" [57, 58] and the role they play in clinical trials than the more obvious conflicts represented by industry sponsorship. Knowledgeable reviewers are the major defense against bias, and all readers should be cautious in accepting what they read, "remembering that the ultimate validation for any scientific observation is replication" [58].

Publication bias is another important source of bias in the literature. Unfavorable RCT results are sometimes not published or are pooled with favorable RCTs to produce a favorable publication, and the hazards of interpreting the results of clinical trials when negative results remain undisclosed have received increasing attention in both the medical and lay literature. In addition, favorable RCT results are sometimes published multiple times. In one example, a total of 15 RCTs were conducted to assess the efficacy of an antidepressant for major depression; three of these were never published, yet a total of 20 publications describing the RCTs appeared in the literature, including duplicate publications of the same trial but with different authors [43]. Various efforts are underway to encourage investigators, from both industry and academia, to register trials at their inception so that a public record is available of all clinical trials that have been conducted [59]. Although clinical trial registration is a very positive development, its effectiveness remains to be established. To ensure that the development of improved clinical trial research methods and the identification of efficacious treatments are not impeded, the publication of negative trials by sponsors, investigators, and journal editors must therefore be strongly encouraged.

Conclusion

Advances in clinical trial designs used to study treatments for chronic pain must keep pace with the rapid evolution in understanding pain mechanisms that is taking place [60]. A major focus of ongoing research is to identify the mechanisms of different pain conditions, devise methods for reliably identifying these mechanisms in individual patients, and develop treatments that target these mechanisms. The ultimate goal of these efforts is to provide the foundation for a mechanism-based treatment approach in which therapeutic interventions target the specific mechanisms of a patient's chronic pain. Such increased knowledge of genetic, pathophysiologic, and psychosocial mechanisms of chronic pain and its response to different treatments will require major modifications in the clinical trial designs that we have discussed in this chapter. To the extent that individualized treatments are developed, study designs in which treatments are matched to particular patient characteristics will be needed [61, 62], and patients in clinical trials will not only be more homogeneous but may also respond more favorably to such mechanism-based treatments. RCTs of mechanism-based treatments will be complicated by the need for sophisticated subject assessments to identify pain mechanisms and potentially large numbers of patients who fail to meet the eligibility criteria of trials targeting specific mechanisms. Fortunately, not only are efforts being made to identify factors that influence whether trials succeed in demonstrating efficacy [63, 64], but alternatives to the standard parallel group RCT are also receiving increasing attention, including, for example, various enrichment and adaptive allocation designs [65–67].

References

1. World Health Organization. International Clinical Trials Registry Platform (ICTRP). www.who.int/ictrp/en/
2. Merskey H, Bogduk N (eds) *Classification of Chronic Pain: Descriptions of Chronic Pain Syndromes and Definitions of Pain Terms.* IASP Press, Seattle, WA, 1994.
3. Treede R-D, Jensen TS, Campbell JN, *et al.* Neuropathic pain: redefinition and a grading system for clinical and research purposes. *Neurology* 2008; **70**(18): 1630–1635.
4. Max MB, Portenoy RK, Laska EM (eds) *The Design of Analgesic Clinical Trials.* Raven Press, New York, 1991.
5. McQuay H, Moore AA. *An Evidence-Based Resource for Pain.* Oxford University Press, Oxford, 1998.
6. Bandolier. Bandolier Bias Guide, 2001. www.jr2.ox.ac.uk/bandolier/learnzone.html.
7. Bandolier. Critical Appraisal, 2001. www.jr2.ox.ac.uk/bandolier/learnzone.html.
8. Turk DC, Melzack R (eds) *Handbook of Pain Assessment,* 2nd edn. Guilford Press, New York, 2001.
9. Max MB. Small clinical trials. In: Gallin JI, Ognibene F (eds) *Principles and Practice of Clinical Research,* 2nd edn. Elsevier, New York, 2007: 219–235.
10. Max MB. Clinical trials of pain treatment; the design of clinical trials of treatments for pain. In: Max MB, Lynn J (eds) *Symptom Research: Methods and Opportunities.* Bethesda, MD: National Institute of Dental and Craniofacial Research, National Institutes of Health. http://symptom-research.nih.gov.
11. Dunn CM, Chadwick GL. *Protecting Study Volunteers in Research: A Manual for Investigative Sites,* 3rd edn. Thomson CenterWatch, Boston, MA, 2004.
12. Max, MB. Neuropathic pain syndromes. In: Max M, Portenoy R, Laska E (eds) *The Design and Analysis of Analgesic Trials.* Raven Press, New York, 1991: 193–219.
13. Max MB. Divergent traditions in analgesic clinical trials. *Clin Pharmacol Ther* 1994; **56**: 237–241.
14. Schwartz D, Lellouch J. Explanatory and pragmatic attitudes in therapeutical trials. *J Chron Dis* 1967; **20**: 637–648.
15. Piantadosi S. *Clinical Trials: A Methodologic Perspective.* John W0iley, New York, 1997.
16. Layton D, Pearce GL, Shakir SA. Safety profile of tolterodine as used in general practice in England: results of prescription-event monitoring. *Drug Saf* 2001; **24**: 703–713.
17. Raja SN, Haythornthwaite JA, Pappagallo M, *et al.* Opioids versus antidepressants in postherpetic neuralgia: a randomized, placebo-controlled trial. *Neurology* 2002; **59**: 1015–1021.
18. Sindrup SH, Bach FW, Madsen C, Gram LF, Jensen TS. Venlafaxine versus imipramine in painful polyneuropathy: a randomized, controlled trial. *Neurology* 2003; **60**: 1284–1289.
19. Gilron I, Bailey JM, Tu D, Holden RR, Weaver DF, Houlden RL. Morphine, gabapentin, or their combination for neuropathic pain. *N Engl J Med* 2005; **352**: 1324.
20. Khoromi S, Cui L, Nackers L, Max MB. Morphine, nortriptyline and their combination vs. placebo in patients with chronic lumbar root pain. *Pain* 2007; **130**: 65–75.
21. Henanff AL, Giraudeau B, Baron G, Ravaud P. Quality of reporting of noninferiority and equivalence randomized trials. *JAMA* 2006; **295**: 1147–1151.
22. Kaul S, Diamond GA. Good enough: a primer on the analysis and interpretation of noninferiority trials. *Ann Intern Med* 2006; **145**: 62–69.
23. Piaggio G, Elbourne DR, Altman DG, Pocock SJ, Evans SJW. Reporting of noninferiority and equivalence randomized trials: an extension of the CONSORT statement. *JAMA* 2006; **295**: 1152–1160.
24. Temple R, Ellenberg SS. Placebo-controlled trials and active-control trials in the evaluation of new treatments: part 1: ethical and scientific issues. *Ann Intern Med* 2000; **133**: 455–463.
25. Ellenberg SS, Temple R. Placebo-controlled trials and active-control trials in the evaluation of new treatments: part 2: practical issues and specific cases. *Ann Intern Med* 2000; **133**: 464–470.
26. Friedman LM, Furberg CD, DeMets DL. *Fundamentals of Clinical Trials,* 3rd edn. Springer, New York, 1998.
27. Jadad AR, Moore RA, Carroll D, *et al.* Assessing the quality of randomized clinical trials: is blinding necessary? *Control Clin Trial* 1996; **17**: 1–12.

28. Moscucci M, Byrne L, Weintraub M, Cox C. Blinding, unblinding, and the placebo effect: an analysis of patients' guesses of treatment assignment in a double-blind clinical trial. *Clin Pharmacol Ther* 1987; **41**: 259–265.

29. Max MB, Kishore-Kumar R, Schafer SC, *et al.* Efficacy of desipramine in painful diabetic neuropathy: a placebo-controlled trial. *Pain* 1991; **45**: 3–9.

30. Max MB, Lynch SA, Muir J, Shoaf SF, Smoller B, Dubner R. Effects of desipramine, amitriptyline, and fluoxetine on pain in diabetic neuropathy. *N Engl J Med* 1992; **326**: 1250–1256.

31. Quitkin F. Placebos, drug effects, and study design: a clinician's guide. *Am J Psychiatry* 1999; **156**: 829–836.

32. Dworkin RH, Katz J, Gitlin MJ. Placebo response in clinical trials of depression and its implications for research on chronic neuropathic pain. *Neurology* 2005; **65**(suppl 4): S7–S19.

33. Morello CM, Leckband SG, Stoner CP, Moorhouse DF, Sahagian GA. Randomized double-blind study comparing the efficacy of gabapentin with amitriptyline on diabetic peripheral neuropathy pain. *Arch Intern Med* 1999; **159**: 1931–1937.

34. Freynhagen R, Strojek K, Griesing T, Whalen E, Balkenohl M. Efficacy of pregabalin in neuropathic pain evaluated in a 12-week, randomized, double-blind, multicentre, placebo-controlled trial of flexible- and fixed-dose regimens. *Pain* 2005; **115**: 254–263.

35. Rowbotham MC, Twilling L, Davies PS, Reisner L, Taylor K, Mohr D. Oral opioid therapy for chronic peripheral and central neuropathic pain. *N Engl J Med* 2003; **348**: 1223–1232.

36. Wasan AD, Davar G, Jamison R. The association between negative affect and opioid analgesia in patients with discogenic low back pain. *Pain* 2005; **117**: 450–461.

37. Turk DC, Dworkin RH, Allen RR, *et al.* Core outcome domains for chronic pain clinical trials: IMMPACT recommendations. *Pain* 2003; **106**: 337–345.

38. Dworkin RH, Turk DC, Farrar JT, *et al.* Core outcome measures for chronic pain clinical trials: IMMPACT recommendations. *Pain* 2005; **113**: 9–19.

39. Dworkin RH, Nagasako EM, Hetzel RD, Farrar JT. Assessment of pain and pain-related quality of life in clinical trials. In: Turk DC, Melzack R (eds) *Handbook of Pain Assessment*, 2nd edn. Guilford Press, New York, 2001: 659–692.

40. Begg C, Cho M, Eastwood S, *et al.* Improving the quality of reporting of randomized controlled trials: the CONSORT statement. *JAMA* 1996; **276**: 637–639.

41. Altman DG, Schulz KF, Moher D, *et al.* The revised CONSORT statement for reporting randomized trials: explanation and elaboration. *Ann Intern Med* 2001; **134**: 663–694.

42. Moher D, Schulz KF, Altman DG. The CONSORT Statement: revised recommendations for improving the quality of reports of parallel-group randomised trials. *Lancet* 2001; **357**: 1191–1194.

43. Melander H, Ahlqvist-Rastad J, Meijer G, *et al.* Evidence b(i)ased medicine – selective reporting from studies sponsored by pharmaceutical industry: review of studies in new drug applications. *BMJ* 2003; **326**: 1171–1175.

44. Sheiner LB, Rubin DB. Intention-to-treat analysis and the goals of clinical trials. *Clin Pharmacol Ther* 1995; **57**: 6–15.

45. Sheiner LB. Is intent-to-treat analysis always (ever) enough? *Br J Clin Pharmacol* 2002; **54**: 203–211.

46. United States Food and Drug Administration, Center for Drug Evaluation and Research. Medical review: NDA 21-445 Lyrica (pregabalin). www.fda.gov/cder/foi/nda/2004/021446_LyricaTOC.htm.

47. Safer DJ. Design and reporting modifications in industry-sponsored comparative psychopharmacology trials. *J Nerv Ment Dis* 2002; **190**: 583–92.

48. Farrar JT, Young JP, LaMoreaux L, Werth JL, Poole RM. Clinical importance of changes in chronic pain intensity measured on an 11-point numerical pain rating scale. *Pain* 2001; **94**: 149–158.

49. Farrar JT, Dworkin RH, Max MB. Use of the cumulative proportion of responders analysis graph to present pain data over a range of cut-off points: making clinical trial data more understandable. *J Pain Symptom Manage* 2006; **31**: 369–377.

50. Juurlink DN, Mamdani MM, Lee DS, *et al.* Rates of hyperkalemia after publication of the Randomized Aldactone Evaluation Study. *N Engl J Med* 2004; **351**: 543–551.

51. Vickers A, Goyal N, Harland R, Rees R. Do certain countries produce only positive results? A systematic review of controlled trials. *Controlled Clin Trials* 1998; **19**: 159–166.

52. Gross CP, Mallory R, Heiat A, Krumholz HM. Reporting the recruitment process in clinical trials: who are these patients and how did they get there? *Ann Intern Med* 2002; **137**: 10–16.

53. van Spall HGC, Toren A, Kiss A, Fowler RA. Eligibility criteria of randomized controlled trials published in high-impact general medical journals: a systematic sampling review. *JAMA* 2007; **297**: 1233–1240.

54. Lexchin J, Bero LA, Djulbegovic B, Clark O. Pharmaceutical industry sponsorship and research outcome and quality: systematic review. *BMJ* 2003; **326**: 1167–1170.

55. Chan A-W, Hrobjartsson A, Haahr MT, Gøtzsche PC, Altman DG. Empirical evidence for selective reporting of outcomes in randomized trials: comparison of protocols to published articles. *JAMA* 2004; **291**: 2457–2465.

56. Als-Nielsen B, Chen W, Gluud C, Kjaergard LL. Association of funding and conclusions in randomized drug trials: a reflection of treatment effect or adverse events? *JAMA* 2003; **290**: 921–928.

57. Lewinsky NG. Nonfinancial conflicts of interest in research. *N Engl J Med* 2002; **347**: 759–761.

58. Schwid SR, Gross RA. Bias, not conflict of interest, is the enemy. *Neurology* 2005; **64**: 1830–1831.

59. Laine C, Horton R, DeAngelis CD, *et al.* Clinical trial registration. *BMJ* 2007; **334**: 1177–1178.

60. Campbell JN, Basbaum AI, Dray A, Dubner R, Dworkin RH, Sang CN (eds) *Emerging Strategies for the Treatment of Neuropathic Pain*. IASP Press, Seattle, WA, 2006.

61. Turk DC. Customizing treatment for chronic pain patients: who, what, and why. *Clin J Pain* 1990; **6**: 255–270.

62. Woolf CJ. Pain: moving from symptom control toward mechanism-specific pharmacologic management. *Ann Intern Med* 2004; **140**: 441–451.

63. Katz N. Methodological issues in clinical trials of opioids for chronic pain. *Neurology* 2005; **65**(suppl 4): S32–S49.

64. Katz J, Finnerup NB, Dworkin RH. Clinical trial outcome in neuropathic pain: relationship to study characteristics. *Neurology* 2008; **70**(4): 250–251.

65. Temple RJ. Special study designs: early escape, enrichment, studies in non-responders. *Commun Stat Theory Methods* 1994; **23**: 499–531.

66. Krishnan KRR. Efficient trial designs to reduce placebo requirements. *Biol Psychiatry* 2000; **47**: 724–726.

67. Berry DA. Bayesian clinical trials. *Nature Rev Drug Discov* 2006; **5**: 27–36.

CHAPTER 3

Introduction to evaluation of evidence

Eija Kalso

Department of Anaesthesia and Intensive Care Medicine, Helsinki University Central Hospital, Helsinki, Finland

What is evidence-based medicine?

Evidence-based medicine (EBM) is an approach to patient care that promotes the collection, interpretation, and integration of valid, important and applicable patient-reported, clinician-observed, and research-derived evidence. The best available evidence, moderated by patient circumstances and preferences is applied to improve the quality of clinical judgment.

The best available evidence is based on well-designed, randomized, double-blind and controlled trials (RCT) that have been diligently carried out (Table 3.1). RCTs are not always feasible, e.g. if the condition is very rare. Pharmacologic interventions are easier to perform as RCTs compared with, for example, invasive interventions. The latter are challenging regarding the control groups. The problem of the placebo effect (or expectation) is particularly acute regarding invasive treatments. An ethical concern is to decide how invasive a control treatment can be.

It is important to differentiate between lack of evidence (no controlled trials have been performed) and evidence for lack of effect (there is enough evidence to indicate that the treatment is not effective). Another question is whether the evidence is valid regarding an individual patient. This important question will be discussed later.

Randomization is important to minimize selection bias as inadequate concealment of treatment allocation overestimates the treatment effect by 41% [1] and nonrandomized studies can give wrong answers [2]. Each patient should have the same

Table 3.1 Type and strength of efficacy evidence

I	Strong evidence from at least one systematic review of multiple well-designed randomized controlled trials
II	Strong evidence from at least one properly designed randomized controlled trial of appropriate size
III	Evidence from well-designed trials without randomization, single group pre-post, cohort, time series or matched case–control studies
IV	Evidence from well-designed nonexperimental studies from more than one center or research group
V	Opinions of respected authorities, based on clinical evidence, descriptive studies or reports of expert committees

Four levels of scientific evidence for the effectiveness of a certain intervention on a certain condition.

Level A	Strong reserach-based evidence provided by generally consistent findings in multiple high-quality RCTs
Level B	Moderate research-based evidence provided by generally consistent findings in one high-quality RCT plus one or more low-quality RCTs, or generally consistent findings in multiplelow-quality RCTs
Level C	Limited or conflicting research-based evidence provided by one RCT (either high or low quality) or inconsistent findings in multiple RCTs
Level D	No research-based evidence, i.e. no RCTs

Evidence-Based Chronic Pain Management. Edited by C. Stannard, E. Kalso and J. Ballantyne. © 2010 Blackwell Publishing.

31

probability of being included in each study group and the allocation should be concealed. Randomization should be performed by someone who has no direct relationship to the study participants using tables of random numbers or numbers generated by computers.

Lack of double blinding will overestimate the treatment effect by roughly 17% [1] and this can lead to completely different answers, as with acupuncture in back pain [3]. Double blinding is achieved if at least the study subject and those making the observations are unaware of the treatment. Patients and observers can decode blinding because of adverse effects (and informed consents). Blinding can be tested by asking the participants which treatment they thought was given.

The control group is important as it indicates what the natural course of the disease is and/or how the new treatment compares with an established treatment. Figure 3.1 shows what effects different control groups can have. Patients with painful diabetic polyneuropathy showed a large "placebo" response. This could indicate that the patients either expected a large effect (the way the study was run enhanced the therapeutic effect of the treatment given) or the tendency for clinical improvement was greater in this group of neuropathic pain patients.

An ideal protocol should include an inactive control (placebo) and an active control (a gold standard if such exists), and the study drug in more than one dose. This means several groups and large numbers of patients need to be recruited. Thus the size of the trial may be compromised and the study will lack power to show any difference. Studies to demonstrate

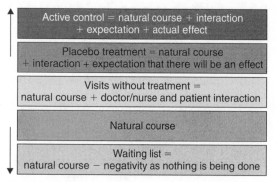

Figure 3.1 Different components of the "placebo" effect in different control groups.

unequivocally that there is no difference have to be very large, many times greater than standard analgesic trials. This is why an inactive control is important.

Quantitative systematic reviews or meta-analyses

According to the *Dictionary of Evidence-Based Medicine* [4], meta-analysis refers to the systematic quantitative pooling of available evidence on a particular research question with the use of appropriate statistical methods. As such, it forms part of many systematic reviews. In the context of drug efficacy, clinical trial evidence is sought systematically and the relevant efficacy data extracted. The data are then pooled using suitable weights such as sample variance or sample size. The pooled estimate of efficacy is then presented with the appropriate confidence bounds to define its precision.

Various statistical methods can be applied. The results of a meta-analysis are usually presented graphically with confidence interval (typically 95%) estimates for the individual as well as the pooled estimates of effect. Figure 3.2 shows the effect in individual studies and pooled effect of perioperative ketamine on the amount of morphine consumed in the ketamine versus placebo groups. In a cumulative meta-analysis the trials are arranged sequentially in order of publication date to provide a pooled estimate for the first two trials and then to update it with each subsequent trial [5].

The most "user-friendly" is number needed to treat (NNT), a term is used to define the reciprocal of the risk or rate difference. In a comparative study of two treatments A (analgesic) and P (placebo), suppose that the numbers of patients having at least 50% less pain after receiving treatments A and P are 80/100 and 60/100 respectively. Then the difference in rate of 50% pain relief is equal to 20/100. The reciprocal of this value, 5, is the NNT. This is interpreted as "on average, five patients need to be treated with treatment A for one more patient to achieve at least 50% pain relief than would be the case if they received treatment P."

The formula to calculate NNT:

$$1/[(A_{improved}/A_{total}) - (P_{improved}/P_{total})]$$
$$= 1/[(80/100) - (60/100)] = 5.$$

NNTs are "easy" to understand and to compare across studies. It is important that those who calculate and

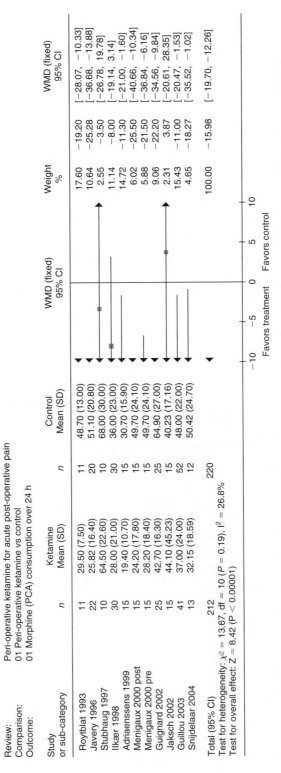

Figure 3.2 Meta-analysis of the 24 h-consumption of morphine via patient controlled analgesia as an outcome for the efficacy of perioperative ketamine vs. placebo. Reproduced from Bell *et al.* [5].

use NNTs understand both the problems and benefits when applying them. Pharmacologic studies in acute pain relief offer the highest quality data for meta-analyses in pain research (see Chapter 2). NNT is treatment specific. It describes the difference between active treatment and control in achieving a certain clinical outcome.

The NNTs shown in Figure 3.3 are based on randomized and placebo-controlled studies where the baseline pain intensities have been at least moderate. The pain-relieving effect of a single dose of the studied drug and placebo is assessed over 4–6 hours. If rescue medication is given during this period, the last value before rescuing is used for the remaining time points. The area under the time–analgesic effect curve for pain relief (TOTPAR) from time point 0 to 6 hours is calculated. The calculation of NNTs is based on data that cover a period of 4–6 hours postoperatively. The calculation of NNTs requires dichotomous data. In this case, the end-point for improvement is set at >50% pain relief, meaning that the TOTPAR shows that pain has decreased by at least 50% from the baseline pain intensity.

As all the data for the analgesic league table shown in Figure 3.3 are based on single dose studies in acute postoperative pain over a period of 6 hours, all conclusions should be restricted within these limits. A similar TOTPAR can be produced by a very effective but short-lasting analgesic and a less effective analgesic that has a longer duration of action. The time to onset of analgesia is not shown, so analgesics with slow onset but long duration of action or those with fast onset and fast offset may seem to underperform.

Figure 3.3 shows that nonsteroidal anti-inflammatory drugs (NSAIDs) compare well with opioids and that increasing the dose will improve the effectiveness of both NSAIDs and opioids. Higher doses will increase the risk for adverse effects. These are very different for the two groups of drugs. Figure 3.3 also shows that combination analgesics are effective. The combination analgesic is more effective than the opioid component alone. Two examples are paracetamol versus paracetamol plus codeine [6] and tramadol versus tramadol plus paracetamol [7]. This is important when trying to minimize adverse effects.

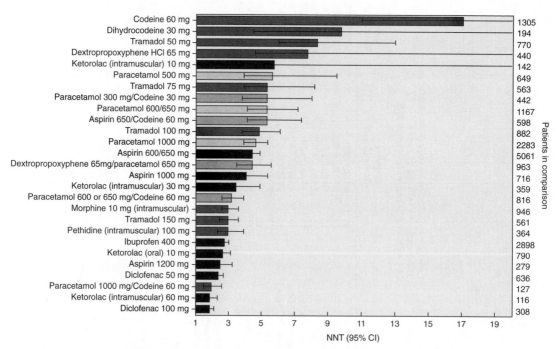

Figure 3.3 Oxford League Table of Analgesic Efficacy: NNT for at least 50% pain relief in patients with moderate to severe postoperative pain over 4–6 hours. Information was from randomized, double-blind, placebo-controlled trials. All doses oral except where indicated. The lower the NNT, the more effective the analgesic.

The number of patients included in the calculation of the NNT is important. The number of patients required in each group for a clinically relevant NNT (NNT within ±0.5 of true value) depends on the experimental event rate (EER = the proportion of patients given the active drug experiencing at least 50% pain relief). Based on single-dose acute pain analgesic trials in over 5000 patients, the control event rate (CER = proportion of patients experiencing at least 50% pain relief with placebo) is roughly 16%. Most common analgesics have EERs in the range of 40–60%. The group size required to obtain a probability of 0.95 would be >500 if the EER is 40% and about 180 if the EER is 60% [8].

The L'Abbé plot displays individual trial results so that the reader can easily identify which of the trials show benefits in favor of the test treatment and which do not (Fig. 3.4). The two axes of the plot represent the response of interest (e.g. percentage of patients having at least 50% pain relief) for the two treatment groups. Identical scales are chosen for each group's response (y axis for the test treatment, e.g. ibuprofen, and x axis for the control treatment, e.g. placebo) and the plane subdivided into two equal areas separated by a 45° diagonal line of equality.

Trials which show results in favor of the test treatment fall in the region above the diagonal while those which favor the control treatment fall below the diagonal. The symbol (circle) chosen to represent the individual trial may be sized to reflect the sample size or inverse variance of the estimate and hence the weight which should be attached to each of the trials [9].

Qualitative systematic reviews

The *Dictionary of Evidence-Based Medicine* [4] defines a systematic review as a review of a particular subject undertaken in such a systematic way that the risk of bias is reduced. The review objectives are defined precisely and formal and explicit methods are used to retrieve the available evidence as comprehensively as possible. Inclusion and exclusion criteria for studies are defined. In the evaluation of medical interventions, outcomes to be used for efficacy or safety are identified and the relevant data extracted using explicit methods. Appropriate statistical methods are used for pooling any suitable quantitative data (meta-analysis) to provide an estimate of efficacy or safety and the clinical significance of the results discussed.

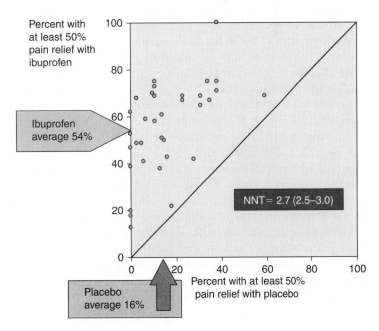

Figure 3.4 Ibuprofen 400 mg vs. placebo. Each point represents one trial with the proportion of patients achieving at least 50% pain relief on the study drug plotted on the y-axis, and the proportion of patients achieving the same endpoint with placebo on the x-axis. The drugs were given for postoperative pain when the pain was at least moderate in severity. All circles above the line of equality indicate that ibuprofen was more effective than placebo. Modified from McQuay HJ, Moore RA. *Oral ibuprofen and diclofenac in postoperative pain in. An evidence-based resource for pain relief.* Oxford University Press, Oxford: 1998.

It is often not possible to combine (pool) data, resulting in a qualitative rather than a quantitative systematic review. Combining data is not possible if:

- no quantitative information is available in the component trials of the review
- trials had different clinical outcomes
- patients were followed for different lengths of time
- combining continuous rather than dichotomous data may be difficult.

Narrative (nonsystematic) reviews are important as they are often used as a source for references. They can easily be biased, however, as both inclusions and conclusions may be determined by the author's own opinion rather than by systematic methodology. Setting criteria for inclusion, assessing quality and vote counting, i.e. determining how many studies show that the intervention works or does not work, requires at least three authors. Vote counting can lead to wrong results if more weight is not given to studies of higher quality and validity.

Quality and validity

Quality scales (Table 3.2) score trials for randomization, double blinding and description of withdrawals and drop-outs. A trial must be of a certain quality to be included in a review. Nonrandomized and randomized studies can show completely different results. A review of transcutaneous electrical nerve stimulation (TENS) for postoperative pain relief [2] analyzed 17 randomized and 19 nonrandomized studies. Seventeen of the 19 nonrandomized studies showed that TENS was more effective than placebo while 15 of the 17 randomized studies showed that it was less effective than placebo.

Nonblinded studies may also overestimate treatment effects. A review of acupuncture for back pain [3] included both blinded and nonblinded studies. The blinded studies showed that 57% of patients improved with acupuncture and 50% with control. The five nonblinded studies, however, showed a significant difference from control as 67% improved with acupuncture and only 37% with control.

In general, studies with low quality score (Table 3.2) show greater effects of treatment than higher quality studies. A systematic review analyzed 50 trials with 2394 patients for the effectiveness of acupuncture in chronic pain [10]. Most high-quality studies showed either no benefit or that acupuncture was worse than

Table 3.2 Quality scoring. From Jadad *et al.* [45]

	Score
Randomized?	
• Yes	1
• Appropriate?	
– yes (table)	1
– no (alternate)	−1
Double-blind?	
• Yes	1
• Appropriate	1
– yes (double-dummy)	1
– no	−1
Withdrawals described?	
• Yes	1

control. From 40% to 50% of the low-quality trials showed acupuncture to be better than control.

However, this does not necessarily mean that the trial is of adequate design to answer the question it posed. The issue of validity is thus different from that of quality. An analgesic trial with a high quality score would not be valid if the trial investigated patients with insufficient baseline pain to show an analgesic effect. Adequate baseline pain intensity [6] and adequate numbers of patients in each group [8] are two of the most important inclusion criteria based on assessment of validity (Table 3.3). In pre-emptive studies where the analgesic is given before the pain appears, it is not possible to assess baseline pain and new methodologic approaches need to be developed [11]. This is particularly important considering the current interest in preventing acute pain becoming chronic (see Chapter 16).

It is essential that the authors are familiar with the clinical setting in order to appreciate the specific questions of validity. Assessment of validity may require tailor-made criteria for different settings, e.g. in dental [12] or back problems [13]. Valid outcomes should also be considered carefully. Simple pain intensity or pain relief scales may not be the most appropriate outcomes in chronic pain, particularly if they are used as the only measures. Several interventions may improve the quality of life, physical functioning or coping strategies of the patients with little effect on pain itself.

Systematic reviews do not carry quality control labels apart from Cochrane reviews that have been

Table 3.3 Oxford Pain Validity Scale (OPVS). From Smith *et al.* [46]

Item	Score
Blinding	
• The trial was convincingly double blind	6
• The trial was convincingly single blind or unconvincingly double blind	3
• The trial was not blind/blinding is unclear	0
Size of trial groups	
• Group size ≥40	3
• Group size 30–39	2
• Group size 20–29	1
• Group size 10–19	0
Outcomes	
• The paper included results for at least one *pre-hoc* desirable outcome, and used it appropriately	2
• No results for any of the *pre-hoc* desirable outcomes/a *pre-hoc* desirable outcome was used inappropriately	0
Baseline pain and internal sensitivity	
• For all treatment groups, there was enough baseline pain to detect a difference between baseline and post-treatment levels/the trial demonstrated sensitivity	1
• For all treatment group, baseline levels were insufficient to be able to measure a change following the intervention/baseline levels could not be assessed/internal sensitivity was not demonstrated	0
Data analysis	
a. Definition of outcomes	
• The paper defined the relevant outcomes clearly	1
• The paper failed to define the outcomes clearly	0
b. Data presentation: location and dispersion	
• The paper presented mean data ± SD/dichotomous outcomes/median + range/sufficient data to enable extraction of any of these	1
• The paper presented none of the above	0
c. Statistical testing	
• Appropriate statistical test with correction for multiple tests where relevant were used	1
• Inappropriate statistical test and/or multiple testing without correction/no statistics were used	0
d. Handling of drop-outs	
• The drop-out rate was either ≤10%, or was >10% and includes an ITT analysis in which drop-outs were included appropriately	1
• The drop-out rate was >10% and drop-outs were not included in the analysis/it is not possible to calculate drop-out rate presented in the paper	0
The maximum total score is	16

approved by editors of the Cochrane Collaboration. The following list of quality control checks has been suggested by Oxman & Guyatt [14].

- Were the questions and methods stated clearly?
- Were the search methods used to locate relevant studies comprehensive?
- Were explicit methods used to determine which articles to include in the review?
- Was the methodologic quality of the primary studies assessed?
- Were the selection and assessment of the primary studies reproducible and free from bias?
- Were differences in individual study results explained adequately?
- Were the results of the primary studies combined appropriately?
- Were the reviewers' conclusions supported by the data cited?

A major concern regarding validity is also the relevance of the RCT for current practice. Medicine develops rapidly and therefore studies performed 10–20 years apart from each other are hardly comparable.

Systematic reviews do not compete with original research; rather, they complement each other. The greatest benefit of systematic reviews is the lessons they have taught us about trial methodology. They provide a means of quality control over clinical trials and help us to develop and apply better research methodology and to produce more reliable data. The Consolidated Standards of Reporting Trials (CONSORT) Statement was first published in 1996 and was revised in 2001 for improving the quality of reports of parallel group randomized trials [16] cluster randomized trials [17], noninferiority and equivalence trials [18], herbal interventions [19] and nonpharmacologic treatments [20]. Most high impact factor medical journals currently endorse the CONSORT statement [21]. Standards for improving the quality for reporting on meta-analyses of RCTs were published in 1999 [22].

Evaluating adverse effects

There is a profound need to recognize the importance of adverse events. In the USA, adverse drug reactions (ADRs) have been found to be involved with large numbers of deaths, with fatal ADRs ranking as the fourth to sixth leading cause of death after heart disease, cancer, and stroke, and similar to pulmonary disease and accidents [23]. A recent Swedish study showed that fatal drug reactions account for approximately 3% of all deaths in the general population [24]. In hospitals, analgesics are associated with the single largest number of adverse effects, with opioids particularly a concern [25]. As well as the human dimension, adverse events are expensive. Studies of the cost of gastrointestinal bleeding due to NSAIDs across countries are consistent, and in the UK the estimate was a conservative £250 million (410 million euros) a year [26].

Adverse events can be common or rare, minor or major, reversible or permanent, and mild or severe. They generally fall into two distinct groups: they tend to be common, minor and reversible, on the one hand, or rare, major and permanent on the other. Examples of the two groups might be dry mouth with antidepressants and upper gastrointestinal bleeding with NSAIDs. How we examine evidence on adverse events depends to a large extent on which group the adverse event belongs to.

Information on common, minor and reversible adverse events may be present in clinical trial reports, but these are frequently matters of secondary importance to efficacy, and consequently they are poorly reported [27]. In a review of adverse event reporting in 192 randomized trials in seven clinical areas, the number of discontinuations was most commonly reported in 75% of trials, though the reason was reported in only 46% [28].

Adverse events can be collected in systematic reviews. This is not always done, however, and the reporting is commonly not done in any standard way in clinical trials. Adverse events are usually reported as:
- patients reporting any adverse event: this collects information on all patients who had any complaint, of any severity
- particular adverse events: this collects patient information about specific (hopefully well-defined) adverse events
- severe adverse events: if there is a definition of an adverse event that has a clinically evident severe consequence.

Information on adverse events can be dealt with in the same way as with efficacy, using L'Abbé plots, statistical tests, numbers needed to harm (NNH), and percentage of patients with the event. Adverse events often occur less frequently than do the efficacy events of interest, and that means amounts of information available are often inadequate for a sensible answer. Trials are usually powered for efficacy, not adverse events. Adverse events are also more complicated to assess and analyze because there may be several different types of adverse events with different severity. The importance of an adverse event also depends on the patient (cannot possibly put up with a dry mouth or inability to drive a car) and his/her condition (constipation after bowel surgery).

Information on adverse events in a single-dose analgesic trial is of limited value. Information from pooling of several studies can produce more useful information about adverse effects though numbers may still be low. The meta-analysis of tramadol in postoperative pain [29] showed that increasing the dose of tramadol also increased the incidence of adverse events.

The method of assessment (spontaneous report, checklist, patient diary) and data provided by the informed consent form affect the reported incidence of adverse events, and that complicates the comparison of results across trials. If adverse event rates are very similar in the active and control (placebo) groups, this indicates that most "adverse events" are probably not due to the analgesic itself but could be related to the underlying disease (e.g. nausea in cancer). This makes it difficult to identify an adverse event that is solely due to the analgesic being used because of the background "noise" due to other interventions or diseases.

Rare, major and permanent adverse events pose even trickier territory because, being so rare, they are unlikely to be seen in randomized trials, and therefore in systematic reviews. Information on rare and serious adverse events will usually be found in epidemiologic studies. Examples are studies that examined the relationship between NSAID use and upper gastrointestinal bleeding [30, 31], NSAID use and renal failure [32] and heart failure [33].

Studies have been specifically designed and powered to analyze gastrointestinal safety when comparing COX-2-selective drugs with nonselective NSAIDs. A total of 8000 patients were enrolled in two large randomized trials [34, 35] and they and the meta-analyses of randomized trials [36, 37] showed that COX-2 selectivity decreased the risk for GI complications by about 50%.

These large studies estimate the annual risk of a gastrointestinal bleeding to be 1–2%, without indication of the severity, which could include death. Tramèr et al. [38] introduced a new model to quantitatively estimate rare adverse events that follow a biologic progression. They searched systematically for any report of chronic (≥2 months) use of NSAIDs that gave information on gastroduodenal ulcer, bleed or perforation, death due to these complications, or progression from one level of harm to the next. In addition to 15 RCTs (nearly 20,000 patients exposed to NSAID), three cohort studies (over 215,000 patients), six case–control studies (about 3000 cases), 20 case series (7400 cases) and 4450 case reports were analyzed.

In RCTs the incidence of bleeding/perforation was 0.69% with two deaths. Of the over 11,000 patients with bleeding/perforation with or without NSAID exposure across all reports, an average of 12% died. The risk was lowest in RCTs and highest in case reports. Death from bleeding/perforation in all controls not exposed to NSAIDs occurred in 0.002%.

From these numbers, the authors calculated the NNT for one patient to die due to gastroduodenal complications with chronic NSAID as 1/[0.69 [mult] (12%–0.002%)] = 1220. On average, one in 1200 patients taking NSAIDs for at least 2 months will die from gastroduodenal complications who would not have died had they not taken NSAIDs.

The CONSORT Group published an update of the CONSORT Statement for better reporting of harms in randomized trials in 2004 [39].

Balancing benefit and harm

Balancing benefit and harm by comparing NNT and NNH is justified only if both values are reliable. Single-dose analgesic studies (2898 patients, 1606 receiving ibuprofen, 1292 placebo) in postoperative pain suggest an NNT of about 3 for 50% pain relief after 400 mg of oral ibuprofen. The respective NNH for any patient experiencing any minor adverse event is about 25. We know that roughly 16% of patients have at least 50% pain relief with placebo (CER is 16%) and that most common analgesics have EERs in the range of 40–60%. The group size required to obtain a probability of 0.95 would be >500 if the EER is 40% [8]. The CER for adverse events is 15% and the common analgesics cause an adverse event in 19% of the patients. The group size to obtain a probability of 0.95 would be >2000 [7]. With sufficient information, plots of NNT versus NNH might be useful aids in making clinical or policy decisions.

Patient withdrawal from a study due to adverse events is considered as major harm and is reported commonly [28]. The drop-out figures in clinical trials may not reflect the real-life situation, as patient compliance may be better during short clinical trials than in long-term use. One method of achieving more realistic estimates of patient preference may be to ask the patient to balance benefit and harm: how much and what adverse events are an acceptable price for a certain amount of pain relief? Studies on drugs affecting the CNS (e.g. antidepressants and anticonvulsants) often have to use a design where the patient titrates him/herself to the dose that gives adequate pain relief or the highest tolerated dose even if pain relief is not adequate. If the design of an RCT has not used individual titration, the results on major harm may be flawed as they do not reflect a real-life situation.

If we have seen no serious adverse event in 1500 exposed patients, we can be 95% sure that they do not occur more frequently than 1 in 500 patients. Few new drugs have been tested in more than a few thousand patients when they first become commercially available. This makes case reports, yellow cards, and properly done postmarketing surveillance important. Pharmacogenomics may provide information in the future that will make estimation of adverse drug reactions easier.

Using evidence for the individual patient

The evidence that we have from systematic reviews and meta-analyses tells us how an intervention works in general in the average patient. This is important when large-scale estimates are made regarding, for example, the cost-effectiveness of drugs. However, when making treatment plans for an individual patient, this kind of evidence forms only one part of the information that is needed for appropriate decision making. The patient (e.g. age, gender, other diseases and medications, organ function, financial capacity) will form the framework within which various treatment options are balanced for benefit and harm. It is well known that patients do generally better in RCTs than in normal clinical practice. This may be due to the usually strict entrance criteria. However, there are many factors in the RCTs (patient information, regular appointments and other contacts, true patient participation, encouragement) that could be used to improve clinical outcomes.

Future of evidence?

There are two important developments that should, at least theoretically, change the way we collect evidence for interventions. One is the introduction of electronic patient reports and the other is genomics research. Structured reporting and assessment of, for example, drug effects could be performed in the clinic and the data could be used not only for the benefit of the individual patient but also for the almost online compilation of evidence. Some pharmacologic interventions (e.g. drugs metabolized via CYP enzymes) will be connected to pharmacogenetic analyses (e.g. assessment of CYP 2D6 metabolizer status). This will

also mean that future RCTs will be more targeted and have genomics-based entrance criteria.

Acknowledgment

This chapter is based on a series of essays, "Five easy pieces on evidence-based medicine" [40–44]. I wish to thank Jayne Edwards, Henry McQuay and Andrew Moore, the co-authors of the easy pieces, and the *European Journal of Pain* for the permission to use this material.

References

1. Schultz KF, Chalmers I, Hayes RJ, Altman DG. Empirical evidence of bias: dimesions of methodological quality associated with estimates of treatment effects in controlled trials. *JAMA* 1995; **273**: 408–412.
2. Carroll D, Tramèr M, McQuay H, Nye B, Moore A. Randomization is important in studies with pain outcomes: systematic review of transcutaneous electrical nerve stimulation in acute postoperative pain. *Br J Anaesth* 1996; **77**: 798–803.
3. Ernst E, White AR. Acupuncture for back pain: a meta-analysis of randomised controlled trials. *Arch Intern Med* 1998; **158**: 2235–2241.
4. Li Wan Po A. A practical guide to undertaking a systematic review. *Pharmaceut J* 1997; **258**: 518–520.
5. Bell RF, Dahl JB, Moore RA, Kalso E. Peri-operative ketamine for acute postoperative pain. A quantitative and qualitative systematic review (Cochrane review). *Acta Anaesthesiol Scand* 2005; **49**: 1405–1428.
6. Moore A, Collins S, Carroll D, McQuay H. Paracetamol with and without codeine in acute pain: a quantitative systematic review. *Pain* 1997; **70**: 193–201.
7. Edwards JE, McQuay HJ, Moore RA. Combination analgesic efficacy: individual patient data meta-analysis of single-dose oral tramadol plus acetaminophen in acute postoperative pain. *J Pain Symptom Manage* 2002; **23**(2):121–30.
8. Moore RA, Gavaghan D, Tramèr, MR, Collins SL, McQuay HJ. Size is everything – large amounts of information are needed to overcome random effects in estimating direction and magnitude of treatment effects. *Pain* 1998; **78**: 209–216.
9. L'Abbé KA, Detsky AS, O'Rourke K. Meta-analysis in clinical research. *Ann Intern Med* 1987; **107**: 224–233.
10. Ezzo I, Berman B, Hadhazy VA, Jadad AR, Lao L, Singh BB. Is acupuncture effective for the treatment of chronic pain? A systematic review. *Pain* 2000; **86**: 217–225.
11. Kalso E, Smith L, McQuay HJ, Moore RA. No pain, no gain: clinical excellence and scientific rigour – lessons learned from IA morphine. *Pain* 2002; **98**: 269–275.
12. Antczak AA, Tang J, Chalmers TC. Quality assessment of randomized controlled trials in dental research. I. Methods. *J Peridontal Res* 1986; **21**: 305–314.
13. van Tulder MW, Assendelft WJ, Koes BW, *et al*. Method guidelines for systematic reviews in the Cochrane Collaboration Back Review Group for Spinal Disorders. *Spine* 1997; **22**: 2323–2330.

14. Oxman AD, Guyatt GH. Guidelines for reading literature reviews. *Can Med Assoc J* 1988; **138**: 697–703.

15. Begg C, Cho M, Eastwood S, *et al*. Improving the quality of reporting of randomized controlled trials: the CONSORT statement. *JAMA* 1996; **276**: 637–639.

16. Moher D, Schulz KF, Altman DG, for the CONSORT Group. The CONSORT statement: revised recommendations for improving the quality of reports of parallel-group ransomised trials. *Lancet* 2001; **357**: 1191–1194.

17. Campbell MK, Elbourne DR, Altman DG, for the CONSORT Group. CONSORT statement: extension to cluster randomised trials. *BMJ* 2004; **328**: 702–708.

18. Piaggio G, Elbourne DR, Altman DG, Pocock SJ, Evans SJW, for the CONSORT Group. Reporting of noninferiority and equivalence randomized trials: an extension of the CONSORT statement. *JAMA* 2006; **295**: 1152–1160.

19. Gagnier JJ, Boon H, Rochon P, Moher D, Barnes J, Bombardier C, for the CONSORT Group. Reporting randomized, controlled trials of herbal interventions: an elaborated CONSORT statement. *Ann Intern Med* 2006; **144**: 364–367.

20. Boutron I, Moher D, Altman DG, Schulz K, Ravaud P, for the CONSORT Group. Extending the CONSORT statement to randomized trials of nonpharmacologic treatment: an explanation and elaboration. *Ann Intern Med* 2008; **148**: 295–309.

21. Hopewell S, Altman DG, Moher D, Schulz KF. Endorsement of the CONSORT Statement by high impact factor medical journal: a survey of journal editors and journal "Instructions to Authors". *Trials* 2008; **9**: 1–7.

22. Moher D, Cook DJ, Eastwood S, Olkin I, Rennie D, Stroup DF. Improving the quality of reports of meta-analyses of randomised controlled trials: the QUORUM statement. Quality of Reporting Meta-analyses. *Lancet* 1999; **354**: 1896–1990.

23. Lazarou J, Pomeranz BH, Corey PN. Incidence of adverse drug reactions in hospitalized patients. *JAMA* 1998; **279**: 1200–1205.

24. Wester K, Jönsson AK, Spigset O, Druid H, Hägg S. Incidence of fatal adverse drug reactions: a population based study. *Br J Clin Pharmacol* 2008; **65**: 573–579.

25. Bates DW, Cullen DJ, Laird N, *et al*. Incidence of adverse drug events and potential adverse drug events. *JAMA* 1995; **274**: 29–34.

26. Moore RA, Phillips CJ. Cost of NSAID adverse effects to the UK National Health Service. *J Med Econ* 1999; **2**: 45–55.

27. Edwards JE, McQuay HJ, Moore RA, Collins SL. Reporting of adverse effects in clinical trials should be improved. Lessons from acute postoperative pain. *J Pain Symptom Manage* 1999; **81**: 289–297.

28. Ioannidis JPA, Lau J. Completeness of safety reporting in randomized trials: an evaluation of 7 medical areas. *JAMA* 2001; **285**: 437–443.

29. Moore RA, McQuay HJ. Single-patient data meta-analysis of 3453 postoperative patients: oral tramadol versus placebo, codeine and combination analgesics. *Pain* 1997; **69**: 287–294.

30. Henry D, Dobson A, Turner C. Variability in the risk of major gastrointestinal complications from nonaspirin nonsteroidal anti-inflammatory drugs. *Gastroenterology* 1993; **105**: 1078–1088.

31. Hernandez-Diaz S, Rodridguez LAG. Association between nonsteroidal anti-inflammatory drugs and upper gastrointestinal tract bleeding/perforation. *Arch Intern Med* 2000; **160**: 2093–2099.

32. Henry D, Page J, Whyte I, *et al*. Consumption of nonsteroidal anti-inflammatory drugs and the development of functional renal impairment in elderly subjects. Results of a case–control study. *Br J Clin Pharmacol* 1997; **44**: 85–90.

33. Page J, Henry D. Consumption of NSAIDs and the development of congestive heart failure in elderly patients. *Arch Intern Med* 2000; **160**: 777–784.

34. Bombardier C, Laine L, Reicin A, *et al*. Comparison of upper gastrointestinal toxicity of rofecoxib and naproxen in patients with rheumatoid arthritis. *N Engl J Med* 2000; **343**: 1520–1528.

35. Silverstein FE, Faich G, Golstein JL, *et al*. Gastrointestinal toxicity with celecoxib vs nonsteroidal anti-inflammatory drugs for osteoarthritis and rheumatoid arthritis. The CLASS study: a randomised controlled trial. *JAMA* 2000; **284**: 1247–1255.

36. Langman MJ, Jensen DM, Watson DJ, *et al*. Adverse upper gastrointestinal effects of rofecoxib compared with NSAIDs. *JAMA* 1999; **282**: 1929–1933.

37. Bensen WG, Zhao SZ, Burke T, *et al*. Upper gastrointestinal tolerability of celecoxib, a COX-2 specific inhibitor, compared to naproxen and placebo. *J Rheumatol* 2000; **27**: 1876–1883.

38. Tramèr MR, Moore RA, Reynolds DJ, McQuay HJ. Quantitative estimation of rare adverse events which follow a biological progression: a new model applied to chronic NSAID use. *Pain* 2000; **85**: 169–182.

39. Ioannidis JP, Evans SJ, Gotzsche PC, *et al*. for the CONSORT Group. Better reporting of harms in randomized trials. An extension of the CONSORT statement. *Ann Intern Med* 2004; **141**: 781–788.

40. Kalso E. Five easy pieces on evidence-based medicine (1): Introduction. *Eur J Pain* 2000; **4**: 217–219.

41. Kalso E, Moore RA. Five easy pieces on evidence-based medicine (2): Why randomized and (placebo) controlled? *Eur J Pain* 2000; **4**: 321–324.

42. Kalso E, Edwards J, McQuay HJ, Moore RA. Five easy pieces on evidence-based medicine (3): Quantitative systematic reviews. *Eur J Pain* 2001; **5**: 227–230.

43. Kalso E, Edwards J, McQuay HJ, Moore RA. Five easy pieces on evidence-based medicine (4): Qualitative systematic reviews. *Eur J Pain* 2002; **6**: 89–93.

44. Kalso E, Edwards J, McQuay HJ, Moore RA. Five easy pieces on evidence-based medicine (5): trading benefit against harm – pain relief vs. adverse effects. *Eur J Pain* 2002; **6**: 409–412.

45. Jadad AR, Moore RA, Carroll D, *et al*. Assessing the quality of reports of randomized clinical trials: is blinding necessary? *Control Clin Trials* 1996; **17**: 1–12.

46. Smith LA, Oldman AD, McQuay HJ, Moore RA. Teasing apart quality and validity in systematic reviews: an example from acupuncture trials in chronic neck and back pain. *Pain* 2000; **86**: 119–132.

CHAPTER 4

Neurobiology of pain

Victoria Harvey and Anthony Dickenson

Department of Pharmacology, University College London, London, UK

Introduction

Pain is a sensation related to potential or actual damage in some tissue of the organism. At the dawn of time, the first organisms developed systems that allowed them to move away from a painful (nociceptive) stimulus. This alarm sign represents the beginning of a chain of biological events one purpose of which is to provide a warning to the organism. Thus, the activation of the pathways involved in coding, transmitting and interpreting pain are involved in sensory perception of the stimulus, but other systems activate muscles to enable active avoidance of the painful stimulus. In fact, it is thought that there are general similarities in the pattern of acute nociceptive behavior observed in the marine snail, *Aplysia californica*, with those from more evolved phyla, such as rats and humans, suggesting that common nocifensive responses such as injury detection, escape and recuperation are shared in genetically diverse species [1].

Pain perception in higher order species, including humans, also involves the activation of areas of the brain associated with emotions, such that we feel anxiety, anger, and fear as a result of pain [2, 3]. The mechanisms underlying the transmission and perception of pain are numerous and diverse in nature, including sophisticated neuronal networks involving thousands of nerve cells and multiple chemical factors (Fig. 4.1). Pain is not simply a

Evidence-Based Chronic Pain Management. Edited by C. Stannard, E. Kalso and J. Ballantyne. © 2010 Blackwell Publishing.

neurophysiologic problem; in fact, pain perception is a highly complicated process that can be modulated by gender, age, and psychological, psychosocial and genetic factors [4, 5].

Despite the knowledge gained over the last few years on the mechanisms of pain and analgesia, the problem of pain is still not fully resolved, particularly when the signals that pain promotes remain over long periods of time, generating chronic pain. In this situation, the survival or warning action of pain has an unclear function. In the same way, neuropathic pain generated as a consequence of a lesion in neuronal pathways should predictably only lead to numbness but patients frequently have pain as well. This is probably due to our having systems that can enhance, amplify and prolong pain as a further warning mechanism but with chronic neuropathic pain, these become dysfunctional or outlast their usefulness in the short term.

Chronic pain can be broadly categorized into three types: inflammatory, neuropathic and dysfunctional pain. We have used the terms inflammatory and neuropathic pain in this account to distinguish these major types of pain on the basis of the involvement of tissue damage or disease process. Some authors use the term nociceptive pain to reflect inflammatory pain. All pain is nociceptive and we feel that the designation of tissue damage within the term inflammatory is more apt. Inflammatory pain can arise from an insult to the integrity of tissues either by trauma or infection, and associated conditions include headaches, arthritis and appendicitis. Neuropathic pain, defined by trauma to or pathological changes in the central or peripheral nervous systems, often responds poorly to standard pain treatments. Examples of neu-

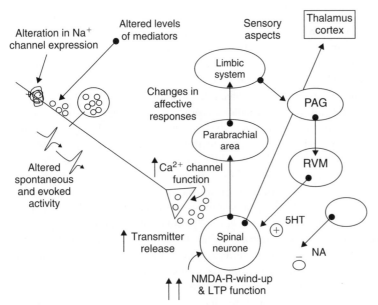

Figure 4.1 Some of the pathways of pain. Inputs from the periphery activate spinal systems and then engage supraspinal circuits. The plasticity in signaling in various pain states is depicted. 5HT, 5 hydroxytryptamine; NA, noradrenaline; NMDA, N-methyl-D-aspartate; LTP, long-term potentiation; PAG, periaqueductal gray; RVM, rostroventral medulla.

ropathic pain, amongst others, include pain arising from nerve degeneration as a consequence of diabetes, stroke, ischemia or multiple sclerosis, nerve infection from viral agents such as shingles or HIV, entrapment neuropathy underlying the commonly reported carpal tunnel syndrome, and alcoholism which can cause neuropathy through nutritional deficiencies. The third type of pain can be ascribed to nerve dysfunction and is thought to underlie conditions such as fibromyalgia, irritable bowel syndrome (IBS) and migraine, and is often poorly characterized by nonlocalized diffuse pain which is not accompanied by overt tissue inflammation or nerve pathology.

By classifying the type of pain a patient is suffering, the first essential step in pain management has been taken. However, some chronic pain states are heterogeneous conditions and cannot always be categorized unequivocally; for example, osteo-arthritis is a chronic degenerative disorder characterized by inflammation within the joint and potential neuropathy resulting from joint deformity. Similarly, cancer pain involves inflammatory pain aspects and neuropathic pain resulting from nerve compression or distension or engendered by chemotherapy-induced neurotoxicity leading to atypical neuronal functionality.

Pain can be spontaneous, existing without a stimulus, or can be triggered by stimuli. Spontaneous pain can be either constant or intermittent, and most patients describe having both (e.g. constant "burning" pain plus intermittent "shooting" or "electric shock-like pain"). Evoked pains often include allodynia where normally non-noxious stimuli such as cooling, gentle touch, movement and pressure now evoke pain. In addition, abnormal sensations including crawling, numbness, itching, and tingling are often reported, suggesting changes in the nervous system as a result of the insult. The symptoms are similar despite the many causes of nerve injury. In a recent study, 26% of patients with type 2 diabetes were found to have neuropathic pain [6], and it has also been reported to occur in more than one-third of HIV patients [7]. Moreover, the severity and prevalence of pain vary with the type and stage of the disease. In cancer pain, for example, 30–45% of patients on average experience moderate to severe pain at the time of diagnosis and at intermediate stages this rises to nearly 75% of patients with advanced stage cancer [8].

The mechanisms underlying aberrant behavioral and neuronal signs in animal models of peripheral neuropathic pain can be divided into peripheral and central. Four main mechanisms have been suggested to be relevant: changes in ion channels (mainly sodium channels) at and around the site of injury, changes in transmitter release through calcium channels, central spinal hyperexcitability and finally, increases in descending facilitations. They are universal to different models of neuropathy and not only do these mechanisms have some supporting evidence from humans but often the mechanisms relate to clinically effective drugs.

Peripheral events

The first stage in the transmission of acute pain involves activation of specialized sensory receptors on a certain set of peripheral nerves called C-fibers – the nociceptors. These receptors include mechano, chemo- and thermoreceptors, so the nociceptors associated with C-fibers are often termed polymodal since they can respond to a variety of painful stimuli [9]. C-fibers are responsive to such a range of peripheral painful stimuli since nociceptors are not single entities but comprise a number of receptors or channels that sense and respond to a variety of stimuli. It has long been known that capsaicin, the hot ingredient in chilli peppers, evokes a sensation of burning pain thought to occur from the activation of the vanilloid receptor 1 (VR1/TRPV1), a receptor thought to represent the molecular identity of our heat sensor [10]. More recently, two members of the transient receptor potential (TRP) family, TRPM8 and TRPA1, have been associated with the transduction of cool and noxious cold signaling, respectively [11]. The epithelial Na^+ channel (ENaC) [12] and the K^+ channel TRAAK [13] are thought to open or close in response to mechanical stimuli. The ongoing discovery of receptors and mechanisms associated with pain perception reflects the complexity of the processes which underlie it. By identifying the sensors involved in the transduction of noxious stimuli, novel therapies could arise from drugs that block these sensors.

Tissue damage

The peripheral terminals of small-diameter neurones, especially in conditions of tissue damage, may be excited by a number of endogenous chemical mediators. These chemical mediators then interact to cause a sensitization of nociceptors so that afferent activity to a given stimulus is increased by the presence of inflammation. This has been called primary hyperalgesia.

Chronic inflammation arises when C-fibers, which normally transmit noxious information, become activated by chronically inflamed tissue and thus sensitized nociceptors now transmit low-threshold signals to the spinal cord as pain. One of the most important components in inflammation is the production of arachidonic acid metabolites, giving rise to a large number of prostaglandins. These chemicals do not normally activate nociceptors directly but, by contrast, reduce the C-fiber threshold and so sensitize the nociceptors to other mediators and stimuli. Thus the use of both steroids and the nonsteroidal anti-inflammatory (NSAID) drugs is based on their ability to block the enzyme cyclo-oxygenase (COX) which catalyzes the conversion of arachidonic acid to these mediators. The main action of the NSAID is to inhibit COX-1 but as this form is the constitutive enzyme, COX-1 inhibition results in varied gastrointestinal complications ranging in severity from dyspepsia to serious ulcer bleeds and perforations. Importantly, a second inducible form of COX, COX-2, has been described, displaying a different pattern of distribution and activity from COX-1 [14]. This has led to the hypothesis that the selective blockade of COX-2 would improve the therapeutic profile of this class of drugs by avoiding the undesired gastropathy associated with COX-1 inhibition [15]. However, two selective COX-2 inhibitors, Vioxx (rofecoxib) and Bextra (valdecoxib), have been removed from the market following reports indicating an increased risk of heart attack or stroke among patients, and serious cutaneous adverse reactions respectively [16,17]. This effect of these second-generation NSAID has called into question their improved therapeutic gain.

Bradykinin, hydrogen ions and serotonin, 5-hydroxytryptamine (5HT) accumulate in damaged tissue and further excitation of nociceptive afferents can occur via the activation of its large number of receptors [18]. These same chemicals cause a number of effects including vasodilation and plasma extravasation so that blood vessels become leaky and plasma seeps out, so causing edema that often accompanies tissue damage. The key role, but not the exact mechanisms of action, of 5HT in the pain associated with migraine [19] and other headaches is well established but little is known about the actions of this mediator in other nonheadache pains.

Nerve damage

Neuropathic pain states are characterized by both negative symptoms (sensory loss, numbness) and the positive symptoms of allodynia, hyperalgesia and ongoing pain that are unlike the consequences of damage to our other sensory systems. These positive symptoms strongly suggest changes within the nervous system that are excessive attempts to compensate for sensory loss. The initial events of neuropathic pain are thought to be generated in the peripheral sensory neurones within the nerve itself at the site of damage and so are independent of peripheral nociceptor activation. Following damage to peripheral nerves, a number of changes can be produced, in terms of activity, properties and transmitter content. Damaged nerves may start to generate ongoing "ectopic" activity where patterns of excitability and conduction in primary afferent fibers (PAF) are markedly altered. Nerve endings may also seal off and sometimes unsuccessfully attempt to sprout, resulting in the formation of a neuroma which can often lead to abnormal mechanosensitivity [20].

The causes of the spontaneous ectopic activity are thought to involve sodium channel receptor accumulation and clustering in the PAF neuroma [21], but may also involve changes of the density or functional properties of calcium and potassium channels [22–25]. These changes may also be dependent on the type of nerve damage encountered since the expression of tetrodotoxin (TTX)-resistant sodium channels, for example, is downregulated following axonal lesions but upregulated following inflammation [26]. This aberrant activity can then start to spread rapidly to the cell body in the dorsal root ganglia (DRG). In addition to changes within the nerve, sympathetic efferents become able to activate sensory afferents. These peripheral ectopic impulses can cause spontaneous pain and hyperalgesia. This peripheral activity may be a rational basis for the use of systemic local anesthetics, such as lignocaine, in neuropathic states since damaged nerves have been shown to be highly sensitive to systemic sodium channel blockers

[27–29]. This too is probably part of the basis for the mechanisms of established effective anticonvulsants that block sodium channels, such as carbamazepine [30] and phenytoin [31].

The potential for a systemic drug that blocks pain-related sodium channels has now gained impetus as at least two sodium channels with either unique (Nav 1.8) or selective (Nav 1.7) localization in small afferents have been validated [32, 33]. The former has a selective blocker, effective in preclinical models [34], and the latter has been shown to be implicated in human familial pain disorders [35, 36]. If effective in humans, these agents could provide truly novel approaches to pain control.

Gabapentin and pregabalin are drugs licensed for neuropathic pain that have analgesic activity in neuropathic pain states from varying origins. In randomized controlled trials both gabapentin and pregabalin have demonstrated their value in the treatment of pain associated with diabetic peripheral neuropathy and postherpetic neuralgia [37–39]. The mechanism of action of gabapentin and pregabalin is now clearly established; although both drugs are lipophilic analogs of GABA, their analgesic action is attributed to their interaction with the auxiliary-associated protein $\alpha_2\delta$ subunit, common to all voltage-gated calcium channels [40, 41]. In animals, gabapentin displays state-dependent analgesia inasmuch as it selectively inhibits altered neuronal function resulting from neuropathy whilst leaving normal activity unaffected [41–44]. This ability to alter abnormal activity in a somewhat selective manner may partly result from the fact that the spinal cord $\alpha_2\delta$ subunit is upregulated after nerve injury accompanied by functional changes in the roles of a number of calcium channels [24].

However, this is not the only factor that governs this state dependency, with pathways from midbrain hyperalgesic systems also participating. A likely pathway involves spinal lamina I substance P-responsive neurones which project to the parabrachial region and subsequently the rostroventral medulla (RVM) where descending serotonergic pathways can become activated, modulating spinal excitability through spinal neurones with substance P-saporin (SP-SAP), or intrathecal administration of the 5HT antagonist ondansetron, attenuates mechanical and tactile hypersensitivity and aberrant neuronal coding following spinal nerve injury. Furthermore, in these animals, gabapentin efficacy can be switched on and off by interference with these 5HT-3 systems [45].

This descending facilitatory serotonergic drive is thought to play only a minor role under normal conditions compared with pathophysiological conditions [46] and may be important not only in neuropathy but also in dysfunctional pains where not only is 5HT implicated but these pathways provide a route by which abnormal central processing can diffusely increase spinal sensitivity. Human imaging studies have verified these circuits in non-neuropathic pains and shown an interaction with gabapentin [47, 48].

Central excitatory systems

The arrival of action potentials in the dorsal horn (DH) of the spinal cord, carrying the sensory information either from nociceptors in inflammation or generated both from nociceptors and intrinsically after nerve damage, produces yet greater complexity in pain and analgesia. Within the CNS, not only are excitatory mechanisms of prime importance but in contrast to much of the peripheral signalling, the role of controlling inhibitory transmitter systems is of paramount importance. Within our spinal cords and brains, not only are the sensory and emotional aspects of pain generated but there are also mechanisms that can make the pain signals stronger (descending facilitation) or weaker (descending inhibition). The main issue here is that the former predominate in most conditions since an absence of pain after trauma is a rare event confined to the short term in situations such as combat or sports events.

A large majority of nocisponsive PAF and many projection neurones contain the major excitatory neurotransmitter glutamate. Glutamate acts at both metabotropic (mGlu) receptors (G-protein coupled) and the ionotropic AMPA, Kainate and NMDA receptors (coupled directly to ion channels). During persistent pain, C-fibers are stimulated repetitively at a high frequency, resulting in wind-up, an amplification and prolongation of the response of spinal DH neurones. In particular, NMDA receptors are thought to play a central role in this sensitization of DH neurones by increasing the synaptic efficacy of nociceptive pathways (long-term potentiation, LTP) and hence underpin hyperalgesia and allodynia [49].

Spinal LTP therefore presents one likely mechanism by which acute pain becomes chronic [50].

The development of NMDA receptor antagonists for the treatment of pain has been hampered since the NMDA receptor is essential for normal neuronal function [51]. First-generation NMDA antagonists include ketamine, memantine and dextromethorphan. This class of low-affinity uncompetitive open channel blockers is thought to inhibit only tonic pathophysiological NMDA receptor activity, leaving phasic physiological activity unaffected [52–55]. Ketamine, originally clinically used as a dissociative anesthetic, can be used at low subanesthetic analgesic doses in a wide range of pain states. When administered at a low dose perioperatively, ketamine spares opioid consumption and reduces opioid-related side effects such as nausea and vomiting [56], and is also effective as a "rescue analgesic" in acute pain that is poorly responsive to morphine [57]. The use of ketamine in the treatment of chronic pain, however, is more limited since long-term abuse engenders cognitive impairments of memory, attention and judgment and there is a paucity of data about issues such as tolerance, dependence and withdrawal. However, low-dose intravenous ketamine has proved effective in reducing allodynia associated with post-traumatic pain [58] and spinal cord injury pain [59], and patients suffering refractory cancer pain responded well to short-term "burst" treatment [60].

The long-term increase in pain sensitivity frequently seen following injury or peripheral nerve damage is thought to be due to both alterations in transmission within the spinal cord and to changes in descending controls that run back to the spinal cord from the brainstem. Within this circuit, nociceptive information is also relayed to higher centers in the brain via projection neurones. The neuroanatomy of these ascending pain pathways is highly complex, and supraspinal contacts include centers involved with the sensory-discriminative aspects of pain such as the intensity, location and duration of the stimulus as well as centers involved in the affective-cognitive aspects including anxiety, emotion and memory [61]. Importantly, these are the same areas of the brain that modulate descending serotonergic and noradrenergic inputs from the brainstem that regulate nociceptive processing at spinal levels. Thus, a network of spinal and brain circuits can change spinal sensitivity to peripheral inputs, and regulation of this by descending pathways from the brain can link the level of cord sensitivity to the behavioral and environmental context. For example, pain can cause anxiety and sleep deficits, and the sensation of pain becomes more intense as a result of this reciprocal regulation. Conversely, "fear conditioning," whereby anticipation in response to re-exposure to a situation previously associated with a noxious stimulus, can activate the endogenous antinociceptive descending pathways and thus provides an important survival response in mammals [62].

Several classes of antidepressant including serotonin and noradrenaline reuptake inhibitors (SSRIs, SNRIs), and tricyclic antidepressants, in particular amitriptyline, have proved effective in the treatment of certain types of neuropathic pain [63, 64]. The analgesic mechanism of action of antidepressants is not fully understood but it is thought to be independent of their antidepressant effect. Since these agents increase synaptic levels of noradrenaline and 5HT, their central analgesic action is likely to involve either presynaptic mechanisms reducing nociceptive transmission or postsynaptic mechanisms enhancing the endogenous descending inhibitory pathways. Likely targets include the activation of central inhibitory $\alpha 2$-adrenoreceptors and members of the inhibitory 5HT-1 receptor family as well-known analgesics such as the antihypertensive drug clonidine and the triptan family, used in the treatment of migraine, exert their analgesic effects through these receptors respectively [65, 66]. Given that facilitatory 5HT-3 receptors are also present in the dorsal horn [67], the improved efficacy of SNRIs over SSRIs observed in the treatment of neuropathic pain [68] may be accredited to this. More recently, a horde of peripheral analgesic targets has also been proposed [69]; at these sites it is unlikely that the increased availability of 5HT and noradrenaline is accountable since these agents are thought to be pronociceptive at this level.

Central inhibitory systems

The role of inhibitory systems is important in the control of events following C-fiber stimulation. Opioids are the major inhibitory controls on pain and all clinically used opioid drugs act on the μ receptor, the receptor for morphine which is thought to be responsible for both the analgesic and adverse effects of morphine [70]. The actions of clinically used opioids can now be explained in terms of their acting as agonists at one of the four opioid receptors found in the brain, spinal cord and peripheral nervous system. All opioid receptors are inhibitory. The receptors are for the endogenous opioid peptides that function as transmitters in the nervous system. Like all other peptides, they are synthesized as large inactive precursors in the neuronal cell body and transported to the terminal, with processing *en route* yielding the active fragment which is then released into the synapse and activates the appropriate receptors. Morphine activates opioid receptors to a much greater extent than the opioid peptides and so produces profound analgesia.

The opioid receptors are found on postsynaptic sites but presynaptic locations predominate so that activation of the receptors can control the release of a number of neurotransmitters. The endogenous peptides are rapidly degraded so that nonpeptide agonists are needed. Side effects are due to the peripheral and central receptors whereas the analgesic effects are due to the interaction of opioid with central receptors. The degree of analgesia can be limited by the side effects. All clincially important opioids act on the mu receptor and hopes for other opioids acting on the other opioid receptors have not yet been fulfilled.

μ Receptors are located in the periphery, where their transportation from the DRG is upregulated following inflammation [71], and at pre- and postsynaptic sites in the spinal cord and in the brain. The actions of opioids are best understood in the DH of the spinal cord, where their analgesic mechanisms involve reduced transmitter release from nociceptive C-fibers following noxious stimulation [72], and postsynaptic inhibitions resulting from K^+ hyperpolarization of projection neurones conveying information from the spinal cord to the brain. The opioid receptors in the spinal cord are predominantly of the μ and δ types and are found in the C-fiber terminal zone (the substantia gelatinosa) in the superficial dorsal horn. Up to 75% of the opioid receptors are found presynaptically on the C-fiber terminals and when activated, inhibit neurotransmitter release. Their opening of potassium channels will reduce calcium flux. The remaining postsynaptic receptors hyperpolarize and so inhibit projection neurones and interneurones; the net result is further inhibition of the C-fiber induced activity. This spinal action of opioids can be targeted by using the intrathecal or epidural routes of administration which have an advantage over systemic application of avoiding the side effects mediated by opioid receptors in the brain and periphery. Complete C-fiber inhibition can be produced and so complete analgesia can be achieved but opioids do not always act so effectively when the pain arises from nerve damage. Reasons for this are suspected to be excessive transmitter release and spinal NMDA-mediated activity which are hard to inhibit.

There are other important sites of opioid actions located in the 5HT and noradrenergic nuclei of the brainstem and midbrain, including the raphe nuclei (RVM), the periaqueductal gray matter (PAG) and the locus coeruleus. These areas of the brain are important in sleep, anxiety and fear and explain how these functions interact with and are altered by pain. Opioid receptors in these zones, when activated, alter the level of activity in descending pathways from these zones to the spinal cord that in turn reduces activity of spinal cord neurones. The relative roles of the 5HT receptors in the spinal cord are unknown but the spinal target for noradrenaline (NA) released from descending pathways is α2 receptors which have similar actions and distribution to the opioid receptors. Sedation and hypotension with α2 agonists presently limit their use as analgesics but they are useful veterinary drugs.

Most of the data concerning morphine analgesia have been derived from studies of patients with cancer pain, since its therapeutic potential for the treatment of neuropathic pain has been limited [73]. However, opioid therapy for chronic noncancer pain (CNCP) is now becoming more acceptable where long-term consumption can be therapeutically beneficial [74, 75]. Moreover, methadone, normally associated with the treatment of opioid addiction, may provide an appropriate replacement when side effects have limited dose escalation [76]. Tramadol, which displays both serotonergic and opioidergic mechanisms, has proved effective in the treatment of painful diabetic peripheral neuropathy [77] and relieved ongoing pain and reduced allodynia in patients with polyneuropathy [78], and offers a treatment option with lower abuse liability [79].

The ORL1 receptor (also known as nociceptin, orphanin FQ or NOP receptor) is structurally related to μ opioid receptors but resistant to classic opioid agonists such as morphine [80]. The endogenous ligand for ORL1 receptors, nociceptin, is thought to be important in spinal nociceptive transmission [81–83] and displays antinociceptive effects in animal models of neuropathic and inflammatory pain [84, 85]. Recently, a likely mechanism has been proposed involving ORL1 receptor-mediated internalization of calcium channels leading to decreased neuronal excitability [86].

Conclusion

We now have a good understanding of the basic mechanisms of pain transmission and analgesia and can say that hyperexcitability can be set up both peripherally and centrally. The latter means that minor peripheral inputs may cause severe pain, if, for example, wind-up is established centrally. However, there are many areas in which our understanding is still inadequate. For example, individual differences in levels of pain, in the transition from acute to chronic pain, differences in susceptibility to neuropathic pain after nerve damage and in analgesic effectiveness may have a genetic basis. In order for pain to be better controlled, our knowledge of mechanisms needs to be translated into therapy.

References

1. Walters ET, Alizadeh H, Castro GA. Similar neuronal alterations induced by axonal injury and learning in Aplysia. *Science* 1991; **253**(5021): 797–799.
2. Gaskin ME, Greene AF, Robinson ME, Geisser ME. Negative affect and the experience of chronic pain. *J Psychosom Res* 1992; **36**(8): 707–713.
3. Keefe FJ, Rumble ME, Scipio CD, Giordano LA, Perri LM. Psychological aspects of persistent pain: current state of the science. *J Pain* 2004; **5**(4): 195–211.
4. Riley JL 3rd, Robinson ME, Wise EA, Myers CD, Fillingim RB. Sex differences in the perception of noxious experimental stimuli: a meta-analysis. *Pain* 1998; **74**(2–3): 181–187.
5. Overmeer TBK, Linton SJ. Psychosocial factors in back pain: a comparison of factors listed by health care providers with the evidence. In: Herta Flor EK, Dostrovsky JO (eds) 11th World Congress on Pain, 2006. IASP Press, Sydney, 2006.
6. Davies M, Brophy S, Williams R, Taylor A. The prevalence, severity, and impact of painful diabetic peripheral neuropathy in type 2 diabetes. *Diabetes Care* 2006; **29**(7): 1518–1522.

7. Schifitto G, McDermott MP, McArthur JC, *et al.* Markers of immune activation and viral load in HIV-associated sensory neuropathy. *Neurology* 2005; **64**(5): 842–848.

8. Daut RL, Cleeland CS. The prevalence and severity of pain in cancer. *Cancer* 1982; **50**(9): 1913–1918.

9. Dickenson AH. *Pain and Analgesia.* John Wiley, Chichester, 2001.

10. Caterina MJ, Schumacher MA, Tominaga M, Rosen TA, Levine JD, Julius D. The capsaicin receptor: a heat-activated ion channel in the pain pathway. *Nature* 1997; **389**(6653): 816–824.

11. McKemy DD. How cold is it? TRPM8 and TRPA1 in the molecular logic of cold sensation. *Molec Pain* 2005; **1**(1): 16.

12. Fricke B, Lints R, Stewart G, *et al.* Epithelial Na^+ channels and stomatin are expressed in rat trigeminal mechanosensory neurons. *Cell Tissue Res* 2000; **299**(3): 327–334.

13. Maingret F, Fosset M, Lesage F, Lazdunski M, Honore E. TRAAK is a mammalian neuronal mechano-gated K^+ channel. *J Biol Chem* 1999; **274**(3): 1381–1387.

14. Burian M, Geisslinger G. COX-dependent mechanisms involved in the antinociceptive action of NSAIDs at central and peripheral sites. *Pharmacol Ther* 2005; 107(2): 139–154.

15. Needleman P, Isakson PC. The discovery and function of COX-2. *J Rheumatol* 1997; **49**(suppl): 6–8.

16. European Medicines Agency. EMEA press release: European Medicines Agency concludes action on COX-2 inhibitors EMEA/207766/2005. European Medicines Agency, London, 2005.

17. Food and Drug Administration. Food and Drug Administration announces series of changes to the class of marketed non-steroidal anti-inflammatory drugs (NSAIDs). Food and Drug Administration, Rockville, MD, 2005.

18. Wood JN, Docherty R. Chemical activators of sensory neurons. *Annu Rev Physiol* 1997; 59: 457–482.

19. Ramadan NM, Buchanan TM. New and future migraine therapy. *Pharmacol Ther* 2006; **112**(1): 199–212.

20. Babbedge RC, Soper AJ, Gentry CT, Hood VC, Campbell EA, Urban L. In vitro characterization of a peripheral afferent pathway of the rat after chronic sciatic nerve section. *J Neurophysiol* 1996; **76**(5): 3169–3177.

21. Devor M, Govrin-Lippmann R, Angelides K. Na^+ channel immunolocalization in peripheral mammalian axons and changes following nerve injury and neuroma formation. *J Neurosci* 1993; **13**(5): 1976–1992.

22. Abdulla FA, Smith PA. Ectopic alpha2-adrenoceptors couple to N-type Ca^{2+} channels in axotomized rat sensory neurons. *J Neurosci* 1997; **17**(5): 1633–1641.

23. Amir R, Devor M. Spike-evoked suppression and burst patterning in dorsal root ganglion neurons of the rat. *J Physiol* 1997; **501**(Pt 1): 183–196.

24. Li CY, Zhang XL, Matthews EA, *et al.* Calcium channel alpha(2)delta(1) subunit mediates spinal hyperexcitability in pain modulation. *Pain* 2006; **125**(1–2): 20–34.

25. Xiao WH, Bennett GJ. Synthetic omega-conopeptides applied to the site of nerve injury suppress neuropathic pains in rats. *J Pharmacol Exper Therapeut* 1995; **274**(2): 666–672.

26. Waxman SG, Dib-Hajj S, Cummins TR, Black JA. Sodium channels and pain. *Proc Natl Acad Sci USA* 1999; **96**(14): 7635–7639.

27. Kastrup J, Petersen P, Dejgard A, Angelo HR, Hilsted J. Intravenous lidocaine infusion – a new treatment of chronic painful diabetic neuropathy? *Pain* 1987; **28**(1): 69–75.

28. Mao J, Chen LL. Systemic lidocaine for neuropathic pain relief. *Pain* 2000; **87**(1): 7–17.

29. Tremont-Lukats IW, Challapalli V, McNicol ED, Lau J, Carr DB. Systemic administration of local anesthetics to relieve neuropathic pain: a systematic review and meta-analysis. *Anesthes Analges* 2005; **101**(6): 1738–1749.

30. Blom S. Trigeminal neuralgia: its treatment with a new anticonvulsant drug (G-32883). *Lancet* 1962; 1: 839–840.

31. Kuo CC, Bean BP. Slow binding of phenytoin to inactivated sodium channels in rat hippocampal neurons. *Molec Pharmacol* 1994; **46**(4): 716–725.

32. Nassar MA, Stirling LC, Forlani G, *et al.* Nociceptor-specific gene deletion reveals a major role for Nav1.7 (PN1) in acute and inflammatory pain. *Proc Natl Acad Sci USA* 2004; **101**(34): 12706–12711.

33. Matthews EA, Wood JN, Dickenson AH. Nav 1.8-null mice show stimulus-dependent deficits in spinal neuronal activity. *Molec Pain* 2006; **2**: 5.

34. Jarvis MF, Honore P, Shieh CC, *et al.* A-803467, a potent and selective Nav1.8 sodium channel blocker, attenuates neuropathic and inflammatory pain in the rat. *Proc Natl Acad Sci USA* 2007; **104**(20): 8520–8525.

35. Cox JJ, Reimann F, Nicholas AK, *et al.* An SCN9A channelopathy causes congenital inability to experience pain. *Nature* 2006; **444**(7121): 894–898.

36. Yang Y, Wang Y, Li S, *et al.* Mutations in SCN9A, encoding a sodium channel alpha subunit, in patients with primary erythermalgia. *J Med Genet* 2004; **41**(3): 171–174.

37. Backonja M, Beydoun A, Edwards KR, *et al.* Gabapentin for the symptomatic treatment of painful neuropathy in patients with diabetes mellitus: a randomized controlled trial. *JAMA* 1998; **280**(21): 1831–1836.

38. Freynhagen R, Strojek K, Griesing T, Whalen E, Balkenohl M. Efficacy of pregabalin in neuropathic pain evaluated in a 12-week, randomised, double-blind, multicentre, placebo-controlled trial of flexible- and fixed-dose regimens. *Pain* 2005; **115**(3): 254–263.

39. Rowbotham M, Harden N, Stacey B, Bernstein P, Magnus-Miller L. Gabapentin for the treatment of postherpetic neuralgia: a randomized controlled trial. *JAMA* 1998; **280**(21): 1837–1842.

40. Gee NS, Brown JP, Dissanayake VU, Offord J, Thurlow R, Woodruff GN. The novel anticonvulsant drug, gabapentin (Neurontin), binds to the alpha2delta subunit of a calcium channel. *J Biol Chem* 1996; **271**(10): 5768–5776.

41. Stanfa LC, Singh L, Williams RG, Dickenson AH. Gabapentin, ineffective in normal rats, markedly reduces C-fiber evoked responses after inflammation. *Neuroreport* 1997; **8**(3): 587–590.

42. Chapman V, Suzuki R, Chamarette HL, Rygh LJ, Dickenson AH. Effects of systemic carbamazepine and gabapentin on

spinal neuronal responses in spinal nerve ligated rats. *Pain* 1998; **75**(2–3): 261–272.

43. Field MJ, Oles RJ, Lewis AS, McCleary S, Hughes J, Singh L. Gabapentin (neurontin) and S-(+)-3-isobutylgaba represent a novel class of selective antihyperalgesic agents. *Br J Pharmacol* 1997; **121**(8): 1513–1522.

44. Tanabe M, Takasu K, Kasuya N, Shimizu S, Honda M, Ono H. Role of descending noradrenergic system and spinal alpha2-adrenergic receptors in the effects of gabapentin on thermal and mechanical nociception after partial nerve injury in the mouse. *Br J Pharmacol* 2005; **144**(5): 703–714.

45. Suzuki R, Rahman W, Rygh LJ, Webber M, Hunt SP, Dickenson AH. Spinal-supraspinal serotonergic circuits regulating neuropathic pain and its treatment with gabapentin. *Pain* 2005; **117**(3): 292–303.

46. Suzuki R, Rahman W, Hunt SP, Dickenson AH. Descending facilitatory control of mechanically evoked responses is enhanced in deep dorsal horn neurones following peripheral nerve injury. *Brain Res* 2004; **1019**(1–2): 68–76.

47. Dickenson AH, Bee LA, Suzuki R. Pains, gains, and midbrains. *Proc Natl Acad Sci USA* 2005; **102**(50): 17885–17886.

48. Iannetti GD, Zambreanu L, Wise RG, *et al.* Pharmacological modulation of pain-related brain activity during normal and central sensitization states in humans. *Proc Natl Acad Sci USA* 2005; **102**(50): 18195–18200.

49. Dickenson AH. Mechanisms of central hypersensitivity: excitatory amino acid mechanisms and their control. In: *The Pharmacology of Pain. Handbook of Experimental Pharmacology.* Springer-Verlag, Berlin, 1997.

50. Rygh LJ, Svendsen F, Fiska A, Haugan F, Hole K, Tjolsen A. Long-term potentiation in spinal nociceptive systems – how acute pain may become chronic. *Psychoneuroendocrinology* 2005; **30**(10): 959–964.

51. Cull-Candy S, Brickley S, Farrant M. NMDA receptor subunits: diversity, development and disease. *Curr Opin Neurobiol* 2001; **11**(3): 327–335.

52. Chen HS, Pellegrini JW, Aggarwal SK, *et al.* Open-channel block of N-methyl-D-aspartate (NMDA) responses by memantine: therapeutic advantage against NMDA receptor-mediated neurotoxicity. *J Neurosci* 1992; **12**(11): 4427–4436.

53. Kornhuber J, Weller M. Psychotogenicity and N-methyl-D-aspartate receptor antagonism: implications for neuroprotective pharmacotherapy. *Biol Psychiatry* 1997; **41**(2): 135–144.

54. Parsons CG, Danysz W, Quack G. Memantine is a clinically well tolerated N-methyl-D-aspartate (NMDA) receptor antagonist – a review of preclinical data. *Neuropharmacology* 1999; **38**(6): 735–767.

55. Rogawski MA. Therapeutic potential of excitatory amino acid antagonists: channel blockers and 2,3-benzodiazepines. *Trends Pharmacol Sci* 1993; **14**(9): 325–331.

56. Bell RF, Dahl JB, Moore RA, Kalso EA. Perioperative ketamine for acute postoperative pain. *Cochrane Database of Systematic Reviews* 2006, Issue 1. Art. No.: CD004603. DOI: 10.1002/14651858.CD004603.pub2.

57. Weinbroum AA. A single small dose of postoperative ketamine provides rapid and sustained improvement in morphine analgesia in the presence of morphine-resistant pain. *Anesthes Analges* 2003; **96**(3): 789–795.

58. Max MB, Byas-Smith MG, Gracely RH, Bennett GJ. Intravenous infusion of the NMDA antagonist, ketamine, in chronic posttraumatic pain with allodynia: a double-blind comparison to alfentanil and placebo. *Clin NeuroPharmacol* 1995; **18**(4): 360–368.

59. Eide PK, Jorum E, Stubhaug A, Bremnes J, Breivik H. Relief of post-herpetic neuralgia with the N-methyl-D-aspartic acid receptor antagonist ketamine: a double-blind, crossover comparison with morphine and placebo. *Pain* 1994; **58**(3): 347–354.

60. Jackson K, Ashby M, Martin P, Pisasale M, Brumley D, Hayes B. "Burst" ketamine for refractory cancer pain: an open-label audit of 39 patients. *J Pain Symptom Manage* 2001; **22**(4): 834–842.

61. Millan MJ. The induction of pain: an integrative review. *Prog Neurobiol* 1999; **57**(1): 1–164.

62. Watkins LR, McGorry M, Schwartz B, Sisk D, Wiertelak EP, Maier SF. Reversal of spinal cord non-opiate analgesia by conditioned anti-analgesia in the rat. *Pain* 1997; **71**(3): 237–247.

63. Gidal BE. New and emerging treatment options for neuropathic pain. *Am J Manag Care* 2006; **12**(9 suppl): S269–278.

64. Watson CP, Evans RJ, Reed K, Merskey H, Goldsmith L, Warsh J. Amitriptyline versus placebo in postherpetic neuralgia. *Neurology* 1982; **32**(6): 671–673.

65. Saxena PR, Ferrari MD. 5-HT(1)-like receptor agonists and the pathophysiology of migraine. *Trends Pharmacol Sci* 1989; **10**(5): 200–204.

66. Yaksh TL. Pharmacology of spinal adrenergic systems which modulate spinal nociceptive processing. *Pharmacol Biochem Behav* 1985; **22**(5): 845–858.

67. Kia HK, Miquel MC, McKernan RM, *et al.* Localization of 5-HT3 receptors in the rat spinal cord: immunohistochemistry and in situ hybridization. *Neuroreport* 1995; **6**(2): 257–261.

68. Mattia C, Paoletti F, Coluzzi F, Boanelli A. New antidepressants in the treatment of neuropathic pain. A review. *Minerva Anestesiol* 2002; **68**(3): 105–114.

69. Mico JA, Ardid D, Berrocoso E, Eschalier A. Antidepressants and pain. *Trends Pharmacol Sci* 2006; **27**(7): 348–354.

70. Kieffer BL. Opioids: first lessons from knockout mice. *Trends Pharmacol Sci* 1999; **20**(1): 19–26.

71. Hassan AH, Ableitner A, Stein C, Herz A. Inflammation of the rat paw enhances axonal transport of opioid receptors in the sciatic nerve and increases their density in the inflamed tissue. *Neuroscience* 1993; **55**(1): 185–195.

72. Yaksh TL, Jessell TM, Gamse R, Mudge AW, Leeman SE. Intrathecal morphine inhibits substance P release from mammalian spinal cord in vivo. *Nature* 1980; **286**(5769): 155–157.

73. Arner S, Meyerson BA. Lack of analgesic effect of opioids on neuropathic and idiopathic forms of pain. *Pain* 1988; **33**(1): 11–23.

74. American Pain Society. Consensus Statement from the American Academy of Pain Medicine and the American

Pain Society. The use of opioids for the treatment of chronic pain. *Pain Forum* 1997; 77–79.

75. McQuay H. Opioids in pain management. *Lancet* 1999; **353**(9171): 2229–2232.

76. Toombs JD, Kral LA. Methadone treatment for pain states. *Am Fam Physician* 2005; **71**(7): 1353–1358.

77. Harati Y, Gooch C, Swenson M, *et al.* Double-blind randomized trial of tramadol for the treatment of the pain of diabetic neuropathy. *Neurology* 1998; **50**(6): 1842–1846.

78. Sindrup SH, Andersen G, Madsen C, Smith T, Brosen K, Jensen TS. Tramadol relieves pain and allodynia in polyneuropathy: a randomised, double-blind, controlled trial. *Pain* 1999; **83**(1): 85–90.

79. Preston KL, Jasinski DR, Testa M. Abuse potential and pharmacological comparison of tramadol and morphine. *Drug Alcohol Depend* 1991; **27**(1): 7–17.

80. Knoflach F, Reinscheid RK, Civelli O, Kemp JA. Modulation of voltage-gated calcium channels by orphanin FQ in freshly dissociated hippocampal neurons. *J Neurosci* 1996; **16**(21): 6657–6664.

81. Carpenter KJ, Vithlani M, Dickenson AH. Unaltered peripheral excitatory actions of nociceptin contrast with enhanced spinal inhibitory effects after carrageenan inflammation: an electrophysiological study in the rat. *Pain* 2000; **85**(3): 433–441.

82. Maie IA, Dickenson AH. Cholecystokinin fails to block the spinal inhibitory effects of nociceptin in sham operated and neuropathic rats. *Eur J Pharmacol* 2004; **484**(2–3): 235–240.

83. Stanfa LC, Chapman V, Kerr N, Dickenson AH. Inhibitory action of nociceptin on spinal dorsal horn neurones of the rat, in vivo. *Br J Pharmacol* 1996; **118**(8): 1875–1877.

84. Yamamoto T, Nozaki-Taguchi N, Kimura S. Analgesic effect of intrathecally administered nociceptin, an opioid receptor-like1 receptor agonist, in the rat formalin test. *Neuroscience* 1997; **81**(1): 249–254.

85. Yamamoto T, Nozaki-Taguchi N, Kimura S. Effects of intrathecally administered nociceptin, an opioid receptor-like1 (ORL1) receptor agonist, on the thermal hyperalgesia induced by carageenan injection into the rat paw. *Brain Res* 1997; **754**(1–2): 329–332.

86. Altier C, Khosravani H, Evans RM, *et al.* ORL1 receptor-mediated internalization of N-type calcium channels. *Nat Neurosci* 2006; **9**(1): 31–40.

CHAPTER 5

Intractable pain and the perception of time: every patient is an anecdote

David B. Morris

University of Virginia, Charlottesville, VA, USA

What distinguishes intractable pain is less its intensity or even its resistance to treatment than its persistence over time [1]. Time matters in chronic pain, however, far beyond the persistence or duration implied in the concept of chronicity. Time seemed to stop for 13 chronic pain patients, according to a phenomenologic study, and the future was unfathomable [2]. This distinctive relation to time not only separates intractable pain from many other chronic illnesses, such as diabetes [3]. It raises important questions about the treatment of chronic pain, because different perceptions of time by doctors and by patients may reduce quality in healthcare [4]. In general, patients and physicians differ in their perceptions of what constitutes *timely* access to care [5]. In particular, low back pain patients in primary care (according to a study conducted in the western United States) develop their own beliefs about their back pain, about what it means for them, and such beliefs remained "very stable" over the 6-month period studied [6].

Temporal stability matters here especially because the beliefs correlated with predictable positive or negative outcomes. In short, time is far more complex and significant for patients and for their physicians than textbooks imply in designating a conventional number of months that supposedly divides pain into its chronic and nonchronic states. It is thus worth reflecting broadly, in what follows, on how the

Evidence-Based Chronic Pain Management. Edited by C. Stannard, E. Kalso and J. Ballantyne. © 2010 Blackwell Publishing.

distinctive perceptions of time help redefine, even reconstitute, the person in chronic pain.

Many people undergo a jolting, destructive injury, in an automobile accident, say, but 6 months later they are back at work, rehab complete, free from pain and apparently healed. In such fortunate outcomes, the time between injury and healing marks the full trajectory of trauma – beginning, middle, end – like a classic drama. Intractable pain, however, follows a different temporal arc: unfinished, protracted, repetitive. It is a liminal state, blurring the traditional borders that demarcate health and illness, a void that swallows up healing. Illness of course always takes place over time and may even follow a predictable timetable or natural history, but temporality has a marginal impact on many medical conditions. Temporality, however, remains both central to intractable pain – inseparable from it – and difficult to transform into evidence-based data, since objective clock time differs from subjective duration (time as a personal, psychologic perception). A concert pianist facing permanent hand injury may experience time not by the calendar but by subjective fears of a pain that destroys any conceivable future. Intractable pain has an atypical time signature built into its structure. Its most alien feature, separating it from the familiar and somewhat reassuring model of acute pain, is the threat of endlessness: pain that never stops.

We know very little, as it happens, about how patients with intractable pain perceive time. Perceptions of time clearly differ across cultures, just as the cultural invention of railroads altered space/time relations and changed human ideas of punctuality [7].

Rural or indigenous cultures tend to experience time in leisurely cycles and seasons, unlike the high-speed, do-it-now urban pace of the proverbial New York minute. Age and illness also alter the perception of time. A healthy child experiences time differently from how it is experienced by a geriatric cancer patient. In the absence of meta-analyses or randomized double-blind studies, I'd like to tell a story.

The other day, at age 64, I noticed that my garden-variety chronic low back pain, a constant unwelcome companion for the past 20 years, had disappeared. Not completely – I don't want to call down Nemesis. Still, as I pulled on my socks one morning I was surprised to notice that my back wasn't, as usual, pressed for support against the closet door. It was like the old days: one foot on the floor, one foot airborne, wobbly but pain free. This is a dull story, I admit, except if it were *your* back. A doctor's son, I had long resisted medical help after depending on medicine to rule out catastrophic low-back trauma. Waiting rooms frustrate me more than pain does, and I enjoyed inventing *work-arounds* in which I accomplished ordinary tasks (say, making the bed) without bending at the waist. My pain, I decided, could be reconfigured as a badge of honor – like a combat wound – or, honorable in its own twisted way, writer's cramp. I didn't like the pain, I didn't like the two daily 600 mg ibuprofen caplets that my saintly primary care physician prescribed, but so it goes. Then, after 20 years, the pain disappeared. I keep wondering if it will return tomorrow in a firestorm of hot, aching soreness, or maybe the next day. Right now, at the computer keyboard, I feel a small steady belt of tiredness behind me, but nothing serious, nothing to bother about. I can't quite believe my good luck. That's my story.

The perception of time, like chronic pain, is undoubtedly a function of complex brain networks. The cortical links responsible for the perception of time are evident mainly through their disruption in various neurodegenerative dementias. Brain-damaged patients, for example, often experience temporal-spatial disorientation, losing track of hours, days, months or years. French philosopher Paul Ricoeur, in his magisterial three-volume *Time and Narrative* (1983–1985), argues that time achieves meaningful human status only "to the extent that it is articulated through a narrative mode ..." [8]. From Hesiod's *Works and Days* to Proust's *Remembrance of Time Past,* from ancient myth to modern cinema, narrative is a machine for the co-production of temporality. In fact, researchers across several fields are beginning to make the case, drawing upon recent neurologic data, that humans possess a "narrative brain" [9]. That is, our brains predispose us to create narrative structures with their implicit temporal ordering. Confabulation, another product of brain damage, suggests that a neurobiologic narrative drive persists even in the absence of conscious control [10]. Wherever such research leads, the human perception of time owes less to calendars and clocks (which our ancestors invented rather late in the game) than to brains and stories. The perception of time is what allows us to make sense of (not just inhabit) a planet that rotates on its axis every 24 hours and that once each year revolves around the sun. Narrative thus holds special importance for studies that seek to understand how chronic pain patients experience the crucial human dimension of time.

Patient stories may be dull or fascinating – an esthetic matter – but as a clinical matter they constitute evidence, often neglected evidence. Anecdote of course occupies the bottom rung in the hierarchy of evidence-based medicine. It is often dismissed out of hand as unscientific, especially when patients claim to receive benefits from therapies that physicians distrust, as with conventional and alternative medicine. "Such testimonials are worthless as evidential support," as one EBM textbook puts it [11]. Anecdote is evidence nonetheless, not always or automatically worthless, and at times it may be the best evidence available. Certainly, despite the recent boom in clinical practice guidelines, the percentage of healthcare based on high-quality or gold-standard evidence is "always very low" [12]. In a classic study, physician Eric Cassell asks how a clinician can know when the patient is suffering. His iconoclastic answer: "Ask the patient" [13]. Suffering often accompanies intractable pain – both conditions linked to an altered sense of time – and *asking the patient* may well produce evidence about temporality. Some evidence will surely take the form of anecdote, possibly a humdrum, pointless account of no clinical value, but how do you *know* it's valueless unless you ask and listen?

The value of anecdotal evidence lies in its particularity. An irreducible particularity is what in fact excludes anecdotes from the best evidence of typical clinical guidelines. When it comes to understanding an individual patient, however, the patient's particular first-person speech and story, in all its possibly tedious subjectivity, constitutes relevant evidence. Not the *only* evidence, certainly. Some patients confabulate; some are confused; some cling to patently erroneous beliefs. Anecdotal evidence must be judged alongside other evidence, including better evidence such as lab tests and objective observation. If contradictions emerge, the anecdotal evidence has helped to uncover a patient-centered problem that might need to be addressed. An "n of 1" obviously makes no sense as the population for a valid scientific study. On the other hand, each patient is an "n of 1" – distinctive if not unique – endowed with personal experience and possibly with genetic traits that may confound expectations based on vast statistical studies. Statistical studies, in any case, have great difficulty taking account of qualitative data, and (as pain specialist Daniel B. Carr argues) qualitative data expose the inherent limits of biomedical assumptions about objectivity that theory-based sciences have abandoned or modified [14]. There is yet another argument, however, for taking the clinical care required to gather relevant anecdotal evidence. Stories, from this point of view, are not just bits of evidence, raw data somehow detachable from the person, like a broken tooth or fMRI. Physician, therapist, author, and medical educator Rachel Naomi Remen puts the strongest medical argument for anecdotal evidence this way: "Everybody is a story" [15].

Thus, people do not *possess* stories the way they possess, say, a virus or a suitcase. As Remen carefully phrases it, people do not "have" stories, they *are* stories. As one loosely affiliated group of psychologists puts it, human experience and human identity are inherently "storied." If you subtract my stories from my personal identity, so this argument runs, you get zero. Zero includes a living organism, but nothing that most patients would recognize as fully human. Remen's assertion, presumably based upon observation inside and outside the clinic, draws support from various investigators looking into the construction of human consciousness. Together such lines of thought suggest that it makes good sense to weigh the evidence provided by patient narratives, especially in cases of intractable pain. Where causes are often elusive and treatment vexed, anecdote constitutes not just

evidence but indispensable, irreplaceable evidence. In this sense, anecdotes, however flawed or imperfect their status, are never irrelevant. Indeed, they offer a vital point of connection between evidence-based medicine and a value-based medicine that integrates objective data with subjective, patient-perceived quality-of-life improvement [16].

An attention to patient *narrative*, to substitute a less pejorative term for *anecdote*, allows clinicians to understand better what is distinctive in the experience of each particular patient [17]. Because evidence-based treatment depends for its benefit upon statistical generalizations about large populations, its clinical effectiveness can only be improved, in the sense of sharpened in its focus on the individual, by incorporating narrative data from a singular patient who speaks with a singular clinician (also equally storied) in a professional exchange that, despite its resemblance to everyday speech, has not occurred before in the history of the planet [18]. This is the claim I'd like to address.

Illness tends to divide time into a before-and-after structure. "I want the old me," writes breast cancer patient and poet-novelist Audre Lorde following her mastectomy [19]. Time has not changed for the rest of the world; it still goes by in minutes, hours, days. For Lorde, however, time has split in half, and the new bipartite structure extends to her sense of self: a former stable identity is replaced by an unstable (fractured or divided) identity, no longer whole or self-consistent across time. "When pain is no longer useful as a symptom," as one recent study reports, "identity is challenged, weakened and at risk ..." [20]. Chronic pain, like a serious illness, splits time and splits being. Audre Lorde's account of the changes that followed her mastectomy is unusual only in its articulate explicitness: "This event called upon me to re-examine the quality and texture of my entire life, its priorities and commitments, as well as the possible alterations that might be required in the light of that re-examination" [21]. Certainly, not every breast cancer patient will choose Lorde's subsequent 1970s identity as warrior-activist, just as few might share her self-definition as a black, lesbian, feminist poet. A narrative-based focus, however, is exactly what is needed to produce evidence relevant to her particular treatment: evidence missed in a checklist of psychosocial categories based on job, family, alcohol, and tobacco.

Temporality may divide again if healing or recovery occurs, as it did for Lorde. The initial bipartite "before-and-after" structure of serious illness yields to a retrospective tripartite structure: *before* ("the stable old self"), *during* ("self in crisis"), and *after* ("a stable new self"). American novelist Reynolds Price struggled with intractable pain associated with spinal cancer and radiation therapy, and the memoir of his illness, *A Whole New Life: An Illness and a Healing* (1994), offers a vivid instance of tripartite temporality. "The kindest thing anyone could have done for me, once I'd finished five weeks' radiation," he writes from the retrospective position of someone able to live successfully with intractable pain, "would have been to look me square in the eye and say this clearly, 'Reynolds Price is dead. Who will you be now? Who *can* you be and how can you get there, doubletime?" [22]. Price wishes in effect that someone had advised him to move instantly across time, to cut out the middle stage of a tripartite structure, so he could move directly from before (the old Price) to after (the new Price). He could not be clearer about the need to construct a new identity. The construction of identity, however, occurs only over time, through the medium of temporality, and Price's memoir tells the story of his slow, idiosyncratic healing process, materially aided by pain specialists who recognized how his distinctive strengths as a novelist might aid in recovery.

Patients who experience intractable pain enter a life-world (as phenomenologists call it) where temporality is important to assess. It is a life-world where clear diagrammatic bipartite *before/after* structures or tripartite *before/during/after* structures may prove inadequate to the patient's lived experience of time, while nonetheless offering clinicians a rough instrument for assessing the impact of divided time and divided identities. Such diagrammatic structures are useful to recognize not only because they underwrite very different stories of illness but also because patients who tell these stories also *live* the stories, for better or for worse.

The experience of temporality that Lorde and Price write about, even if completely eccentric and wholly subjective, matters from a clinical perspective as evidence relevant to providing patients with the best possible treatment. All narrative, as philosopher and novelist Richard Kearney describes it, shares the common function of "someone telling something to someone about something ..." [23]. Even lyric poetry fulfills the function of telling someone about something, and poet Emily Dickinson tells readers something clinically useful about temporality and pain:

> Pain - has an Element of Blank -
> It cannot recollect
> When it begun - or if there were
> A time when it was not -
>
> It has no Future-but itself -
> Its Infinite contain
> Its Past - enlightened to perceive
> New Periods - of pain. [24]

Enlightenment, if we construe the poem as spoken by someone in pain, here leads only to the grim truth that pain obliterates ordinary time. Any reassuring before/after structure collapses because, to the person in pain, nothing ever changes: it is all a drab, blank, infinite sameness. The poem offers a means of understanding that the unit of time most consequential to chronic pain patients, as one study concludes, is "the moment." It is a paradoxical moment – "a lengthy, heavy one that does not correspond to customary notions of clock time" – precisely because it appears endless: "The moment contains not only the pain now but also the perceived possibility of an eternity of suffering ..." [2]. No future but itself. No future except as enlightened to see its unity with the past. Hope, always oriented to future time, yields to an undifferentiated, present-tense hopelessness.

It is possible to construe Dickinson's poem differently, less as a lyrical cry than as an impersonal description, in which case intractable pain appears as an almost eternal force, outside history, unchanged from the dawn of time. Enlightenment here, ironically, means something exactly opposite to a conventional semantics designating the 18th-century ideology of empirical science with its optimistic expectations of technologic progress. Hers is an anti-Enlightenment geologic time with no Precambrian or Mesozoic, merely one undifferentiated Period of Pain. The slight differences in these two interpretations, lyric or impersonal, never approach contradiction, but the divergences emphasize that narrative is never transparent. That is, meanings are often undecidable and contested. Stories, including patient narratives, regularly arouse disagreements about meaning, as happens also in medicine, where second opinions nonetheless do not fatally undermine confidence in the possibility of beneficial treatment or of general consensus. The main point is that Dickinson's poem, despite possible disagreements, depicts pain as inseparable from a skewed temporality that plays havoc with typical optimistic expectations of future improvement.

Intractable pain skews temporality, then, in ways that demand clinical attention. A recent European study concludes that pain intensity has less impact on quality of life, for chronic pain patients, than do beliefs about pain [25]. The most harmful pain belief is what specialists call catastrophizing. A catastrophe is, etymologically, a down-turn (Greek *kata* = down + *strophein* = to turn). Its earliest use in English comes from formalist literary theory, where the *catastrophe* in a drama designates the change (often unhappy) that produces a final conclusion. Chronic pain patients who catastrophize do not consciously invoke the formal structures of drama, but clinicians might reflect on a life-world that appears to take a final, conclusive downturn.

Catastrophizing is more than unjustified fear of disaster. For patients, it involves a largely unthought experience of temporality in which the varied narrative arc of an individual life turns toward flatline. Here intractable pain makes contact with yet another structure of time. The blank, atemporal dimension that Emily Dickinson described now permits the glimmer of a future, but it is always the same disastrous future, the opposite of recovery. Fear is a present-tense experience, of course, and we fear what hasn't yet happened: a future if imminent event. This uncanny future-present time is the site of catastrophe. Attention to catastrophizing pain beliefs can do more than predict a narrative arc of negative outcomes or difficulties ahead. It might allow interventions targeted to change patient beliefs about relations between pain and temporality, reducing pain by reducing anxiety, and thus measurably improving quality of life.

The temporality of intractable pain, as my dull opening story indicates, is not always a site of catastrophe, and a narrative that strikes pain specialists as dull may not bore pain patients, especially not the specific teller. Significantly, the story of my disappearing low back pain depicts temporality neither as changeless misery nor as impending disaster.

It might even count as a modest success story [26]. Success is defined variously, of course, and what counts as success for a particular patient may emerge only through the give-and-take of narrative conversations. My particular success story entails my resistance to accepting the category of patient, a refusal that some other people in pain share. Medicine knows very little about such people, people who resist a self-definition or medical definition as patients, who manage to live successfully (on their own terms) with chronic pain. These are not people who *cope* or *manage*, which are medical terms applied to patients, but people who *live* with pain as nonpatients, who exist outside the structure of medicalization (which is also a temporal structure, as the term "waiting" room deftly indicates). Arguably, one measure of success for medicine would be fewer people with low back pain who present as patients, especially patients who accept or seek medical certification as disabled. I recognize that my respite from back pain may be – again to invoke time – temporary, a false summer, the prelude to its heartbreaking, unremitting return. Equally possible, I have simply reached the tipping point at which I stumble into the side benefits of senior citizenship. Chronic pain is well known as being less prevalent among the elderly. Of course, my story predicts that I will reject a medical explanation of my passage into a possibly less toxic elder pain, which doesn't mean that the explanation is incorrect. It is simply a story I don't want to hear. The relevant pain narratives that we can't tell or refuse to hear may be as crucial as the stories we can't help repeating.

What matters most about success stories is that some patients find them a helpful source of hope. While evidence-based medicine offers facts about populations, it does not provide a basis for infallible predictions about individuals, who may defy the odds. Should population-based statistical evidence possess the unintended authority to banish hope? Success stories, in my view, have a valid place as a limited form of evidence, within a careful, ethical explanation of all the relevant facts, especially as they offer hope based on the perception that someone else in a similar dilemma managed to find a way out. Success stories certainly alter the patient's perception of time. They point toward a time to come that differs from both present and past. They crack open a static temporality – transform "the moment" in its frozen, monolithic hopelessness – so that the glimmer of an unfolding, differentiated future reappears. It may be in some cases that individual success stories, such as Reynolds Price recounts in his personal illness narrative, offer patients incentive to create or discover (as he tells readers that he did) not only a new life but also almost a new identity.

The significance of time in intractable pain goes far beyond the possible therapeutic value of success stories. An attention to temporality emphasizes that what matters in intractable pain is not time but the patient's *perception* of time. Perception is open to change, even if pain is not, even if nerve endings and neurotransmitters may be permanently unresponsive to treatment. John Loeser, neurosurgeon and distinguished pain specialist, writes that the brain is the organ responsible for all pain [27]. The brain is also the organ responsible for our perception of time. Effective therapies might well re-educate the brain in its experience of temporality, but first it is necessary to understand that temporality is a possible locus of re-education. Especially in a condition such as intractable pain, where the best evidence may not be very good, good evidence about the role of temporality in chronic pain should not be hard to come by, including good evidence about the role of brains and cultures in creating our perceptions of time. Meanwhile, I offer my "n-of-one" anecdote about how one morning I woke up and noticed, with an amazement as if time had flipped open like a venetian blind, that the pain was gone. I can now report, alas, that after a few months of respite the pain has returned. Lingered. Settled right into its old slot in the low back. A downturn, sure, but not a catastrophe. Or so my story goes. It is, like all stories, a narrative that deliberately or nonconsciously enfolds a sense of time. To be continued.

Acknowledgment

The poem on p. 55 is reprinted by permission of the publishers and the Trustees of Amherst College from *The Poems Of Emily Dickinson*, Thomas H. Johnson, ed., Cambridge, Mass.: The Belknap Press of Harvard University Press, Copyright © 1951, 1955, 1979, 1983 by the President and Fellows of Harvard College.

References

1. Complex regional pain syndrome, type I (reflex sympathetic dystrophy). In: Merskey H, Bogduk N (eds) *Classifications of Chronic Pain*, 2nd edn. IASP Press, Seattle, WA, 1994: 41–42.

2. Thomas SP, Johnson M. A phenomenologic study of chronic pain. *Western J Nursing Res* 2000; **22**: 683–705.

3. Levneh H, Martz E. Reactions to diabetes and their relationship to time orientation. *Int J Rehab Res* 2007; **30**: 127–136.

4. Ortendahl M. Different time perspectives of the doctor and the patient reduce quality in health care. *Quality Manage Health Care* 2008; **17**: 136–39.

5. Barry DW, Melhado TV, Chacko KM, *et al*. Patient and physician perceptions of timely access to care. *J Gen Intern Med* 2006; **21**: 130–133.

6. Foster NE, Bishop A, Thomas E, *et al*. Illness perceptions of low back pain patients in primary care: what are they, do they change and are they associated with outcome? *Pain* 2008; **136**: 177–187.

7. Schivelbusch W. *The Railway Journey: The Industrialization and Perception of Time and Space*. University of California Press, Berkeley, CA, 1987.

8. Ricoeur P. *Time and Narrative, I* (trans. McLaughlin K, Pellauer D). University of Chicago Press, Chicago, IL, 1984: 52.

9. See, for example, McVay TE Jr, Flannigan OJ. *Narrative and Consciousness: Literature, Psychology, and the Brain*. Oxford University Press, New York, 2003. Newman K. The case for the narrative brain. In: *Proceedings of the Second Australasian Conference on Interactive Entertainment*, ACM International Conference Proceeding Series, vol. 123, Creativity and Cognition Studios Press, Sydney, 2005: 145–149.

10. Hirstein W. *Brain Fiction: Self-Deception and the Riddle of Confabulation*. MIT Press, Cambridge, MA, 2006.

11. Jenicek M, Hitchcock DL. *Evidence-Based Practice: Logic and Critical Thinking in Medicine*. AMA Press, Chicago, IL, 2005: 126. For a different approach to anecdote, see two essays by Kathryn Montgomery Hunter: "There was this guy…": the uses of anecdotes in medicine. *Perspect Biol Med* 1986; **29**: 619–630; and An N of 1: syndrome letters in the New England Journal of Medicine. *Perspect Biol Med* 1990; **33**: 237–251. See also Montgomery K. *How Doctors Think: Clinical Judgment and the Practice of Medicine*. Oxford University Press, New York, 2006: 129–130.

12. Goodman KW. *Ethics and Evidence-Based Medicine: Fallibility and Responsibility in Clinical Science*. Cambridge University Press, Cambridge, MA, 2003: 6.

13. Cassell EJ. The nature of suffering and the goals of medicine. *N Engl J Med* 1982; **306**: 639–645.

14. Carr DB. Memoir of a meta-analyst: on the silent 'I' in qualitative. In: Carr DB, Loeser JD, Morris DB (eds) *Narrative, Pain, and Suffering*. IASP Press, Seattle, WA, 2005: 325–354.

15. Remen RN. *Kitchen Table Wisdom: Stories That Heal*. Riverhead Books, New York, 1996: xxvii.

16. Brown MM, Brown GC, Sharma S. *Evidence-Based to Value-Based Medicine*. AMA Press, New York, 2005: 5.

17. Charon R. Narrative medicine: a model for empathy, reflection, profession, and trust. *JAMA* 2001; **286**: 1897–1902.

For an expanded discussion see Charon's *Narrative Medicine: Honoring the Stories of Illness*. Oxford University Press, New York, 2006.

18. Greenhalgh T, Hurwitz B (eds). *Narrative Based Medicine: Dialogue and Discourse in Clinical Practice*. BMJ Press, London, 1998.

19. Lorde A. *The Cancer Journals*, 2nd edn. Aunt Lute Books, San Francisco, CA, 1980: 12.

20. Eccleston C, Williams AC, Rogers WS. Patients' and professionals' understandings of the causes of chronic pain: blame, responsibility and identity protection. *Soc Sci Med* 1997; **43**(5): 699–709.

21. Lorde A. *The Cancer Journals*, 2nd edn. Aunt Lute Books, San Francisco, CA, 1980: 61.

22. Price R. *A Whole New Life: An Illness and A Healing*. Atheneum, New York, 1994: 184.

23. Kearney R. *On Stories*. Routledge, London, 2002: 5. Kearney continues: "it is this crucially intersubjective model of discourse which ... marks narrative as a quintessentially *communicative* act".

24. Johnson TH (ed). *The Complete Poems of Emily Dickinson*. Little, Brown, Boston, MA, 1960: no. 650.

25. Lame IE, Peters ML, Vlaeyen JW, Kleef M, Patijn J. Quality of life in chronic pain is more associated with beliefs about pain, than with pain intensity. *Eur J Pain* 2005; **9**: 15–24.

26. Morris DB. Success stories: narrative, pain, and the limits of storylessness. In: Carr DB, Loeser JD, Morris DB (eds) *Narrative, Pain, and Suffering*. IASP Press, Seattle, WA, 2005: 269–285.

27. Loeser JD. What is chronic pain? *Theoret Med* 1991; **12**: 213–225.

CHAPTER 6

Psychology of chronic pain and evidence-based psychological interventions

Christopher Eccleston

Centre for Pain Research, University of Bath, Bath, UK

Understanding the psychology of pain and the psychology of analgesic behavior can improve your practice as a pain clinician, enrich your experience of dealing day to day with suffering, and provide you with new ways of thinking about working in pain. I start with the fundamental aspects, exploring the psychological factors that influence and structure the experience of pain, introduce specific psychological models that help one understand patient behavior, and finally focus on the evidence base for psychological interventions for pain.

A primer in psychology

Psychology as an academic subject was born from physiology and philosophy. It has been influenced in its short history by political developments in social science, methodological advancements in biological science, and fashionable attempts to make itself an applied science, offering opinions and expertise in subjects that range from marketing and business to individual change through psychotherapy. It is instructive to bear in mind when reading anything about psychology that as a science it (a) occupies territory not occupied by any other science; that is, the explanation, prediction and control of behavior, (b) its theories draw on a wide range of other sciences, so such explanations can sometimes be based in the behavior of molecules, and other times based

in the behavior of populations, and (c) that it slips between deductive and inductive methods, often without comment. What this means is that to the nonpsychologist it can sometimes appear to be free-floating; at its worse it operates only to state the obvious, at its best it displays astonishing perspicacity, providing explanations that enable people to act.

Applied to pain, what this means is that it is unhelpful to think of a unitary psychology of pain. There are at least three psychologies that are useful to consider in this chapter. The first we call "cognitive" because it relates to private mental events, experiences of thought or perception. The second we call "social" because it relates to influences on behavior that arise from our evolutionary imperative to behave collectively. The third we call clinical, because it relates to specific attempts to intervene with individuals or groups for a desired health-related outcome. I will briefly introduce what we know about the cognitive, social, and clinical psychologies of pain. Next, the evidence for psychological interventions in acute and chronic non-malignant pain is reviewed. Finally, we focus on what we don't know that we really need to know, in order to move forwards.

First, it is important to revisit briefly the definition of pain, from a psychological perspective.

A definitional interlude

Pain was defined by committee as "an unpleasant sensory and emotional experience, associated with actual or potential tissue damage, or described in terms of such damage" [1]. I repeat this here, even though

Evidence-Based Chronic Pain Management. Edited by C. Stannard, E. Kalso and J. Ballantyne. © 2010 Blackwell Publishing.

you will be familiar with it, because it is important to reflect on it from a psychological point of view.

First, it recognizes that pain is fundamentally an unpleasant or aversive experience. Pain is different from other sensations in which the emotional content can be considered an association to the primary sensory experience, occurring sequentially after the sensation. Instead pain is immediately emotional. Pain that is not aversive is not pain.

Second, it recognizes that pain is only loosely related to tissue damage. There is now ample evidence that the relationship between pain and damage is weak. Of course, they often occur together but the objective extent of physical damage is a poor predictor of pain report, and pain is a poor predictor of the extent of tissue damage. The intrapersonal, interpersonal, and contextual variability of pain reporting is where psychological explanations operate.

Third, it recognizes that pain is a communicative event that relies often on its description. This aspect of the definition has two elements. When in pain, people typically communicate it, verbally or nonverbally, intentionally and unintentionally. In addition, for those who are capable, people seek to make sense of the experience by symbolically representing it in language. Commonly, this language will revolve around descriptions of bodily damage and violence.

Missing from this definition is any attention to the function of pain, what it operates to achieve. Recently, I have argued that pain is fundamentally an affective-motoric event to be understood in a context of an evolved social warning system. In other words, pain functions to warn oneself, and others in one's group, of real or potential danger. This is not the space to expand this argument, which can be found elsewhere [2], but it is important to recognize that pain is fundamentally threatening: it alarms, it promotes avoidance and escape. Further, one learns, and is motivated to learn more about, what the cause of pain is and how to avoid it in the future. This functional account of pain is at the heart of an understanding of the cognitive, social and clinical psychologies of pain. From this perspective, pain is fundamentally an alarm system that imposes new behavioral priorities. Cognitively, it is an attentional interrupt that brings a forced disengagement with other thought processes, and imposes new thoughts and behaviors. Socially, its communication is shaped by social forces, and has consequences for other people in one's social group. Clinically, when we attempt to help people "cope" with pain nonpharmacologically, we need to understand that we are often asking them to behave counterintuitively, and counterculturally, in ignoring a strong alarm.

Cognitive psychology and pain: private mental experience and pain

Pain is commonly explained as the result of a series of specific sensory processes in the nervous system. The results of these sensory processes are presented to conscious awareness. Cognitive psychology is concerned with the interaction between environment, the emergence of pain into awareness, and the consequences of being aware of pain. Pain acts to interrupt current concerns with a danger signal. We have a good understanding of the interruptive characteristics of the pain stimulus. The more intense, novel, unpredictable, and associated with danger a pain is, the more interruptive it is. Similarly, pain stimuli that are more associated with threat, due to either learning or the immediate context, will be more interruptive.

Two critical aspects of the context in which pain emerges will govern the threat value of pain. One is the environmental. If there are no other competing demands for attention then pain will emerge more easily (e.g. at night). Similarly, if one is predisposed to being anxious about pain then threatening pain will be identified more easily. This predisposition, or sensitivity, to identify pain-relevant cues has been investigated in a number of ways, and we know that those who are highly somatically aware are more likely to be interrupted, as are those given to catastrophic thinking about pain and those who have a heightened vigilance to pain-relevant information [3–5].

Social psychology and pain: collective experience

Pain has typically been described as the archetypal existential experience. It is immediately personal, private, fundamental, and closed to external scrutiny or validation. However, in its ubiquity it is also an archetypal common, collective, and fundamentally social experience. Although there are arguments that pain is "language-stealing" or even a prelinguistic experience [5], in coming to make sense of pain, it is in social linguistic exchange that people seek meaning for their pain. There is much study on the beliefs that are held about the meaning of pain, in particular as to the cause, consequence, treatment, and broader abstract meaning. In acute pain, much of which is common everyday pain, such as headache, or is accident related, the meaning is often either clear or diagnostically useful. However, in chronic nonmalignant conditions the meaning of pain is typically neither of these things, and often becomes contested.

Psychologists are interested in the beliefs that people hold about their pain, and their negotiation, because these beliefs are implicated in patient behavior. For example, those who believe that back pain is caused by a medical condition will resist treatment attempts aimed at movement despite pain and a therapeutic focus on stress-related factors. Similarly, those who cannot accept that a valuable life can be led without analgesia will not benefit from attempts to teach self-management, without addressing those beliefs. Matching belief to adaptive behavior is a socially mediated process. For a recent example, worrying thoughts and beliefs about the meaning of pain can lead people to seek medical support, which when appropriate is adaptive. However, when a medical cure is pursued in opposition to unhelpful, unchanged beliefs about the cause of pain, this pursuit can fuel anxiety, depression and disability [6].

Clinical psychology: applications of psychological knowledge

Psychology is most commonly, although not exclusively, applied in the clinical task of helping people adapt to a chronic persistent pain and its widespread negative consequences. Its primary activities are (a) assessment and formulation, (b) treatment planning and intervention, and (c) evaluation of outcome. There is a plethora of measurement tools available for use with patients in pain, and excellent guidance exists on the optimal methods of selection [7]. Perhaps less advice is available on the common activity of case formulation although guidance can be found [8]. There is, however, no shortage of data available on treatment interventions, from the first cognitively orientated manuals and tasks [9] to the recent focus on acceptance and commitment therapy

[10]. Clinical psychology, despite a relatively short history, has a variety of schools within it that can confuse the casual observer or visitor. However, common across its schools of thought is a concern with understanding how people's behavior in context confines or shapes their future behavior, recognizing that a critical aspect of that context is other people's behavior. The most common form of applied clinical psychology is known as "cognitive behavioral therapy" or CBT. CBT has a dual focus, as its name suggests: first, on the patterns and habits of behavior, their antecedents, contingencies, and consequences; and second, on the private mental experience, in particular on the thoughts and feelings that are associated with a life lived in pain.

Cognitive behavioral therapy for chronic pain management

Cognitive behavioral therapy or CBT has emerged as the treatment of choice for chronic pain [11]. CBT comes in a variety of forms and it is probably wise to consider it a family of different techniques and interventions [12]. The phrase has proven so popular as to now invoke reference to a broad set of principles concerned with the general practice of taking into account beliefs about cause and consequence of disease and treatment, and a focus on habit and lifestyle as possible factors in the maintenance of suffering. CBT, however, is more than this general set of principles. Here, in describing CBT, I refer specifically to a psychotherapeutic intervention; that is, the use of specific psychological techniques in the service of sustained behavior change.

Specific techniques include skills of self-regulation such as relaxation and mindfulness meditation, biofeedback, attentional control, and hypnosis, graded exposure to fear-related stimuli, cognitive therapy focused on examining the veracity of belief, control of catastrophic thinking, problem solving and habit reversal. The targets of CBT can be specific, for example in reducing the frequency of headache, reducing the number of times one sleeps in the daytime, or increasing the length of time one engages in meaningful social exchange. The targets can also be general, for example, in increasing the subjective sense of global well-being, or reducing the subjective sense of struggling with one's values.

Cognitve behavioral therapy is more commonly offered as a program of therapeutic techniques delivered in a specific order, with a specific dose, and held together with a defined model of therapeutic change. The smallest dose I know of was reported by Turner and colleagues who ran a 16-hour intervention, of 2 hours a week for 8 weeks with homework [13]. The largest dose was reported by Williams and colleagues who for many years ran the INPUT pain management unit in London, a 4-week residential program [14]. Targets of outcome will be multiple. Typical targets include: self-report of pain-related depression, anxiety, and coping, and objective report of improvement in engagement with social activity such as work. Often there is some attempt to capture achievement in goals that are personal or that are valued by the individual.

Perhaps the most common form of CBT is referred to as coping skills training. The content typically involves education aimed at providing rationale for self-management and an understanding of the biological bases of pain, skills of pain control such as attentional based methods, and skills practice, in particular activity pacing, and relaxation in stressful environments. Some programs of therapy are focused on specific problems. For example, common additions are a focus on social problem solving by teaching communication skills, a focus on sleep and fatigue, or more recently a focus on addiction control, and a withdrawal from use of prescribed medicines.

Recent developments have also focused on specific aspects of treatment or treatment outcome. For example, Keefe and colleagues at Duke University in the USA have for over 10 years been studying the potential role of partners and spouses. Spouse-assisted CBT makes use of the presence and involvement of the spouse as carer and trainer. Spouses are significant influences on one's behavior, and if one can use this influence positively it may improve patient outcomes. Working with patients with osteo-arthritis of the knees who report pain, distress, and disability, these authors conducted a trial of spouse-assisted CBT compared with normal CBT compared with an education-only control intervention. Six months following therapy, they reported that both the CBT interventions were superior over education alone, and that those patients in the spouse-assisted CBT showed more coping attempts and greater marital satisfaction [15]. Delivering this therapy with an exercise intervention is superior over one without [16].

Another significant development in CBT has been the introduction of assistive electronic technology to deliver healthcare education and behavior change messages remotely. Typically these have been introduced where significant geographic or resource barriers exist in accessing healthcare. This is a growing field of research and a recent review has highlighted that for common management problems associated with older age, remotely assisted care could significantly reduce their impact [17]. Medicine in general has been slow to grasp the possibilities of information and computing technologies. Psychological interventions are no different as they have remained largely untouched by technological influences. Face-to-face therapy, with an individual or a group, remains the dominant mode of delivery. There has been greater advance in the fields of CBT for anxiety and depression, but in pain we are only beginning. Technology can simply assist by replacing or allowing an aspect of therapy, as with the telephone. Or technology can be a key part of a therapy designed to make use of novel features of the therapy, a good example being the case of virtual reality interventions [18].

Despite its popularity, or perhaps because of it, CBT has attracted criticism. First, there has been from its inception a resistance to its reductionist tendencies, a seemingly uncritical attachment to computing metaphors reified into psychological processes, and mechanistically applied. Some theorists would argue that much of what emerges into awareness and determines mental life is the end product of largely unconscious influences that are personal. Understanding, analyzing and assessing the whole of one's psychological history in a personal relationship with a therapist is argued to be more relevant and potentially useful than attempting to control or banish the products. There is a range of psychological therapies that offer such a personalized approach. To date, there is insufficient evidence for the effectiveness or lack of effectiveness of psychoanalytic or psychodynamic therapies for chronic pain management.

Second, CBT has been criticized for a lack of theoretical fidelity or in some cases any relationship to theory at all. CBT is not alone in this as an applied clinical science, but it can sometimes seem to operate without a coherent model of action, without a strong understanding of the reasons why certain choices within therapy can and should be made. Some of its main components remain unevidenced.

Third, CBT can fail because it most often operates, like many psychotherapeutic interventions, without attention to any mechanism of quality control. Each therapist manufactures the intervention in the moment (normally real time). Essential, but rarely seen, is attention to whether the content of therapy was correct, delivered appropriately, or had a desired effect.

Finally, within the psychological community there is reference to a "third wave" of psychological therapy based on acceptance and commitment therapy, which itself emerges from a different trajectory of behavior therapy. In chronic pain management, a focus on the context in which people struggle to escape inescapable pain has led to novel developments in therapeutic methods [10]. The early evidence is promising, and the therapeutic model is attractive to clinicians and patients alike. However, to date there is insufficient evidence for the effectiveness or lack of effectiveness of acceptance-based CBT for chronic pain management.

The evidence base

I reviewed the evidence base by searching for all published randomized controlled trials of interventions described as psychological in nature, principally those described as examining behavior therapy or cognitive behavior therapy for adults with chronic pain [11]. For this particular review trials of headache treatments were excluded. Thirty-three papers were recovered that described 30 trials; 25 had data that could be entered into a meta-analysis.

Because pain has multiple and widespread effects on patients, I expected to find multiple treatment targets and measurement tools across the 25 trials analyzed. In total, over 200 separate measurement tools were employed in these trials. For clarity, all these measurement tools were classified into a domain of measurement. These were: pain experience, mood/affect, cognitive coping and appraisal, pain behavior, biological/physical fitness, social role functioning, and use of healthcare systems. Not all trials had measurement tools in each domain, and some trials used numerous measures within a domain. The most psychometrically sound measure used in each domain was selected for analysis.

Working across domains allows aggregation and summary of data. The findings were quite clear. Compared with doing nothing, in this case a traditional waiting list control arm in which patients were randomly assigned to waiting for treatment, patients who were randomly assigned to a psychological therapy had positive outcomes across the domains. The overall median effect size of treatment improvements across trials was 0.5. For behavior therapy, the effect sizes ranged from 1.41 for the effects of behavior therapy (BT) on cognitive coping and appraisal to −0.03 for behavior therapy on mood. For CBT, the effect sizes ranged from 0.61 for the effect on social role functioning to 0.33 for pain experience.

Although doing nothing has some ecological validity in that many chronic pain patients receive no care, it is not the most robust comparison. In part, this is because patients entering these trials will have been aware that they were randomly assigned away from a treatment that may have helped. They would be blind to the assignment but not to the outcome of the assignment. The ideal comparator would be a placebo treatment. Placebic psychological treatments are uncommon but not impossible. In essence, one would have to hold delivery characteristics of the treatment stable (e.g. therapist contact time) and maintain a belief that therapy was being delivered (i.e. deceive patients that they were being treated with an active intervention). Essentially, this involves engaging patients in neutral, nondirective, untherapeutic conversation. This is not commonly used because it is difficult to maintain the deception over a long contact period, difficult to keep patients from withdrawing from such an inert treatment, and some have questioned the possible adverse effects of prolonged engagement with inert sham therapy.

A common comparator, and one that was analyzed in this 1999 meta-analysis, is comparison with another active treatment or treatment as usual. When comparing with treatment as usual, the effects of BT and CBT are not as strong. Fewer trials contribute to these summary data. The overall median effect size of treatment improvements across trials was 0.17. For BT, the effect sizes ranged from 0.62 for the effects of BT on mood to −0.4 for the effects of BT on cognitive coping and appraisal. For CBT, the effect sizes ranged from 0.55 for the effects on cognitive coping and appraisal and 0.14 for the effects on mood.

Overall, there are positive effects of psychological therapies on enabling people with chronic pain to cope, improve mood, return to social function and reduce pain. However, for the development of psychological therapies for chronic pain, the picture is somewhat unclear. The effects of BT alone appear highly variable and contradictory. This is most likely caused by the number of small and underpowered trials entering the analyses. CBT has more consistent trial support. However, the lack of effect of CBT on mood/affect in trials that used an active comparator should be cause for concern. One of the primary goals of most CBT is to alter mood. Taken together with the robust finding that patients report changes in their cognitive appraisal of their disability and their perception of their ability to cope, I suspect that the content of the therapies may have drifted toward a more mechanistic and prescriptive coping skills training model, and away from more fundamental concern with disordered affect – the traditional domain of psychotherapy. It may, however, be a function of a dilution of therapy content and/or skill in its delivery. Morley *et al.* [11], commenting on the poor reporting of therapy content in trials, suggested that "…. It is possible that expediency and economy of reporting is a product of external pressures (e.g. editorial demands), but this does not account for what appear to be brief interventions delivered by relatively inexperienced therapists to chronically distressed patients for any realistic expectation of change to take place" (p 10). This review has recently been updated [19].

A more recent review of psychological interventions focused on the specific case of low back pain of various origin [20]. Hoffman and colleagues deliberately adopted a wider definition of psychological therapy, extending it to include social support and education with a psychological flavor. They identified 39 articles, of which 25 provided extractable data on 22 randomized or quasi-randomized controlled trials. They measured outcomes of interventions in pain intensity, pain interference, depression, anxiety, health-related quality of life, healthcare utilization (doctor visits), healthcare utilization (medication usage), healthcare utilization (costs), work disability, and compensation status. Given that these categories were from the ideal set established by IMPAACT [21], rather than arising from what was published, most trials did not have measurement tools in each of these domains.

In the main analysis in which they pooled all effect sizes of all psychological treatments, on all outcomes, they had an omnibus significant result of treatment effectiveness of 0.48 when compared with control conditions. The effect sizes ranged from 0.50 for pain intensity to nonsignificant changes for depression from CBT. Again, there is a concerning finding emerging from the literature that traditional CBT for chronic pain may not be effective at changing depression status in patients. Of course, to some extent this finding is not additive because some of the same trials entered the analysis. However, the scope of this review was different, being more narrowly focused on chronic low back pain and more broadly focused on all therapies purporting to be psychological. The authors raise this issue as a challenge to the field, writing that "… Inconsistent effects of these interventions on emotional functioning underscore a challenge to the field" (p 8), although they do not discuss possible reasons for these inconsistencies.

One other meta-analysis of trial data is worth mentioning here. Dixon and colleagues from the Duke University lab reviewed data from trials of psychological therapy for the management of pain from arthritis-related conditions [22]. Arthritis is the most common cause of disability, and pain is reported as the most prominent symptom. As with other chronic pain conditions, it is associated with significant disability, distress, and life interference. In this review, the authors expanded their definition of psychological therapy beyond CBT and coping skills training to include hypnosis, psychodynamic psychotherapy, and emotional disclosure. They identified 37 publications of which 31 provided extractable data on 27 randomized or quasi-randomized controlled trials, comparing pre–post treatment effects. Outcomes were grouped into four broad categories: pain, psychological functioning, physical functioning, and biological functioning. The overall effect size (ES) for the effects of psychological interventions on pain intensity was 0.177. This held when taking account of heterogeneity in studies, and study quality. Unpacking psychological functioning, five studies reported a positive effect on anxiety (ES = 0.28), seven reported a positive effect on depression (ES = 0.21), six reported a positive effect on psychological disability (ES = 0.25), and five reported an improvement in coping (ES = 0.72). The overall ES for the effects of psychological interventions on improvements in physical functioning was 0.15. Finally, the overall ES for the effects of psychological functioning on biological functioning, principally joint swelling, was 0.35.

Psychological therapies, and in particular CBT, are perhaps in most common use in the service of musculoskeletal pain problems such as low back pain or osteo-arthritis. In part, this may be due to the high prevalence of these conditions and the growing recognition of interventions aimed at self-management rather than cure. CBT, however, has wider applicability in pain associated with malignancies [23, 24]. For just one example, Tatrow & Montgomery recently reported a meta-analysis of CBT therapy techniques on the pain and distress reported by women with breast cancer [25]. Distress and pain associated with the diagnosis and treatment of breast cancer are reported as severe by half of those with breast cancer. The psychological effects can be extensive and debilitating, and are characterized by fear and the cognitive dominance of catastrophic ideation. The scope of the review was limited to CBT but included studies focusing on one component of CBT. Outcomes were focused on the report of pain and the report of distress. Sixty-one papers were recovered from the search strategy, which yielded 20 studies allowing data synthesis. The overall effect size for CBT on pain was 0.49, and for distress was 0.31. Interestingly, the data allowed for further analyses of delivery format. The authors found that CBT delivered to an individual has a greater effect (ES = 0.48) than when delivered to groups (ES = −0.06). This finding should be treated with some caution given that the overall data set revealed a sample bias such that the larger the sample, the less likely the studies were to show a significant effect, and group treatments had larger samples. Finally, the authors also attempted an analysis of breast cancer severity, based on a dichotomous variable of metastatic versus nonmetastatic disease. There were no significant differences between the effect sizes for both pain and distress, both showing a positive effect of CBT on reports of pain and distress regardless of the stage of disease.

In summary, there is now a great deal of evidence from randomized controlled trials in support of the effectiveness of CBT for the treatment of patients reporting chronic pain. These findings appear to be significant not only for pain outcomes, but also for psychological, physical, and biological outcomes. The evidence base extends beyond the traditional domain of nonspecific or idiopathic pain syndromes such as chronic low back pain, with evidence for its effectiveness in pain and its associated disability and distress for patients with malignant and nonmalignant disease.

Extending the evidence base

So, overall, the evidence base appears to be very strong and in general supportive of CBT for chronic pain. This has been an active field of clinical research. The tools and techniques of CBT, both in isolation and in a programmatic multidisciplinary form, have been subject to evaluation with randomized controlled trials for the last 30 years. If we stand back to admire this picture it will all appear relatively well constructed and attractive. Closer examination, however, reveals some problems.

We should consider these trials perhaps as first-generation trials, which have a number of problems. First, many were designed to answer specific questions in specific settings, and were designed prior to the development of guidelines and standards of trials design and reporting such as CONSORT (see www. consort-statement.org/) who have recently introduced a revised statement to extend to trials concerned with nondrug interventions [26], and prior to the guidance offered by the Cochrane Collaboration (www. cochrane.org/). As a consequence, most of the individual trials entering the various meta-analyses reported above are small, bringing all the biases associated with small trials, most concerningly a lack of control over both type I and type II errors. Second, many of the trials are overcomplicated, comparing too many variations or types of therapy, and examining their effects on too many outcomes. In part, this arises from the complexity of the patient group, presenting with many disabilities that cannot meaningfully be captured in a primary outcome. Third, many of the trials have inadequate bias control mechanisms built into the design. In particular, infrequently reported are any attempts to control for the treatment quality: the training of the therapist, the allegiance of the therapist, the content of the therapy, whether it was delivered adequately, and its credibility with the patients. Fourth, the reliance on waiting list and no treatment controls rather than placebo controls causes problems of interpretation. Fifth, and related to this, the small numbers of patients and use of waiting list controls mean that it is difficult to maintain patients into trial beyond immediate post-treatment assessment. Therefore, the longer term effects of CBT remain largely a mystery. Although this is not a specific problem of trials of psychological therapy, it will become important to have some consideration of long-term effects for therapies that are aimed at self-management of lifelong health conditions. Finally, a serious problem for the discipline of psychology and first-generation trials has been the wholesale ignorance and avoidance of any concern with adverse effects of therapy. Rarely are adverse effects reported or discussed. It is not plausible that they do not exist, and the absence of their consideration undermines the credibility of psychotherapy as a clinical discipline.

Next steps

Methods of evaluation of therapies will evolve. Guidance is available on how to undertake a trial of psychological therapy, and how to judge the quality of a trial of psychological therapy in chronic pain [27]. Knowledge of how to produce an excellent trial is available. Meeting it will remain a challenge. In addition, even with good trial data, understanding how to translate the findings into real-world settings will become an important focus [28]. Beverly Thorn and her colleagues, commenting on the development of evidence-based practice, address these wider issues [29]. What commissioners of treatments need from an evidence base, which is to know whether it works or not and whether it should be made available, is different from what practitioners need. Evidence-based practice will be enhanced if the evidence of effectiveness is complemented with access to treatment manuals, guidance on how to tailor treatments to different client groups, and multisite audit and evaluation of methods of therapy delivery.

Other challenges remain for the development of effective psychotherapy for chronic pain management. First, although the evidence base is very strong, there remain critical gaps: there are client groups that I have not discussed in this selective review. For example, we know that psychological techniques are highly effective for the management of headache in childhood but know very little about other childhood presentations [30]. Second, psychological interventions can operate pragmatically and without theoretical coherence. Although such pragmatism is sometimes celebrated as a necessary part of real therapy delivery, it brings problems to the discipline as a whole. I would argue that understanding and allying oneself to a single school of therapy, whatever it may be, from radical behaviorism to psychoanalysis, at least allows for a coherent direction for development. Despite the large number of trials of therapy, the development of new and improved therapies has been very slow. There are few new inventions. The cognitive model is being extended to account for the work on catastrophic thinking and worry, third-wave CBT is being developed for chronic pain and, as we have seen above, a number of groups are working on new methods of delivery to solve problems of access or are studying the influence of family members. However, development in this field has slowed to a creeping pace. Third, I stress that attempts to improve therapy are as important as evaluating existing therapies because better therapy is needed. At present, for example, it appears that we may have seriously underestimated the extent of affective disorder in chronic pain patients, and need to improve its treatment.

In conclusion, if we accept that chronic pain often means that patients also present with complex and multiple problems of pain-associated disability and distress, then we can allow for the role of psychological interventions in promoting self-management and rehabilitation. There is a strong tradition of psychotherapy, in particular of CBT, in chronic pain management in both idiopathic and disease-related pain. Overall, the evidence for the effectiveness of CBT is very strong, and it should be considered a standard treatment option for any chronic pain service. The next generation of psychotherapy promises greater maturity. Innovation will come not only in the development of more effective techniques for addressing severe affective distress, but also in increasing patient access to these effective treatments.

References

1. Merskey H, Bogduk N. *Classification of Chronic Pain*, 2nd edn. IASP Press, Seattle, WA, 1994.
2. Chapman CR, Gavin J. Suffering: the contributions of persistent pain. *Lancet* 1999; **353**: 2233–2237.

3. Eccleston C, Crombez G. Pain demands attention: a cognitive-affective model of the interruptive function of pain. *Psychol Bull* 1999; **125**: 356–366.

4. Crombez G, van Damme S, Eccleston C. Hypervigilance to pain: an experimental and clinical analysis. *Pain* 2005; **116** (1–2): 4–7.

5. Scarry E. *The Body in Pain: The Making and Unmaking of the World*. Oxford University Press, New York, 1985.

6. Eccleston C, Crombez G. Worry and chronic pain: a misdirected problem solving model. *Pain* 2007; **132**: 233–236.

7. Williams A. Selecting and applying pain measures. In: Breivik H, Campbell W, Eccleston C (eds) *Clinical Pain Management: Practical Applications and Procedures*. Arnold, London, 2003: 3–14.

8. Turk DC, Melzack R. *Handbook of Pain Assessment*, 2nd ed. Guilford Press, New York, 2001.

9. Turk DC, Meichenbaum D, Genest M. *Pain and Behavioral Medicine*. Guilford Press, New York, 1983.

10. McCracken L. *Contextual Cognitive Behavioral Therapy for Chronic Pain*. IASP Press, Seattle, WA, 2005.

11. Morley S, Eccleston C, Williams A. Systematic review and meta-analysis of randomized controlled trials of cognitive behaviour therapy and behaviour therapy for chronic pain in adults, excluding headache. *Pain* 1999; **80**: 1–13.

12. Gaudiano BA. Cognitive-behavioural therapies: achievements and challenges. *Evidence Based Mental Health* 2008; **11**: 5–7.

13. Turner JA, Clancy S. Comparison of operant behavioral and cognitive behavioral group treatment for chronic low-back pain. *J Consult Clin Psychol* 1988; **56**: 261–266.

14. Williams A, Richardson PH, Nicholas MK, *et al*. Inpatient versus outpatient pain management: results of a randomised controlled trial. *Pain* 1996; **66**: 13–22.

15. Keefe FJ, Blumenthal J, Baucom D, *et al*. Effects of spouse-assisted coping skills training and exercise training in patients with osteoarthritic knee pain: a randomized controlled study. *Pain* 2004; **110**: 539–549.

16. Keefe FJ, Caldwell DS, Baucom D, *et al*. Spouse-assisted coping skills training in the management of knee pain in osteoarthritis: long-term followup results. *Arthritis Care Res* 1999; **12**: 101–111.

17. Brownsell S, Aldred H, Hawley MS. The role of telecare in supporting the needs of elderly people. *J Telemed Telecare* 2007; **13**: 293–297.

18. Wiederhold MD, Wiederhold BK. Virtual reality and interactive simulation for pain distraction. *Pain Med* 2007; S182–S188.

19. Eccleston C, Williams AC de C, Morley S. Psychological therapies for the management of chronic pain (excluding headache) in adults. *Cochrane Database of Systematic Reviews*. 2009, Issue 2. Art. No.: CD003968. DOI: 10.1002/14651858 .CD003968.pub2.

20. Hoffman BM, Papas RK, Chatkoff DK, Kerns RD. Meta-analysis of psychological interventions for chronic low back pain. *Health Psychol* 2007; **26**: 1–9.

21. Dworkin RH, Turk DC, Farrar JT, *et al*. Core outcome measures for chronic pain clinical trials: IMMPACT recommendations. *Pain* 2005; **113**: 9–19.

22. Dixon KE, Keefe FJ, Scipio CD, Perri LM, Abernathy AP. Psychological interventions for arthritis pain management in adults: a meta-analysis. *Health Psychol* 2007; **26**: 241–250.

23. Graves KD. Social cognitive theory and cancer patients' quality of life: a meta-analysis of psychosocial intervention components. *Health Psychol* 2003; **22**: 210–219.

24. Leubert K, Dahme B, Hasenbring M. The effectiveness of relaxation training in reducing treatment-related symptoms and improving emotional adjustment in acute nonsurgical cancer treatment: a meta-analytical review. *Psycho-oncology* 2001; **10**: 490–502.

25. Tatrow K, Montgomery GH. Cognitive behavioral therapy techniques for distress and pain in breast cancer patients: a meta-analysis. *J Behav Med* 2006; **29**: 17–27.

26. Boutron I, Moher D, Altman DG, Schulz KF, Ravaud P. Extending the Consort statement to randomized controlled trials of nonpharmacologic treatment: explanation and elaboration. *Ann Intern Med* 2008; **148**: 295–309.

27. Yates S, Morley S, Eccleston C, Williams A. A scale for rating the quality of trials of psychological trials for pain. *Pain* 2005; **117**: 314–325.

28. Glasgow RE, Green LW, Klesges LM, *et al*. External validity: we need to do more. *Ann Behav Med* 2006; **31**: 105–108.

29. Thorn BE, Cross TH, Walker BB. Meta-analyses and systematic reviews of psychological treatments for chronic pain: relevance to evidence based practice. *Health Psychol* 2007; **26**: 10–12.

30. Eccleston C, Yorke L, Morley S, Williams A, Mastroyannopoulou K. Psychological therapies for the management of chronic and recurrent pain in children and adolescents. *Cochrane Database of Systematic Reviews* 2003, Issue 1. Art. No.: CD003968. DOI: 10.1002/14651858.CD003968.

PART 2

Clinical pain syndromes: the evidence

CHAPTER 7

Chronic low back pain

Maurits van Tulder[1,2] *and Bart Koes*[3]

[1]EMGO Institute for Health and Care Research, VU University Medical Centre, Amsterdam, The Netherlands
[2]Department of Health Sciences, Faculty of Earth and Life Sciences, VU University, Amsterdam, The Netherlands
[3]Department of General Practice, Erasmus MC-University Medical Center Rotterdam, Rotterdam, The Netherlands

Background

Many randomized controlled trials have been conducted and published on conservative and complementary treatments for nonspecific low back pain. A substantial number of systematic reviews have also been published, in which the evidence from these trials has been summarized [1, 2]. Recently, the evidence from trials and reviews has formed the basis for clinical practice guidelines on the management of low back pain that have been developed in various countries around the world [3]. This chapter on evidence-based medicine for chronic low back pain provides an overview of the evidence on diagnosis and treatment of chronic nonspecific low back pain and summarizes how this evidence has been translated into guideline recommendations.

The current underst nding of relevant pathophysiology

Low back pain is usually defined as pain, muscle tension or stiffness localized below the costal margin and above the inferior gluteal folds, with or without leg pain (sciatica). Low back pain is typically classified as being "specific" or "non-specific." Specific low back pain refers to symptoms caused by

a specific pathophysiologic mechanism, such as hernia nucleus pulposus (HNP), infection, inflammation, osteoporosis, rheumatoid arthritis, fracture or tumor. Only in about 10% of the patients can specific underlying diseases be identified [4]. The vast majority of patients (up to 90%) are labeled as having nonspecific low back pain, which is defined as symptoms without clear specific cause, i.e. low back pain of unknown origin. Spinal abnormalities on X-rays and magnetic resonance imaging (MRI) are not strongly associated with nonspecific low back pain, because many people without any symptoms also show these abnormalities [5, 6].

Nonspecific low back pain is usually classified according to duration as acute (less than 6 weeks), subacute (between 6 weeks and 3 months) or chronic (longer than 3 months) [7]. In general, prognosis is good and most patients with an episode of nonspecific low back pain will recover within a couple of weeks. However, back pain among primary care patients is often a recurrent problem with fluctuating symptoms. The majority of back pain patients will have experienced a previous episode and acute exacerbations of chronic low back pain are common [8].

Prevalence figures/epidemiology

Epidemiological data reported in the literature usually have been collected in different populations. Incidence and prevalence data need to be reported for specific populations.

Evidence-Based Chronic Pain Management. Edited by
C. Stannard, E. Kalso and J. Ballantyne. © 2010 Blackwell
Publishing.

Incidence

Incidence in general practice

A large epidemiological study in The Netherlands included data from a random sample of 161 general practitioners in 103 practices with a total population of 335,000 patients [9]. The registration period was from April 1987 to April 1988 using the ICPC classification. The incidence of low back pain was 28.0 episodes per 1000 persons per year. The reported incidence of low back pain with sciatica was 11.6 per 1000 per year. The incidence of low back pain was higher for men (32.0) than for women (23.2) and was highest for people between 25 and 64 years of age.

Another epidemiological study from The Netherlands reported data collected by 59 general practitioners in 21 practices with a population of 41,000 patients [10]. The ICPC was used for classification. The incidence of low back pain (ICPC code L03) was 30 episodes per 1000 persons per year. The incidence of low back pain with sciatica (ICPC code L86, including herniated disk and diskopathy) was six episodes per 1000 persons per year. The incidences of both low back pain and low back pain with sciatica were highest for patients between 45 and 64 years of age.

The South Manchester Back Pain Study in the UK included 2715 adults who were free of low back pain during the month prior to the baseline survey. Subsequently, all primary care consultations were prospectively monitored [11]. The 12-month cumulative incidence of new consulting episodes was 3% in men and 5% in women. Those with a history of previous low back pain had twice the rate of new episodes compared to those with no low back pain in the past.

Incidence in the general population

The South Manchester Back Pain Study also included a follow-up survey after 1 year to determine new episodes that had not led to consultation (nonconsulting episodes) during that 1-year period. The 12-month cumulative incidence of new nonconsulting episodes was 31% in men and 32% in women. Those with a history of previous low back pain and those with widespread pain had a much higher incidence than those with no low back pain in the past [11].

Prevalence

Reported lifetime prevalence ranges widely, from 49% to 70%, as does point prevalence from 12% to 30%, and period prevalence from 25% to 42%. A large epidemiological study on low back pain among the general population in The Netherlands was conducted from 1993 to 1995 [12]. The study population consisted of a sample of 13,927 men and women aged 20–59 years. Almost half of the respondents (49.2%, of whom 45.5% men and 52.4% women) reported low back pain in the previous year. More than 40% of the respondents reported that the episode lasted for more than 12 weeks (7.1%) or that the low back pain was continuously present (34.7%). Chronic low back pain was more common among women (22.6%) than men (18.3%) and increased with age from 12% at 20–29 years of age to 27.1% at 50–59 years of age.

In general, the conclusion from these prevalence estimates is quite clear: low back pain is a common disorder in Western countries. The estimates of prevalence may vary because of national variations, age or gender of the population and sampling method used.

Risk factors

Many epidemiological studies have been conducted evaluating the association between risk factors and the occurrence of nonspecific low back pain. Relatively little is known about risk factors for the transition from acute to chronic low back pain. Usually variables associated with nonspecific low back pain are classified as individual, psychosocial or occupational factors. Risk factors are summarized in Table 7.1.

Risk factors for occurrence

Individual risk factors

Although results of epidemiological studies are not necessarily consistent, factors that have been reported to be associated with low back pain are age, physical fitness, and strength of back and abdominal muscles. There seems to be no association between low back pain and other individual factors such as gender, length, weight, Body Mass Index, flexibility/mobility and structural deformities of the spine.

Recent systematic reviews found that smoking and body weight should be considered weak risk indicators and not causes of low back pain [13, 14], and

Table 7.1 Risk factors for occurrence and chronicity

	Occurrence	Chronicity
Individual factors	Age Physical fitness Strength of back and abdominal muscles Smoking	Obesity Low educational level High levels of pain and disability
Psychosocial factors	Stress Anxiety Mood/emotions Cognitive functioning Pain behavior	Distress Depressive mood Somatization
Occupational factors	Manual material handling Bending and twisting Whole-body vibration Job dissatisfaction Monotonous tasks Work relations/social support Control	Job dissatisfaction Unavailability of light duties on return to work Job requirement of lifting for ¾ of the day

that alcohol consumption [68], standing or walking, sitting, sports, and total leisure-time physical activity [15] do not seem to be associated with low back pain.

Psychosocial risk factors

Psychosocial factors that traditionally have been reported to be associated with low back pain are anxiety, depression, emotional instability, and alcohol or drug abuse [16]. A recent systematic review of observational studies of psychosocial factors for the occurrence of back pain found insufficient evidence for an effect of psychosocial factors in private life, such as family support, presence of a close friend or neighbor, social contact, social participation, instrumental support and emotional support [17].

A prospective cohort study provided evidence that psychologic distress at 23 years of age more than doubled the risk of low back pain onset 10 years later, while other factors (e.g. social class, childhood emotional status, Body Mass Index, job satisfaction) did not increase the risk [18]. Another systematic review found a clear link between psychologic variables and low back pain [19]. Psychologic variables that are associated with low back pain are stress, distress or anxiety as well as mood and emotions, cognitive functioning, and pain behavior.

Occupational risk factors

Occupational factors such as physically heavy work, lifting, bending, twisting, pulling and pushing (or the combination of these last three with lifting), and vibrations have often been associated with low back pain [20].

A systematic review of aspects of physical load found strong evidence that manual materials handling, bending and twisting, and whole-body vibration are risk factors for back pain [17]. Two systematic reviews of psychologic workplace variables in back pain found strong evidence that job dissatisfaction, monotonous tasks, work relations, social support in the workplace, demands, stress, and perceived ability to work were associated with the occurrence of low back pain [17, 21]. Moderate evidence was found for work pace, control, emotional effort at work, and the belief that work is dangerous, and insufficient evidence was found for a high work pace, high qualitative demands [21], low job content and low job control [17].

Studies on the association between occupational risk factors and low back pain are hampered by the difficulties of measuring exposure to specific factors. Exposure to specific risk factors may vary among employees with the same job, but also the task they perform may vary. Also, the "healthy worker effect" may considerably affect results of epidemiologic studies in occupational settings. That is, healthy workers may stay on the same job or perform the same task for years, while workers with low back pain may have moved to another job or function or their tasks may have been adjusted.

Risk factors for chronicity

It is important to identify early those low back pain patients at risk for long-term disability and sick leave, because early and specific interventions may be developed and used in this subgroup of patients. As stated before, most patients are likely to recover within a couple of days or weeks, but recovery for those who develop chronic low back pain and disability becomes increasingly less likely the longer the problems continue. The small group of patients with long-term severe low back pain also account for substantial healthcare utilization and sick leave, and associated costs.

Evidence suggests that psychosocial factors are important in the transition from acute to chronic low back pain and disability [19]. A systematic review of prospective cohort studies found that some psychologic factors (distress, depressive mood, and somatization) are associated with an increased risk of chronic low back pain [22].

Individual and workplace factors, such as job dissatisfaction, low educational level, and high levels of pain and disability, have also been reported to be associated with the transition to chronic low back pain [23, 24]. A prospective cohort study found that severe leg pain, obesity, functional disability, poor general health status, unavailability of light duties on return to work, and a job requirement of lifting for three-fourths of the day or more were associated with the transition from acute to chronic occupational back pain [25]. Job dissatisfaction or poor workplace relations were not associated with chronic low back pain [25]. Another prospective cohort study of 328 employees identified prognostic factors for return to work of employees with 3–4 months sick leave due to low back pain [26]. Risk factors included poor general health status, low job satisfaction, not being a bread winner, lower age and higher pain intensity. The authors concluded that psychosocial aspects of health and work in combination with economic aspects have a significantly larger impact on return to work when compared to relatively more physical aspects of disability and physical requirements of the job [26].

The transition from acute to chronic low back pain seems complicated and many individual, psychosocial and workplace factors may play a role. As the identification of patients at risk of chronicity will depend on identification of these factors, the implication for clinical management is still unclear. Although psychosocial yellow flags are at present expected to play an important role in screening of high-risk patients with acute and subacute low back pain [27] and a screening instrument has been suggested for use in clinical practice [28], future research is definitely needed to test the predictive value of these factors and instruments in clinical practice.

Diagnosis

The diagnosis of nonspecific low back pain is based on the exclusion of relevant specific causes. When searching for specific causes, the physician should first focus on features of serious spinal pathology (so called "red flags"; see Table 7.2). Such pathology may be suspected primarily on the basis of history and physical examination and can be confirmed with additional diagnostic procedures. However, in most cases of acute low back pain it is not possible to arrive at a diagnosis based on detectable pathologic changes. Several classification systems of diagnosis have been suggested, in which low back pain is categorized based on, for example, pain distribution, pain behavior, functional disability or clinical signs. However, none of these systems of classification has been critically validated. A simple and practical classification, which has gained international acceptance, divides acute

Table 7.2 "Red flags": warning signs and symptoms indicating an increased likelihood of serious spinal pathology

Age of onset <20 or >55 years
Violent trauma
Constant progressive, nonmechanical pain (no relief with bedrest)
Thoracic pain
Past medical history of malignant tumor
Prolonged use of corticosteroids
Drug abuse, immunosuppression, HIV
Signs of systemic disease
Unexplained weight loss
Widespread neurology (including cauda equina syndrome)
Structural deformity
Fever

low back pain into three categories – the so-called "diagnostic triage":

• serious spinal pathology
• nerve root pain/radicular pain
• nonspecific low back pain.

The priority in the examination procedure follows this line of clinical reasoning. First, the patient's age and history should be considered. Second, a standard history should include considering the distribution and severity of the pain and the relation with time and posture. Third, a standard phsyical examination is conducted including inspection of posture and movement, and local anatomic derangements, assessment of spinal tenderness on percussion over the spinal processes or axial pressure and palpation of the abdomen. In some patients, nerve root disorders may be suspected on the basis of pain distribution and pattern. Then, provocation of pain on coughing, sneezing or straining, weakness, sensory loss and micturition disturbance (incontinence) should be queried. Also, the diagnostic process should include a neurologic examination looking for typical radiating pain in the leg during straight-leg raising, and anteflexion, paresis (at least requesting the patient to walk on toes and heels), and reflex disturbance.

The initial examination also serves other important purposes besides reaching a "diagnosis." Through a thorough history taking and physical examination, it is possible to evaluate the degree of pain and functional disability. This enables the healthcare professional to outline a management strategy that matches the magnitude of the problem. Finally, the careful initial examination serves as a basis for imparting credible information to the patient regarding diagnosis, management and prognosis and may help in reassuring the patient.

History taking

One systematic review of nine studies evaluated the accuracy of history in diagnosing low back pain in general practice [29]. The review found that history taking does not have a high sensitivity and high specificity for radiculopathy and ankylosing spondylitis. The combination of history and erythrocyte sedimentation rate had a relatively high diagnostic accuracy in vertebral cancer.

Physical examination

One systematic review of 17 studies found that the pooled diagnostic odds ratio (OR) for straight-leg raising (SLR) for nerve root pain was 3.74 (95% confidence interval (CI) 1.2–11.4); sensitivity for nerve root pain was high (1.0–0.88), but specificity was low (0.44–0.11) [30]. All included studies were surgical case series at nonprimary care level. Most studies evaluated the diagnostic value of SLR for disk prolapse. The pooled diagnostic OR for the crossed straight-leg raising test was 4.39 (95% CI 0.74–25.9), with low sensitivity (0.44–0.23) and high specificity (0.95–0.86). The authors concluded that the studies do not enable a valid evaluation of diagnostic accuracy of the SLR test [30].

Diagnostic imaging

One systematic review was found that included 31 studies on the association between X-ray findings of the lumbar spine and nonspecific low back pain [6]. The results showed that degeneration, defined by the presence of disk space narrowing, osteophytes and sclerosis, is consistently and positively associated with nonspecific low back pain with OR ranging from 1.2 (95% CI 0.7–2.2) to 3.3 (95% CI 1.8–6.0). Spondylolysis/listhesis, spina bifida, transitional vertebrae, spondylosis and Scheuermann's disease did not appear to be associated with low back pain. There is no evidence on the association between degenerative signs at the acute stage and the transition to chronic symptoms.

A review of the diagnostic imaging literature (MRI, radionuclide scanning, computed tomography, radiography) concluded that for adults younger than 50 years of age with no signs or symptoms of systemic disease, diagnostic imaging does not improve treatment of low back pain. For patients 50 years of age and older or those whose findings suggest systemic disease, plain radiography and simple laboratory tests can almost completely rule out underlying systemic diseases. The authors concluded that advanced imaging should be reserved for patients who are considering surgery or those in whom systemic disease is strongly suspected [31].

A randomized controlled trial (RCT) of 380 patients aged 18 years or older whose primary physicians had ordered that their low back pain be evaluated by radiographs determined the clinical and economic consequences of replacing spine radiographs with rapid MRI [32]. Although physicians and patients preferred the rapid MRI, there was no difference between rapid MRIs and radiographs in outcomes for primary care patients with low back pain. The authors concluded that substituting rapid MRI for radiographic evaluations in the primary care setting may offer little additional benefit to patients, and it may increase the costs of care because of the increased number of spine operations that patients are likely to undergo.

Treatment

Various healthcare providers may be involved in the treatment of low back pain in primary care. Although there may be some variations between countries, general practitioners, physiotherapists, manual therapists, chiropractors, exercise therapists, McKenzie therapists, orthopedic surgeons, neurologists/neurosurgeons, rheumatologists and others may all be involved. The primary care physician has a central role in the management of nonspecific low back pain. The therapeutic management of specific spinal disorders is generally the domain of medical specialists. It is important that information and treatment are consistent across professions, and that healthcare providers collaborate closely with each other.

Within the framework of the Cochrane Back Review Group, systematic reviews of RCTs on therapeutic interventions for back pain are promoted, conducted, and disseminated [33, 34]. In 1997, the Cochrane Back Review Group developed and published method guidelines for systematic reviews in this field. These method guidelines were updated in 2003 [35]. The aim of these guidelines is to improve the quality of reviews, to facilitate comparison across reviews, and to enhance consistency among reviewers. The evidence on treatment of acute and chronic low back pain is summarized below. Cochrane and other systematic reviews are used and a recent edition of *Clinical Evidence*, in which these reviews have been updated with additional trials [1, 2]. The evidence from systematic reviews on chronic low back pain is summarized in Box 7.1.

Evidence of effectiveness of treatments for chronic low back pain

Acupuncture

A recent Cochrane review of 32 RCTs on chronic low back pain found evidence of pain relief and functional improvement for acupuncture compared to

---

Box 7.1   Evidence of treatments for chronic low back pain

Interventions supported by evidence
Exercise therapy
Intensive multidisciplinary treatment programs
Muscle relaxants
Analgesics
Acupuncture
Antidepressants
Back schools
Behavioral therapy
Nonsteroidal anti-inflammatory drugs
Spinal manipulation

Commonly used interventions currently unproven
Epidural steroid injections
Electromyographic biofeedback
Lumbar supports
Massage
Transcutaneous electrical nerve stimulation (TENS)
Traction
Local injections

Interventions refuted by evidence
Facet joint injections

---

no treatment or sham therapy. These effects were only observed immediately after the end of the sessions and at short-term follow-up. There is evidence that acupuncture, added to other conventional therapies, relieves pain and improves function better than the conventional therapies alone. However, effects are only small. Dry-needling appears to be a useful adjunct to other therapies for chronic low back pain. No clear recommendations could be made about the most effective acupuncture technique [36].

Analgesics

One RCT found that tramadol versus placebo decreased pain and increased functional status. A second RCT found that paracetamol versus diflunisal increased the proportion of people who rated the treatment as good or excellent [37].

Antidepressants

One systematic review found that antidepressants versus placebo provided significantly better pain relief, but no consistent difference in functioning or depression [38, 39].

Back schools

A Cochrane review of 19 RCTs found moderate evidence suggesting that back schools have better short- and intermediate-term effects on pain and functional status than other treatments for recurrent and chronic LBP. There is moderate evidence suggesting that back schools for chronic LBP in an occupational setting are more effective than other treatments and placebo or waiting list controls on pain, functional status and return to work during short- and intermediate-term follow-up.

Behavioral therapy

A Cochrane review of 21 RCTs found strong evidence that a combined respondent-cognitive therapy reduced pain more than a waiting list, and moderate evidence that progressive relaxation reduced pain and improved behavioral outcomes more than waiting list (short term only). There were no differences between operant treatment and waiting list on general functional status and behavioral outcomes (short term only). There is limited evidence that a graded activity program in an industrial setting is more effective than usual care for early return to work and reduced long-term sick leave. There is also limited evidence that there are no differences between behavioral treatment and exercises. Finally, there is moderate evidence that there are no significant differences in short-term and long-term effectiveness when behavioral components are added to usual treatment programs (i.e. physiotherapy, back education) on pain, generic functional status and behavioral outcomes [40].

Electromyographic (EMG) biofeedback

One systematic review found no difference in pain relief or functional status between electromyographic biofeedback and placebo or waiting list control, but found conflicting results on the effects of EMG biofeedback compared with other treatments [37].

Epidural steroid injections

A Cochrane review found no significant difference between epidural steroid injections and placebo or between epidural steroid injections and saline injections in pain relief after 6 weeks or 6 months [41]. Most of these trials included patients with sciatica.

Exercise

A Cochrane review found evidence of effectiveness in chronic populations relative to comparisons at all follow-up periods; pooled mean improvement was 7.3 points (95% CI 3.7–10.9) for pain (out of 100), 2.5 points (1.0–3.9) for function (out of 100) at earliest follow-up. In studies investigating patients (i.e. presenting to healthcare providers) mean improvement was 13.3 points (5.5–21.1) for pain, 6.9 (2.2–11.7) for function, representing significantly greater improvement over studies where participants included those recruited from a general population (e.g. with advertisements) [42, 43].

Facet joint injections

A Cochrane review found no significant difference in pain relief between facet joint injections and placebo or facet joint nerve blocks [41]. Most of these trials included patients with sciatica.

Functional restoration

A Cochrane review has found that functional restoration programs with a cognitive behavioral approach plus physical training for workers with back pain reduced sick days but not the risk of being off work at 12 months compared with usual general practitioner care or with other interventions [44].

Local injections

A Cochrane review found that four out of five trials indicated that injection therapy was more effective than placebo injection, irrespective of the medication used. However, the meta-analysis showed that there was no significant difference in pain relief. Two trials did not show any differences between local injection with bupivacaine and lignocaine or bupivacaine and methylprednisolone [41]. Most of these trials included patients with sciatica.

Lumbar supports

A Cochrane review found insufficient evidence on the effects of lumbar supports [45]. Three studies included solely patients with chronic LBP [46-48]. One study [47] found limited evidence that lumbar supports are not more effective than no intervention on short-term pain and functional status for patients with chronic LBP. The same study found limited evidence that a flexible corset is not more effective than a semi-rigid corset regarding short-term pain and functional status for patients with chronic LBP [47]. Another RCT found limited evidence that a lumbar corset with back support is more effective on short-term pain and back-specific functional status than a lumbar support alone for patients with chronic LBP [48]. One RCT found limited evidence that lumbar support as supplement to a muscle-strengthening program is not more effective on short- and long-term pain and back pain-specific functional status than a muscle training program alone [46].

Massage

A Cochrane review found that massage combined with exercises and education is more effective than soft tissue massage only, remedial exercises and education only, and sham laser therapy. The review found conflicting evidence about the effects of massage compared with other treatments [49].

Multidisciplinary treatment programs

A Cochrane review found that intensive multidisciplinary biopsychosocial rehabilitation with functional restoration reduces pain and improves function compared with inpatient or outpatient nonmultidisciplinary treatments or usual care. The review found no significant difference between less intensive multidisciplinary treatments and nonmultidisciplinary treatment or usual care in pain or function [50].

Muscle relaxants

A Cochrane review found better short-term pain relief and overall improvement with muscle relaxants compared to placebo. One RCT found that adverse effects in people using muscle relaxants are common and include dependency, drowsiness, and dizziness [51].

Nonsteroidal anti-inflammatory drugs

A Cochrane review found that the pooled standardized mean difference of four studies comparing nonstercidal anti-inflammatory drugs (NSAIDs) with placebo for chronic low back pain was –0.48 (95% CI –0.61 to –0.36), indicating a statistically significant effect in favor of NSAIDs compared to placebo. The pooled relative risk (RR) for side effects was 1.24 (95% CI 1.07–1.43), indicating statistically significantly fewer side effects in the placebo group.

One high-quality study found limited evidence that NSAIDs are more effective for pain relief than paracetamol in patients with chronic low back pain [52].

Paracetamol was associated with fewer side effects compared with NSAIDs.

Two RCTs found conflicting evidence on the effects of NSAIDs versus other analgesics [53–55]. One study reported equal effectiveness for an NSAID compared to a herbal medicine (*Harpagophytum procumbens/doloteffin*) [56]. One study found moderate evidence that there were no differences in pain relief between COX-2 and traditional NSAIDs for chronic low back pain [57].

Spinal manipulation

One systematic review identified 16 comparisons in 13 RCTs. The review found that spinal manipulation versus placebo did not improve pain and function [58].

Traction

One systematic review found no significant difference between traction and placebo or between traction and other treatments on any outcome [59].

Transcutaneous electrical nerve stimulation

A Cochrane review found no significant difference in pain relief and function between transcutaneous electrical nerve stimulation and sham stimulation [60].

Guidelines and implementation

During the last decade, various clinical guidelines on the management of acute low back pain in primary care have been published [3, 61]. At present, guidelines on acute low back pain exist in at least 12 different countries: Australia, Denmark, Finland, Germany, Israel, The Netherlands, New Zealand, Norway, Sweden, Switzerland, the United Kingdom and the United States. However, recently the first guidelines on chronic low back pain were published [62]. To increase consistency in the management of nonspecific low back pain across countries in Europe, the European Commission has approved a program for the development of European guidelines for the management of low back pain, called "COST B13." The main objectives of this COST action were:

- developing European guidelines for the prevention, diagnosis and treatment of nonspecific low back pain.
- ensuring an evidence-based approach through the use of systematic reviews and existing clinical guidelines

- enabling a multidisciplinary approach; stimulating collaboration between primary healthcare providers and promoting consistency across providers and countries in Europe
- promoting implementation of these guidelines across Europe.

Representatives from 13 countries participated in this project that was conducted between 1999 and 2004. The experts represented all relevant health professions in the field of low back pain: anatomy, anesthesiology, chiropractic, epidemiology, ergonomy, general practice, occupational care, orthopedic surgery, pathology, physiology, physiotherapy, psychology, public healthcare, rehabilitation, and rheumatology. Besides guidelines for the management of chronic low back pain, guidelines were also developed on acute low back pain, prevention of low back pain, and pelvic girdle pain.

Development and dissemination of guidelines do not automatically mean that healthcare providers will read, understand and use the guidelines. Passive dissemination of information is generally ineffective and specific implementation strategies are necessary to establish changes in practice. Systematic reviews have shown that a clear and strong evidence base, clear messages, consistent messages across professions, clear sense of ownership, communication with all relevant stakeholders, charismatic leadership, continuity of care, continuous education, and continuous evaluation are successful ingredients for the implementation of guidelines [63–65].

Guidelines should have a clear and strong evidence base and be based on systematic reviews. Guidelines that are not based on sound scientific evidence might effectively implement the wrong evidence. Also, there should be an explicit link between recommendations and evidence. Messages should be clear, specific and unambiguous. Inconsistent recommendations across health professions may be confusing. Therefore, messages of the various healthcare providers involved in the management of low back pain should be consistent.

Several barriers to the implementation of guidelines have been identified. The practice behavior of health professionals may be influenced by a lack of knowledge, a shortage of time, disagreement with the guideline content or reluctance of colleagues to adhere to the guideline. Furthermore, health professionals may get lost in the large number of different guidelines received. A priority in getting evidence into practice is identifying barriers to change the behavior of health professionals.

However, changing behavior is complex and difficult and interventions developed to change the behavior of health professionals have shown only limited effects. Identifying efficient implementation strategies to increase the uptake of evidence-based guideline recommendations will be a major challenge for the future.

How to produce evidence of effectiveness in the future

A promising strategy is trying to identify relevant subgroups that may benefit more from a specific intervention. A recently published RCT found that patients with acute or subacute low back pain had significantly better functional outcomes when they received a matched treatment versus an unmatched treatment [66] The authors examined all patients before treatment and assigned them to one of three groups (manipulation, stabilization exercises, or specific exercise) thought most likely to benefit the patients. Patients were subsequently randomized irrespective of this subgroup assignment into one of the three interventions groups with the same treatments. The analyses were focused on matched versus unmatched treatment according to their baseline subgroup assignment.

Previous studies also found better results of matched treatments in subgroups of patients with nonspecific low back pain. For example, one study showed that it was possible to identify a subgroup of patients likely to benefit from spinal manipulation [67]. These types of studies may further improve the management of patients with low back pain and better tailor treatment options to the needs of individual patients. It might be recommended to further investigate which subgroups of patients with chronic low back pain (e.g. based on their psychosocial yellow flags) will especially benefit from exercise therapy or cognitive behavioral therapy.

Authors' recommendations

- Current evidence mostly favors active treatment approaches compared to passive treatments in acute as well as chronic low back pain.
- Evidence-based guidelines for the management of low back pain are available in many countries, but implementation needs more effort.
- The main challenge is the early identification (e.g. based on psychosocial risk factors) of patients at risk for chronicity and subsequently preventing the chronicity.

References

1. Van Tulder MW, Koes BW. Acute low back pain and sciatica. *Clin Evid* 2003; **9**: 1245–1259.

2. van Tulder MW, Koes BW. Chronic low back pain and sciatica. *Clin Evid* 2003; **9**: 1260–1276.

3. Koes BW, van Tulder MW, Ostelo R, Kim BA, Waddell G. Clinical guidelines for the management of low back pain in primary care: an international comparison. *Spine* 2001; **26**: 2504–2513.

4. Deyo RA, Rainville J, Kent DL. What can the history and physical examination tell us about low back pain? *JAMA* 1992; **268**: 760–765.

5. Jensen MC, Brant-Zawadzki MN, Obuchowski N, Modic MT, Malkasian D, Ross JS. Magnetic resonance imaging of the lumbar spine in people without back pain. *N Engl J Med* 1994; **331**: 69–73.

6. van Tulder MW, Assendelft WJJ, Koes BW, Bouter LM. Spinal radiographic findings and nonspecific low back pain: a systematic review of observational studies. *Spine* 1997; **22**: 427–434.

7. Frymoyer JW. Back pain and sciatica. *N Engl J Med* 1988; **318**: 291–300.

8. von Korff M, Saunders K. The course of back pain in primary care. *Spine* 1996; **21**: 2833–2837.

9. van den Velden J, de Bakker DH, Claessens A, Schellevis FG. Een nationale studie naar ziekten en verrichtingen in de huisartspraktijk. NIVEL, Utrecht, 1991.

10. Lamberts H. In het huis van de huisarts. Verslag van het Transitieprojekt. Meditekst, Lelystad, 1991.

11. Papageorgiou AC, Croft PR, Thomas E, Ferry S, Jayson MI, Silman AJ. Influence of previous pain experience on the episode incidence of low back pain: results from the South Manchester Back Pain Study. *Pain* 1996; **66**: 181–185.

12. Picavet HSJ, Schouten JSAG, Smit HA. Prevalences and consequences of low back pain in the MORGEN-project 1993–1995. Rijksinstituut voor volksgezondheid en milieu, Bilthoven, 1996.

13. Leboeuf-Yde C. Smoking and low back. A systematic literature review of 41 journal articles reporting 47 epidemiologic studies. *Spine* 1999; **24**: 1463–1470.

14. Leboeuf-Yde C. Body weight and low back pain. A systematic literature review of 56 journal articles reporting on 65 epidemiologic studies. *Spine* 2000; **25**: 226–237.

15. Hoogendoorn WE, van Poppel MNM, Bongers PM, Koes BW, Bouter LM. Physical load during work and leisure time as risk factors for back pain. *Scand J Work Environ Health* 1999; **25**: 387–403.

16. Andersson GBJ. The epidemiology of spinal disorders. In: Frymoyer JW (ed) *The Adult Spine: Principles and Practice.* Lippincott-Raven, Philadelphia, 1997: 93–141.

17. Hoogendoorn WE, van Poppel MNM, Bongers PM, Koes BW, Bouter LM. Systemic review of psychosocial factors at work and private life as risk factors for back pain. *Spine* 2000; **25**: 2114–2125.

18. Power C, Frank J, Hertzman C, Schierhout G, Li L. Predictors of low back pain onset in a prospective British study. Am J Pub Health 2001; **91**: 1671–1678.

19. Linton SJ. A review of psychological risk factors in back and neck pain. *Spine* 2000; **25**: 1148–1156.

20. Bongers PM, de Winter CR, Kompier MAJ, Hildebrandt VH. Psychosocial factors at work and musculoskeletal disease: a review of the literature. *Scand J Work Environ Health* 1993; **19**: 297–312.

21. Linton SJ. Occupational psychological factors increase the risk for back pain: a systematic review. *J Occup Rehabil* 2001; **11**: 53–66.

22. Pincus T, Burton AK, Vogel S, Field AP. A systematic review of psychological factors as predictors of chronicity/disability in prospective cohorts of low back pain. *Spine* 2002; **27**: E109–E120.

23. Cats-Baril WL, Frymoyer JW. Identifying patients at risk of becoming disabled because of low back pain: the Vermont Rehabilitation Engineering Center predictive model. *Spine* 1991; **16**(6): 605–607.

24. Gatchel RJ. The dominant role of psychosocial risk factors in the development of chronic low back pain disability. *Spine* 1995; **20**: 2702–2709.

25. Fransen M, Woodward M, Norton R, Coggan C, Dawe M, Sheridan N. Risk factors associated with the transition from acute to chronic occupational back pain. *Spine* 2002; **27**: 92–98.

26. van der Giezen AM, Bouter LM, Nijhuis FJ. Prediction of return-to-work of low back pain patients sicklisted for 3–4 months. *Pain* 2000; **87**: 285–294.

27. Kendall N, Linton S, Main C. *Guide to Assessing Psychosocial Yellow Flags in Acute Low Back Pain: Risk Factors for Long-Term Disability and Work Loss.* National Advisory Committee on Health and Disability, and ACC (Accident Rehabilitation and Compensation Insurance Corporation), Wellington, 1997.

28. Linton SJ, Hallden K. Can we screen for problematic back pain? A screening questionnaire for predicting outcome in acute and subacute back pain. *Clin J Pain* 1998; **14**: 209–215.

29. van den Hoogen HMM, Koes BW, van Eijk JThM, Bouter LM. On the accuracy of history, physical examination and erythrocyte sedimentation rate in diagnosing low back pain in general practice. A criteria-based review of the literature. *Spine* 1995; **20**: 318–327.

30. Deville WL, van der Windt DA, Dzaferagic A, Bezemer PD, Bouter LM. The test of Lasegue: systematic review of the accuracy in diagnosing herniated discs. *Spine* 2000; **25**: 1140–1147.

31. Jarvik JG, Deyo RA. Diagnostic evaluation of low back pain with emphasis on imaging. *Ann Intern Med* 2002; **137**: 586–597.

32. Jarvik JG, Hollingworth W, Martin B, *et al.* Rapid magnetic resonance imaging vs radiographs for patients with low back pain: a randomized controlled trial. *JAMA* 2003; **289**: 2810–2818.

33. Bombardier C, Esmail R, Nachemson AL, Back Review Group Editorial Board. The Cochrane Collaboration Back Review Group for spinal disorders. *Spine* 1997; **22**: 837–840.

34. Bouter LM, Pennick V, Bombardier C; The Editorial Board of the Back Review Group. Cochrane back review group. *Spine* 2003; **28**: 1215–1218.

35. van Tulder M, Furlan A, Bombardier C, Bouter L, Editorial Board of the Cochrane Collaboration Back Review Group. Updated method guidelines for systematic reviews in the Cochrane Collaboration Back Review Group. *Spine* 2003; **28**: 1290–1299.

36. Furlan AD, van Tulder M, Cherkin D, *et al.* Acupuncture and dry-needling for low back pain: an updated systematic review within the framework of the Cochrane Collaboration. *Spine* 2005; **30**(8): 944–963.

37. van Tulder MW, Koes BW, Bouter LM. Conservative treatment of acute and chronic non-specific low back pain: a systematic review of randomized controlled trials of the most common interventions. *Spine* 1997; **22**: 2128–2156.

38. Browning R, Jackson JF, O'Malley PG. Cyclobenzaprine and back pain. *Arch Intern Med* 2001; **161**: 1613–1620.

39. Salerno SM, Browning R, Jackson JL. The effect of antidepressant treatment in chronic back pain: a meta-analysis. *Arch Intern Med* 2002; **162**: 19–24.

40. Ostelo RW, van Tulder MW, Vlaeyen JW, Linton SJ, Morley SJ, Assendelft WJ. Behavioural treatment for chronic low-back pain. Cochrane Database Syst Rev. 2005 Jan 25;(1): CD002014.

41. Nelemans PJ, de Bie RA, de Vet HCW, *et al.* Injection therapy for subacute and chronic benign low back pain. The Cochrane Library, Issue 3, 2002. Update Software, Oxford.

42. Hayden JA, van Tulder MW, Tomlinson G. Systematic review: strategies for using exercise therapy to improve outcomes in chronic low back pain. *Ann Intern Med* 2005; **142**(9): 776–785.

43. Hayden JA, van Tulder MW, Malmivaara AV, Koes BW. Meta-analysis: exercise therapy for nonspecific low back pain. *Ann Intern Med* 2005; **142**(9): 765–775.

44. Schonstein E, Kenny DT, Keating J, Koes BW. Work conditioning, work hardening and functional restoration for workers with back and neck pain (Cochrane Review). The Cochrane Library, Issue 1, 2003. Update Software, Oxford.

45. van Tulder MW, Scholten RJPM, Koes BW, Deyo RA. Nonsteroidal anti-inflammatory drugs for low back pain: a systematic review within the framework of the Cochrane Collaboration. *Spine* 2000; **25**: 2501–2513.

46. Dalichau S, Scheele K. Effects of elastic lumbar belts on the effect of a muscle training program for patients with chronic back pain [German]. *Z Orthopädie Grenzgebiete* 2000; **138**: 8–16.

47. Gibson JNA, Ahmed M. The effectiveness of flexible and rigid supports in patients with lumbar backache. *J Orthop Med* 2002; **24**: 86–9.

48. Million R, Nilsen KH, Jayson MIV, Baker RD. Evaluation of low-back pain and assessment of lumbar corsets with and without back supports. *Ann Rheumatic Disorders* 1981; **40**: 449–54.

49. Furlan AD, Brosseau L, Imamura M, Irvin E. Massage for low-back pain: a systematic review within the framework of the Cochrane Collaboration Back Review Group. *Spine* 2002; **27**: 1896–1910.

50. Guzman J, Esmail R, Karjalainen K, Malmivaara A, Irvin E, Bombardier C. Multidisciplinary rehabilitation for chronic low back pain: systematic review. *BMJ* 2001; **322**(7301): 1511–1516.

51. van Tulder MW, Touray T, Furlan AD, Solway S, Bouter LM, Cochrane Back Review Group. Muscle relaxants for nonspecific low back pain: a systematic review within the framework of the Cochrane Collaboration. *Spine* 2003; **28**(17): 1978–1992.

52. Hickey RF. Chronic low back pain: a comparison of diflunisal with paracetamol. NZ Med J 1982; **95**(707): 312–314.

53. Famaey JP, Bruhwyler J, Vandekerckhove K, *et al.* Open controlled randomised multicenter comparison of nimesulide and diclofenac in the treatment of subacute and chronic low back pain. *J Drug Assess* 1998; **1**: 349–368.

54. Veenema KR, Leahey N, Schneider S. Ketorolac versus meperidine: ED treatment of severe musculoskeletal low back pain. *Am J Emerg Med* 2000; **18**: 404–407.

55. van Tulder MW, Scholten RJ, Koes BW, Deyo RA. Nonsteroidal anti-inflammatory drugs for low back pain: a systematic review within the framework of the Cochrane Collaboration Back Review Group. *Spine* 2000; **25**(19): 2501–13.

56. Chrubasik, Model S, Black A, Pollak A, S. A randomized double-blind pilot study comparing Doloteffin and Vioxx in the treatment of low back pain. *Rheumatology (Oxford)* 2003; **42**: 141–148.

57. Zerbini C, Ozturk ZE, Grifka J, *et al.* Efficacy of etoricoxib 60 mg/day and diclofenac 150 mg/day in reduction of pain and disability in patients with chronic low back pain: results of a 4-week, multinational, randomized, double-blind study. *Curr Med Res Opin* 2005; **21**: 2037–2049.

58. Assendelft WJJ, Morton SC, Yu EI, Suttorp MJ, Shekelle PG. Spinal manipulative therapy for low back pain. A meta-analysis of effectiveness relative to other therapies. *Ann Intern Med* 2003; **138**: 871–881.

59. Clarke JA, van Tulder MW, Blomberg SE, *et al.* Traction for low-back pain with or without sciatica. Cochrane Database Syst Rev. 2007 Apr 18; (2): CD003010.

60. Milne S, Welch V, Brosseau L, Saginur M, Shea B, Tugwell P, Wells G. Transcutaneous electrical nerve stimulation (TENS) for chronic low back pain. Cochrane Database Syst Rev. 2001; (2): CD003008.

61. van Tulder MW, Tuut M, Pennick V, Bombardier C, Assendelft WJ. Quality of primary care guidelines for acute low back pain. *Spine* 2004; **29**(17): E357–62.

62. Airaksinen O, Brox JI, Cedraschi C, *et al.*, on behalf of the COST B13 Working Group on Guidelines for Chronic Low Back Pain. European guidelines for the management of chronic nonspecific low back pain. *Eur Spine J* 2006; **15**(suppl 2): S192–300.

63. Bero LA, Grilli R, Grimshaw JM, Harvey E, Oxman AD, Thomson MA. Closing the gap between research and practice: an overview of systematic reviews of interventions to promote the implementation of research findings.

The Cochrane Effective Practice and Organization of Care Review Group. *BMJ* 1998; **317**: 465–468.

64. Grol R. Beliefs and evidence in changing clinical practice. *BMJ* 1997; **315**: 418–421.

65. Grimshaw J, Shirran L, Thomas R. Changing provider behavior: an overview of systematic reviews of interventions. *Med Care* 2001; **29**: II2–II45.

66. Brennan GP, Fritz JM, Hunter SJ, Thackeray A, Delitto A, Erhard RE. Identifying subgroups of patients with acute/subacute "nonspecific" low back pain. Results of a randomized clinical trial. *Spine* 2006; **31**: 623–631.

67. Childs JD, Fritz JM, Flynn TW, *et al.* Validation of a clinical prediction rule to identify patients with low back pain likely to benefit from spinal manipulation. *Ann Intern Med* 2004; **141**: 920–928.

68. Leboeuf-Yde C. Alcohol and low-back pain: a systematic literature review. *J Manip Physiol Ther* 2000; **23**: 343–346.

CHAPTER 8

Chronic neck pain and whiplash

Allan Binder

Lister Hospital, E & N Hertfordshire NHS Trust, Stevenage, UK

Introduction

Most patients who present with chronic neck symptoms fit into the category of nonspecific neck pain, which includes a variety of conditions having a postural or mechanical basis. Etiology is usually multifactorial and includes poor posture, anxiety, depression, neck strain and occupational or sporting activities. It also includes pain following a "whiplash" injury provided there is no bony injury or objective neurologic deficit. Where mechanical factors are prominent, the condition is often called "cervical spondylosis" although this term is loosely applied to all patients with nonspecific neck pain.

Whiplash syndrome is very common throughout the world, but the incidence of reported symptoms and patients who go on to chronic disability or seek compensation varies greatly between countries, and even different social groups within the same country [1]. As the dynamics associated with whiplash differ so much from other causes of neck pain, there is a need to differentiate these patients from other patients with nonspecific neck pain [2]. Unfortunately, many studies of neck pain do not specify the type of patients included.

The duration of symptoms before presentation might also influence outcome, and in practice, most therapeutic studies of nonspecific pain are carried out in patients with chronic disease (>4 months duration), with study of acute symptoms (<4 weeks) being confined to whiplash.

Evidence-Based Chronic Pain Management. Edited by C. Stannard, E. Kalso and J. Ballantyne. © 2010 Blackwell Publishing.

Background

Pathophysiology of nonspecific neck pain

Nontraumatic causes

Many patients with nonspecific neck pain show degenerative changes in the cervical disks with osteophyte formation and involvement of adjacent soft tissue structures. However, similar degenerative changes in the cervical spine are common in asymptomatic people over the age of 30 years, with changes being evident both on plain X-rays [3] and MRI scanning [4]. As there is such a poor correlation between symptoms and radiological findings, the boundary between "normal" aging and disease is difficult to define, and diagnosis is usually made on clinical grounds alone.

Whiplash

Patients develop symptoms soon after a sudden acceleration-deceleration of the neck, as occurs in road traffic or sporting accidents. While symptoms are often severe, the source of the pain is uncertain, and no specific pathology can be identified on detailed clinical or radiological investigation. While soft tissue injury is considered likely, this is difficult to confirm even using MRI scanning. In some patients with chronic whiplash, facet joint abnormality [5] or brachial plexus involvement has been identified [6]. It is not clear whether pre-existing degenerative change in the cervical spine influences outcome in these patients.

Epidemiology of nonspecific neck pain

Epidemiological studies of neck pain are based on questionnaires and surveys, which may overestimate the frequency of the condition. Nevertheless, it is clear that nonspecific neck pain including whiplash places a heavy burden on individuals, employers, and healthcare services.

Nontraumatic causes

About two-thirds of the population will experience neck pain at some time in their lives [7, 8], with the condition being most common in middle age, and in women [9]. The reported prevalence of neck pain varies widely between studies, but has a mean point prevalence of 7.6% (range 5.9–38.7%) and a mean lifetime prevalence of 48.5% (range 14.2–71%) [9]. A UK survey found that 18% of 7669 adults had neck pain at the time of the survey, but when symptomatic people were re-questioned 1 year later (58% responded), half were still symptomatic [10]. A Norwegian survey of 10,000 adults also reported that 34% of responders had experienced neck pain in the previous year [11]. Neck pain is second only to back pain in frequency of musculoskeletal consultation in primary care.

Whiplash

Although whiplash injury is very common throughout the world, the incidence of reported symptoms and patients who go on to chronic disability or to seek compensation varies greatly between countries and even between different regions or social groups within the same country. There is no consistency in the literature about the epidemiology and natural history of whiplash, partially because of the poor quality of studies [12, 13]but more specifically because of the complex interactions between the individual, legal, economic, and societal factors, which may influence presentation and outcome [12, 13]. In some countries, like Lithuania and Greece where there is no litigation or compensation culture, chronic whiplash is very rare and outcome is universally favorable [14, 15]. In other countries like the USA, Canada, The Netherlands, Australia and the UK, much higher proportions of patients develop chronic whiplash and suffer prolonged disability [16]. Internationally, whiplash lasting for over 6 months varies between 2% and 58% [13, 17] but typically lies between 20% and 40% [18].

Risk factors

Natural history of nonspecific neck pain and whiplash with factors associated with chronic disability

Nontraumatic causes

Nonspecific neck pain usually resolves within days or weeks, but can recur or become chronic. Once pain becomes persistent, outcome is more unpredictable, and there is little consistency in the literature regarding the duration of symptoms and factors that influence outcome. A systematic review of the clinical course and prognostic factors in nonspecific neck pain found little consensus as to outcome or relevant prognostic factors, although this was based on poor-quality studies [19]. The systematic review found evidence that in patients with chronic pain treated in secondary care or an occupational setting, 20–78% (median 54%) of patients remained symptomatic, irrespective of the therapy given. Six of the included studies documented prognostic factors, and the severity of pain at presentation was the best predictor of a poor outcome, although previous episodes of neck pain were also important. Three subsequent studies also considered the factors at presentation which might influence outcome at 1 year, and found older age, and concomitant low back pain [10, 20] and severity and duration of the pain [21] to be significant. Patients with chronic spinal conditions were also found to have other chronic pain syndromes (69%), chronic physical conditions (55%) or psychologic problems (35%)[22, 23].

Neck pain with neurological complications

Many patients with neurological abnormality as a result of nonspecific neck pain will require MRI scanning of the cervical spine at an early stage, particularly if there is progressive myelopathy or intractable pain. Radiculopathy generally has a favorable outcome, although recovery can be slow. The result of decompressive surgery for myelopathy complicating nonspecific neck pain is often disappointing. While the rate of progression of the neurological loss may be slowed by the surgery, the lost function may not recover or symptoms may progress at a later date. The poor outcome following surgery may reflect the irreversible damage to the cervical cord or compromise to the vascular supply to the cord immediately or subsequently.

Whiplash

The prognosis for whiplash is also generally favouable [12] but as already mentioned, shows great variability as to the frequency, severity and duration of disability. This variability in outcome is at least in part related to the culture of litigation and compensation [1] but this cannot explain all the differences, particularly within the same population. Two comprehensive systematic reviews [12, 13] found little consistency as to factors influencing outcome, although societal factors like litigation and compensation culture were most important [1, 24, 25]. How other societal factors influence outcome is complex and even more poorly understood [26]. Systematic reviews of prognostic factors following whiplash injury [12, 13, 17] found conflicting evidence for pre-existing physical or psychologic factors, or crash-related factors. The most consistent predictors of an unfavorable outcome from the systematic reviews and subsequent studies were severity of pain, headache and disability at presentation.

Therapeutic interventions for neck pain

Methods

Literature searches on therapeutic options for treating mechanical neck pain were carried out using the following databases: Chirolars (now called Mantis), Bioethicsline, CINAHL, Current Contents, and Medline, with data being used to prepare and update an article in *Clinical Evidence* [2]. I will summarize the evidence on treatment modalities currently in use, with an indication of questions which still need to be answered. Studies relating to specific conditions like fibromyalgia and disk prolapse will not be discussed.

Data on therapy will be considered for patients with (uncomplicated) nonspecific neck pain, neck pain plus radiculopathy, and whiplash. Therapies will then be categorized as "likely to be effective," where there is at least one high-quality RCT suggesting benefit and reasonable consensus from other studies; "likely to be ineffective," where there is at least one high-quality study suggesting a lack of benefit from the treatment; and "unknown effectiveness," where there is insufficient or conflicting evidence without a consensus (Boxes 8.1–8.3). Relevant systematic

---

Box 8.1 Therapeutic options for nonspecific neck pain

Likely to be effective
Exercise
Manual therapy (mobilization or manipulation)
Exercise plus manual therapy

Likely to be ineffective
Patient education
Heat

Unknown effectiveness
Multimodal therapy
Traction
Acupuncture
Pulsed electromagnetic field therapy
Transcutaneous electrical nerve stimulation
Drug treatments
Soft collar and special pillows
Biofeedback
Spray and stretch

Box 8.2 Therapeutic options for neck pain complicated by radiculopathy

Unknown effectiveness
Epidural injection
Physical therapies
Immobilization in a collar

Box 8.3 Therapeutic options for acute and chronic whiplash

Acute whiplash
Likely to be effective
Early exercise or mobilization

Unknown effectiveness
Early return to normal activities
Early home exercise
Pulsed electromagnetic field therapy
Multimodal therapy
Drug treatments

Chronic whiplash
Unknown effectiveness
Percutaneous radiofrequency neurotomy
Multimodal therapy
Physical therapies

reviews with be mentioned, but with data mainly from the higher quality RCTs.

Most neck pain appears to respond to conservative measures, although the effect size is often quite small, and the optimal therapeutic approach for uncomplicated neck pain has yet to be established. Even where an initial benefit is shown, this advantage is not sustained. Few modalities of treatment have been assessed in high-quality randomized studies, but I will try to present the best available evidence for the most commonly used modalities. The evidence is often contradictory because of the poor quality of many of the studies, use of interventions in combination, and diverse patient groups. The lack of consistency in study design makes it difficult to identify which intervention may be of use in which type of patients.

Nonspecific neck pain (see Box 8.1)

Therapies likely to be effective
1. Exercise
Systematic reviews [2,27-30] identified RCTs using different exercise strategies, but none of the reviews could perform a meta-analysis because of heterogeneity among the trials in types of exercise and study designs.

Positive studies
- **Proprioceptive and strengthening exercise versus usual care:** one RCT (60 people with chronic neck pain) [31] found a proprioceptive and strengthening exercise program to be significantly more effective (P < 0.004) at reducing pain at 10 weeks when compared with usual care (analgesics, nonsteroidal anti-inflammatory drugs or muscle relaxants).
- **Endurance exercise versus strengthening exercise versus no specific exercise program:** an RCT (180 female office workers with chronic neck pain) [32] compared a program of "endurance" (dynamic) or "strength" (isometric) exercises to a control group (no specific exercise), with exercise being carried out three times a week for 1 year. Both endurance and strength exercises significantly improved neck pain and disability after 12 months compared to the control therapy (P < 0.001 for exercise groups versus control).
- **Strength training versus endurance training versus co-ordination exercises versus stress**

management: an RCT (103 women with chronic work-related neck pain) [33] compared three exercise regimens (strength training, endurance training, co-ordination exercises) compared to stress management over 10 weeks. It found that any type of exercise significantly reduced pain compared with stress management after 10–12 weeks (P < 0.05), but there was no significant difference in outcomes between the different exercise programs. There was also no significant difference in neck pain among the four groups after 3 years [34]. Another RCT (180 women with chronic neck pain) assessed the rate of change in neck strength, pain and disability of a 1-year training program comparing high-intensity strength training or lower intensity endurance training to a control group. The greatest improvement in strength was achieved within the first 2 months for both treated groups, but with improvement continuing to a year. The decrease in pain at 12 months was 69% for strength training, 61% for endurance training and 28% for controls, compared to baseline, all being significant (P < 0.001). The number of patients who were pain free or nearly pain free at 12 months was significantly greater for the treated groups (53% and 49% respectively) compared to the controls (20%) [35]. However, this study does not describe how randomization and blinding were achieved.
- **Exercise plus infrared versus transcutaneous electrical nerve stimulation (TENS) plus infrared versus infrared alone:** one RCT (218 patients with chronic neck pain) [36] compared the effects of twice-weekly therapy for 6 weeks using intensive exercise plus infrared, TENS plus infrared, and infrared alone. The RCT found that the addition of exercise or TENS significantly improved pain compared to infrared alone at 6 weeks (P = 0.02) and 6 months (P = 0.019), but with no difference between the two combination treatment groups.
- **Exercise plus special pillow versus either alone versus control (hot/cold pack plus massage):** an RCT (151 patients with chronic neck pain) [37] compared the effects of exercise plus a special pillow to exercise or a pillow alone or a control group and found a significant advantage for the combination group at 6 weeks, although the difference was small.

Negative study
- **Dynamic muscle training versus relaxation training versus advice to continue with ordinary activity:** one RCT (393 women office workers with chronic neck pain) [38] compared three interventions for 12 weeks: dynamic muscle training, relaxation training, and advice to continue with ordinary activities, and found no significant difference in outcome in pain or disability in the three groups at 3, 6, and 12 months of follow-up. However, the average number of 30-minute training sessions completed by participants over 12 weeks for both treatment groups was only 40% of the maximum available, and this might have influenced the result.

2. Manual therapy (manipulation and mobilization physiotherapy)
Systematic reviews [2, 27, 28, 39–44] identified a number of RCTs comparing manipulation and/or mobilization with each other or with other treatments.

Positive studies
- **Manipulation or mobilization versus other physical treatments, versus usual care versus placebo:** one RCT (256 people with chronic neck and back pain; 64 with neck and 48 with neck and back involvement) [45] compared four treatment groups: manual treatment (mobilization, manipulation or both); physical treatments at the discretion of the physiotherapist; usual GP care; and placebo. It found that manual treatment significantly improved outcomes after 12 months compared with all the other treatments (statistical analysis for people with neck pain alone was not reported). It was not possible to directly compare the effects of mobilization versus manipulation.
- **Manipulation versus mobilization versus exercise:** one RCT (119 people with chronic neck pain) [46] compared three treatments: mobilization, manipulation, and intensive exercise training. It found no significant difference in pain among the three groups by the end of treatment or after 12 months, although pain score improved significantly from baseline in all groups.
- **Manipulation versus mobilization:** three RCTs compared manipulation to mobilization. The first RCT (100 people with acute or chronic neck pain)

[47] compared a single manipulation treatment versus a single mobilization treatment and found no significant difference between them in immediate improvement in pain (85% with manipulation, 69% with mobilization). In this study, there was a transient increase in pain in 5% of people receiving manipulation and 6% receiving mobilization. The second RCT (336 people with acute or chronic neck pain) [48] found no significant difference between manipulation and mobilization in "average" pain, "severe" pain and neck disability scores between a variable number of chiropractic mobilizations and a variable number of manipulations after 6 months. In this RCT, only 35% of eligible people agreed to participate, and this may reduce the external validity of the study. A follow-up questionnaire of adverse effects at 2 weeks [49] found that 30% of the 280 people who responded reported at least one minor adverse effect such as increased pain or headache associated with manipulation and less commonly with mobilization. In the third RCT (70 patients with chronic neck pain) [50], patients received one manipulation or one mobilization with assessment before the therapy and 5 minutes after treatment. Both groups showed significant improvement in pain and range of movement, but with a greater benefit for the manipulation group.
- **Mobilization versus exercise versus usual care:** one RCT (183 people with neck pain for >2 weeks) [51] compared three 6-week courses of treatment with mobilization, exercise or usual care, with treatment "success" being defined as "much improved" or "completely recovered." The RCT found "success" to be significantly more common at 7 weeks with mobilization compared to exercise or usual care, but there was no difference between exercise and usual care. Long-term follow-up of this RCT [52] found that mobilization was still superior at 26 weeks, but not at 1 year.

Negative studies
- **Manipulation versus diazepam, anti-inflammatory drugs or usual care:** one review [40] performed a meta-analysis of three RCTs (155 people with chronic neck and back pain) comparing manipulation to diazepam, anti-inflammatory drugs or usual care. It found no significant difference in improvement

in pain at 3 weeks between manipulation and other treatments, although all treatments improved pain. However, the meta-analysis may have been underpowered to detect a clinically important difference.

- **McKenzie mobilization versus general exercise versus placebo:** one small low-quality RCT (77 people) [53] compared McKenzie mobilization, exercise and placebo, and found no significant difference in pain between the groups at 6 months and 12 months.
- **Adverse events associated with manipulation:** manipulation has been associated with occasional serious neurologic complications and the estimated risk from case reports of cerebrovascular accident is 1–3/million manipulations [54], while the estimated risk of all serious adverse effects (such as death or disk herniation) is 5–10/10 million manipulations [40].

3. Manual therapy plus exercise

Two systematic reviews by the same Cochrane group reviewed exercise therapy [30] and manual therapy [41] in patients with nonspecific neck pain, neck pain with radiculopathy and whiplash, and found the best evidence of efficacy was for the combination of manual therapy (mobilization or manipulation) with exercise when compared with any other treatments. However, the review did not provide a subgroup analysis in people with uncomplicated nonspecific neck pain.

Positive study

- **Manipulation plus strengthening exercises versus either treatment alone:** one RCT (191 people with chronic neck pain) [55] compared three treatments: low-technology strengthening exercises plus manipulation (combined treatment), high-technology MedX strengthening exercises (exercise), and manipulation alone (manipulation). The RCT found that the combined treatment significantly improved patient satisfaction, objective strength, and range of movement (P < 0.05) compared with manipulation after 11 weeks. The RCT also found that both the combined treatment and exercise significantly improved pain and patient satisfaction compared to manipulation after 1 year, although it found no significant difference among treatments in health status, neck disability or medication use. The 2-year follow-up to this RCT (data available for 76% of the original patients) [56]

found superior pain reduction for the combined treatment or exercise groups compared to manipulation (P = 0.04).

Negative study

- **Manipulation, mobilization or shortwave diathermy plus exercise and advice:** one pragmatic multicenter RCT (350 patients with chronic neck pain) [57] found no benefit from the addition of manual therapy (63% had mobilization physiotherapy) or pulsed shortwave diathermy to advice plus exercise at 6 weeks or 6 months.

Therapies likely to be ineffective

1. Patient education alone

Two RCTs in people with chronic neck, back or shoulder pain found no significant benefit from patient education (individual advice, pamphlets or group instruction) with or without analgesics, stress management or cognitive behavioral therapy.

- **Educational pamphlet versus more extensive information versus cognitive behavioral therapy (CBT):** the first RCT (243 people with neck and back pain) [58] compared three interventions: an educational pamphlet, a more extensive information program, and six sessions of CBT, and found no significant difference among treatments. However, *post hoc* analysis suggested that CBT significantly reduced time off work compared with an educational pamphlet (P = 0.05).
- **Individualized education plus exercise program versus stress management versus no intervention:** the second RCT (282 nurses with neck, shoulder or back pain in the preceding 12 months) [59] compared three interventions: an individualized education and exercise program, stress management, and no intervention. The RCT found no significant difference in pain among the groups immediately after treatment, or at 12 and 18 months.

2. Heat

Systematic reviews [2, 27, 28] identified two RCTs suggesting that heat was less effective than other therapies in people with uncomplicated neck pain. One RCT of people with chronic neck and back pain [45] found that heat combined with other physical treatment was less effective in improving outcomes than manipulation or mobilization (see "Manual therapy"). The second RCT [36] found infrared less effective when used alone than when combined with exercise or TENS (see "Exercise").

Therapies of unknown effectiveness

1. Multimodal treatment
Systematic reviews [2, 60] identified two RCTs which provided insufficient evidence to assess the benefit or cost-effectiveness of multimodal treatment in people with uncomplicated neck pain.

- **Multimodal treatment versus CBT versus minimal treatment:** one RCT (185 patients with non-specific neck [87%] and/or back [91%] pain) [61] compared minimal therapy (advice to keep active), CBT (six sessions of structured CBT), and CBT plus physical therapy (same regimen as CBT group plus physical training). The RCT found that minimal treatment significantly increased the risk of being off work for 15 or more days compared with CBT plus physical training. It found no significant difference in sick leave between CBT and CBT plus physical therapy. However, the RCT included people with neck pain, back pain or both, and did not separately report results for those with neck pain alone.
- **Different forms of multimodal therapy:** the second RCT (66 people with chronic neck and shoulder pain) [62] compared exercise plus behavioral modification (patient education and advice, with a psychologist acting as an advisor to other staff) to exercise plus CBT (with CBT administered by a psychologist). It found no significant difference between the interventions in pain or time off work after 6 months.

2. Traction
Systematic reviews [2, 27, 28, 63, 64] identified two RCTs comparing traction versus sham traction, placebo tablets, exercise, acupuncture, heat, collar, and analgesics. The RCTs found no consistent difference in pain between traction and any of the other interventions.

3. Acupuncture
Systematic reviews [2, 27, 28, 65–67] identified 14 RCTs comparing needle or laser acupuncture with different control procedures (sham acupuncture, sham TENS, diazepam, traction, short-wave diathermy, and mobilization) in people with acute or chronic neck pain. None of the reviews was able to perform a meta-analysis, and the RCTs found no consistent difference in pain between acupuncture and any of the other interventions. The quality of the studies was considered "disappointing."

4. Pulsed electromagnetic field treatment (PEMF)
Systematic reviews [2, 27, 28, 68] identified one RCT of moderate quality comparing PEMF versus sham PEMF in people with chronic neck pain. The RCT (81 people with neck pain and 86 people with osteo-arthritis of the knee) [69] compared true to sham PEMF. Subgroup analysis in people with chronic neck pain found that PEMF significantly reduced pain ($P < 0.04$) and pain on passive motion ($P = 0.03$), compared with sham PEMF, but there was no difference in a range of other parameters. Although randomization was conducted appropriately, baseline characteristics of treated and placebo groups were, by chance, different and it is not clear how much of the observed effect was caused by bias introduced by the baseline differences.

5. Transcutaneous electrical nerve stimulation (TENS)
Systematic reviews [2, 27, 28, 68] identified one RCT [36] that found that TENS plus infrared was equally effective to infrared plus exercise, and superior to infrared alone at 6 weeks (see "Exercise").

6. Drug treatments (analgesics, NSAIDs or muscle relaxants, tricyclic antidepressants)
No systematic review or RCTs examining the effects of drug treatments in people with nonspecific neck pain were found.

7. Facet joint injection
Two systematic reviews [70, 71] found moderate evidence of efficacy for facet joint block using medial branch blocks, but no evidence for cervical intra-articular facet joint blocks. One RCT of medial branch blocks of the facet joints (60 patients with facet joint disease confirmed by diagnostic medial branch block) were randomized to receive one of four preparations with the medial branch blocks: bupivacaine alone, bupivacaine plus sarapin, bupivacaine

plus betamethasone, or all three agents together, with the same injections being repeated as required over the next year. Significant pain relief (>50%) and improved disability were observed in 80–87% of all patients at 3 months, 80–93% at 6 months and 87–93% at 12 months, but with no difference between the treatment groups or patients who did or did not receive the steroid. The average number of treatments per patient was 3.8 +/−0.7 in the nonsteroid groups, and 3.4 +/−1.0 in the steroid groups, with no significant difference among the groups [72].

8. Soft collars, special pillows, biofeedback, spray and stretch
There are no data on these measures in patients with nonspecific neck pain.

Neck pain with radiculopathy (see Box 8.2)

Therapies of unknown effectiveness
Neck pain with radiculopathy usually has a favorable prognosis without the need for surgical intervention, but there are very few studies looking at conservative approaches to therapy, like epidural injection or a comparison between conservative and surgical treatments.

1. Cervical epidural injection (interlaminar or transforaminal)
Systematic reviews [2, 73–75] identified two small poor-quality RCTs which provided insufficient evidence on the effects of cervical epidural interlaminar steroid injections for radiculopathy complicating nonspecific neck pain. One RCT (40 patients with radiculopathy confirmed by MRI and diagnostic transforaminal block) had one transforaminal injection of either steroid or saline plus local anesthetic with weekly assessments for 3 weeks. Six of 20 patients in each group reported improvement at 3 weeks, with no difference between the groups for any parameter at any time [76]. Epidural injections are more invasive in the cervical than lumbar region, and need to be used with caution. Complications, such as infection or abscess formation, have been documented following the procedure [73].

- **Cervical epidural versus posterior neck muscle injection of steroid plus lidocaine:** the first RCT

(52 people with chronic cervical brachialgia) [77] compared cervical epidural steroid plus lidocaine injection to similar injection into the posterior neck muscles, and found that more people receiving the epidural injections had reduced pain at 1 year (68% with epidural versus 12% with control), although the significance was not reported.
- **Epidural steroid plus lidocaine versus epidural steroid plus lidocaine plus oral morphine:** the second RCT (24 people with cervical radiculopathy for >1 year) [78] found similar success rates over 1 year for epidural steroid (triamcinolone) alone or when used with oral morphine (78.5% with epidural alone versus 80% with epidural plus morphine).

2. Conservative versus surgical treatment
Systematic reviews [2, 79] identified one RCT (81 people with severe radicular symptoms for at least 3 months) [80] comparing three interventions: surgery, physical treatments, and immobilization. It found no significant difference among treatments in symptoms after 1 year.

Treatment of acute whiplash to prevent chronic disability (see Box 8.3)
The studies of acute whiplash are included to see if early treatment can influence the development of prolonged disability. Although there is some evidence that early active interventions can reduce disability, the studies are insufficiently robust to confirm this [18].

Therapies likely to be effective
1. Early physiotherapy (mobilization and/or exercises) versus immobilization or less active treatment
Systematic reviews [2, 12, 18, 81] identified RCTs comparing early physiotherapy to less active treatments.

Positive studies
- **Early mobilization versus immobilization in a collar:** three studies found early mobilization to be more effective than immobilization in a collar. The first RCT (61 people with acute whiplash) [82] compared early mobilization versus immobilization in a collar plus rest for 14 days followed by gradual mobilization. It found that early mobilization significantly improved pain and range of movement after 4 and 8 weeks compared with immobilization plus less active treatment (P < 0.01). In the second RCT (97

people with acute whiplash) [83], there were early benefits in pain relief and improved movement with early mobilization compared with immobilization in a collar, but similar pain relief after 12 weeks (proportion with neck pain: 2% with mobilization versus 16% with collar). The RCT did not assess the significance of the difference between the groups. In the third RCT (200 people treated within 48 hours of injury) [84], instruction on mobilization (2–5 physiotherapy visits in the first week) was compared to immobilization with a soft collar. Mobilization significantly reduced the proportion of people with neck pain or disability at 6 weeks compared to those treated with a soft collar. However, by 6 weeks, 36% of the collar group and 15% of the exercise group had dropped out, and an intention-to-treat analysis was not carried out.

- **Physical treatments versus advice on early mobilization versus rest for 7–14 days followed by mobilization:** this RCT (247 people with acute whiplash) [85] compared three interventions: advice on early mobilization, physical treatments, or rest for 7–14 days followed by gentle mobilization. All participants were given a soft collar and analgesics. Follow-up at 2 years of 167 people responding to a questionnaire found that advice on early mobilization significantly reduced the proportion of people who still had symptoms compared with physical treatments or rest (P = 0.02 for early mobilization versus other treatments).
- **Immediate mobilization versus mobilization after 96 hours delay versus rest plus a collar:** one RCT (97 people with acute whiplash) [86] found that mobilization (home mobilization and exercise) significantly improved pain compared with rest plus a collar (P < 0.001), but only if mobilization was started immediately after injury. If mobilization was delayed by more than 96 hours, there was no significant difference between treatments after 6 months. However, a 3-year follow-up of this RCT [87] found that mobilization significantly reduced pain and sick leave (P < 0.05) compared with rest plus a neck collar, even if it was delayed for 2 weeks, although only people who had received active intervention within 96 hours had a total cervical range similar to matched controls.

Negative study
- **Active physiotherapy versus GP care:** this RCT (80 patients with whiplash persisting to 4 weeks) [88]

compared active physiotherapy (exercise or mobilization) to GP care, with both groups receiving advice on graded activity. There was substantial improvement in both groups over time, but no statistically significant differences between the two groups for pain, headache or work disability at 8, 12, 26 or 52 weeks. However, treatment was delayed for up to 4 weeks after the injury and this might have influenced the result.

Therapies of unknown effectiveness

1. Early return to normal activity
Systematic reviews [2, 18, 81] identified one RCT (201 people with acute whiplash) [89] which compared advice to "act as usual" versus immobilization plus 14 days' sick leave. The RCT found that advice to "act as usual" significantly improved some symptoms (pain, neck stiffness, headache, poor memory and concentration) after 6 months compared with immobilization. However, there was no difference in neck range or length of sick leave between the treatment groups. Furthermore, a similar proportion of people had severe neck pain after 6 months (11% with "act as usual" versus 15% with immobilization).

2. Early home exercise
Systematic reviews [2, 18, 29, 81] identified one RCT (59 people with acute whiplash) [90] which compared two home exercise regimens: regular exercise versus the same exercise regimen plus isometric exercises at least three times daily. The RCT found no significant difference between treatments in disability or pain after 3 or 6 months.

3. Pulsed electromagnetic field treatment (PEMF)
Systematic reviews [2, 12, 18, 81] identified one small RCT (40 people with acute whiplash) [91] which compared PEMF with sham PEMF, and found the active therapy significantly more effective after 4 weeks (P < 0.05), but not after 3 months.

4. Multimodal treatment
Systematic reviews [2, 18, 81] identified one RCT (60 people with whiplash in the previous 2 months) [92] which compared multimodal treatment (postural training, psychologic support, eye fixation exercises, and manual treatment) with physical treatments. The RCT found that multimodal treatment significantly reduced pain by the end of treatment (P < 0.05) and

after 1 and 6 months (P < 0.001) compared with physical treatments. There was a similar benefit for time to return to work. Further study is necessary to determine if multimodal treatment is a cost-effective approach.

5. Drug treatments (analgesics, NSAIDs, antidepressant drugs, muscle relaxants)

Systematic reviews [2, 12, 18] identified no studies of efficacy of drug therapies in acute whiplash. One RCT (40 patients with acute whiplash of less than 8 hours) treated with IV methylprednisolone or placebo led to a significant reduction in pain at 1 week and less sick leave for the steroid-treated group compared to placebo, but this benefit was not sustained to 6 months [93].

Treatment of chronic whiplash (see Box 8.3)

Few RCTs have considered treatment for chronic whiplash, but many of these people are included in RCTs of chronic nonspecific neck pain.

Therapies of unknown effectiveness

1. Percutaneous radiofrequency neurotomy

- **Percutaneous radiofrequency neurotomy versus sham treatment:** systematic reviews [2, 73, 81, 94] identified one small RCT (24 people with chronic whiplash) [5], which found that radiofrequency neurotomy significantly increased the proportion of people who were free from pain compared with sham treatment after 27 weeks (58% with active treatment versus 8% with sham treatment). The neurotomy also significantly increased the pain-free period (median time for more than half of the pain to return – 263 days with neurotomy versus 8 days with sham treatment; P = 0.04). Although this high-quality RCT suggested benefits from this therapy, the trial was very small and there is no supporting evidence of efficacy.

2. Physical and multimodal treatment

- **Multimodal treatment versus physical treatment:** systematic reviews [2, 81] identified one RCT (33 people with chronic whiplash) [95], which compared physical treatments alone with multimodal treatment and found no significant difference between treatments in pain, disability or range of movement at the end of treatment or at 3 months. However, significantly more people treated with

multimodal treatment were satisfied with pain control at the end of treatment and their ability to perform activities at 3 months (P < 0.05).

- **Exercise plus advice versus advice alone:** one RCT (134 patients with whiplash of 3–12 months' duration) compared three advice sessions to exercise (12 sessions over 6 weeks) plus advice. Exercise resulted in a significant benefit at 6 weeks, but not at 12 months. Exercise was more effective for patients with higher pain scores. However, 56% of advice patients and 29% of exercise patients sought further treatment between 6 weeks and 12 months, and could have biased the results [96].

Future research

The lack of consistency in study design, patient population, outcome measures and durations of follow-up and the use of multiple interventions in the same study complicate comparison between studies. Large well-designed randomized prospective studies using standardized protocols should clarify efficacy and cost-effectiveness of individual treatment modalities.

The benefit of most therapeutic interventions for nonspecific neck pain is small, and many patients improve with limited or even no treatment [97]. It is therefore important that future studies set predetermined minimum differences, which are considered to be clinically relevant. This approach should avoid the current difficulty that many studies, while showing statistically significant differences in outcome, may have little clinical importance.

If patient groups are more homogeneous, meta-analyses may be possible to provide more robust guidance on cost-effective approaches to therapy for specific patient groups.

Discussion

Nonspecific neck pain including whiplash is a very common cause of disability, and places a heavy burden on individuals, employers and society. However, there are many aspects regarding etiopathogenesis and treatment which remain poorly understood. Furthermore, if the factors that influence the progression from acute to chronic pain were better understood, it might be possible to reduce the frequency and severity of chronic disability for both whiplash and other causes of nonspecific neck pain. Most studies of acute neck pain are in patients following whiplash injury, and it is not clear if the findings from those studies can be generalized to neck pain from nontraumatic causes.

There have been some higher quality randomized controlled trials of therapy in patients with nonspecific neck pain, which suggest that exercise [32, 33] and manual therapy (mobilization physiotherapy or manipulation) [45, 46, 48] are the treatments of choice, and are more effective than less active therapies, but the relative cost-effectiveness of these modalities has not been studied. One high-quality study suggests additional benefits if exercise is used in combination with mobilization or manipulation [55, 56], and this approach has been advocated by a Cochrane systematic review group [30, 41] but needs further study.

Cervical radiculopathy usually has a favorable outcome, and there is increasing interest in conservative approaches. However, there have only been a few poor-quality studies of epidural injection [77, 78] or conservative approaches [80] and further study is required.

There is some evidence that early mobilization can influence outcome following whiplash injury [82–86] but a recent systematic review that included 23 studies (2344 participants) questioned the quality of the data and robustness of the evidence for early active interventions [18]. Whether there is a window of opportunity for preventing chronic pain in patients with traumatic and nontraumatic neck pain remains uncertain.

Many commonly used first-line strategies such as analgesic, anti-inflammatory agents, tricyclic antidepressants, reduction in the number of pillows, stress management, and postural advice have not been studied but remain mainstays of treatment. Other modalities such as acupuncture, traction, electrotherapy, and psychotherapy are of uncertain value and also need further study [2].

Author recommendation: a pragmatic approach to the treatment of nonspecific neck pain, including untested measures

It is not currently possible to treat neck pain solely on the basis of proven evidence-based measures, as many aspects of therapy have not been adequately tested. While exercise, mobilization, and manipulation are mainstays of therapy, any regime must address postural factors identified in individual patients. Reduction in the number of pillows at night is often important, but there is no evidence to suggest that "special" pillows justify the additional cost. Stress management, yoga, Pilates and the Alexander Technique all improve neck posture and are useful, but require further study.

Low-dose tricyclic antidepressants seem to be more effective than simple analgesics or anti-inflammatory drugs in reducing pain, particularly at night, but have not been subjected to controlled study.

Comment

I have outlined the evidence for commonly used therapeutic modalities used to treat nonspecific neck pain with or without radiculopathy, and following whiplash injury, highlighted the shortcomings of the studies presented and the current state of our knowledge. As the studies are so disparate, meta-analyses were not possible, and I have presented the individual studies.

Acknowledgment

Data on therapy included in contribution by the author to the publication *Clinical Evidence*.

References

1. Ferrari R, Russell AJ. Epidemiology of whiplash: an international dilemma. *Ann Rheum Dis* 1999; **58**: 1–5.
2. Binder AI. Neck pain syndromes. *Clinical Evidence*, Issue 18, Dec 2007. BMJ Publishing Group, London.
3. Gore DR, Sepic SB, Gardner GM. Roentgenographic findings of the cervical spine in asymptomatic people. *Spine* 1986; **11**: 521–524.
4. Boden SD, McCowin PR, Davis DO, Dina TS, Mark AS, Wiesel S Abnormal magnetic–resonance scans of the cervical spine in asymptomatic subjects. A prospective investigation. *J Bone Jt Surg* 1990; **72A**: 1178–1184.
5. Lord SM, Barnsley L, Wallis BJ, McDonald GJ, Bogduk N. Percutaneous radio-frequency neurotomy for chronic cervical zygapophyseal-joint pain. *N Engl J Med* 1996; **335**: 1721–1726.
6. Sterling M, Treleaven J, Jull G. Responces to a clinical test of mechanical provocation of nerve tissue in whiplash associated disorder. *Manual Ther* 2002; **7**: 89–94.
7. Mäkelä M, Heliövaara M, Sievers K. Prevalence, determinants, and consequences of chronic neck pain in Finland. *Am J Epidemiol* 1991; **134**: 1356–1367.

8. Cote P, Cassidy D, Carroll L. The Saskatchewan health and back pain survey: the prevalence of neck pain and related disability in Saskatchewan adults. *Spine* 1998; **23**: 1689–1698.

9. Fejer R, Kyvik KO, Hartvigsen J The prevalence of neck pain in the world population: a systematic clinical review of the literature. *Eur Spine J* 2006; **15**: 834–848.

10. Hill J, Lewis M, Papageorgiou AC, Dziedzic K, Croft P. Predicting persistent neck pain: a 1-year follow-up of a population cohort. *Spine* 2004; **29**: 1648–1654.

11. Bovim G, Schrader H, Sand T. Neck pain in the general population. *Spine* 1994; **19**: 1307–1309.

12. Spitzer WO, Skovron ML, Salmi LR, Cassidy JD, Duranceau J, Suissa S, Zeiss E. Scientific monograph of the Quebec Task Force on whiplash-associated disorders: redefining "whiplash" and its management. *Spine* 1995; **20**(suppl 8): 1–73. (Erratum in *Spine* 1995; **20**: 2372.)

13. Cote P, Cassidy JF, Carroll L, Frank JW, Bombardier C. A systematic review of the prognosis of acute whiplash and a new conceptual framework to synthesize the literature. *Spine* 2001; **26**(19): E445–E458.

14. Obelieniene D, Schrader H, Bovim, G, Miseviciene I, Sand T. Pain after whiplash: a prospective controlled inception cohort study. *J Neurol Neurosurg Psych* 1999; **66**: 279–283.

15. Partheni M, Constantoyannis C, Ferrari R, Nikiforidis G, Voulgaris S, Papadakis N. A prospective cohort study of the outcome of acute whiplash injury in Greece. *Clin Exper Rheum* 2000; **18**: 67–70.

16. Suissa S, Harder S Veilleux. The relation between initial symptoms and signs and the prognosis of whiplash. *Eur Spine J* 2001; **10**: 44–49.

17. Scholten-Peeters GGM, Verhagen AP, Bekkering GE, *et al*. Prognostic factors of whiplash-associated disorders: a systematic review of prospective cohort studies. *Pain* 2003; **104**: 303–322.

18. Verhagen AP, Scholten-Peeters GGGM, van Wijngaarden S, de Bie R, Bierma-Zeinstra SMA. Conservative treatments for whiplash. Cochrane Database of Systematic Reviews 2007, Issue 2. Art. No.: CD003338. DOI: 10.1002/14651858. CD003338.pub3.

19. Borghouts JA, Koes BW, Bouter LM. The clinical course and prognostic factors of nonspecific neck pain: a systematic review. *Pain* 1998; **77**: 1–13.

20. Hoving JL, de Vet HCW, Twisk JWR, *et al*. Prognostic factors for neck pain in general practice. *Pain* 2004; **110**: 639–645.

21. Kjellman G, Skargren E, Oberg B. Prognostic factors for perceived pain and function at one year follow-up in primary care patients with neck pain. *Disabil Rehabil* 2002; **24**: 364–370.

22. Cote P, Cassidy JD, Carroll L. The treatment of neck and low back pain: who seeks care? Who goes where? *Med Care* 2001; **39**: 956–967.

23. Carroll LJ, Cassidy JD, Cote P. Depression as a risk factor for onset of an episode of troublesome neck and low back pain. *Pain* 2004; **107**: 134–139.

24. Cassidy JD, Carroll LJ, Cote P, Lemstra M, Berglund A, Nygren A. Effect of eliminating compensation for pain and suffering on the outcome of insurance claims for whiplash injury. *N Engl J Med* 2000; **342**: 1179–1186.

25. McDermott FT. Reduction in cervical "whiplash" after new motor vehicle accident legislation in Victoria. *Med J Aust* 1993; **158**: 720–721.

26. Virani SN, Ferrari R. Russell AS. Physician resistance to the late whiplash syndrome. *J Rheumatol* 2001; **28**: 2096–2099.

27. Aker PD, Gross AR, Goldsmith CH, *et al*. Conservative management of mechanical neck pain: systematic overview and meta-analysis. *BMJ* 1996; **313**: 1291–1296.

28. Kjellman GV, Skargren EI, Oberg BE. A critical analysis of randomised clinical trials on neck pain and treatment efficacy. A review of the literature. *Scand J Rehabil Med* 1999; **31**: 139–152.

29. Sarig-Bahat, H. Evidence for exercise therapy in mechanical neck disorders. *Manual Ther* 2003; **8**: 10–20.

30. Kay TM, Gross A, Goldsmith CH, Hoving JL, Brønfort G. Exercises for mechanical neck disorders. Cochrane Database of Systematic Reviews 2005, Issue 3. Art. No.: CD004250. DOI: 10.1002/14651858.CD004250.pub3.

31. Revel M, Minguet M, Gregory P, *et al*. Changes in cervicocephalic kinesthesia after a proprioceptive rehabilitation program in patients with neck pain: a randomised controlled study. *Arch Phys Med Rehabil* 1994; **75**: 895–899.

32. Ylinen J, Takala E, Nykanen M, *et al*. Active neck muscle training in the treatment of chronic neck pain in women: a randomized controlled trial. *JAMA* 2003; **289**: 2509–2516.

33. Waling K, Sundelin G, Ahlgren C, *et al*. Perceived pain before and after three exercise programs – a controlled clinical trial of women with work–related trapezius myalgia. *Pain* 2000; **85**: 201–207.

34. Waling K, Jaörvholm B, Sundelin G. Effects of training on female trapezius myalgia: an intervention study with a 3–year follow-up period. *Spine* 2002; **27**: 789–796.

35. Ylinen JJ, Hakkinen AH, Takala EP, *et al*. Effects of neck muscle training in women with chronic neck pain: one year follow-up study. *J Strength Cond Res* 2006; **20**: 6–13.

36. Chiu TT, Hui-Chan CW, Chein G. A randomized clinical trial of TENS and exercise for patients with chronic neck pain. *Clin Rehabil* 2005; **19**: 850–860.

37. Helewa A, Goldsmith CH, Smythe HA, Lee P, Obright K, Stitt L. Effect of therapeutic exercise and sleeping neck support on patients with chronic neck pain: a randomised clinical trial. *J Rheumatol* 2007; **34**: 151–158.

38. Viljanen M, Malmivaara A, Uitti J, *et al*. Effectiveness of dynamic muscle training, relaxation training, or ordinary activity for chronic neck pain: randomised controlled trial. *BMJ* 2003; **327**: 475–477.

39. Koes BW, Assendelft WJ, van der Heijden GJ, *et al*. Spinal manipulation and mobilization for back and neck pain: a blinded review. *BMJ* 1991; **303**: 1298–1303.

40. Hurwitz EL, Aker PD, Adams AH, *et al*. Manipulation and mobilization of the cervical spine: a systematic review of the literature. *Spine* 1996; **21**: 1746–1760.

41. Gross A, Hoving JL, Haines T, *et al*., Cervical Overview Group. Manipulation and mobilization for mechanical neck disorders. Cochrane Database of Systematic Reviews 2004, Issue 1. Art. No.: CD004249. DOI: 10.1002/14651858. CD004249.pub2.

42. Bronfort G, Haas M, Evans RL, *et al.* Efficacy of spinal manipulation and mobilization for low back pain and neck pain: a systematic review and best evidence synthesis. *Spine J* 2004; **4**: 335–356.

43. Canadian Chiropractic Association, Canadian Federation of Chiropractic Regulatory Boards, Clinical Practice Guidelines Development Initiative, Guidelines Development Committee (GDC). Chiropractic clinical practice guideline: evidence-based treatment of adult neck pain not due to whiplash. *J Can Chiropr Assoc* 2005; **49**(3): 158–209.

44. Vernon H, Humphreys K, Hagino C. Chronic mechanical neck pain in adults treated by manual therapy: a systemic review of change scores in randomised clinical trials. *J Manip Physiol Therapeut* 2007; **30**: 215–227.

45. Koes BW, Bouter LM, van Mameren H, *et al.* Randomised clinical trial of manipulative therapy and physiotherapy for persistent back and neck complaints: results of one year follow up. *BMJ* 1992; **304**: 601–605.

46. Jordan A, Bendix T, Nielsen H, *et al.* Intensive training, physiotherapy, or manipulation for patients with chronic neck pain. A prospective, single-blinded, randomized clinical trial. *Spine* 1998; **23**: 311–319.

47. Cassidy JD, Lopes AA, Yong-Hing K. The immediate effect of manipulation versus mobilization on pain and range of motion in the cervical spine: a randomised controlled trial. *J Manip Physiol Therapeut* 1992; **15**: 570–575.

48. Hurwitz EL, Morgenstern H, Harber P, *et al.* A randomized trial of chiropractic manipulation and mobilization for patients with neck pain: clinical outcomes from the UCLA neck-pain study. *Am J Public Health* 2002; **92**: 1634–1641.

49. Hurwitz EL, Morgenstern H, Vassilaki M, *et al.* Adverse reactions to chiropractic treatment and their effects on satisfaction and clinical outcomes among patients enrolled in the UCLA Neck Pain Study. *J Manip Physiol Therapeut* 2004; **27**: 16–25.

50. Martinez-Segura R, Fernandez-de-las-Penas C, Ruiz-Saez M, Lopez-Jimenez C, Rodriguez-Blanco C. Immediate effects on neck pain and active range of motion after a single cervical high velocity low amplitude manipulation in subjects presenting with mechanical neck pain: a randomised controlled trial. *J Manip Physiol Therapeut* 2006; **29**: 511–517.

51. Hoving J, Koes B, de Vet H, *et al.* Manual therapy, physical therapy, or continued care by a general practitioner for patients with neck pain. A randomized, controlled trial. *Ann Intern Med* 2002; **136**: 713–722.

52. Korthals-de Bos I, Hoving J, van Tulder, M, *et al.* Cost effectiveness of physiotherapy, manual therapy, and general practitioner care for neck pain: economic evaluation alongside a randomised controlled trial. *BMJ* 2003; **326**: 911–914.

53. Kjellman G, Oberg B. A randomised clinical trial comparing general exercise, McKenzie treatment and a control group in patients with neck pain. *J Rehabil Med* 2002; **34**: 183–190.

54. Dabbs V, Lauretti WJ. A risk assessment of cervical manipulation vs NSAIDS for the treatment of neck pain. *J Manip Physiol Therapeut* 1995; **18**: 530–536.

55. Bronfort G, Evans R, Nelson B, *et al.* A randomized clinical trial of exercise and spinal manipulation for patients with chronic neck pain. *Spine* 2001; **26**: 788–797.

56. Evans R, Bronfort G, Nelson B, *et al.* Two-year follow-up of a randomized clinical trial of spinal manipulation and two types of exercise for patients with chronic neck pain. *Spine* 2002; **27**: 2383–2389.

57. Dziedzic K, Hill J, Lewis M, *et al.* Effectiveness of manual therapy or pulsed shortwave diathermy in addition to advice and exercise for neck disorders: a pragmatic randomized controlled trial in physical therapy clinics. *Arthritis Care Res* 2005; **53**: 214–222.

58. Linton SJ, Andersson T. Can chronic disability be prevented? A randomized trial of a cognitive-behaviour intervention and two forms of information for patients with spinal pain. *Spine* 2000; **25**: 2825–2831.

59. Horneij E, Hemborg B, Jensen I, *et al.* No significant differences between intervention programmes on neck, shoulder and low back pain: a prospective randomized study among home-care personnel. *J Rehabil Med* 2001; **33**: 170–176.

60. Karjalainen KA, Malmivaara A, van Tulder MW, *et al.* Multidisciplinary biopsychosocial rehabilitation for neck and shoulder pain among working age adults. Cochrane Database of Systematic Reviews 2003, Issue 2. Art. No.: CD002194. DOI: 10.1002/14651858. CD002194.

61. Linton SJ, Boersma K, Jansson M, *et al.* The effects of cognitive-behavioral and physical therapy preventive interventions on pain-related sick leave: a randomized controlled trial. *Clin J Pain* 2005; **21**: 109–119.

62. Jensen I, Nygren A, Gamberale F, *et al.* The role of the psychologist in multidisciplinary treatments for chronic neck and shoulder pain: a controlled cost-effectiveness study. *Scand J Rehabil Med* 1995; **27**: 19–26.

63. van der Heijden GJ, Beurskens AJ, Koes BW, *et al.* The efficacy of traction for back and neck pain: a systematic, blinded review of randomized clinical trial methods. *Phys Ther* 1995; **75**: 93–104.

64. Graham N, Gross AR, Goldsmith C, and the Cervical Overview Group. Mechanical traction for mechanical neck disorders: a systemic review. *J Rehabil Med* 2006; **38**: 145–152.

65. White AR, Ernst E. A systematic review of randomized controlled trials of acupuncture for neck pain. *Rheumatology* 1999; **38**: 143–147.

66. Smith LA, Oldman AD, McQuay HJ, *et al.* Teasing apart quality and validity in systematic reviews: an example from acupuncture trials in chronic neck and back pain. *Pain* 2000; **86**: 119–132.

67. Trinh K, Graham N, Gross A, *et al.*, Cervical Overview Group. Acupuncture for neck disorders. Cochrane Database of Systematic Reviews 2006, Issue 3. Art. No.: CD004870. DOI: 10.1002/14651858.CD004870.pub3.

68. Kroeling P, Gross A, Goldsmith CH, Houghton PE, Cervical Overview Group. Electrotherapy for neck disorders. Cochrane Database of Systematic Reviews 2005, Issue 2. Art. No.: CD004251. DOI: 10.1002/14651858.CD004251.pub3.

69. Trock DH, Bollet AJ, Markoll R. The effect of pulsed electromagnetic fields in the treatment of osteoarthritis of

the knee and cervical spine. Report of randomized double-blind placebo controlled trials. *J Rheumatol* 1994; **21**: 1903–1911.

70. Boswell MV, Colson JD, Spillane WF. Therapeutic facet joint intervention in chronic spinal pain: a systematic review of effectiveness and complications. *Pain Physician* 2005; **8**: 101–114.

71. Boswell MV, Colson JD, Sehgal N, *et al.* A systematic review of therapeutic facet joint interventions in chronic spinal pain. *Pain Physician* 2007; **10**: 229–253.

72. Manchikanti L, Damron K, Cash K, Manchukonda R, Pampati V. Therapeutic cervical medial branch blocks in managing chronic neck pain: a preliminary report of randomised, double-blind, controlled trial NCT0033272, *Pain Physician* 2006; **9**: 333–346.

73. Boswell MV, Hansen HC, Trescot AM, *et al.* Epidural steroids in the management of chronic spinal pain and radiculopathy. *Pain Physician* 2003; **6**: 319–334.

74. Abdi S, Datta S, Lucas LF. Role of epidural steroids in the management of chronic spinal pain: a systematic review of effectiveness and complications. *Pain Physician* 2005; **8**: 127–143.

75. Abdi S, Datta S, Trescot AM, *et al.* Epidural steroids in the management of chronic spinal pain: a systematic review. *Pain Physician* 2007; **10**: 185–212.

76. Anderberg L, Annertz M, Persson L, Brandt L, Saveland H. Transforaminal steroid injections for the treatment of cervical radiculopathy: a prospective and randomised study. *Eur Spine J* 2007; **16**: 321–328.

77. Stav A, Ovadia L, Sternberg A, *et al.* Cervical epidural steroid injection for cervicobrachialgia. *Acta Anaesthesiol Scand* 1993; **37**: 562–566.

78. Castagnera L, Maurette P, Pointillart V, *et al.* Long-term results of cervical epidural steroid injection with and without morphine in chronic cervical radicular pain. *Pain* 1994; **58**: 239–243.

79. Fouyas IP, Statham PF, Sandercock PA. Cochrane review on the role of surgery in cervical spondylotic radiculomyelopathy. *Spine* 2002; **27**: 736–747.

80. Persson LC, Carlsson CA, Carlsson JY. Long-lasting cervical radicular pain managed with surgery, physiotherapy, or a cervical collar: a prospective randomised study. *Spine* 1997; **22**: 751–758.

81. Seferiadis A, Rosenfeld M, Gunnarsson R. A review of treatment interventions in whiplash-associated disorders. *Eur Spine J* 2004; **13**: 387–397.

82. Mealy K, Brennan H, Fenelon GC. Early mobilization of acute whiplash injuries. *BMJ* 1986; **292**: 656–657.

83. Bonk AD, Ferrari R, Giebel GD, Edelmann M, Huser R. Prospective, randomized, controlled study of activity versus collar, and the natural history for whiplash injury, in Germany. *J Musculoskel Pain* 2000; **8**: 123–132.

84. Schnabel M, Ferrari R, Vassiliou T, *et al.* Randomised, controlled outcome study of active mobilization compared with collar therapy for whiplash injury. *Emerg Med J* 2004; **21**: 306–310.

85. McKinney LA. Early mobilization and outcome in acute sprains of the neck. *BMJ* 1989; **299**: 1006–1008.

86. Rosenfeld M, Gunnarsson R, Borenstein P. Early intervention in whiplash-associated disorders: a comparison of two treatment protocols. *Spine* 2000; **25**: 1782–1787.

87. Rosenfeld M, Seferiadis A, Carlsson J, *et al.* Active intervention in patients with whiplash-associated disorders improves long-term prognosis: a randomized controlled clinical trial. *Spine* 2003; **28**: 2491–2498.

88. Scholten-Peeters GGM, Neeleman-van der Steen CW, van der Windt DA, *et al.* Education by general practitioners or education and exercises by physiotherapists for patients with whiplash-associated disorders? A randomized clinical trial. *Spine* 2006; **31**: 723–731.

89. Borchgrevink GE, Kaasa A, McDonagh D, *et al.* Acute treatment of whiplash neck sprain injuries: a randomised trial of treatment during the first 14 days after a car accident. *Spine* 1998; **23**: 25–31.

90. Söderlund A, Olerud C, Lindberg P. Acute whiplash-associated disorders (WAD): the effects of early mobilization and prognostic factors in long-term symptomatology. *Clin Rehab* 2000; **14**: 457–467.

91. Foley-Nolan D, Moore K, Codd M, *et al.* Low energy high frequency pulsed electromagnetic therapy for acute whiplash injuries. A double blind randomised controlled study. *Scand J Rehabil Med* 1992; **24**: 51–59.

92. Provinciali L, Baroni M, Illuminati L, *et al.* Multimodal treatment to prevent the late whiplash syndrome. *Scand J Rehabil Med* 1996; **28**: 105–111.

93. Pettersson K, Toolanen G. High-dose methylprednisolone prevents extensive sick leave after whiplash injury. A prospective randomised double-blind study. *Spine* 1998; **23**: 984–989.

94. Niemisto L, Kalso EA, Malmivaara A, Seitsalo S, Hurri H. Radiofrequency denervation for neck and back pain. Cochrane Database of Systematic Reviews 2003, Issue 1. Art. No.: CD004058. DOI: 10.1002/14651858.CD004058.

95. Söderlund A, Lindberg P. Cognitive behavioural components in physiotherapy management of chronic whiplash associated disorders (WAD) – a randomised group study. *Physiother Theory Pract* 2001; **17**: 229–238.

96. Stewart MJ, Maher CG, Refshauge KM, Herbert RD, Bogduk N, Nicholas M. Randomized controlled trial of exercise for chronic whiplash-associated disorders. *Pain* 2007; **128**: 59–68.

97. Vernon H, Humphreys BK, Hagino C. The outcome of control groups in clinical trials of conservative treatments for chronic mechanical neck pain: a systematic review. *BMC Musculoskel Disord* 2006; **7**: 58.

CHAPTER 9

Pain associated with osteo-arthritis

David L. Scott

Department of Rheumatology and Weston Education Centre, Kings College London School of Medicine, London, UK

Background

Pathophysiology

Osteo-arthritis involves joint cartilage, subchondral bone and synovium. It is characterized by loss of articular cartilage, new bone formation both subchondrally and at the joint margins, and variable amounts of synovial inflammation. Its clinical features comprise pain, stiffness, bony joint swelling and reduced joint movement. With time, these impair quality of life. The eventual outcome of osteo-arthritis is joint failure [1, 2].

Osteo-arthritis is mechanically driven and chemically mediated. It involves attempted but aberrant repair of the joint cartilage. In the early stages there is an imbalance between the destructive and reparative processes in articular cartilage. Its development is linked with a range of genetic, environmental, metabolic and biochemical factors. So far, the search for a single identifiable cause of osteo-arthritis has not been fruitful, and many believe it is a family of disorders and not a single disease entity.

In early osteo-arthritis a number of "triggering factors" activate the division and multiplication of chondrocytes. The most important trigger is excessive force. As a consequence, the chondrocytes multiply and become metabolically active. Initially the chondrocytes produce increased amounts of proteoglycans and collagen. However, these overproduced proteoglycans are immature. Over time the collagen fibers are altered and the proteoglycans break down

faster than they are synthesized. The decreased proteoglycan content and altered collagen matrix result in deterioration in the physiologic features of cartilage.

The early stages of cartilage damage are characterized by microfractures and fibrillations. With time there is gross damage to articular cartilage. The initially smooth surface of the cartilage becomes rough and eroded with cracks. It often shows ulceration. Many of these early cartilage changes are mediated by proteolytic enzymes, in particular metalloproteases. Key roles are played by collagenase, which is responsible for collagen degradation, and stromelysin, which is responsible for proteoglycan degradation.

Changes in the cartilage matrix are accompanied by synovial inflammation, with the involvement of a range of inflammatory mediators. Proinflammatory cytokines, such as tumor necrosis factor α, are important, though there is a balance between cytokine-driven anabolic and catabolic processes. A range of cytokines have been implicated, including interleukin-1 and interleukin-6.

Many other small molecular mediators are involved in the development of osteo-arthritis. Examples include nitric oxide, which is involved in many inflammatory conditions in which there are vascular changes, and a range of prostaglandins. These small mediators not only regulate cytokines but also result in pain and inflammation and changes in blood vessels.

Classification

Osteo-arthritis can be classified based on its symptoms, findings on examination and radiographic assessment. In most patients there is not a discrete onset, there are no specific laboratory abnormalities

Evidence-Based Chronic Pain Management. Edited by C. Stannard, E. Kalso and J. Ballantyne. © 2010 Blackwell Publishing.

and no pathognomonic features. Osteo-arthritis covers a broad spectrum of clinical features. Consequently both its classification and epidemiology are highly varied.

Osteo-arthritis can be classified by the joints involved (such as knee or hip), and by whether it is primary or secondary related to metabolic, anatomic, traumatic or inflammatory conditions. Primary generalized osteo-arthritis is a recognised subtype in which there is involvement of the distal and proximal interphalangeal joints of the hand, the first carpometacarpal joint, knees, hips and the metatarsophalangeal joints. Most patients have a less well-defined pattern.

The American College of Rheumatology has developed classification criteria for knee osteo-arthritis [3]. These criteria, which depend on expert physical examination and X-rays, are used in reporting clinical trials but are rarely applied in epidemiological studies or used in everyday clinical practice.

Epidemiology

In epidemiological studies, osteo-arthritis is most commonly defined by radiological criteria. However, many patients with radiographically defined changes in the knee have no symptoms. Radiographic criteria proposed by Kellgren and Lawrence over 40 years ago remain the principal method for defining osteo-arthritis. An alternative approach is to assess the frequency of knee pain in later life, usually considered as over 55 or 60 years of age. Osteo-arthritis is found at some sites in most people older than 65 years, and over 80% of those over the age of 75 years.

Autopsy studies show pathological features of osteo-arthritis are very common. Almost everyone over the age of 65 years will have autopsy evidence of cartilage damage. Cartilage erosions, subchondral bone changes and osteophytes in the knees are seen in over 60% of people who die in their seventh and eighth decades.

A North American study – the National Health and Nutrition Examination Survey – reported that knee osteo-arthritis is rare (0.1%) in people aged 25–34. It rises to over 30% in those aged 75 years or older [4]. Another large North American study – the Framingham Study – found the prevalence of knee osteo-arthritis was 30% among those aged 65–74 years. The prevalence of radiographic osteo-arthritis rises steeply with age [5]. Overall population-based studies in the USA and Europe show about 1% of the population have knee osteo-arthritis under 35 years of age and this rises to over 30% above the age of 75 years.

The natural history of osteo-arthritis of the knee is not well characterized. A substantial number of patients show radiological progression and up to 25% of osteo-arthritic knees with initially normal joint space show major damage after 10 years. However, there is no close relationship between X-ray progression and clinical features. People with osteo-arthritis requiring specialist referral usually have bad outcomes with high levels of physical disability. The extent to which this reflects the disease itself or associated co-morbidities is debatable.

Risk factors

Age is the dominant risk factor for osteo-arthritis, and in many ways the disorder can be viewed as an inevitability of aging. Sex is also important; about twice as many women get osteo-arthritis, mainly after the menopause. Whether this increased incidence is due to specific hormonal factors remains uncertain. Overall, there is limited evidence to suggest that female sex hormones have a definite effect on osteo-arthritis.

Osteo-arthritis runs in families, particularly generalized osteo-arthritis. There is less genetic involvement in knee than hand osteo-arthritis. Candidate genes for osteo-arthritis include the vitamin D receptor gene, insulin-like growth factor 1 genes, cartilage oligomeric protein genes, and the HLA region. It seems likely that genes affecting osteo-arthritis will influence its occurrence in many joints. Along with these genetic risks are racial differences in the development of the disease. For example, in North America the frequency of osteo-arthritis is higher in black women.

Weight is a very important risk factor for knee osteo-arthritis. It is thought that overloading knee joints leads to cartilage breakdown and failure of ligamentous and other structural support. The effect of weight on osteo-arthritis is particularly important because obesity is a serious and growing public health problem in the Western world. In persons who are overweight, weight loss can reduce the risk for osteo-arthritis.

Some occupations increase the risk of osteo-arthritis. For example, heavy physical labor, especially lifting, may increase the risk of developing osteo-arthritis of the knee, as can kneeling and squatting. Some sports, especially high-impact sports, also increase the risk of osteo-arthritis. Participation in some competitive sports is associated with the subsequent development of knee osteo-arthritis. However, moderate regular running has low, if any, risk. Sports that increase risks are those that demand high-intensity, acute, direct joint impact as a result of contact with other participants, playing surfaces or equipment, for example injuries to the knees of soccer players.

Finally, there is incomplete evidence that continuous exposure to oxidants contributes to the development of osteo-arthritis as well as other common age-related diseases. As micronutrient antioxidants provide defense against tissue injury, high dietary intake of such micronutrients might protect against osteo-arthritis, though the evidence for this is incomplete.

Interventions

Assessing benefit in osteo-arthritis

The primary goals of treatment are reducing pain, stiffness and disability. Associated aims are to improve the quality of life and ensure adverse effects are minimal. All treatments achieve these goals to a greater or lesser extent. A long-term goal is to reduce progressive joint damage, though no treatment yet achieves this.

The medical management of pain in osteo-arthritis is by definition nonsurgical. However, it is important to appreciate that surgical intervention in osteo-arthritis can be particularly important in overcoming pain as well as having positive effects in reducing disability and specifically improving mobility. Joint replacement surgery is particularly effective, but it lies outside the themes explored in this review.

Most trials use simple assessments of pain and disability. Pain is recorded using visual analog scales or five-point Likert scales. Pain can be recorded globally or in specific situations such as at rest or during exercise. There are also specific scales that record pain, stiffness and function in osteo-arthritis; the most widely used is the Western Ontario and McMaster Osteo-Arthritis (WOMAC) Scale [6].

As virtually all trials assess global pain, changes in this measure are the focus of the treatment reviews that follow. The benefit of this assessment has been counterbalanced by an assessment of adverse events. In all cases the most recent systematic review has been the basis for judging efficacy. In some situations efficacy and adverse events have been assessed separately, for example with oral nonsteroidal anti-inflammatory drugs (NSAIDs). This is because no single review examines both. The overall benefits of effective treatments are summarized in Table 9.1.

Table 9.1 Strength of evidence for treatments in knee osteo-arthritis: largest systematic reviews compared for effective treatments

Treatment	Placebo-controlled trials	Patients	Effectiveness	Adverse effects	Overall value
Paracetamol	7	1966	SMD −0.13	Minimal	Low efficacy compensated by few adverse effects
Oral NSAID/COXIBs	23	10,845	Pooled effect size 0.32	Multiple serious adverse effects	Efficacy limited by high rates of adverse effects
Local NSAIDs	7	976	Pooled effect size 0.41	Minimal	Efficacy only in short term
Opioids	18	4856	Pooled effect size 0.79	Multiple unpleasant adverse effects	Efficacy limited by high rates of adverse effects
Local steroid injections	28	1973	Mean weighted difference 21.9	Uncommon	Efficacy only in short term
Hyaluronic acid injections	40	2542	Mean weighted difference 9.0	Uncommon	Sustained efficacy but limited by need for repeated injections

Interventions supported by evidence

Simple analgesia with paracetamol

Paracetamol is the most commonly used analgesic. A single 1000 mg dose of paracetamol provides >50% pain relief over 4–6 hours in moderate or severe pain compared with placebo. There are virtually no contraindications, significant drug–drug interactions or side effects at the recommended dosage. It is well tolerated by patients with peptic ulcers. Despite many years of use, the mechanism of action of paracetamol is not well understood. It may be centrally active, producing analgesia by elevating the pain threshold through prostaglandin synthetase inhibition in the hypothalamus. At therapeutic dosages it does not inhibit prostaglandin synthetase in peripheral tissues, so has no anti-inflammatory activity.

A systematic review (seven randomized controlled trials (RCTs), 1966 people with osteo-arthritis) [7] compared paracetamol with placebo. Five of the RCTs reviewed reported that paracetamol was superior to placebo. Two showed no benefit of paracetamol over placebo. Overall, paracetamol was significantly better than placebo in several assessments of pain including pain response, pain on motion, and overall pain, and also physician and patient global assessment. Dichotomous outcomes were recorded in a single study and the number needed to treat (NNT) for a pain response was 4 (95% confidence interval (CI) 2–24) and for an improvement in patient global assessment was 2 (95% CI 2–13). Overall pain, recorded as a continuous variable in five studies, showed a standard mean difference (SMD) of −0.13 (95% CI −0.22 to −0.04) with a NNT of 16.

In terms of toxicity, the total number of patients reporting any adverse event, the relative risk of paracetamol to placebo was 1.02 (95% CI 0.89–1.17). For the toxicity outcome of total number of withdrawals due to toxicity, the relative risk was 1.24 (95% CI 0.87–1.77). Consequently, there were no significant differences in toxicity between paracetamol and placebo in these trials.

The overall assessment of paracetamol is that it is beneficial, with a favorable ratio of benefits to risks. However, its effect is minor and therefore only a small number of patients will wish to take it. It has one specific disadvantage: it needs to be taken in substantial amounts on a regular basis and most patients are reluctant to take 1 g paracetamol four times daily.

Opioid analgesics

Opioid analgesics, particularly mild opioids, have been widely suggested to be both effective and relatively safe for treating moderate to severe osteoarthritis that does not respond to first-line treatment. The effects are mainly mediated centrally by changing pain perceptions in the brain. There is some evidence for peripheral effects of opioids in arthritis. The disadvantage of opioids is their significant adverse effects including both gastrointestinal problems like nausea and central problems like drowsiness.

A systematic review (18 RCTs, 4856 people with osteo-arthritis) [8] compared opioid analgesics with placebo. The opioids included oxycodone, fentanyl and morphine, tramadol, tramadol with paracetamol, and codeine. The pooled effect sizes of all opioids compared to placebo on pain intensity was −0.79 (95% CI −0.98 to −0.59). The heterogeneity of these trials was substantial; however, there was no evidence to suggest that the conclusions differed for type of opioid, the way in which pain was measured and the methodologic quality of the study. The most frequent adverse events with opioids were nausea, constipation, dizziness, somnolence and vomiting. The average treatment discontinuation rate for toxicity was 25% with opioids and 7% with placebos. The number needed to harm (NNH) for all opioids compared to placebo was 5; for strong and weak opioids it was 4 and 9, respectively.

Another systematic review specifically evaluated tramadol and tramadol and paracetamol combinations (11 RCTs, 1939 people with osteo-arthritis) [9]. Three trials included placebo controls and they showed a weighted mean difference in favor of tramadol of −8.5 (95% CI −12.1 to −4.9). Two placebo-controlled studies reported data on pain relief from 216 participants who received active treatment and 218 participants who received placebo, and showed that tramadol increased by 53% the likelihood of a moderate improvement compared to placebo. This improvement was equivalent to a number needed to benefit of 8 (95% CI 5–25). Common adverse events with tramadol included vomiting, dizziness, constipation, somnolence, tiredness and headache. In placebo-controlled trials minor adverse events occurred 2.2 times more often with tramadol, and the NNH was 5 (95% CI 4–7). For adverse events that were severe enough for treatment to be withdrawn, the NNH was 8 (95% CI 7–12).

Oral NSAIDs

Nonsteroidal anti-inflammatory drugs are a diverse group. Their name distinguishes them from anti-inflammatory steroids (glucocorticoids) and non-narcotic analgesics. NSAIDs are one of the most frequently used groups of drugs overall, although their benefits must be set against significant, sometimes fatal, gastrointestinal and renal toxicity and also the recently described cardiovascular risks with cyclo-oxygenase-2 (COX-2) inhibitors.

COX was originally purified in the 1970s. By 1990 it was realized that the enzyme had two isoforms. The COX-1 isoform is responsible for the production of "housekeeping" prostaglandins critical for normal renal function, gastric mucosal integrity and vascular hemostasis. By contrast, COX-2 is an inducible enzyme. It is upregulated in macrophages, monocytes and other inflammatory cells by various stimuli including IL-1 and other cytokines. NSAIDs can be classified according to their relative effect on COX-1 and COX-2. Generally, the risk of gastrointestinal adverse effects is reduced with increasing COX-2 selectivity. However, other factors are involved in the causation of gastrointestinal toxicity because, paradoxically, certain NSAIDs that are relatively COX-2 selective have been associated with a higher incidence of gastrointestinal adverse events. NSAIDs have many actions other than their effect on COX. These include uncoupling oxidative phosphorylation; inhibiting lysosomal enzyme release; inhibiting complement activation; antagonizing the generation of activity in kinins; inhibiting free radicals.

The most recent large systematic review of efficacy of oral NSAIDs compared them against placebo (23 trials, 10,845 people with osteo-arthritis) [10]. This review found that NSAIDs significantly reduced pain compared with placebo. The pooled effect size for a reduction in pain was 0.32 (95% CI 0.24–0.39). Those trials that used short durations of treatment of less than 6 weeks showed no difference in effect sizes for reduced pain.

The disadvantage of conventional oral NSAIDs (such as ibuprofen, naproxen and diclofenac) and newer COX-2 specific drugs, which have been termed COXIBs (such as celecoxib, lumiracoxib and etoricoxib) is their propensity to cause adverse effects. These include upper gastrointestinal ulcers and bleeding, small bowel problems, cardiac problems such as myocardial infarction and renal problems. Older conventional NSAIDs had a substantial risk of upper gastrointestinal adverse events, many of which were serious, and the newer COXIBs such as celecoxib reduced these significantly. However, COXIBs have resulted in other problems, particularly the onset of myocardial infarctions when used for prolonged periods of time at high dosages. The older clinical trials were short term and did not investigate cardiac risks in detail. However, recent trials of COXIBs have almost entirely used conventional NSAIDs as comparators. Consequently it is difficult to estimate the overall risks of conventional NSAIDs and COXIBs.

In a long-term randomized trial lasting up to 4 years, 61–63% of patients receiving oral NSAIDs and 50% of those receiving placebo reported adverse events [11]. One systematic review evaluated the ability of COXIBs and other gastroprotective strategies with conventional NSAIDs to reduce upper gastrointestinal risks [12]. There was strong evidence that COXIBs, in comparison to conventional NSAIDs, reduce events by about 50% in meta-analyses of randomized trials (52, 474 patients) and large observational studies in clinical practice (3093 bleeding events). Evidence on the efficacy of NSAIDs plus gastroprotection with acid suppressants (proton pump inhibitors and histamine antagonists), based on the surrogate measure of endoscopic ulcers, suggested that NSAIDs with added protection was more damaging than COXIBs. Another systematic review evaluated thrombotic cardiovascular adverse events [13] and reported that in placebo studies, COXIBs gave a 42% relative increase in the incidence of serious vascular events, which was chiefly attributable to an increased risk of myocardial infarction. Overall, the incidence of serious vascular events was similar between a selective COX-2 inhibitor and any traditional NSAIDs (1.0%/year versus 0.9%/year).

Topical NSAIDs

Two systematic reviews have compared topical NSAIDs with placebo. The first systematic review (seven RCTs, 976 people with osteo-arthritis) [14] found that topical NSAIDs significantly reduced pain compared with placebo in weeks 1 and 2 (effect size 0.41, 95% CI 0.18–0.63) but not in weeks 3 and 4 (effect size +0.08, 95% CI −0.04 to +0.2. The second systematic review (three RCTs, 790 people with osteo-arthritis) [15] evaluated trials involving topical diclofenac. Compared with placebo, topical diclofenac significantly reduced pain scores with a standardized mean difference –0.33 (95% CI –0.48 to –0.18). The main adverse effect of topical treatment is local skin irritation; systemic adverse effects were no more common than with placebo.

Corticosteroid injections

Local steroids have been widely used for almost 50 years in arthritis. A number of formulations are available including hydrocortisone and methylpred-nisolone; most clinicians favor longer-acting steroids such as methylprednisolone.

One systematic review (28 RCTs, 1973 people with osteo-arthritis) compared intra-articular corticoster-oids with placebo and other treatments [16]. It found that intra-articular corticosteroids significantly reduced pain at 1 week compared with placebo; the weighted mean difference was –21.9 (95% CI –29.9 to –13.9). There was some evidence of benefit at 2 and 3 weeks but no evidence for a sustained effect beyond 4 weeks. Adverse effects are uncommon; symptom flare, tissue atrophy, fat necrosis, calcifica-tion and vascular necrosis have all been reported and there is a theoretical risk of infection but virtually no evidence that it is a relevant issue.

Hyaluronic acid injections

Hyaluronic acids are large glucosaminoglycans in synovial fluid. They have high but variable molecu-lar weight and viscosity. The reason why they may improve knee osteo-arthritis is uncertain and a number of mechanisms have been suggested, includ-ing providing lubrication and shock absorption. The usual source is avian and there may be some protein contamination that can cause allergic reactions. Some products are produced from bacterial sources and so avoid this potential problem. The degree of cross-linking of the hyaluronic acid is variable. Usually 3–5 weekly injections comprise a course of treatment. Recent research is aiming to reduce this to a single injection.

Two systematic reviews have compared various formulations of hyaluronic acid to placebo. The first systematic review (40 trials, 2542 people with osteo-arthritis) compared intra-articular hyaluronan and hyaluronan derivatives with placebo [17]. Hyaluronan significantly improved pain compared to placebo for up to 6 months post injection. The weighted mean dif-ference in the first 3 months after injection was –7.7 (95% CI –11.3 to –4.1). In the second 3 months after injection the weighted mean difference in pain was –9.0 (95% CI –14.8 to –3.2). The second systematic review (11 RCTs, 1443 people with osteo-arthritis) compared hyaluronan injection with placebo [18]. It showed that hyaluronic acid injections were moderately effective in relieving knee pain in patients with osteo-arthritis up to 10 weeks post injection, but not thereafter. Local skin reactions are reported with hyaluronic acid prepa-rations but there is no evidence of a significant increase compared to placebo treatment.

Interventions refuted by evidence

Antioxidant vitamin and selenium supplements

One systematic review evaluated antioxidants (nine trials, 567 patients) [19]. Seven trials examined vita-min E and other trials examined selenium ACE, vitamin A and vitamin C. The authors found no con-vincing evidence that selenium, vitamin A, vitamin C or the combination product selenium ACE was effec-tive in the treatment of osteo-arthritis.

Other alternative treatments

A detailed recent systematic review of alternative treatments in osteo-arthritis [20] found no evidence to support the use of homeopathy, magnet therapy, tai chi, leech therapy, music therapy, yoga, imagery and therapeutic touch. For these various treatments the evidence was weak and contradictory.

Commonly used interventions currently unproven

Glucosamine

Glucosamine is a sugar, a sulfated amino-monosac-charide. It is one constituent of the disaccharide units in cartilage proteoglycans. Experimentally it can alter chondrocyte metabolism, and this was part of the rationale underlying its clinical use, though whether or not oral glucosamine reaches chondrocytes in the joint is uncertain. Its classification as a drug, food supplement, nutriceutical or complementary therapy is debatable.

One systematic review of glucosamine (15 trials, 2613 people with osteo-arthritis) found that glucosamine hydrochloride was not effective, but there was some evidence supporting the use of glucosamine sulfate [21]. The pooled effect size of glucosamine hydrochloride on pain was 0.06 (95% CI −0.08 to +0.20) and the pooled effect size of glucosamine sulfate on pain was 0.44 (95% CI 0.18–0.70). However, there was considerable heterogeneity amongst trials and therefore the overall impact of glucosamine was uncertain.

Adverse reactions to glucosamine sulfate were evaluated in an earlier systematic review of 12 trials; only seven of 1486 patients receiving glucosamine sulfate were withdrawn for glucosamine-related toxicity and only 48 reported any glucosamine-related adverse reactions [22].

Chondroitin

Chondroitin is a glycosaminoglycan that is found in the proteoglycans of articular cartilage. It is an ingredient found commonly in dietary supplements used to treat osteo-arthritis. It is commonly combined with glucosamine. Most chondroitin is made from extracts of cartilaginous cow and pig tissues; other sources such as shark cartilage are also used. Since chondroitin is not a uniform substance, and is naturally present in a wide variety of forms, the composition of each supplement varies. Only a minority of chondroitin taken by mouth is absorbed.

One systematic review of chondroitin (20 trials, 3846 people with osteo-arthritis) found the symptomatic benefit of chondroitin is minimal or nonexistent [23]. The initial meta-analysis showed a large effect size on pain of −0.75 (95% CI −0.99 to −0.50). However, there was not only a substantial degree of heterogeneity between trials but the results also showed that the benefit of chondroitin was high in early trials and fell to nonexistent in larger, more recent trials. Overall, the authors dismissed its impact as being not clinically relevant. The overall risk of adverse events was small; the pooled relative risk was 0.99 (95% CI 0.76–1.31).

Herbal treatments

Hundreds of herbal remedies are used for osteo-arthritis, but very few have any evidence supporting their use. A review of systematic reviews in this area [24], using data from two systematic reviews [25, 26],

concluded there was some evidence to support the use of avocado/soybean unsaponifiables, topical capsaicin, and devil's claw. For example, an analysis of three trials involving capsaicin showed that the odds ratio favoring capsaicin affecting pain was 4.36. However, the numbers of trials and their size were insufficient to determine a definite benefit from any of these specific herbal treatments.

Comparison of treatments

The short-term effects of different treatments for osteo-arthritis have been compared in a single systematic review of placebo-controlled trials (63 trials, 14,060 people with osteo-arthritis) [27]. Opioids and oral NSAID therapy in patients with moderate to severe pain had maximum efficacies compared to placebo at 2–4 weeks with improvements in 100 mm visual analog pain scores of 10.5 mm (95% CI 7.4–13.7) and 10.2 mm (95% CI 8.8–11.2) respectively. There was some evidence that the efficacy of opioids was inflated by high withdrawal rates and "'best-case'" scenarios reported in intention-to treat analyses. By comparison, intra-articular steroid injections and topical NSAIDs had maximum efficacies at 1–3 weeks of 14.5 mm (95% CI 9.7–19.2) and 11.6 mm (95% CI 7.4–15.7), respectively. Paracetamol, glucosamine sulfate and chondroitin sulfate had maximum mean efficacies of 4.7 mm or less. These effects are summarized in Figure 9.1. The benefits of treatments other than NSAIDs, opioids and local steroids appear highly questionable in the short term.

Future research to improve management of pain in osteo-arthritis

Ideally we need new drugs that are more effective in controlling pain in osteo-arthritis. The problem with this goal is that very few such treatments have been introduced over the last 25 years, with the exception of new NSAIDs, including the COXIBs. There have been some improvements in how conventional drugs are delivered, particularly focusing on transdermal routes of administration which reduce adverse events. However, given the size of the problem, these advances have been disappointingly small.

One innovation that in the medium term may improve pain control is the imaging of pain using

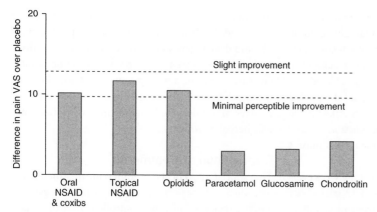

Figure 9.1 Changes in pain over 2–4 weeks in placebo-controlled trials in osteo-arthritis. VAS, visual analog scale. Reproduced from Bjordal *et al.* [27] with permission from Elsevier.

functional magnetic resonance imaging (fMRI). The approach has been applied to chronic pain because, unlike in acute pain, the central nervous system (CNS) is involved through pain centralization. The resulting neural activity causes changes in capillary blood flow which can be visualized by fMRI. Positron emission tomography and fMRI studies using experimental pain models in arthritis and other conditions have demonstrated the existence of the CNS pain matrix – the changes in CNS activity which accompany chronic pain. fMRI has helped to define the neurobiology of acupuncture and has been used to assess fibromyalgic pain, chronic back pain and response to NSAIDs in arthritis. Borsook & Becerra [28] believe fMRI may revolutionize the understanding of pain, help evaluate different pain states and develop new treatments. Although no research has yet been undertaken in osteo-arthritis, it is inevitable that fMRI will be a powerful instrument in assessing pain in these patients and for identifying and evaluating new treatment strategies.

The other key need is to integrate physical and drug treatments. Pain control in osteo-arthritis is not just a matter of better drugs. Improved fitness and regular exercise are equally if not more important. As well as prescribing drug treatment, clinicians ought to prescribe exercise regimens for patients as these appear equally effective.

Author recommendations

There is no single simple treatment for osteo-arthritis, and therapy needs to be individually tailored. Equally, the disease is variable and over time patients will need a range of different treatments.

I prefer to use simple analgesics and topical NSAIDs in mild disease, NSAIDs in patients in whom there is an inflammatory component, and injections of hyaluronic acid in patients in whom there has been little improvement with these simpler medical treatments. In terms of balancing benefits with risks of adverse events, my own perspective is that the advantages of therapy invariably outweigh its risks.

Many patients like to take self-prescribed glucosamine and chondroitin. My views are invariably neutral on whether this is sensible, though if asked I personally think they are very safe but regrettably ineffective. Not every expert has reached the same conclusion on the published evidence and I try to respect the views of other clinicians on this complex problem.

References

1. Dieppe PA, Lohmander LS. Pathogenesis and management of pain in osteoarthritis. *Lancet* 2005; **365**: 965–973.
2. Felson DT. An update on the pathogenesis and epidemiology of osteoarthritis. *Radiol Clin North Am* 2004; **42**: 1–9.
3. Altman R, Asch E, Bloch D, *et al.* Development of criteria for the classification and reporting of osteoarthritis. Classification of osteoarthritis of the knee. Diagnostic and Therapeutic Criteria Committee of the American Rheumatism Association. *Arthritis Rheum* 1986; **29**: 1039–1049.
4. Dillon CF, Rasch EK, Gu Q, Hirsch R. Prevalence of knee osteoarthritis in the United States: arthritis data from the Third National Health and Nutrition Examination Survey 1991–94. *J Rheumatol* 2006; **33**: 2271–2279.
5. Felson DT, Zhang Y, Hannan MT, *et al.* The incidence and natural history of knee osteoarthritis in the elderly. The Framingham Osteoarthritis Study. *Arthritis Rheum* 1995; **38**: 1500–1505.
6. Bellamy N, Buchanan WW, Goldsmith CH, Campbell J, Stitt LW. Validation study of WOMAC: a health status

instrument for measuring clinically important patient relevant outcomes to antirheumatic drug therapy in patients with osteoarthritis of the hip or knee. *J Rheumatol* 1988; **15**: 1833–1840.

7. Towheed T, Maxwell L, Judd M, Catton M, Hochberg MC, Wells GA. Acetaminophen for osteoarthritis. Cochrane Database of Systematic Reviews 2006, Issue 1. Art. No.: CD004257. DOI: 10.1002/14651858.CD004257.pub2.

8. Avouac J, Gossec L, Dougados M. Efficacy and safety of opioids for osteoarthritis: a meta-analysis of randomized controlled trials. Osteoarthritis Cartilage 2007; **15**(8): 957–965.

9. Cepeda MS, Camargo F, Zea C, Valencia L. Tramadol for osteoarthritis: a systematic review and metaanalysis. *J Rheumatol* 2007; **34**: 543–555.

10. Bjordal JM, Ljunggren AE, Klovning A, Slordal L. Non-steroidal anti-inflammatory drugs, including cyclo-oxygenase-2 inhibitors, in osteoarthritic knee pain: meta-analysis of randomised placebo controlled trials. *BMJ* 2004; **329**: 1317.

11. Scott DL, Berry H, Capell H, *et al*. The long-term effects of non-steroidal anti-inflammatory drugs in osteoarthritis of the knee: a randomized placebo-controlled trial. *Rheumatology (Oxford)* 2000; **39**: 1095–1101.

12. Moore RA, Derry S, Phillips CJ, McQuay HJ. Nonsteroidal anti-inflammatory drugs (NSAIDs), cyxlooxygenase-2 selective inhibitors (coxibs) and gastrointestinal harm: review of clinical trials and clinical practice. *BMC Musculoskelet Disord* 2006; **7**: 79.

13. Kearney PM, Baigent C, Godwin J, Halls H, Emberson JR, Patrono C. Do selective cyclo-oxygenase-2 inhibitors and traditional non-steroidal anti-inflammatory drugs increase the risk of atherothrombosis? Meta-analysis of randomised trials. *BMJ* 2006; **332**: 1302–1308.

14. Lin J, Zhang W, Jones A, Doherty M. Efficacy of topical non-steroidal anti-inflammatory drugs in the treatment of osteoarthritis: meta-analysis of randomised controlled trials. *BMJ* 2004; **329**: 324–326.

15. Towheed TE. Pennsaid therapy for osteoarthritis of the knee: a systematic review and metaanalysis of randomized controlled trials. *J Rheumatol* 2006; **33**: 567–573.

16. Bellamy N, Campbell J, Welch V, Gee TL, Bourne R, Wells GA. Intraarticular corticosteroid for treatment of osteoarthritis of the knee. Cochrane Database of Systematic Reviews 2006, Issue 2. Art. No.: CD005328. DOI: 10.1002/14651858.CD005328.pub2.

17. Bellamy N, Campbell J, Welch V, Gee TL, Bourne R, Wells GA. Viscosupplementation for the treatment of osteoarthritis of the knee. Cochrane Database of Systematic Reviews 2006, Issue 2. Art. No.: CD005321. DOI: 10.1002/14651858.CD005321.pub2.

18. Modawal A, Ferrer M, Choi HK, Castle JA. Hyaluronic acid injections relieve knee pain. *J Fam Pract* 2005; **54**: 758–767.

19. Canter PH, Wider B, Ernst E. The antioxidant vitamins A, C, E and selenium in the treatment of arthritis: a systematic review of randomized clinical trials. *Rheumatology (Oxford)* 2007; 46(8): 1223–1233.

20. Ernst E. Complementary or alternative therapies for osteoarthritis. *Nat Clin Pract Rheumatol* 2006; **2**: 74–80.

21. Vlad SC, Lavalley MP, McAlindon TE, Felson DT. Glucosamine for pain in osteoarthritis: why do trial results differ? *Arthritis Rheum* 2007; **56**: 2267–2277

22. Towheed TE, Anastassiades TP. Glucosamine therapy for osteoarthritis. *J Rheumatol* 1999; **26**: 2294–2297.

23. Reichenbach S, Sterchi R, Scherer M, *et al*. Meta-analysis: chondroitin for osteoarthritis of the knee or hip. *Ann Intern Med* 2007; **146**: 580–590.

24. Soeken KL. Selected CAM therapies for arthritis-related pain: the evidence from systematic reviews. *Clin J Pain* 2004; **20**: 13–18.

25. Little CV, Parsons T, Logan S. Herbal therapy for treating osteoarthritis. Cochrane Database of Systematic Reviews 2000, Issue 4. Art. No.: CD002947. DOI: 10.1002/14651858. CD002947.

26. Long L, Soeken KL, Ernst E. Herbal medicines for the treatment of osteoarthritis: a systematic review. *Rheumatology* 2001; **40**: 779–793.

27. Bjordal JM, Klovning A, Ljunggren AE, Slordal L.Short-term efficacy of pharmacotherapeutic interventions in osteoarthritic knee pain: a meta-analysis of randomised placebo-controlled trials. *Eur J Pain* 2007; **11**: 125–138.

28. Borsook D, Becerra LR. Breaking down the barriers: fMRI applications in pain, analgesia and analgesics. *Mol Pain* 2006; **2**: 30.

CHAPTER 10

Pain associated with rheumatoid arthritis

Paul Creamer[1] and Sarah Love-Jones[2]

[1]Southmead Hospital, Bristol, UK
[2]Frenchay Hospital, Bristol, UK

Background

Rheumatoid arthritis (RA) is a multisystem inflammatory disorder principally affecting the synovial linings of joints and tendons (Fig. 10.1).

Pain is the most common symptom of RA and is primarily located in and around affected joints. Early disease commonly affects metacarpophalangeal (MCP), metatarsophalangeal (MTP), wrist and proximal interphalangeal (PIP) joints, with knees, shoulders and hips also involved in many patients. Affected joints are painful, swollen, warm and tender. The other cardinal sign of inflammation, redness (erythema), is unusual in RA and should alert the doctor to the possibility of super-added infection. Other synovial joints can be affected, including, for example, temporomandibular (TMJ), giving jaw pain, or cricoarytenoid, giving throat pain and hoarse voice. Neck pain is common in RA and usually reflects facet joint inflammation: however, an important complication is atlantoaxial disease, which can result in subluxation and potentially cervical cord compression. In addition to joints, other structures lined by synovium, such as tendons and bursae, can also become inflamed and painful. It is important to consider the anatomic source of pain, since that directs treatment. "Wrist pain" may therefore be due to synovitis of the wrist joint itself or tenosynovitis of the extensor tendons; "elbow" pain may arise from the elbow joint or the olecranon bursa, and so on. Muscle pain and stiffness, similar to that seen in polymyalgia

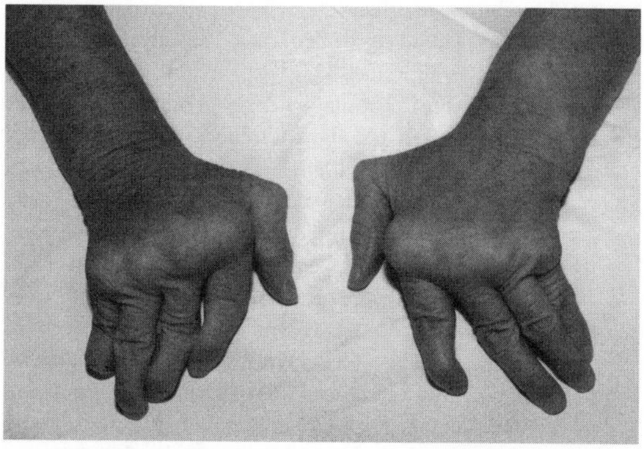

Figure 10.1 Rheumatoid hands, showing typical deformities associated with advanced disease.

rheumatica, can be a presenting symptom, especially in the elderly.

Other symptoms of RA include stiffness, especially morning stiffness. The duration of early morning stiffness is a good measure of the degree of inflammation or "disease activity." Systemic symptoms such as fatigue, fever, anemia and weight loss also occur, especially during inflammatory episodes. Extra-articular involvement may affect eyes, nervous system, heart, lungs and skin.

Rheumatoid arthritis is a phasic disease. Periods of inflammation (often described by the patient as "flares") are interspersed with quiescent phases in which the inflammatory response is reduced. Joints may still be painful at these times, due to damage that has already been done. Although RA rarely becomes completely "burnt out" or noninflammatory, as disease duration increases the cause of pain becomes predominantly mechanical or due to secondary osteo-arthritis. Assessment of pain in RA must attempt to determine

Evidence-Based Chronic Pain Management. Edited by C. Stannard, E. Kalso and J. Ballantyne. © 2010 Blackwell Publishing.

Table 10.1 Differentiation between inflammatory and noninflammatory pain in RA

	Inflammatory	Noninflammatory
Pain	++	++
Swelling	++ (soft tissue)	+/− (bony)
Stiffness	++ (early morning)	+/− (inactivity/gelling)
Extra-articular features	+++	−
Fatigue, malaise, weight loss	+++	−
ESR, CRP	Raised	Normal
Response to analgesia	+++	+++
Response to DMARDs	+++	−

CRP, C-reactive protein; DMARDs, disease-modifying antirheumatic drugs; ESR, erythrocyte sedimentation rate.

if the pain is inflammatory or noninflammatory, as the treatment for these will be different. Some clues to aid differentiation are listed in Table 10.1.

Pathophysiology

The primary site of change in RA is the synovium, which becomes swollen, hypertrophic and inflamed. Lymphocytes and plasma cells invade the tissue and excess synovial fluid production leads to joint swelling and effusion. Erosion of bone, due to local pressure from inflamed tissue or the effects of destructive cytokine release, occurs at the periarticular regions of the joint. These changes are first seen on X-ray at the MCP, MTP and PIP joints and around the ulna styloid at the wrist (Fig. 10.2). It is now clear that X-ray is a relatively insensitive way of detecting erosions and MRI or ultrasound can detect lesions at a preradiographic stage (potentially allowing earlier, more aggressive treatment). Untreated, continued bone and cartilage destruction leads to irreversible deformity and secondary osteo-arthritis.

Mechanisms of pain in RA

Primary articular nerves consist of unmyelinated (IV, C fibers 80%) and myelinated (III, Aδ and II Aβ, 20%) fibers. Aβ fibers end in corpuscles. Aδ and C fibers are free nerve endings; in the normal joint these are widely distributed throughout the synovium, capsule, ligaments and bone. The synovial membrane is not only richly innervated with C fibers but also with sympathetic nerves, whereas cartilage has no innervation at all. In RA there is a loss of C fibers from the synovium, possibly due to the rapid growth of

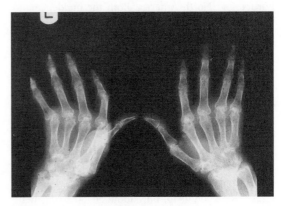

Figure 10.2 X-ray changes of RA.

synovial tissue outstripping the capacity of the nerve supply. This results in a drop-out in laminae I and II of the dorsal horn. Aβ (proprioceptive) fibers replace the pain fibers in these laminae so normal joint movement can be perceived as pain.

Inflammation, such as that seen in RA, has little effect on Aβ fibers but Aδ and C become sensitized with an increased response to movement or pressure. Previously "silent" fibers develop mechanically sensitive fields so that simply moving the joint results in stimulation of pain afferents. The mechanisms responsible for this sensitization are complex and involve many mediators such as bradykinin and prostaglandins; hence the effect is blocked by aspirin and other NSAIDs. Peripheral sensitization also results in spinal cord changes, leading to expanded receptive fields so that a spinal neurone responds to stimuli from a wider area. Opioid receptors are found in the synovium and their expression may be increased with inflammation of the joint.

Epidemiology

The epidemiology of RA pain closely reflects that of RA itself. RA is the most common inflammatory joint disease, with an annual incidence in males of between 0.15 and 0.46 per 1000 and in females between 0.24 and 0.88 per 1000 [1], different incidence rates reflecting the different methods used to detect disease. Although peak age presenting to secondary care is 30–50 years, community studies suggest that incidence increases with age until the seventh decade. In all except the oldest age groups, women are affected more than men. The overall prevalence of RA in the UK is about 1% [2], with similar levels found across Europe and North America. Both the incidence and severity of RA may be declining over time, particularly in females.

The cause of RA is unknown but, as for most diseases, represents an interaction between genetic and environmental causes. There is increased familial aggregation and greater concordance in monozygotic (12–15%) than dizygotic (4%) twins. The most clearly associated genetic link is with the major histocompatibility complex antigen HLA DR4, presence of which conveys a sixfold increase in risk of incidence of RA (and also increased disease severity). However, HLA-DR4 accounts for only about 30–50% of genetic susceptibility and other, as yet undetermined genes must be involved. The mechanism by which this gene acts as a susceptibility factor for autoimmune events remains unclear.

Environmental triggers for RA have not been clarified, despite extensive searches for infectious organisms. Many patients blame their RA on a stressful event; though this is unlikely to be causal, there is increasing evidence that stress may modify the immune system and be associated with exacerbations of RA. Hormones clearly play a role in RA. Before the menopause, there is an excess of females affected but this gender difference disappears after the menopause. Pregnancy usually results in amelioration of symptoms though a postpartum flare is often seen. Finally, the contraceptive pill may be weakly protective against RA.

Risk factors

The long-term joint consequences of RA (pain, disability and need for total joint replacement) are secondary to the development of permanent damage or erosions in the joints. This change is irreversible so treatment is directed not only at alleviating the patient's symptoms but also at reducing the chance of erosive progression. No single drug is capable of halting progression.

Of the 600,000 people in the UK with RA, 10,000–12,500 will have severe disease, which has failed to respond to current therapy. RA is not a benign disease, but carries significant morbidity and a standardized mortality ratio of over 1.5 [3]. Survival rates for patients with RA are comparable with Hodgkin's disease, diabetes mellitus, stroke and triple-vessel coronary artery disease [4]. Functional disability (reflecting disease activity) and low socio-economic status are major contributors to early mortality.

Even in the early stages of the disease, patients experience significant morbidity. One study of patients with a mean of 3 years' disease duration found that over half reported significant impact on three or more areas (work, income, daytime rest, leisure, mobility, housing and social support) while 42% were registered work disabled [5]. Radiographic damage (which predicts disability) occurs mostly in the first years of the disease [6]. Early effective treatment is therefore vital to control symptoms, prevent joint damage and improve function.

A number of risk factors have been identified which are associated with an unfavorable prognosis in terms of pain as well as function and joint destruction. These include:
- evidence of joint damage (erosions on plain X-ray) at baseline
- persistently raised inflammatory markers (CRP, ESR)
- functional disability at baseline (as measured, for example by Health Assessment Questionnaire)
- presence of extra-articular features such as nodules
- psychosocial problems
- rheumatoid factor seropositivity
- presence of susceptibility genes (HLA-DR4 0401, 0404 or 0405).

Rheumatoid arthritis is an expensive disease to treat [1, 4]. Using various models [7], it is estimated that the annual cost of treating RA in the UK is £0.8–£1.3 billion [1]; 50% of this is accounted for by hospitalization and long-term care, affecting only those with most severe disease. Five percent of patients (mostly those requiring total joint replacement) account for more than 25% of the total costs [7].

Although the primary aim in treating RA is first to reduce symptoms, especially pain, there is good evidence that early aggressive treatment can reduce long-term complications and is highly cost-effective in the long term.

Assessing pain in rheumatoid arthritis

Pain is almost universal in RA and is usually bilateral, symmetric and involves multiple joint sites.

Several techniques have been used to measure pain in RA, including numerical rating scales, verbal rating scales, visual analog scales (VAS), questionnaires and behavioral observation methods. The Arthritis Impact Measurement Scales (AIMS) pain questions are valid and sensitive to change [8]. A simple 100 mm horizontal VAS with anchors of "no pain" at 0 mm and "worst possible pain" at 100 mm is probably the simplest and most sensitive tool [9]. Other pain assessment scales include the Brief Pain Inventory [10] and the McGill Pain Questionnaire [11].

The overall pain experience in RA appears similar to that of osteo-arthritis (OA) [12,13]. The words used to describe the pain are similar in both – "aching," "sharp," "stabbing" – hence pain descriptors are not helpful in distinguishing OA from RA. In both conditions the affective component is more intense than the sensory component, indicating the importance of emotional factors in the pain experience. Overall pain intensity increases with disease duration. RA pain may differ from that of fibromyalgia in that fibromyalgia patients report a greater variety of pain descriptors and the pain is less clearly localized to joints, though the overall intensity is similar [14].

Management of rheumatoid arthritis pain

As in other conditions, effective therapy of pain in RA should combine optimum analgesia with enhanced function and minimal side effects. Decisions regarding pain control should take into account type of pain (inflammatory versus mechanical, central versus peripheral) and the patient's psychosocial situation.

Given that pain is the direct result of either the inflammatory process underlying RA or of joint damage consequent on that inflammation, management of RA pain is essentially the management of RA itself. The rest of this chapter, therefore, considers the management of RA with special reference to pain, but it should be appreciated that therapies that treat the disease will also relieve pain (for evidence base see Box 10.1).

The need for early referral

Early referral to a hospital specialist is desirable in all patients presenting with a persistent inflammatory polyarthritis. Although RA is the most likely diagnosis, there is a differential including viral, reactive, seronegative and crystal arthritis. Early accurate diagnosis enables the correct management to be instituted without delay. A vital part of early management is referral to other members of the multidisciplinary team for advice and education on joint protection, splinting, exercises and consideration of work- and family-related issues. For most patients, RA is a life-long diagnosis and care will be shared by

---

Box 10.1 Evidence base for pain-reducing interventions in RA

Interventions supported by evidence

Simple analgesia: paracetamol, codeine and other opiates, cannabinoids

NSAIDs

DMARDs

Steroids: oral, intra-articular

Biologic therapy

Education

Physiotherapy

Hydrotherapy

Orthotics

Fish oils

Surgery

Commonly used interventions currently unproven

Glucosamine

Hot and cold

Ultrasound

Hydrotherapy

the consultant, GP and members of the multidisciplinary team.

One of the major reasons for early referral is to ensure optimal pharmacologic treatment. The aims of treatment are to improve symptoms, reduce disease progression and prevent disability. Drug therapy consists of analgesics, nonsteroidal anti-inflammatory drugs (NSAIDs), disease-modifying antirheumatic drugs (DMARDs) and steroids. Early intra-articular aspiration and injection with corticosteroid are often extremely effective. Management paradigms for RA have changed considerably in the last 10 years with the knowledge that early use of disease-modifying therapy can reduce joint damage and, hence, long-term disability. Early diagnosis and prompt intervention with disease modifying drugs have become standard.

Economic evaluation of managing early arthritis suggests that costs are high in the first few months of disease, with approximately half the cost being associated with work absence. Aggressive treatment of disease in the early stages is therefore likely to be cost-effective.

To fully understand the clinical results to be presented, it may be helpful to describe how severity is defined in RA. The standard method of assessing disease activity and response to treatment is the American College of Rheumatology (ACR) response criteria [15]. The following variables are measured at baseline and at set intervals after commencement of therapy.
- Number of tender joints (of 28 assessed)
- Number of swollen joints (of 28 assessed)
- Health Assessment Questionnaire
- Patient assessment of disease activity (VAS)
- Patient assessment of pain (VAS)
- Physician global assessment (VAS)
- Erythrocyte sedimentation rate or C-reactive protein

If a 20% or greater reduction is seen in the number of tender joints, the number of swollen joints and at least three of the remaining five variables, the patient is said to have achieved an "ACR 20" response. An ACR 20 response is defined as the minimal acceptable response to be achieved for a patient to have responded to a drug and may mean that a patient becomes independent in an activity of daily living such as bathing, which can have a large impact on quality of life. An "ACR 50" response is a 50% or greater reduction. An ACR 50 response usually means

that a patient will have a larger improvement in functional status, for example will cease to be housebound or be able to return to work.

The Disease Activity Scale (DAS) is a similar weighted composite score of disease activity in RA, developed by a group of European rheumatologists

Modalities of pain relief

Pharmacologic
Analgesics
Although there is little controlled evidence regarding efficacy of analgesics in RA [16], it is widely believed that simple analgesics such as paracetamol are very helpful, providing quick pain relief with generally low risk of toxicity. Simple analgesics are often used in combination with NSAIDs and DMARDs.

Analgesic compounds with central opioid agonist activity, such as pentazocine and oxycodone, have been available clinically for a number of years for treatment of RA pain but they have not been utilized extensively due to their dysphoric side effects and concerns about dependence. Mild opioids such as codeine are frequently used to supplement other therapy in controlling pain despite a paucity of data from controlled studies, particularly on long-term use.

A retrospective study of 640 patients with chronic arthritis (including RA) found that 290/640 patients had used opiates (codeine or oxycodone) in the past 3 years [17]. Although this was an uncontrolled study, opioids significantly reduced pain severity scores, from 8.2 to 3.6 (on a 0–10 scale) (P < 0.001). Mild side effects were reported in 38%; nausea, dyspepsia, constipation, and sedation were the most common. The mean ±SD initial dosage was 2.1 ± 1.7 30 mg codeine equivalent/day. Dosage escalations occurred in 32 patients and were attributable to worsening of the underlying arthritis in all but four patients, who also displayed other abuse behaviors. The authors concluded that prolonged treatment of rheumatic disease pain with mild opiates reduces pain severity and is associated with only mild toxicity. Development of tolerance, requiring dose escalation, is rarely seen. This study and others suggest that concerns about opioid efficacy, toxicity, tolerance, and abuse or addiction should no longer be used to justify with-holding opioids from patients with well-defined rheumatic disease pain.

The use of opioid medication in RA patients enrolled in Tennessee's Medicaid program was analyzed [18] and found to increase from 38% to 55% (P < 0.001) in the study period of 1995–2004. This study also showed an increase in the use of DMARD and a decrease in the use of glucocorticoids in RA patients.

The consensus statement of an international expert panel focused on the six WHO step III opioids – buprenorphine, fentanyl, hydromorphone, methadone, morphine and oxycodone – most often used in the management of chronic severe pain in the elderly [19]. This population included those with RA. The panel concluded that opioids are efficacious in noncancer pain (treatment data mostly level Ib or IIb) but needed individual dose titration and consideration of their respective tolerability profiles.

A recent review of the evidence of efficacy of opioids for chronic pain is relevant for RA patients and concludes that there is strong evidence to support the initial effectiveness of opioids for the treatment of chronic pain, with much less clarity about the long-term effectiveness [20].

Opioid receptors are also present in periperhal tissue [21], where opiates may exert an anti-inflammatory effect. Compared with standard therapy of an intra-articular dexamethasone application, intra-articular morphine resulted in greater pain reduction and a significant reduction of the leukocyte count in the synovial fluid in patients with OA and RA [22]. This analgesic effect is due only in part to interaction with opioid receptors. The prolonged analgesic effect can also be explained by other mechanisms, such as opioid-mediated inhibition of inflammation. Expression of opiate receptors is increased with inflammation [23] and in experimental arthritis, administration of peripherally acting opioids shows antinociceptive activity. Other animal studies have confirmed that opiates are anti-inflammatory in a dose-dependent, time-dependent, stereoselective and antagonist reversible manner [24]. The potential for opiates to reduce inflammation in human RA has not been studied.

Two cannabinoid receptors (CB1 and CB2) are expressed on neurones and immune cells, particularly in inflammation. Receptor agonists such as anandamide are analgesic. In the only double-blind placebo-controlled study of its kind [25], a 5-week study of 58 patients with RA, a cannabis-based medicine was found to be well tolerated and to significantly reduce pain and disease activity (as measured by DAS). Further studies are required to define the role of cannabinoids in RA.

NSAIDs

There is good evidence that NSAIDs are effective at reducing pain in RA and are usually the first drugs prescribed following symptom onset, often prior to referral to a rheumatologist. Most patients will experience about a 50% reduction in pain following introduction of NSAIDs. One placebo-controlled study of etoricoxib and naproxen found that the percentage of patients who achieved an ACR 20 responder criteria response was 41% in the placebo group, 59% in the etoricoxib group, and 58% in the naproxen group [26].

Many NSAIDs are available. Although there is no evidence that one NSAIDs is consistently more effective than another at relieving RA pain, there is individual variation and it is worth switching NSAIDs in an attempt to find one that suits a particular patient. In general, a long-acting preparation is preferred, often given at night to maximize relief of early morning pain and stiffness. Selective COX-2 inhibitors (COXIBS) are more effective than placebo in RA [27,28] though they are no more effective than traditional NSAIDs [29, 30].

The efficacy of NSAIDs at relieving pain can present a diagnostic difficulty in that symptoms and signs of inflammation may be masked, leading to a delay in diagnosis and hence initiating disease-modifying therapy [30]. Sometimes, therefore, it is necessary to withdraw NSAIDs temporarily to fully assess the degree of disease-related inflammation.

Nonsteroidal anti-inflammatory drugs are associated with significant toxicity, notably on the gastrointestinal (GI) system. The addition of cytoprotective drugs such as misoprostil or proton pump inhibitors may allow patients with RA to continue to take NSAIDs, although it should be remembered that the correlation between GI symptoms and serious GI toxicity (perforation, ulcers, bleeds) is poor and addition of cytoprotection does not fully protect against serious complications. COXIBS are probably associated with lower GI risks in RA [18] though this effect may relatively small [31]. Other side effects which may limit use of NSAIDs include effects on the liver and renal system [32]. About 15% of patients with asthma experience worsening on starting an NSAID; patients should be warned about this and may have to discontinue the drug if they are adversely affected but asthma should not be regarded as an absolute contraindication to NSAIDs.

Recently it has become clear that while attention on toxicity has focused on GI problems, there is likely to be a small but detectable risk of increased heart attacks and strokes in people taking coxibs. This problem was particularly linked to rofecoxib and this drug has now been withdrawn. Several subsequent studies have considered whether other COX-2 drugs and also nonselective NSAIDs might carry a similar increased risk. Data are conflicting [33, 34] but it seems likely that a small increase in cardiac risk is seen with all NSAIDs [35] though there are theoretical reasons, backed up by some data, to suggest that this is greater with coxibs than with nonselective NSAIDs. Current guidelines suggest that all NSAIDs should be used with caution in patients with cardiac disease.

Corticosteroids

There is good evidence that corticosteroids can achieve rapid control of symptoms, including pain and maintenance of function [36], and are particularly useful during flares of disease activity. Oral doses from 7.5 mg to 20 mg daily prednisolone are often used, as are intravenous infusions of between 500 mg and 3 g methylprednisolone. Local injection of inflamed joints, using a long-acting steroid such as triamcinolone, is an excellent and safe way to relieve pain rapidly. Steroids can also be given as an intramuscular depot injection, for example methylprednisolone 120 mg (3 ml). This delivers the equivalent of about 4 mg prednisolone daily for about 6 weeks. Although the average daily dose is small, some patients find such injections more effective than oral prednisolone, possibly because the drug is released continuously rather than in the pulsatile fashion of oral therapy.

Evidence for a long-term disease-modifying effect of prednisolone is conflicting. Combination therapy studies in which high doses of steroids are used initially and then tailed off [37] show greater efficacy than monotherapy. Addition of a fixed dose of prednisolone 7.5 mg daily to standard DMARD results in a reduction in erosive progression [38]. Long-term steroid use is limited by toxicity, though in the short term, harmful effects on, for example, bone mineral density may be outweighed by an increase in strength following reduction in inflammatory mediators and an improvement in patient mobility [39].

Disease-modifying antirheumatic drugs

Disease-modifying antirheumatic drugs differ from NSAIDs in their ability to modify the natural history of the disease and affect disease-related parameters such as systemic markers of inflammation (ESR, CRP) and radiographic progression of erosions [40]. By reducing inflammation, they also reduce pain – hence the "management of RA pain" must include these drugs. The conventional pyramidal approach in which DMARDs are introduced gradually and only if NSAIDs fail to provide adequate symptomatic relief has been superseded by a more aggressive approach, with the early introduction of DMARDs, either singly or in combination, with or without steroids, in the hope of controlling synovitis in the early stages of the disease and preventing joint damage [41, 42]. The patient should be continually assessed clinically, serologically and radiologically to ensure that the chosen therapy is truly suppressing the disease; failure to do this should be an indication to modify DMARDs therapy.

An ideal DMARDs should reduce synovitis, limit joint damage and improve function with minimal toxicity and continued efficacy [43]. Unfortunately, none of the DMARDs currently available fulfill these criteria completely. The most frequently used DMARDs are shown in Table 10.2. Oral gold, penicillamine and cyclophosphamide are used less frequently.

All DMARDs share certain limitations, listed below.

Delayed action. Most DMARDs take 2–3 months to work and are rarely discontinued for lack of effect before 6 months. There is therefore an inevitable window in which inflammation and joint damage may progress unchecked. Further, the delay in response can lead to reduced compliance if the expectations of the patient are unrealistic.

Toxicity. Disease-modifying antirheumatic drugs are toxic. The major problems encountered are listed in Table 10.2. Some side effects resolve but others require cessation of treatment. On average 20–40% of patients

Table 10.2 Disease modifying antirheumatic drugs (DMARD) and their side effects

DMARD	Dose	Common side effects
Methotrexate	7.5 mg po or s/c weekly, increasing up to 25 mg	GI symptoms, teratogenicity, bone marrow suppression, pulmonary hypersensitivity, abnormal liver function tests
Sulfasalazine	1 g bd, increasing to max 1.5 g bd	GI symptoms, rash, headache, abnormal liver function tests, bone marrow suppression (commonest in first 6 months), reversible reduced sperm count
Gold	10 mg IM test dose, 50 mg IM weekly for 12–20 weeks then 50 mg monthly	Rash, pruritus, mouth ulcers, proteinuria, bone marrow suppression, vasomotor injection reactions
Hydroxychloroquine	200–400 mg/day; max 6 mg/kg/day	Rash, retinopathy (rare, much less common than with chloroquine)
Azathioprine	2.5 mg/kg/day	Bone marrow suppression, GI disturbances, flu-like symptoms, increased risk of lymphoproliferative disorders
Cyclosporine	2.5 mg/kg/day in divided 12 hrly doses, max 5 mg/kg/day	Hypertension, raised creatinine, hyperkalemia, hypertrichosis, gum hyperplasia, hepatotoxicity

will need to stop treatment due to toxicity within 2 years. When informed of the risks, many patients elect not to take these drugs, though compliance can be improved by good communication, education and support from other members of the team. It should be stressed, for example, that although there is an undeniable risk of toxicity with DMARDs therapy, it must be remembered that inadequate disease control also carries significant risks in terms of quality of life, disability and mortality.

The need for monthly blood tests can be a disincentive to start or continue treatment and is costly in time and money. The safety of various DMARDs during pregnancy and breastfeeding is an important issue as many patients will be of child-bearing age.

Unpredictable efficacy. Not only are currently available DMARDs relatively toxic but they are also of limited efficacy. Only 70% of patients will respond to a given DMARDs in terms of a noticeable improvement in pain, swelling and function and even this may be lost with time. Data on the ability of DMARDs to limit radiographic damage are also disappointing although this may be improved with earlier introduction of therapy. The results on long-term outcome are also a cause for concern, as levels of disability remain high despite the use of DMARDs therapy for over 20 years.

There is no way of predicting which patients will respond to which DMARDs. It is possible that subsets of patients exist who are more likely to respond to

certain drugs but since the mechanisms of action are poorly understood, it is not possible to target specific parts of the complex inflammatory process responsible for RA.

Current practice is largely with sequential monotherapy until a response is found. The choice of agent is based on familiarity, likely compliance, tolerability of side effects, co-morbidity and concurrent medication as well as consideration of which DMARDs have already been tried and failed. Sometimes changing the route of administration (e.g. subcutaneous injections of methotrexate) can improve efficacy. It is difficult to conclude that a DMARDs is ineffective unless it has been tried at the maximum tolerable dose and for at least 4–6 months.

Biologic therapy

Although early aggressive use of traditional DMARDs, alone or in combination, has proven efficacy in RA, a number of problems remain, as outlined above. The search for novel therapeutic targets has resulted in major breakthroughs in RA treatment.

Cytokines are protein or glycoprotein molecules that deliver important intercellular messages regulating chronic inflammation and tissue damage in RA. Cytokines such as tumor necrosis factor α (TNF-α), interleukin-1 (IL-1), interleukin-6 (IL-6), and granulocyte macrophage-colony stimulating factor (GM-CSF) are abundant in inflamed joints and promote the influx of inflammatory neutrophils and monocytes to the joints.

Tumor necrosis factor α appears to have a pivotal role in perpetuating inflammation and joint damage in RA [44]. Following evidence from animal arthritis models in which antibodies against TNF were shown to prevent or reduce symptoms when administered either before or after the onset of disease, drugs to specifically block the effects of TNF in humans were introduced for the treatment of RA in 1999. Three such drugs are now available: infliximab, etanercept and adalimumab. It is clear that such biologic therapies can produce a dramatic reduction in symptoms and can halt or even reverse the joint damage caused by RA. Anti-TNF-α agents have potent analgesic effect as well as their anti-inflammatory action.

About 40% patients treated with anti TNF-α achieve an ACR 50 at 1 year [45, 46]. Although the ACR 50 measures response to a range of outcomes, it is heavily influenced by pain and a reduction in ACR 50 is inevitably associated with a reduction in pain. For example, the ARMADA trial of adalimumab [47] reported a 55% ACR 50 response rate, with a 47% reduction in self-reported pain levels. Such benefits are sustained for several years. Anti-TNF-α therapy has also been shown capable of reducing erosive progression.

All anti-TNF-α drugs are given by injection: IV infusion every 8 weeks (infliximab), subcutaneous injection every 2 weeks (adalimumab) or twice weekly (etanercept). Although generally well tolerated, anti-TNF-α drugs care associated with side effects, commonly injection site reactions, mild flu-like illness or rash. The rate of infection is probably increased and serious infections such as septic arthritis or tuberculosis are well documented. Current practice includes advice to screen for tuberculosis before starting treatment. There is a theoretical risk of increased malignancy: currently it is unclear whether increased rates observed reflect drug toxicity or simply the greater disease severity of patients in whom these drugs are used. These drugs are expensive, costing about £10,000 per annum, but increasingly these costs will be offset by reduced need for hospital admissions and joint replacement surgery.

If a patient fails to respond to one anti-TNF-α drug, they may respond to another and it is worth switching medication. However, a number of other targets have been identified as contributing to the inflammatory process in RA and drugs have beendesigned specifically to neutralize their effect. A number of these are now available for use in RA.

Abatacept is a selective co-stimulation modulator, which reduces T cell activation [48]. Rituximab selectively depletes B cells from the circulation and is given by infusion every 9–18 months [49].

Cost efficacy of biologic therapies has been examined in detail, for example by the National Institute for Health and Clinical Excellence (NICE) in the UK. Accurate estimates are extremely difficult to obtain since cost savings may not be obtained for many years in the future. Simple assessment of incremental cost-effectiveness ratio gives about £66,000 per quality-adjusted life-year (QALY) for etanercept and £99,000 for infliximab. However, models which attempt to include future cost savings from reduced work loss, reduced need for hospitalization and joint replacement give figures of £16,300 and £29,000 per QALY respectively. It is also arguable that the pain reduction achieved by these drugs has an inherent value over and above that of reduced service utilization.

Tricyclic antidepressants

The tricyclic antidepressants such as amitriptyline are frequently used to treat chronic pain associated with osteo-arthritis and RA. A systematic review [50] of papers published between 1966 and 2007 on antidepressants in rheumatologic conditions looked at 78 clinical studies and 12 meta-analyses from 140 papers. The strongest evidence of an analgesic effect of antidepressants has been obtained in fibromyalgia. A weak analgesic effect is observed for chronic low back pain, with an efficacy level close to that of analgesics such as NSAIDs. Specific comment was difficult to make in relation to RA and ankylosing spondylitis as most trials identified in the review included patients with osteoarthritic conditions. The authors concluded that TCAs have weak analgesic effects in RA patients with or without depressive symptoms. For patients with ankylosing spondylitis, amitriptyline may modify a number of symptoms including pain, fatigue and sleep disorders.

Complementary therapies

Up to 60% patients with arthritis use some form of complementary therapy such as acupuncture, Alexander technique, aromatherapy, massage, homeopathy and reflexology. Many of these may provide relaxation and temporary symptom relief, including pain reduction. They may also improve the patient's general well-being and improve self-efficacy, but a robust evidence base for most of these interventions does not exist.

Many patients also take nutritional supplements (neutriceuticals). Omega-3 fatty acids, found in fish oils and some plant oils, are the first components of a physiologic cascade that results in inhibition of pain-producing mediators such as prostaglandin E2, LTB4 and TNF-α. Fish oils have a modest but clear effect on pain and swollen joints [51] and can reduce the need for NSAID. However, at least 3 g daily are required and many patients find such large doses impractical. Benefit may not be seen for up to 12 weeks.

γ-linolenic acid (GLA) is an omega-6 essential fatty acid found primarily in vegetable oils. Several studies have suggested benefit in RA though trial methodology is variable [52]. There is no evidence that glucosamine or chondroitin have an effect in RA.

Nonpharmacologic
Education
Education is important in providing knowledge to patients about their disease. Other components may include self-help principles, coping with stress and problem solving, nutrition, complementary therapy, physician/patient interaction, pacing skills and so on. Benefits may include: reduction in pain, improved self-efficacy, improved pain behavior, reduced medication and health resource utilization [53]. Education is generally considered to be cost effective, though the evidence base supporting this intervention is very limited. Timing of education is important and the content will differ according to the stage of disease.

Hammond & Freeman [54] found an educational-behavioral training joint protection program to be more effective than a standard arthritis education program: although pain improved in both groups, joint protection adherence, early morning stiffness, function and hand deformities were all better in the education-behavioral group. These benefits persisted 4 years after the intervention.

Physiotherapy and exercise
Three types of exercise may have a role in RA: range of movement (to help maintain or increase flexibility); strengthening exercise (to maintain muscle strength) and aerobic/endurance exercise (to improve cardiovascular function, reduce weight

and improve function). A number of studies have examined the effect of exercise on RA though many are limited by potential bias and limited patient selection. De Jong *et al.* [55] used a program of bi-weekly group exercises involving bicycle training at 70–90% predicted maximum heart rate, nine strengthening exercises and a sporting activity to deliver impact to joints and bones. This program improved function and disability, was safe for patients and did not increase disease activity though a specific effect on pain was difficult to measure. Other aerobic and strengthening programs [56] have confirmed these findings and also demonstrated improved muscle strength. The mechanism for any reduction in pain is unclear but may involve enhanced self-efficacy and modulation of central pain as well as direct effects on muscle and joint. Hydrotherapy is also of value [57]. Many patients use hot and cold treatments – hot water bottles or heated wheat bags for heat; ice packs or a bag of frozen peas for cold – and report pain relief, though firm evidence for benefit is lacking.

Transcutaneous electrical nerve stimulation
Transcutaneous electrical nerve stimulation (TENS) may be of benefit, especially when combined with acupuncture [58]. TENS is a form of electrotherapy and is thought to produce analgesia according to the gate control theory [59]. Conventional TENS (C-TENS) is given at high stimulation frequency with low intensity, whereas acupuncture-like TENS (AL-TENS) is given at low frequency and high intensity. A systematic review [58] included three RCTs, involving 78 people, in which C-TENS and AL-TENS were compared to placebo and each other. Administration of 15 minutes of AL-TENS a week, for 3 weeks, resulted in a significant decrease in rest pain (67% relative benefit, 45 points absolute benefit on 100 mm VAS), but not in grip pain, compared to placebo. AL-TENS did result in a clinical beneficial improvement in muscle power scores with a relative diference of 55%, and an absolute benefit of 0.98, compared to placebo. No significant difference was found between one 20-minute treatment duration of C-TENS versus AL-TENS, or C-TENS versus placebo on decrease in mean scores for rest pain or grip pain, or on the number of tender joints. Results showed a statistically significant reduction in joint tenderness, but no clinical benefit from C-TENS over

placebo in relief of joint tenderness. No statistically significant difference was shown between 15 days of treatment with C-TENS or AL-TENS in relief or joint pain, although there was a clinically important benefit of C-TENS over AL-TENS on patient assessment of change in disease (risk difference 21%, number needed to treat (NNT) 5).

Acupuncture

Acupuncture is used as an adjunct therapy for the treatment of RA pain. A Cochrane Database review [60] evaluated the effects of acupuncture and electroacupuncture on the objective and subjective measures of disease activity in patients with RA. Two comparative controlled studies involving 84 patients were included. One study used acupuncture while the other used electroacupuncture. In the acupuncture study, although not statistically significant, pain in the treatment group improved by four points on a 0–100 mm VAS versus no improvement in the placebo group. In the second, electroacupuncture study, a significant decrease in knee pain was reported in the experimental group, 24 hours post treatment, when compared to the placebo group (weighted mean difference (WMD) -2.0 with 95% CI -3.6 to -4.0). A significant decrease was found also at 4 months post treatment (WMD -0.2, 95% CI -0.36 to -0.04). Although the results show both acupuncture and electroacupuncture may be beneficial to reduce symptomatic knee pain in patients with RA, the reviewers concluded that the poor quality of the trial, including the small sample size, precluded its recommendation.

Occupational therapy

Occupational therapy interventions include advice on joint protection, energy conservation and problem-solving skills, instruction about assistive devices and provision of splints. There is good evidence that "instruction on joint protection" is beneficial and provision of splints (Fig. 10.3) has been shown to decrease pain [61]. As with education, the timing of intervention is important, positive changes being more likely if the patient perceives it as relevant to their needs at the time.

Orthotics

In addition to splints, other forms of orthoses can be very helpful in reducing pain. Simple provision

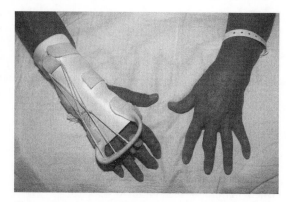

Figure 10.3 Splinting in RA.

of a walking stick can reduce knee pain when held in the contralateral hand by "unloading" the joint. Metatarsalgia (pain over the MTP joint in the forefoot) is a common problem in early RA. Provision of an insole with forefoot support can effectively reduce pain [62].

Surgery

The major indications for surgery in RA are pain and functional loss despite full medical treatment. In well-selected patients surgery is highly effective at relieving pain, even at the expense of some mobility. RA patients are probably at greater risk of complications than other arthritis patients, due to co-morbidity and drug effects. In general, surgery is of benefit to patients with advanced, established RA in which irreversible destructive change has occurred. Exceptions to this might include synovectomy or arthroscopic lavage for persistently inflamed joints but in general inflammation is better treated with drugs.

Synovectomy is a useful way of reducing a large mass of inflammatory tissue and is often combined with another procedure – for example, wrist synovectomy may be combined with excision of the radial head. Tenosynovectomy and tendon reconstruction can also be performed.

Joint fusion (arthrodesis) eliminates joint motion and hence pain though it does increase stress on adjacent joints: wrist, IP joint and talonavicular joints are all amenable to fusion.

Joint replacement (e.g. hip, knee) is highly effective at reducing pain in appropriately selected patients: at 3 years pain decreased by 29% in RA patients having total hip replacemement (compared with 56% in OA). For total knee replacement, a 19% fall in pain in RA was seen compared with 48% in OA [63].

Surgery in RA is often multiple and requires careful advance planning. Some practical rules include:

- stage surgery to avoid immobilization and preserve function
- replace lower limb joint before upper, as rehabilitation using crutches or sticks is much harder on replaced joints
- replace hips before knees as during total hip replacement the knee will be manipulated and stressed
- correct foot problems if possible before large joint replacement.

Future research into pain associated with rheumatoid arthritis

Pain is an almost inevitable consequence of RA: research into better ways of treating the disease will therefore improve outcomes in terms of pain. The introduction of biologic therapies has revolutionized our treatment: future research should continue to identify new components of the immune response that might be amenable to targeted therapy. This is already happening to some extent: B cells, IL-1, IL-6, IL-10, adhesion molecules and co-stimulatory molecules are all being investigated as potential targets for inhibition. New biologic drugs should maximize efficacy whilst minimizing toxicity, especially infection. Data on the long-term effects of these drugs should continue to be collected, for example using national registries such as the BSR Biologics Database. Cost is currently a limiting factor in use of biologics and novel (cheaper) ways of making such drugs would potentially allow extension of their use. Finally, identifying those patients likely to respond to a particular drug would be of great value in reducing the time and money lost by using expensive therapies that are subsequently found to be ineffective in that individual. Genetic study of response to drugs (pharmacogenomics) will offer the potential to, for example, identify whether one particular individual is more likely to respond to anti-TNF whilst another may respond to anti-B cell and a third to anti-IL-10.

Many patients describe flares of RA, with exacerbation of all symptoms including pain, after stressful events such as bereavement or divorce. The relationship between mood, stress and the immune response is another potential area of research. Early work suggests that abnormalities in the hypothalamic-pituitary-adrenal axis may provide a link between psychosocial stress and disease activity in RA.

Personal recommendations for management

Management of pain in RA requires a multidisciplinary team approach and early referral to secondary care is essential [64]. Confirmation of the diagnosis is by clinical assessment supported by simple investigations such as a measure of the acute phase response (CRP or plasma viscosity), measurement of rheumatoid factor (RF) and plain radiography of hands and feet. If there is diagnostic doubt (for example, if a positive RF is found but the patient is clinically atypical for RA, raising the possibility that the RF is false positive), measurement of anti-CCP antibodies and use of more sensitive methods to detect inflammation such as ultrasound of the small joints of the hand should be employed. NSAID should be started early, unless contraindicated. Confirmation of diagnosis should lead to aggressive therapy, with disease-modifying drugs being introduced if signs of inflammation persist 3 months after onset. My preferred drug is methotrexate, initially 7.5 mg weekly, increasing by 2.5 mg every month until disease control is achieved. Alternatives would be sulfasalazine 1 g bd. Prednisolone 7.5 mg daily with appropriate bone protection should be added for the first 2 years in all patients at high risk of progression and others in whom the inflammatory response is inadequately controlled.

Failure to respond to a DMARD (as measured by DAS) should trigger a switch to another DMARD. Failure of three or more DMARDs, alone or in combination, should result in anti-TNF therapy being initiated. Failure of one anti-TNF drug is followed by rituximab or a second anti-TNF drug.

On diagnosis, all patients should be assessed by a physiotherapist, occupational therapist and specialist nurse and the pain-controlling measures outlined above initiated. Surgical referral, ideally to a surgeon with a special interest in surgical management of RA, is undertaken as required.

Potential barriers to implementation of this algorithm include:

- delayed presentation by patients to primary care
- delayed recognition and referral from primary to secondary care
- centrally directed political constraints such as a move to place all rheumatology care in the community
- lack of provision of a multidisciplinary team
- lack of resources to monitor patients closely (essential if lack of response is to be picked up quickly and changes made)
- financial constraints on provision of drugs, especially biologic therapies
- lack of good patient-centered outcome measures.

Conclusion

Pain is the most important symptom of RA: about 50% patients describe themselves as being in "constant pain." Management of RA pain is best achieved by a multidisciplinary approach tailored to the individual and using a variety of drug and nondrug treatments. The introduction of TNF-α blockade has revolutionized the treatment of RA, though cost, nonresponse, increased risk of infection and possible increased risk of malignancy are likely to limit their use to those patients at risk of severe disease. Induction of remission with TNF-α blockade and maintenance with traditional DMARDs is a potentially attractive approach for the future as it may reduce the need for long-term biologic therapy.

Many other biologic therapies are now in development for use in RA (and other autoimmune diseases). With early diagnosis and effective treatment, a complete cure for RA may be a realistic goal within the next 10 years.

References

1. Scott DL, Shipley M, Dawson A, Edwards S, Symmons DP, Woolf AD. The clinical management of rheumatoid arthritis and osteoarthritis: strategies for improving clinical effectiveness. *Br J Rheumatol* 1998; **37**: 546–554.

2. Silman AJ. Epidemiology of rheumatoid arthritis. *APMIS* 1994; **102**: 721–728.

3. Pincus T, Callahan LF. Taking mortality in rheumatoid arthritis seriously – predictive markers, socioeconomic status and comorbidity. *J Rheumatol* 1986; **13**: 841–845.

4. Markenson JA. Worldwide trends in the socio-economic impact and long-term prognosis of rheumatoid arthritis. *Semin Arthritis Rheum* 1991; **110**: 4–12.

5. Albers JM, Kuper HH, van Riel PL, *et al.* Socio-economic consequences of rheumatoid arthritis in the first years of the disease. *Rheumatology* 1999; **38**: 423–430.

6. van der Heijde DMFM, van Leeuwen MA, van Riel PLCM, *et al.* Biannual radiographic assessments of hands and feet in a three year follow up of patients with early rheumatoid arthritis. *Arthritis Rheum* 1992; **35**: 26–34.

7. Gabriel SE, Crowson CS, Luthra HS, *et al.* Modelling the lifetime costs of rheumatoid arthritis. *J Rheumatol* 1999; **26**: 1269–1274.

8. Buchbinder R, Bombardier C, Yeung M, Tugwell P. Which outcome measures should be used in rheumatoid arthritis clinical trials? Clinical and quality-of-life measures, responsiveness to treatment in a randomized controlled trial. *Arthritis Rheum* 1995; **38**: 1568–1580.

9. Bellamy N, Campbell J, Syrotuik J. Comparative study of self-rating pain scales in rheumatoid arthritis patients. *Curr Med Res Opin* 1999; **15**: 121–127.

10. Cleeland CS, Ryan KM. Pain assessment: global use of the Brief Pain Inventory. *Ann Acad Med Singapore* 1994; **2**: 129–138.

11. Melzack R. The McGill Pain Questionnaire. *Pain* 1975: **3**: 277–299.

12. Charter RA, Alexis M, Nehemkis AM, *et al.* The nature of arthritis pain. *Br J Rheumatol* 1985; **24**: 53–60.

13. Helliwell PS. The semeiology of arthritis: discriminating between patients on the basis of their symptoms. *Ann Rheum Dis* 1995; **54**: 924–926.

14. Leavitt F, Katz RS, Golden HE, Glickman PB, Layfer LF. Comparison of pain properties in fibromyalgia patients and rheumatoid arthritis patients. *Arthritis Rheum* 1986; **29**: 775–781.

15. Felson DT, Anderson JJ, Boers M, *et al.* The American College of Rheumatology preliminary definition of improvement in rheumatoid arthritis. *Arthritis Rheum* 1995; **386**: 727–735.

16. Wienecke T, Gøtzsche PC. Paracetamol versus nonsteroidal anti-inflammatory drugs for rheumatoid arthritis. *Cochrane Database of Systematic Reviews* 2004, Issue 1. Art. No.: CD003789. DOI: 10.1002/14651858.CD003789.pub2.

17. Ytterberg SR, Mahowald ML, Woods SR. Codeine and oxycodone use in patients with chronic rheumatic disease pain. *Arthritis Rheum* 1998; **41**: 1603–1612.

18. Grijalva CG, Chung CP, Stein CM, Mitchel Jr EF, Griffin MR. Concise Report: changing patterns of medication use in patients with rheumatoid arthritis in a Medicaid population. *Rheumatology* 2008; **47**: 1061–1064.

19. Pergolizzi J, Boger RH, Budd K, *et al.* Opioids and the management of chronic severe pain in the elderly: Consensus

statement of an International expert panel with focus on the six clinically most often used WHO step III opioids (Buprenorphine, fentanyl, hydromorphone, methadone, morphine, oxycodone). *Pain Pract* 2008; **8**(4): 287–313.

20. Ballantyne JC, Shin NS. Efficacy of opioids for chronic pain: a review of the evidence. *Clin J Pain* 2008; **6**: 469–478.

21. Stein C. Peripheral mechanisms of opioid analgesia. *Anesth Analg* 1993; **76**: 182–191.

22. Stein A, Yassoouridis A, Szopko C, et al. Intraarticular morphine versus dexamethasone in chronic arthritis. *Pain* 1999; **3**: 525–532.

23. Kidd BL, Urban LA. Mechanisms of inflammatory pain. *Br J Anaesth* 2001; **87**: 3–11.

24. Walker JS. Anti-inflammatory effects of opioids. In: Machels H, Stein C (eds) Immune Mechanisms of Pain and Analgesia. Landes Bioscience, Austin, TX, 2002.

25. Blake DR, Robson P, Ho M, Jubb RW, McCabe CS. Preliminary assessment of the efficacy, tolerability and safety of a cannabis-based medicine (Sativex) in the treatment of pain caused by rheumatoid arthritis. *Rheumatology* 2006; **45**: 50–52.

26. Collantes E, Curtis SP, Lee KW. A multinational randomized, controlled, clinical trial of etoricoxib in the treatment of rheumatoid arthritis. *BMC Fam Pract* 2002; **3**: 10.

27. Matsumoto AK, Melian A, Mandel DR, et al. Etoricoxib RA Study Group. A randomized, controlled, clinical trial of etoricoxib in the treatment of RA. *J Rheumatol* 2002; **29**: 1623–1630.

28. Bensen W, Weaver A, Espinoza L, et al. Efficacy and safety of valdecoxib in treating the signs and symptoms of RA: a randomized, controlled comparison with placebo and naproxen. *Rheumatology* 2002; **41**: 1008–1016.

29. Emery P, Zeidler H, Kvien KT, et al. Celecoxib versus diclofenac in long-term management of rheumatoid arthritis: randomized double-blind comparison. *Lancet* 1999; **354**: 2106–2111.

30. Marzo-Ortega H, Green MJ, Karim Z, et al. NSAIDs alter the presentation of early inflammatory arthritis. *Rheumatology* 2000; **39**(suppl 1): 42.

31. Juni P, Rutjes AW, Dieppe PA. Are selective COX 2 inhibitors superior to traditional NSAIDs? *BMJ* 2002; **324**: 1287–1288.

32. Brater DC, Harris C, Redfern JS, Gertz BJ. Renal effects of COX-2-selective inhibitors. *Am J Nephrol* 2001; **21**: 1–15.

33. Solomon DH, Schneeweiss S, Glynn RJ et al. Relationship between selective cyclooxygenase-2 inhibitors and acute MI in older adults. *Circulation* 2004; **109**: 2068–2073.

34. Ray WA, Stein CM, Daugherty JR, et al. COX-2 selective NSAIDs and risk of serious CHD. *Lancet* 2002; **360**: 1071–1073.

35. Graham D, Campen D, Hui R, et al. Risk of acute MI and sudden cardiac death in patients treated with COX 2 selective and non-selective NSAIDs: nested case-control study. *Lancet* 2005; **365**: 475–481.

36. van Everdingen AA, Jacobs J, Siewertsz D, et al. Low-dose prednisone therapy for patients with early active RA: clinical efficacy, disease-modifying properties, and side effects. A randomized, double-blind, placebo-controlled clinical trial. *Ann Intern Med* 2002; **136**: 1–12.

37. Landewé RB, Boers M, Verhoeven A, et al. COBRA combination therapy in patients with early rheumatoid arthritis: long-term structural benefits of a brief intervention. *Arthritis Rheum* 2002; **46**: 347–356.

38. Kirwan JR. The effect of glucocorticoids on joint destruction in rheumatoid arthritis. The Arthritis and Rheumatism Council Low-Dose Glucocorticoid Study Group. *N Engl J Med* 1995; **333**: 142–146.

39. Haugeberg G, Strand A, Kvien T, Kirwan J. Reduced loss of hand bone density with prednisolone in early rheumatoid arthritis. *Arch Intern Med* 2005; **165**: 1293–1297.

40. van der Heijde DM, van Riel PL, Nuver-Zwart IH, Gribnam FW, van de Putte LB. Effects of hydroxychloroquine and sulphasalazine on progression of joint damage in rheumatoid arthritis. *Lancet* 1989; **i**: 1036–1038.

41. van der Heide A, Jacobs JW, Bijlsma JW, et al. The effectiveness of early treatment with "second line" anti-rheumatic drugs. A randomized, controlled trial. *Ann Intern Med* 1996; **124**: 699–707.

42. Boers M, Verhoeven AC, Markusse HM, et al. Randomised comparison of combined step down prednisolone, methotrexare and sulphasalazine with sulphasalazine alone in early rheumatoid arthritis. *Lancet* 1997; **350**: 309–318.

43. Edmonds JP, Scott DL, Furst DE, Brooks PM, Paulus HE. Anti-rheumatic drugs: a proposed new classification. *Arthritis Rheum* 1993; **36**: 336–339.

44. Feldmann M, Brennan FM, Chantry D, et al. Cytokine production in the rheumatoid joint: implications for treatment. *Ann Rheum Dis* 1990; **49**: 480.

45. Lipsky PE, van der Heijde DM, St Clair EW, et al. Infliximab and methotrexate in the treatment of rheumatoid arthritis. *N Engl J Med* 2000; **343**: 1594–1602.

46. Weinblatt ME, Kremer JM, Bankhurst AD, et al. A trial of etanercept, a recombinant tumour necrosis factor receptor:Fc fusion protein in patients with rheumatoid arthritis receiving methotrexate. *N Engl J Med* 1999; **340**: 253–259.

47. Weinblatt ME, Keystone EC, Furst DE, et al. Adalimumab, a fully human anti-tumor necrosis factor monoclonal antibody, for the treatment of rheumatoid arthritis in patients taking concomitant methotrexate: the ARMADA trial. *Arthritis Rheum* 2003; **48**: 35–45.

48. Genovese MC, Becker JC, Schif M, et al. Abatacept for rheumatoid arthritis refractory to tumor necrosis factor α inhibition. *N Engl J Med* 2005; **353**: 1114–1123.

49. Smolen JS, Keystone EC, Emery P, et al., the Working Group on the Rituximab Consensus. Consensus statement on the use of rituximab in patients with rheumatoid arthritis. *Ann Rheum Dis* 2007; **66**: 143–150.

50. Perrot S, Javier R-M, Marty M, LeJeunne C, Laroche F. Is there any evidence to support the use of anti-depressants in painful rheumatological conditions? Systematic review of pharmacological and clinical studies. *Rheumatology* 2008; **47**(8): 1117–1123.

51. Cleland LG, James MJ. Fish oil and rheumatoid arthritis: antiinflammatory and collateral health benefits. *J Rheumatol* 2000; **27**: 2305–2307.

52. Little CV, Parsons T. Herbal therapy for treating rheumatoid arthritis. Cochrane Database of Systematic Reviews 2000, Issue 4. Art. No.: CD002948. DOI: 10.1002/14651858. CD002948.

53. Riemsma RP, Kirwan JR, Taal E, Rasker HJJ. Patient education for adults with rheumatoid arthritis. Cochrane Database of Systematic Reviews 2003, Issue 2. Art. No.: CD003688. DOI: 10.1002/14651858.CD003688.

54. Hammond A, Freeman K The long-term outcomes from a randomized controlled trial of an educational–behavioural joint protection programme for people with rheumatoid arthritis. *Clin Rehabil* 2004; **18**: 520–528.

55. de Jong Z, Munneke M, Zwinderman AH, *et al.* Is a long-term high-intensity exercise program effective and safe in patients with rheumatoid arthritis? Results of a randomized controlled trial. *Arthritis Rheum* 2003; **48**: 2415–2424.

56. van den Ende FC, Breedveld FC, Le Cessie S, *et al.* Effect of intensive exercise on patients with active rheumatoid arthritis: a randomised clinical trial. *Ann Rheum Dis* 2000; **59**: 615–621.

57. Hall J, Skevington SM, Maddison PJ, Chapman K. A randomized and controlled trial of hydrotherapy in rheumatoid arthritis. *Arthritis Care Res* 1996; **9**: 206–215.

58. Brosseau L, Yonge KA, Welch V, *et al.* Transcutaneous electrical nerve stimulation (TENS) for the treatment of rheumatoid arthritis in the hand. Cochrane Database of Systematic Reviews 2003, Issue 2. Art. No.: CD004377. DOI: 10.1002/14651858.CD004377.

59. Melzack R, Wall PD. Pain mechanisms: a new theory. *Science* 1965; **150**: 971–979.

60. Casimiro L, Barnsley L, Brosseau L, Milne S, Welch V, Tugwell P, Wells GA. Acupuncture and electroacupuncture for the treatment of rheumatoid arthritis. Cochrane Database of Systematic Reviews 2005, Issue 4. Art. No.: CD003788. DOI: 10.1002/14651858.CD003788.pub2.

62. Steultjens EM, Dekker J, Bouter LM, *et al.* Occupational therapy for rheumatoid arthritis: a systematic review. *Arthritis Care Res* 2002; **47**: 672–685.

63. Woodburn J, Barker S, Helliwell PS. A randomized controlled trial of foot orthoses in rheumatoid arthritis. *J Rheumatol* 2002; **29**: 1377–1383.

64. Kirwan, JR, Currey H, Freeman M, Snow S, Young P. Overall long term impact of total hip and knee joint replacement surgery on patients with OA and Ra. *Br J Rheumatol* 1994; **33**: 357–360.

65. Luqmani R, Hennell S, Estrach C, *et al.* BSR and BHPR guideline for the management of rheumatoid arthritis (the first 2 years). *Rheumatology* 2006; **45**(9): 1167–1169.

CHAPTER 11

Fibromyalgia

Winfried Häuser[1], *Kati Thieme*[2], *Frank Petzke*[3] *and Claudia Sommer*[4]

[1]Klinikum Saarbrücken, Department of Internal Medicine, Saarbrücken, Germany
[2]Center for Neurosensory Disorders, Thurston Arthritis Research Center,
 University of North Carolina, Chapel Hill, NC, USA
[3]Uniklinik Köln, Department of Anesthesiology, and Postoperative Intensive Care Medicine, Köln, Germany
[4]Universität Würzburg, Department of Neurology, Würzburg, Germany

Background

Many randomized controlled trials have been conducted on the pharmacologic and nonpharmacologic treatment of fibromyalgia syndrome (FMS). A substantial number of systematic reviews have also been published, in which the evidence from these trials has been summarized. Recently, three evidence-based guidelines gave recommendations on the management of FMS. The recommendations of the American Pain Society [1] were based on a systematic search of the literature until April 2004. The European League Against Rheumatism EULAR [2] conducted a systematic search of the literature up to December 2005. The German Association of Pain Therapy, an umbrella organization of the medical and psychological societies involved in the treatment of patients with chronic pain, co-ordinated an interdisciplinary guideline with 10 scientific societies and two patient self-help organizations. The systematic search included literature published up to December 2006 and the recommendations were built following a structured consensus process [3]. This chapter on evidence-based medicine for FMS provides an overview of the current evidence on treatment of FMS and summarizes how this evidence has been translated into the US-American and German guideline recommendations.

Evidence-Based Chronic Pain Management. Edited by
C. Stannard, E. Kalso and J. Ballantyne. © 2010 Blackwell
Publishing.

Definition and classification

According to the criteria of the American College of Rheumatology (ACR), fibromyalgia syndrome is defined as chronic (>3 months) widespread pain (CWP) (including pain on both sides of the body, above and below the waist, and axial pain) and tenderness on manual palpation in at least 11 out of 18 defined tender points [4]. Chronic widespread pain and tender points do not capture the essence of all FMS-associated symptoms [5, 6]. Other key symptoms of FMS are fatigue and nonrestorative sleep. Most patients complain of additional somatic and psychological symptoms [7, 8].

The term "fibromyalgia syndrome" is preferable to "fibromyalgia" because the definition of FMS according to the ACR-criteria is based on a combination of symptoms (CWP) and clinical findings (tenderness). Because no consistent anatomic or specific pathophysiological mechanisms have yet been identified [9], FMS can be classified as a functional somatic syndrome [10, 11]. "Fibromyalgia" is listed in the *International Classification of Diseases* of the World Health Organization within Chapter M, "Diseases of the musculoskeletal system and connective tissue," with the code M 79.7 [12].

Fibromyalgia syndrome is not a distinct nosologic entity like a myocardial infarction following an occlusion within the coronary vasculature. Symptoms of FMS are more like other continuous medical variables such as blood pressure or coronary sclerosis for which clinically relevant limits have been defined to differentiate normal from borderline and pathological conditions. Within this context, FMS can be conceptualized as the extreme of a continuum of distress caused by pain, fatigue, sleeping problems, and cognitive disturbances [13–15]. Chronic pain in different sites of the body and fatigue are common symptoms in the general population as well as in several somatic diseases and mental disorders [16, 17]. CWP has been the focus of independent research and results have been included in this review. Tender points can be found in painful conditions other than FMS as well as in a small percentage of subjects without pain [18]. FMS, according to the ACR criteria, defines a distinct clinical syndrome at the end of a continuum of pain sites, fatigue and tender points[18, 19].

Prevalence

Prevalence in the general population

A review of 10 studies from different Western countries reported a prevalence of FMS according to the ACR criteria in the general adult population of between 0.7% and 3.3%. The prevalence in women was between 1.0% and 4.9%, in men between 0.0% and 1.6%. The sex ratio of women to men was 2–21:1 [20]. Most patients were between 40 and 60 years old but FMS can also be diagnosed in children and adolescents [21].

Prevalence in general practice

Only a few data on the prevalence of FMS in general practice are available. Within the UK General Practice Research Database, an increase of the incidence of FMS from less than 1 per 100,000 in 1990 to 35 per 100,000 in 2001 was found. The rising incidence rates most likely reflect trends in diagnostic labeling rather than true changes in incidence [22]. In a Dutch study using a postal questionnaire, 83% of the GPs reported one or more FMS patients in their practice. The estimated prevalence of FMS as recognized by GPs is low, with 157 patients per 100,000 [23]. The low prevalence in primary care can be explained by the fact that GPs are reluctant to use the tender point examination and the diagnostic category of "FMS" [24].

Prevalence in rheumatologic practices

In a cross-sectional study in a population of patients cared for by rheumatologic practices in public Spanish hospitals, the prevalence of fibromyalgia was 12% (2.2% in men and 15.5% in women) [25].

Prevalence in inpatients

In Israel, the prevalence of FMS in patients hospitalized on internal medicine wards was reported to be 15% [26]. We found no data on the prevalence of FMS in pain clinics. The percentage of inpatients with chronic widespread pain in German pain clinics was reported to be 25–30% [27] (Schiltenwolf, personal communication, 2008). The percentage of inpatients with the primary diagnosis of FMS in a German interdisciplinary secondary care pain clinic was 3.6% (Gockel, personal communication, 2008). The lack of data on FMS in German pain clinics can be explained by the skepticism of most pain therapists about the use of this diagnostic category. Most patients with FMS are coded as "somatoform pain disorder" (Schiltenwolf, personal communication, 2008). The fact that the diagnosis of a somatoform pain disorder and inpatient multidisciplinary treatment leads to higher remuneration than the diagnosis of FMS within the German diagnosis-related system might also explain the coding preferences of German pain therapists.

Course of fibromyalgia syndrome

A review of longitudinal studies on the natural course of FMS demonstrated that the symptoms of FMS persist in the long run. Some patients adapt to the symptoms and the associated restrictions and report a better long-term satisfaction with their health status [11].

Risk factors

A risk factor can be defined as a characteristic, condition or behavior that increases the possibility of a disease. The association between the condition and the disease should be demonstrated not only in clinical populations but also in population-based studies. Risk factors can be assumed to be etiologic factors, if they contribute to the cause of a disease. The causal role of a factor should be demonstrated by prospective studies in the general population. Moreover, pathophysiologic studies should demonstrate an impact of the factor on a pathophysiologic mechanism of the disease. Therefore prospective population-based studies on CWP and FMS have the highest significance for the assessment of risk factors of FMS. The current knowledge on risk factors of FMS is summarized in Table 11.1.

Table 11.1 Risk factors for occurrence and chronicity of chronic widespread pain and fibromyalgia syndrome in adults

	Occurrence	Chronicity
Biologic risk factors	Family aggregation Inflammatory rheumatoid disorder	Physical co-morbidity
Sociodemographic factors	Age Female sex Lower social class index	
Psychologic factors	Depressed mood Family aggregation Mental disorders Occupational psychologic stressors Somatization	Mental co-morbidity Negative life events Psychologic distress Somatization
Occupational factors	Occupational mechanical burdens	

Risk factors for occurrence

Biologic risk factors

Genetics

There is a high aggregation of FMS in families of FMS patients. The mode of inheritance is unknown but is most probably polygenic. There is evidence of polymorphisms of genes in the serotoninergic, dopaminergic, and catecholaminergic systems. These polymorphisms are not specific for FMS and are associated with other functional somatic disorders and depression [28]. An analysis of participants of the Swedish Twin Registry examining probandwise concordance rates and tetrachoric correlations suggested modest genetic influences for both women and men with CWP. Genetic and shared environmental influences explained approximately half of the total variance, with no indication of sex differences in either the type or magnitude of these influences [29].

Inflammatory rheumatoid disorder

An association between FMS and inflammatory rheumatologic disorders (rheumatoid arthritis, systemic lupus erythematosus, Sjögren's syndrome) has been reported in 1–50% of patients [9].

Psychologic risk factors

Mental disorders

Compared with controls, FMS patients show a significantly higher prevalence of depressive and anxiety disorders, reported in 20–80% and 13–63.8% of cases, respectively. This high variability may depend on the psychosocial characteristics of patients, since most of the studies were performed in tertiary care settings. Even referring to the lower percentages, the occurrence of mental disorders is significantly higher in FMS subjects compared to the general population [30]. Co-morbid post-traumatic stress disorders have been reported in 30–60% of FMS patients [9]. Moreover, elevated frequencies of mental disorders have been described in relatives of FMS patients [30, 31]. The FMS/mental disorder aggregation suggests a common pathophysiology, and alterations of neurotransmitter systems may constitute the shared underlying factors [30].

Depressed mood

A prospective Norwegian population-based study found that depressed mood predicted the manifestation of FMS in patients with only local pain on the initial assessment [32].

Functional somatic syndromes

The prevalence of other functional somatic syndromes such as chronic fatigue syndrome or irritable bowel symptoms has been reported as 30–80%, depending on the setting and the diagnostic methods used [33]. The frequent aggregation of functional somatic syndroms suggests a common pathophysiology [17].

Somatization

Two British population-based studies found that somatization predicted the manifestation of CWP [34, 35].

Somatization was a stronger predictor of the manifestation of CWP than work-related mechanical factors [34]. A population-based British study demonstrated that subjects were at substantially increased odds of developing CWP if they displayed features of somatization, healthcare-seeking behavior and poor sleep [36].

Childhood adversities

Numerous retrospective case–control studies have shown that traumatic experiences (maltreatment, sexual abuse, emotional neglect) during childhood are more frequently reported by FMS patients in clinical populations than by medically ill or healthy controls [31]. However, these studies are biased due to recall setting and response bias [37]. A British population-based case–control study found an association between CWP and hospital treatment in childhood, but not with sexual abuse or chronically ill parents [38]. A systematic review of prospective studies on sexal abuse in childhood and chronic pain syndromes in adulthood found no clear evidence for a causal relationship to FMS [37].

Negative life events in adulthood

Although retrospective studies in clinical samples suggest that the onset of FMS is frequently associated with various types of negative life events [31], prospective population-based studies failed to demonstrate an increased risk of FMS-like pain complaints following the World Trade Center terrorist attack [39].

Daily hassles

Workplace bullying, high workload and low decision latitude were associated with an increased incidence of diagnosed FMS within a Finnish prospective population-based study [40].

Sociodemographic factors

Sex

The mechanisms of gender differences in FMS are not fully understood. An interaction between biologic, psychological and sociocultural factors has been postulated [41]. Between puberty and menopause, adult women usually show lower responses of the hypothalamic-pituitary-adrenal axis (HPA) and autonomic responses than men of the same age [42]. Female gender is a risk factor for psychologic distress and some mental disorders (affective and anxiety disorder, PTSD) which are associated with FMS. Functional somatic syndromes

are more common in women than in men [33]. Women tend to report more physical and psychologic symptoms and exhibit a more intensive healthcare-seeking behavior than men [41].

Social class

Within the framework of a German population-based cross-sectional study, subjects with FMS had a 3.6-fold risk of having a lower social class level, when compared to people without chronic pain [43].

Physical and occupational factors

Physical injury

The German FMS guideline group found two prospective studies with conflicting results regarding the occurrence of FMS after a traffic injury with initial neck pain [9].

Occupational factors

A British population-based prospective survey found that pushing/pulling heavy weights, repetitive wrist movements, kneeling and local pain complaints at baseline were associated with new-onset chronic widespread pain. However, the strongest predictor was a high score on the Illness Behavior Scale [44]. Harkness et al. [45] demonstrated in a prospective British study that those who reported low job satisfaction, low social support, and monotonous work had an increased risk of new-onset widespread pain.

Risk factors for chronicity

Somatization

In a British prospective, population-based study, persistent chronic widespread pain was strongly associated with baseline test scores for high psychologic distress and fatigue. In addition, these subjects were more likely to display a pattern of illness behavior characterized by frequent visits to medical practitioners for symptoms disrupting daily activities [46].

Co-morbidities

An American prospective study with FMS patients from both tertiary care and community settings found that poorer health status and more co-morbidity at baseline were predictors of poorer health status 6 months later. After controlling for these co-variates, psychologic distress still contributed significantly to the model [47].

Negative life events

Norwegian FMS patients were followed for 4.5 years. Receiving a permanent disability pension or having experienced an excess of major negative life events predicted a negative outcome [48].

Protective factors

An Australian prospective study with FMS patients from community rheumatologic practices found that regular physical exercise, rather than medication or specific physical therapies, correlated highly with low FMS activity scores. Analysis of mood and coping strategies at the 2-year review showed low correlations with current FMS activity [49]. Norwegian FMS patients were followed for 4.5 years. An adequate physical activity level and increasing age predicted a positive outcome [48]. Another Norwegian study reassessed women with FMS who had participated in exercise and patient education programs after 6 and 8 years. Adjusting to the new situation and distraction from symptoms, as well as frequent participation in physical activities, were associated with a benign long-term outcome [50].

Pathophysiology

Several potential pathophysiologic mechanisms for FMS have been described, but their causal relationship are unclear because of the cross-sectional nature of all these studies. Potential mechanisms include central nervous system (CNS) pain-processing abnormalities, hyporeactivity of the HPA axis, increased systemic proinflammatory and reduced anti-inflammatory cytokine profiles, and disturbances in the dopaminergic and serotonergic systems [9]. Potential linked or underlying genetic mechanisms have been described above. Cross-sectional studies suggested that FMS may be related to hypofunctional stress systems, particularly in the autonomic nervous system (ANS) and the HPA axis. Studies have demonstrated that patients with FMS exhibit lowered sympathoadrenal reactivity to stress [51].

A prospective British population-based study assessed relationships between psychosocial and biologic variables relevant for CWP. Abnormalities of HPA function were more marked in people with established CWP than in those at risk of CWP. Some aspects of the altered function were related to psychosocial distress [52]. Another prospective population-based cohort study of the same study group revealed that dysfunction of the HPA axis (high levels of cortisol post dexamethasone, low levels in morning saliva and high levels in evening saliva) within a group of subjects free of CWP but at future risk based on their psychosocial profile helped to distinguish those who would and would not develop new-onset CWP [35]. Thus, dysfunction of the HPA axis can be triggered by psychosocial distress. On the other hand, coping with psychosocial distress can be impeded by a genetically based hyporeactivity of the HPA axis.

The biopsychosocial model of FMS postulates that there is a heterogeneity in the genetic and psychologic predispositions as well as in the vegetative, endocrine and central nervous system reactions. Different etiologic factors and pathophysiologic mechanisms lead to a common pathway of symptomatology currently classified as FMS [9].

Diagnosis

History taking

Patients presenting with chronic mono- or oligolocular pain should be asked for potential other pain locations. A pain diagram helps to identify patients with CWP. If CWP is diagnosed, other key symptoms of FMS (fatigue/nonrestorative sleep and increased morning stiffness/swelling of the fingers or the hands) should be actively explored. The German interdiscplinary guideline recommends the establishment of a symptom-based diagnosis of FMS if symptoms in all the following three symptom domains are reported by the patient: (1) CWP, (2) fatigue or non-restorative sleep or sleep disturbances, and (3) sensations of stiffness or swelling in the hands or the feet or the face [11].

If the key symptoms of FMS are reported, patients should be screened for symptoms of other functional somatic syndroms and mental disorders as well as current psychosocial stressors. Moreover, restrictions of daily activities and subjective illness attributions should be asked for. Finally all types of medication used by the patient should be assessed since arthralgia, myalgia and fatigue can also be side effects of medication. Misuse of medication should be actively explored [11].

Physical examination

There is an ongoing debate on the utility of the tender point examination in the clinic. The ACR criteria were primarily developed for the classification of FMS [4] to identify a group of patients with similar clinical features for future systematic studies. Their practicability and validity for clinical diagnosis have never been tested outside a rheumatologic setting. Nevertheless, a history of CWP > 3 months and the finding of tenderness in at least 11 of 18 tender points with manual palpation using approximately 4 kg of pressure have become the gold standard of FMS diagnosis in clinical studies. Their use was recently recommended by an editorial in the *Journal of Rheumatology* [18] but the diagnostic use of tender point examination in clinical practice has been criticized by various authors, for the following reasons [53, 54].

- Fibromyalgia syndrome is the only functional somatic syndrome (FSS), which is defined and diagnosed by symptoms and a clinical sign. FSS in other medical disciplines such as irritable bowel syndrome, chronic tension headache, and nonspecific low back pain are "symptoms-only diagnoses."
- The tender point count has been shown to be influenced by the interaction between patient and examiner [55]. Despite efforts to standardize the procedure, such as the manual tender point survey [56], it has not been shown to be reproducible across different clinical settings. It is a poor marker of change in clinical studies and controversial in legal situations.
- There is general agreement that tender points are a marker of psychophysiologic distress [18] and not an objective measure of tenderness [57]. Therefore the limited time of medical consultation should be used to explore psychosocial distress rather than to press on tender points. Most nonrheumatologists are reluctant to use the tender point examination because of the time involved [24].
- A complete physical examination including orthopedic and neurologic examination is recommended to reveal signs of internal or neurologic disorders mimicking the key symptoms of FMS [11].

Questionnaires

Wolfe [58] developed survey criteria for FMS. Here, FMS is simply diagnosed by a questionnaire, the regional pain scale. FMS is diagnosed if the patient indicates pain in at least 11 of 19 pain sites and reports a fatigue score 6 on a 11-point visual analog scale (VAS). The use of standardized somatic symptom scales and questionnaires such as the Patient Health Questionnaire PHQ [59] can be considered in primary care. Restrictions of daily life associated with FMS symptoms can be assessed by the Brief Pain Inventory [60] or the Fibromyalgia Impact Questionnaire [61].

Blood tests and diagnostic imaging

The following routine blood tests are recommended by the German interdisciplinary FMS guideline for patients with CWP (potential differential diagnosis are indicated in parentheses):

- blood sedimentation rate, C-reactive protein, red and white cell blood count (polymyalgia rheumatica, rheumatoid arthritis)
- creatinine kinase (muscle disease)
- calcium (hypercalcemia)
- thyroid-stimulating hormone (hypothyreosis)
- depending on history and examination, further blood tests can be necessary if other differential diagnoses are suspected.

Without cinical signs, routine testing for antibodies associated with inflammatory rheumatologic diseases is not recommended. A Canadian study in outpatient secondary care found no predictive value of the assessment of antibodies associated with inflammatory rheumatologic diseases in patients with a history of CWP and fatigue in the absence of other features such as joint swelling, typical rashes or organ involvement [62]. If no other diseases which require imaging studies for diagnosis are suspected on clinical grounds, X-rays or other diagnostic imaging studies are not recommended. A Norwegian longitudinal study in primary care demonstrated a low diagnostic value of imaging studies in patients with CWP [63].

Referral to specialists

In a case of suspected medical, neurologic or psychiatric disease or the presence of dysfunctional coping styles, referral to a specialist is recommended [24].

Treatment

Problems of evidence-based medicine

The majority of the numerous therapies used in FMS have been systematically reviewed recently, including aerobic exercise [64, 65], complementary and alternative therapy [66], multicomponent therapy [67], patient education [24], physical therapy and physiotherapy [65], pharmacologic therapy [68], and psychotherapy [69]. The reviews demonstrate that there is no therapy that works in every patient. If defined in the study results, responders and non-responders can be found with similar rates in pharmacologci and nonpharmacologic therapies. Overall evidence is limited to middle-aged women with FMS without co-morbidity. The German FMS guideline group found only one RCT in children and adolescents, which demonstrated a superiority of cognitive behavioral therapy over self-monitoring at the end of therapy [70]. Most studies excluded patients with relevant physical and mental co-morbidities [71]. Men were either excluded or no separate analysis for men was performed.

The question of how to manage a life-long disorder remains unanswered by all controlled studies. There is evidence for the short-term effectiveness of some pharmacologic and nonpharmacologic therapies. Most studies lasted between 4 and 12 weeks and assessed the outcomes at the end of the treatment period. There currently is no evidence of a long-term effectiveness (>6 months) of pharmacologic and physical therapies. There is only limited evidence for the long-term effectiveness of aerobic exercise [65], multicomponent therapy [67] and cognitive behavioral therapy (CBT) [69], based on follow-up periods ranging from 6 to 24 months. There is limited evidence of the cost-effectiveness of operant pain therapy and spa therapy [72, 73].

General principles of management of FMS

Self-management

Currently, FMS cannot be cured by any therapy and overall treatment effects are modest at best. According to expert opinion, the aims of therapy are the preservation or improvement of daily functioning and coping with symptoms and disabilities. Coping with symptoms includes both the acceptance of symptoms and of some limitations (e.g. hard physical work) as well as continous self-management (physical activity, stress management) to reduce the impact of the symptoms. Therefore the patient has the major task in FMS therapy[1, 24].

Collaboration

Various healthcare providers may be involved in the treatment of FMS. Although there may be some variations between countries, exercise therapists, general practitioners, neurologists, orthopedic surgeons, pain therapists, psychiatrists, physiotherapists, psychologists, rheumatologists and others may all be involved. The primary care physician has a central role in the co-ordination of the management. It is important that information and treatment are consistent across professions and specialties, and that healthcare providers closely collaborate with each other, with patients and their self-help organizations [24].

Systematic reviews of the effectiveness of treatments for FMS

Interventions strongly supported by evidence

Evidence on the most frequently used treatments of FMS is summarized in Box 11.1. Of the pharmacologic treatments, only duloxetine, milnacipran and pregabalin had been approved for use in FMS in the USA, but not by the EMEA for use in FMS in Europe.

Antidepressants

The German FMS guideline group systematically reviewed 26 RCT on antidepressants. Amitriptyline, studied in 13 RCT, was efficient in reducing pain with a moderate magnitude of benefit (pain reduction by a mean of 26%, improvement in quality of life by 30%). Selective serotonin reuptake inhibitors (SSRI) were studied in 12 RCT, which also gave positive results, except for the two studies on citalopram and one on fluoxetine. Three RCT on the dual serotonin and noradrenaline reuptake inhibitors (SNRI) duloxetine and milnacipran reported positive results at the end of therapy. Results concerning the effectiveness of the monoamine oxidase inhibitor (MAOI) moclobemide (300–600 mg/day) were conflicting [71]. Eighteen RCT (median duration 8 weeks, range 4–38 weeks) involving 1427 subjects were suitable for meta-analysis. There was strong evidence for an association of antidepressants with reduction in pain (standard mean difference (SMD) –0.43, 95% confidence interval (CI) –0.55 to –0.30), fatigue (SMD –0.13, 95% CI –0.26 to –0.01), depressed mood (SMD –0.26, 95% CI –0.3 to –0.12) and sleep disturbances (SMD –0.32, 95% CI –0.46 to –0.18). There was strong evidence

Box 11.1 Evidence of treatments for adult fibromyalgia syndrome

Interventions strongly supported by evidence (systematic reviews)
Aerobic exercise
Amitriptyline
Balneo- and spa therapy
Cognitive behavioral therapy
Cyclobenzaprine
Duloxetine
Fluoxetine
Pregabalin
Multicomponent treatment programs

Interventions supported by evidence (at least two RCT with consistent results)
Homeopathy
Hypnotherapy/guided imagery
Mindfulness meditation
Patient-centered communication
Tramadol
Tropisetron
Vegetarian diet
Whole-body heat therapy
Written emotional disclosure

Commonly used interventions currently unproven (only one RCT with low quality, RCTs with conflicting results or no RCT available)
Acetaminophen
Acupuncture
Body awareness therapy
Lidocaine infusions
Lymph drainage
Massage
Metamizol
Muscle relaxants other than cyclobenzaprine
Osteopathy
Qi-gong
Physiotherapy
Psychodynamic therapy
Tender point injections
Tramadol/acetaminophen

Interventions strongly refuted by evidence (systematic reviews)
Anxiolytics
Biofeedback as single intervention
Citalopram
Corticosteroids
Neuroleptics
Nonsteroidal agents
Patient education as single intervention
Relaxation therapy as single intervention

for an association of antidepressants with improved health-related quality of life (HRQOL) (SMD –0.31, 95% CI –0.42 to –0.20). Effect sizes for pain reduction were large for tricyclic antidepressants (TCA) (SMD –1.64, 95% CI –2.57 to –0.71), medium for MAOI (SMD –0.54, 95% CI –1.02 to –0.07) and small for SSRIs (SMD –0.39, 95% CI –0.77 to –0.01) and SNRIs (SMD –0.36, 95% CI –0.46 to –0.25)[74].

Balneo- and spa therapy

McVeigh et al. [75] systematically reviewed 10 RCT with balneo- or spa therapy or pooled-based exercises. Improvements were demonstrated in pain, health status, anxiety, fatigue, in addition to function and aerobic capacity. However, for the most part, improvements tended to be shor-lived.

Cyclobenzaprine

Tofferi et al. [76] included five RCT with cyclobenzaprine, a muscle relaxant with additional profile of a TCA, in their meta-analysis. The odds ratio (OR) for a global improvement was 3.0 (95% CI 1.6–5.6). Cyclobenzaprine is not licensed in most European countries.

Cognitive behavioral therapy (CBT)

The German FMS guideline group reviewed 14 RCT on CBT. Most studies lasted between 6 and 15 weeks, and most therapies comprised 6–30 hours of intervention. Twelve of the 14 studies found a superiority of CBT in most outcomes at the end of the therapy. Nine of the 14 studies performed follow-ups and 5/9 studies reported a persistant reduction of FMS symptoms after 6–24 months [69]. Twenty-two out of 33 relevant studies investigating 1209 subjects could be meta-analyzed. CBT had large effects on pain, self-efficacy and disability only at follow-up. Hypnotherapy has a large effect on the improvement of self-efficacy pain and a medium effect on the improvement of pain post treatment and at follow-up [77].

Exercise

Busch and co-workers [64] systematically reviewed 34 studies. Meta-analysis of six studies provided moderate-quality evidence that aerobic-only exercise training at American College of Sports Medicine-recommended intensity levels has positive effects on global well-being (SMD 0.49, 95% CI 0.23−0.75) and physical function (SMD 0.66, 95% CI 0.41−0.92) and possibly on pain (SMD 0.65, 95% CI −0.09 to 1.39). Strength and flexibility remain underevaluated; however, strength training may have a positive effect on FMS symptoms.

Multicomponent treatment (MT) programs

There is no internationally accepted definition of multicomponent therapy. The existing systematic reviews on MT agree that MT should include at least one educational or other psychologic therapy and at least one exercise therapy [67, 78]. The German FMS guideline group meta-analyzed 9/14 RCT, with 1119 subjects with a median treatment time of 24 hours included in the meta-analysis. There is strong evidence that MT reduces pain (SMD −0.37, 95% CI −0.62 to −0.13), fatigue (WMD −0.85, 95% CI −1.50 to −0.20), depressive symptoms (SMD −0.67, 95% CI −1.08 to −0.26) and limitations of HRQOL (SMD −0.59, 95% CI −0.90 to −0.27) and improves self-efficacy pain (SMD 0.54, 95% CI 0.26−0.82) and physical fitness (SMD 0.30, 95% CI 0.02−0.57) post treatment. There is no evidence of the efficacy of MT on pain, fatigue, sleep disturbances, depressive symptoms, HRQOL and self-efficacy pain in the long term. There is strong evidence that the positive effects on physical fitness (SMD 0.30, 95% CI 0.09–0.51) can be maintained in the long term (median follow-up 7 months) [79].

Pregabalin

In a meta-analysis of four RCTs with PGB and one RCT with gabapentin with a parallel design there was a strong evidence for the reduction of pain (SMD −0.28, 95% CI −0.36 to −0.20; P < 0.001), improved sleep (SMD −0.39, 95% CI −0.48 to −0.39; P < 0.001), and improved health-related quality of life (HRQOL) (SMD –0.30, 95% CI −0.46 to −0.15; P < 0.001), but not for depressed mood (SMD −0.12, 95% CI –0.30 to 0.06; P = 0.18). There was strong evidence for a not substantial reduction of fatigue (SMD = −0.16, 95% CI −0.23 to −0.09, P < 0.001) and of anxiety (SMD = −0.18, 95% CI −0.27 to −0.10). The external validity was limited because patients with severe somatic and mental disorders were excluded [80].

Interventions supported by evidence

Some further interventions supported by evidence (at least two RCT with consistent results or majority of RCT with consistent results) are listed in Box 11.1. In a systematic search of the literature up to December 2006, the German FMS guideline group found six RCT on balneo- and spa therapy, two studies on home-opathy, five studies on hypnotherapy/guided imagery, three studies on patient-centered communication, two RCT on vegetarian diet, three RCT on whole-body heat therapy, two on written emotional disclosure, three on tropisetron, and three on tramadol (one in combination with acetaminophen), fulfilling the criteria defined above [24, 65, 66, 68, 69]. Since December 2006 further RCT on pharmacologic, psychotherapeutic and physical treatment have been published which support the efficacy of the interventions mentioned above.

Regarding further treatment options, we wish to highlight two RCT with consistent results on mindfulness meditation [81, 82].

Interventions not supported by evidence

It is important to note that evidence is lacking for the effectiveness of frequently used pharmacologic treatments of FMS [7, 11], such as acetaminophen, metamizol, opioids other than tramadol or muscle relaxants other than cyclobenzaprine, as well as for frequently used nonpharmacologic therapies such as massage, osteopathy or lymph drainage.

The German FMS guideline group found inconsistent results in eight RCT on patient education as single intervention and seven studies with massage with conflicting results [24, 65]. Furthermore, inconsistent results of five controlled trials each on biofeedback and relaxation therapy (including autogenic training and progressive muscle relaxation) were found [69].

Interventions strongly refuted by evidence

There is evidence for the noneffectiveness of the most frequently used drug class in FMS, nonsteroidal agents. Furthermore, a systematic review found RCT with negative results for anxiolytics, corticosteroids and neuroleptics [68].

Mayhew & Ernst [83] systematically reviewed five RCT on acupuncture (traditional Chinese acupuncture and electroacupuncture) and concluded because of conflicting results that acupuncture is not effective in FMS therapy.

A stepwise treatment approach to FMS

A graded treatment approach to functional somatic syndromes is recommended [10]. The American Pain Society (APS) [1] and the German Interdisciplinary Guideline Group [24] both recommend a stepwise treatment approach.

Treatment should begin with confirming the diagnosis and patient education. Self-management and patient-centered communication are regarded as key principles of FMS therapy. Both guidelines recommended first, second and third lines of therapy depending on the course of symptoms, the existence of relevant restrictions of daily activities and the response to different treatment modalities. The APS recommended individualized exercise and CBT as first-line therapy. The German guideline recommended aerobic exercise, CBT, amitriptyline and treatment of physical and mental co-morbidities as single interventions or combined as first-line therapies.

In cases of persisting symptoms after first-line treatment, the APS recommended tender point injections, local manual therapies and acupuncture for focal pain, tramadol, SNRI, anticonvulsants for generalized pain, and psychiatric treatment in cases of major mood disorder as second-line therapy. The German guideline recommended multicomponent therapy in cases of persisting restrictions of daily activities as second-line therapy.

Multidisciplinary pain management, psychopharmacology, opioids, experimental therapies and combinations is the third-line therapy recommended by the APS in cases of persisting symptoms. In cases lacking adaptation to symptoms or persistent restrictions of daily functioning, the German guideline recommended either no therapy or self-management (aerobic exercise, stress management, pool-based exercise), or booster multicomponent therapy, or psychotherapy (hypnotherapy, written emotional disclosure), or pharmacologic therapy (duloxetine or fluoxetine or paroxetin or pregabalin, or tramadol with or without acetaminophen), or complementary/alternative therapies (homeopathy, vegetarian diet) as third-line therapy. The choice of treatment options should be based on informed patient consent, the patient's preferences and co-morbidities, and the treatment options locally available [24].

Guidelines and implementation

The development and dissemination of guidelines do not automatically mean that patients and healthcare providers will read, understand and use these guidelines. The following strategies were designed to dissiminate and implement the German guideline.

The results of the systematic reviews and recommendations of the guideline are published in scientific journals and presented at the annual scientific meetings of the societies involved. The scientific version of the guideline (complete and short version) is available on the homepages of the societies involved. The German Society of General and Family Medicine will develop and validate a pocket version of the guideline for primary care physicians. A patient version of the guideline is available on the homepages of the medical scientific societies as well as of the self-help organizations involved and published in the respective journals of the self-help organizations involved. The recommendations were presented and discussed at regional patient–doctor meetings. Thus the strategies aim at modifying not only the practice of healthcare providers but also the knowledge and demands of patients. Patients are accessed by self-help organizations, by regional meetings, the internet and patients' journals. The evaluation of the implementation strategies outlined will be a major challenge for the future.

Producing evidence of effectiveness in the future

Promising strategies include the identification of predictors of a positive treatment outcome [84] and of relevant subgroups that may benefit from more specific intervention tailored to coping strategies and co-morbidity of mental disorders [69, 85]. Furthermore, there is a need to develop strategies to motivate patients for continuous self-management, such as maintaining the benefits of aerobic exercise, CBT, and MT after the end of treatment.

Authors' recommendations

Researchers should take into consideration that causal relationships between FMS, stress/depression, central augmentation of pain processing, and hyporeactivity of the HPA axis might not be linear but recursive. Future research should leave simple linear etiopatho-genetic models and prospectively study the interactions between biologic and psychosocial variables and their underlying genetic factors.

The main therapeutic challenges are the development of cost-effective treatments tailored to defined FMS subgroups and the long-term efficacy of such approaches.

The aim of therapy is to enhance the self-management of the patient to better cope with the symptom load, and to improve daily functioning. Therefore active treatment approaches (aerobic exercise, CBT) should be preferred.

Evidence-based guidelines for the management of FMS should be developed by an interdisciplinary approach and include patients in all stages of development and implementation. It is important to note that many of the recommendations are not based on clinical studies, but rather the agreement of interdisciplinary experts and patients and their joint vision of the management of FMS in a specific health system and societal context.

References

1. Burckhardt CS, Goldenberg D, Crofford L, *et al.* EULAR evidence based recommendations for the management of fibromyalgia syndrome. *Ann Rheum Dis* 2008; **67**: 536–541.
2. Carville SF, Arendt-Nielsen S, Bliddal H, *et al.* EULAR evidence based recommendations for the management of fibromyalgia syndrome. *Ann Rheum Dis* 2008; **67**: 536–541.
3. Bernardy K, Klose P, Üçeyler N, Kopp I, Häuser W. Methodological fundamentals of the development of the guideline. Report of the methodology. *Schmerz* 2008; **22**(3): 244–254. (German)
4. Wolfe F, Smythe HA, Yunus MB, *et al.* The American College of Rheumatology criteria for the classification of fibromyalgia: report of the Multicenter Criteria Committee. *Arthritis Rheum* 1990; **33**: 160–172.
5. Turk DC, Flor H. Primary fibromyalgia is greater than tender points: toward a multiaxial taxonomy. *J Rheumatol* 1989; **19**: 80–86.
6. Mease PJ, Clauw DJ, Arnold LM, *et al.* Fibromyalgia syndrome. *J Rheumatol* 2005; **32**: 2270–2277.
7. Bennett RM, Jones J, Turk DC, Russell IJ, Matallana L. An internet survey of 2569 people with fibromyalgia. *BMC Musculoskelet Disord* 2007; **8**: 27.
8. Häuser W, Zimmer C, Felde E, Köllner V. What are the key symptoms of fibromyalgia? Results of a survey of the German Fibromyalgia Association. *Schmerz* 2008; **22**: 176–183 (German).
9. Sommer C, Häuser W, Gerhold K, *et al.* Etiology and pathophysiology of fibromyalgia syndrome and chronic widespread pain. *Schmerz* 2008; **22**: 267–282 (German).
10. Henningsen P, Zipfel S, Herzog W. Management of functional somatic syndromes. *Lancet* 2007; **369**: 946–955.
11. Eich W, Häuser W, Friedel E, *et al.* Definition, classification and diagnosis of fibromyalgia syndrome. *Schmerz* 2008; **22**: 256–266 (German).
12. World Health Organization. *International Classification of Diseases Version 2007.* www.who.int/classifications/apps/icd/icd10online/?gm70.htm+m797.
13. Croft P, Burt J, Schollum J, Thomas E, Macfarlane G, Silman A. More pain, more tender points: is fibromyalgia just one end of a continuous spectrum? *Ann Rheum Dis* 1996; **55**: 482–485.
14. Ruiz Moral R, Muñoz Alamo M, Pérula de Torres L, Aguayo Galeote M. Biopsychosocial features of patients with

widespread chronic musculoskeletal pain in family medicine clinics. *Fam Pract* 1997; **14**: 242–248.

15. Wolfe F. The relation between tender points and fibromyalgia symptom variables: evidence that fibromyalgia is not a discrete disorder in the clinic. *Ann Rheum Dis* 1997; **56**: 268–271.

16. Brähler E, Schumacher J, Brähler C. First all-Germany standardization of the brief form of the Gissen Complaints Questionnaire GBB-24. *Psychother Psychosom Med Psychol* 2000; **50**: 14–21 (German).

17. Henningsen P, Derra C, Türp JC, Häuser W. Functional somatic pain syndromes: summary of hypotheses of their overlap and etiology. *Schmerz* 2004; **18**: 136–140 (German).

18. Harth M, Nielson WR. The fibromyalgia tender points: use them or lose them? A brief review of the controversy. *J Rheumatol* 2007; **34**: 914–922.

19. Russel IJ. Is fibromyalgia a distinct clinical entity? The clinical investigator's evidence. *Baillière's Best Pract Res Clin Rheumatol* 1999; **13**: 445–454.

20. Gran JT. The epidemiology of chronic generalized musculoskeletal pain. *Best Pract Res Clin Rheumatol* 2003; **17**: 547–561.

21. Michels H, Gerhold K, Häfner R, *et al.* Juvenile fibromyalgia syndrom. *Schmerz* 2008; **22**: 339–345 (German).

22. Gallagher AM, Thomas JM, Hamilton WT, White PD. Incidence of fatigue symptoms and diagnoses presenting in UK primary care from 1990 to 2001. *J R Soc Med* 2004; **97**: 571–575.

23. Bazelmans E, Vercoulen JH, Swanink CM, *et al.* Chronic fatigue syndrome and primary fibromyalgia syndrome as recognized by GPs. *Fam Pract* 1999; **16**: 602–604.

24. Häuser W, Eich W, Herrmann M, Nutzinger DO, Schiltenwolf M, Henningsen P. Fibromyalgia syndrome: classification, diagnosis, and treatment. *Dtsch Arztebl Int* 2009; **106**: 383–391.

25. Gamero RF, Gabriel SR, Carbonell AJ, Tornero MJ, Sánchez MI. Pain in Spanish rheumatology outpatient offices: EPIDOR epidemiological study. *Rev Clin Esp* 2005; **20**: 157–163 (Spanish).

26. Buskila D, Neumann L, Odes LR, Schleifer E, Depsames R, Abu-Shakra M. The prevalence of musculoskeletal pain and fibromyalgia in patients hospitalized on internal medicine wards. *Semin Arthritis Rheum* 2001; **30**: 411–417.

27. Gralow I, Hürter A, Schwerdt C, Hannich HJ, Meyer B, Voss S. Concept of a day hospital. First clinical experience. *Schmerz* 1996; **41**: 242–249 (German).

28. Buskila D, Sarzi-Puttini P, Ablin JN. The genetics of fibromyalgia syndrome. *Pharmacogenomics* 2007; **8**: 67–74.

29. Kato K, Sullivan P, Evengård B, Pedersen N. Importance of genetic influences on chronic widespread pain. *Arthritis Rheum* 2006; **54**: 1682–1686.

30. Fietta P, Fietta P, Manganelli P. Fibromyalgia and psychiatric disorders. *Acta Biomed* 2007; **78**: 88–95.

31. van Houdenhove B, Luyten P. Stress, depression and fibromyalgia. *Acta Neurol Belg* 2006; **106**: 149–156.

32. Forseth KO, Husby G, Gran JT, *et al.* Prognostic factors for the development of fibromyalgia in women with self-reported musculoskeletal pain. A prospective study. *J Rheumatol* 1999; **26**: 2458–2467.

33. Henningsen P, Zimmermann T, Sattel H. Medically unexplained physical symptoms, anxiety, and depression: a meta-analytic review. *Psychosom Med* 2003; **65**: 528–533.

34. Macfarlane GJ, Hunt IM, Silman AJ. Role of mechanical and psychosocial factors in the onset of forearm pain: prospective population based study. *BMJ* 2000; **321**: 676–679.

35. McBeth J, Silman AJ, Gupta A, *et al.* Moderation of psychosocial risk factors through dysfunction of the hypothalamic-pituitary-adrenal stress axis in the onset of chronic widespread musculoskeletal pain: findings of a population-based prospective cohort study. *Arthritis Rheum* 2007; **56**: 360–371.

36. Gupta A, Silman AJ, Ray D, *et al.* The role of psychosocial factors in predicting the onset of chronic widespread pain: results from a prospective population-based study. *Rheumatology (Oxford)* 2007; **46**: 666–671.

37. Raphael KG, Chandler HK, Ciccone DS. Is childhood abuse a risk factor for chronic pain in adulthood? *Curr Pain Headache Rep* 2004; **8**: 99–110.

38. McBeth J, Morris S, Benjamin S, *et al.* Associations between adverse events in childhood and chronic widespread pain in adulthood: are they explained by differential recall? *J Rheumatol* 2001; **28**: 2305–2309.

39. Raphael KG, Natelson BH, Janal MN, *et al.* A community-based survey of fibromyalgia-like pain complaints following the World Trade Center terrorist attacks. *Pain* 2002; **100**: 131–139.

40. Kivimäki M, Leino-Arjas P, Virtanen M, *et al.* Work stress and incidence of newly diagnosed fibromyalgia: prospective cohort study. *J Psychosom Res* 2004; **57**: 417–422.

41. Yunus MB. The role of gender in fibromyalgia syndrome. *Curr Rheumatol Rep* 2001; **3**: 128–134.

42. Kajantie E, Phillips DI. The effects of sex and hormonal status on the physiological response to acute psychosocial stress. *Psychoneuroendocrinology* 2006; **31**: 151–178.

43. Schochat T, Beckmann C. Sociodemographic characteristics, risk factors and reproductive history in subjects with fibromyalgia – results of a population-based case-control study. *Z Rheumatol* 2003; **62**: 46–59 (German).

44. McBeth J, Harkness EF, Silman AJ, *et al.* The role of workplace low-level mechanical trauma, posture and environment in the onset of chronic widespread pain. *Rheumatology (Oxford)* 2003; **42**: 1486–1494.

45. Harkness EF, Macfarlane GJ, Nahit E, *et al.* Mechanical injury and psychosocial factors in the work place predict the onset of widespread body pain: a two-year prospective study among cohorts of newly employed workers. *Arthritis Rheum* 2004; **50**: 1655–1664.

46. McBeth J, Macfarlane GJ, Hunt IM, *et al.* Risk factors for persistent chronic widespread pain: a community-based study. *Rheumatology (Oxford)* 2001; **40**: 95–101.

47. Dobkin PL, de Civita M, Abrahamowicz M, Baron M, Bernatsky S. Predictors of health status in women with fibromyalgia: a prospective study. *Int J Behav Med* 2006; **13**: 101–108.

48. Wigers H. Fibromyalgia outcome: the predictive values of symptom duration, physical activity, disability pension, and critical life events – a 4.5 year prospective study. *J Psychosom Res* 1994; **41**: 235–243.

49. Granges G, Zilko P, Littlejohn GO. Fibromyalgia syndrome: assessment of the severity of the condition 2 years after diagnosis. *J Rheumatol* 1994; **21**: 523–529.

50. Mengshoel AM, Haugen M. Health status in fibromyalgia–a followup study. *J Rheumatol* 2001; **28**: 2085–2089.

51. Okifuji A, Turk DC. Stress and psychophysiological dysregulation in patients with fibromyalgia syndrome. *Appl Psychophysiol Biofeedback* 2002; **27**: 129–141.

52. McBeth J, Chiu YH, Silman AJ, *et al*. Hypothalamic-pituitary-adrenal stress axis function and the relationship with chronic widespread pain and its antecedents. *Arthritis Res Ther* 2005; **7**: R992–R1000.

53. Wolfe F. Stop using the American College of Rheumatology criteria in the clinic. *J Rheumatol* 2003; **30**: 1671–1672.

54. Biewer W, Conrad I, Häuser W. Fibromyalgia. Schmerz 2004; **18**: 118–124.

55. Ohrbach R, Crow H, Kamer A. Examiner expectancy effects in the measurement of pressure pain thresholds. *Pain* 1998; **74**: 163–170.

56. Okifuji A, Turk DC, Sinclair JD, Starz TW, Marcus DA. A standardized manual tender point survey. I. Development and determination of a threshold point for the identification of positive tender points in fibromyalgia syndrome. *J Rheumatol* 1997; **24**: 377–383.

57. Petzke F, Gracely RH, Park KM, Ambrose K, Clauw DJ. What do tender points measure? Influence of distress on 4 measures of tenderness. *J Rheumatol* 2003; **30**: 567–574.

58. Wolfe F. Pain extent and diagnosis: development and validation of the regional pain scale in 12 995 patients. *J Rheumatol* 2003; **30**: 369–378.

59. Spitzer RL, Kroenke K, Williams JB. Validation and utility of a self-report version of PRIME-MD: the PHQ primary care study. Primary Care Evaluation of Mental Disorders. Patient Health Questionnaire. *JAMA* 1999; **282**: 1737–1744.

60. Cleeland CS, Ryan KM. Pain assessment: global use of the Brief Pain Inventory. *Ann Acad Med Singapore* 1994; **23**: 129–138.

61. Burckhardt CS, Clark SR, Bennett RM. The Fibromyalgia Impact Questionnaire: development and validation. *J Rheumatol* 1991; **18**: 728–733.

62. Suarez-Almazor ME, Gonzalez-Lopez L, Gamez-Nava JI, Belseck E, Kendall CJ, Davis P. Utilization and predictive value of laboratory tests in patients referred to rheumatologists by primary care physicians. *J Rheumatol* 1998; **25**: 1980–1985.

63. Lindgren H, Bergman S. The use and diagnostic yield of radiology in subjects with longstanding musculoskeletal pain – an eight year follow up. *BMC Musculoskelet Disord* 2005; **6**: 53.

64. Busch AJ, Schachter CL, Overend TJ, Peloso PM, Barber KA. Exercise for fibromyalgia: a systematic review. *J Rheumatol* 2008; **35**(6): 1130–1144.

65. Schiltenwolf M, Häuser W, Felde E, *et al*. Physiotherapy, exercise and physical therapy in fibromyalgia syndrome. *Schmerz* 2008; **22**: 303–312 (German).

66. Langhorst J, W. Häuser W, Irnich D, *et al*. Complementary and alternative therapies in fibromyalgia syndrome. *Schmerz* 2008; **22**: 324–333.

67. Arnold B, Häuser W, Bernardy K, *et al*. Multicomponent treatment of fibromyalgia syndrome. *Schmerz* 2008; **22**: 334–338 (German).

68. Sommer C, Häuser W, Berliner M, *et al*. Pharmacological therapy of fibromyalgia syndrome. *Schmerz* 2008; **22**: 313–323 (German).

69. Thieme K, Häuser W, Batra A, *et al*. Psychotherapy in patients with fibromyalgia syndrome. *Schmerz* 2008; **22**: 295–302 (German).

70. Kashikar-Zuck S, Swain NF, Jones BA, Graham TB. Efficacy of cognitive-behavioral intervention for juvenile primary fibromyalgia syndrome. *J Rheumatol* 2005; **32**: 1594–1602.

71. Üçeyler N, Häuser W, Sommer C. A systematic review on the effectiveness of treatment with antidepressants in fibromyalgia syndrome. *Arthritis Rheum* 2008; **59**: 1279–1298.

72. Thieme K, Gromnica-Ihle E, Flor H. Operant behavioral treatment of fibromyalgia: a controlled study. *Arthritis Rheum* 2003; **49**: 314–320.

73. Zijlstra TR, Braakman-Jansen LM, Taal E, Rasker JJ, van de Laar MA. Cost-effectiveness of spa treatment for fibromyalgia: general health improvement is not for free. *Rheumatology (Oxford)* 2007; **46**: 1454–1459.

74. Häuser W, Bernardy K, Üçeyler N. Treatment of fibromyalgia syndrome with antidepressants – a meta-analysis. *JAMA* 2009; **301**(2): 198–209.

75. McVeigh JG, McGaughey H, Hall M, Kane P. The effectiveness of hydrotherapy in the management of fibromyalgia syndrome: a systematic review. *Rheumatol Int* 2008; **29**: 119–130

76. Tofferi JK, Jackson JL, O'Malley PG.Treatment of fibromyalgia with cyclobenzaprine: a meta-analysis. *Arthritis Rheum* 2004; **51**: 9–13.

77. Füber N, Bernardy K, Häuser W, Spinath FM. Efficacy of psychotherapy in fibromyalgia syndrome – a metaanalysis. *Schmerz* 2008; **2**(suppl): 165 (German).

78. Burckhardt CS. Multidisciplinary approaches for management of fibromyalgia. *Curr Pharm Des* 2006; **12**: 59–66.

79. Häuser W, Bernardy K, offenbächer M, Arnold B, Schiltenwolf M. Efficacy of multicomponent treatment in fibromyalgia syndrome – a meta-analysis of randomized controlled clinical trials. *Arthritis Rheum* 2009; **61**(2): 216–224.

80. Häuser W, Bernardy K, Üceyler N, Sommer C. Treatment of fibromyalgia syndrome with gabapentin and pregabalin – a meta-analysis of randomized controlled trails. *PAIN* 2009, june 16 epub.

81. Grossman P, Tiefenthaler-Gilmer U, Raysz A, Kesper U. Mindfulness training as an intervention for fibromyalgia: evidence of postintervention and 3-year follow-up benefits in well-being. *Psychother Psychosom* 2007; **76**: 226–233.

82. Sephton SE, Salmon P, Weissbecker I, *et al*. Mindfulness meditation alleviates depressive symptoms in women with fibromyalgia: results of a randomized clinical trial. *Arthritis Rheum* 2007; **57**: 77–85.

83. Mayhew E, Ernst E. Acupuncture for fibromyalgia – a systematic review of randomized clinical trials. *Rheumatology* 2007; **46**: 801–804.

84. Thieme K, Turk DC, Flor H. Responder criteria for operant and cognitive-behavioral treatment of fibromyalgia syndrome. *Arthritis Rheum* 2007; **57**: 830–836.

85. Koulil SV. Cognitive-behavioural therapies and exercise programmes for patients with fibromyalgia: state of the art and future directions. *Ann Rheum Dis* 2007; **66**: 571–581.

CHAPTER 12

Facial pain

Joanna M. Zakrzewska

Division of Diagnostic, Surgical and Medical Sciences, Eastman Dental Hospital, UCLH NHS Foundation Trust, London, UK

Background

Orofacial pain is common and a UK community-based survey showed that 19% of the sample reported some form of orofacial pain, with some 7% being chronic. Just under half seek professional help and up to 17% take time off work or are unable to carry on normal activities because of facial pain [1].

The location of the pain is often the determining factor as to whether a dental or medical professional is consulted and treatment is then determined by this [2]. The majority of orofacial pain will be of dental origin and is well managed by dental practitioners. More chronic oral pains, especially if they also have extraoral features, present a diagnostic dilemma as their management then falls between the dental and medical practitioners.

Woda *et al.* [3] attempted to determine by the technique of cluster analysis whether there were key features that distinguished different types of facial pain. They showed that there are clinical features that differentiate trigeminal neuralgia, migraine and tension headaches into distinct clusters but atypical facial pain, atypical odontalgia and facial arthromylagia (temporomandibular disorders – TMD) differed only in location of pain but otherwise could not be differentiated from each other on symptomatology alone. Burning mouth was closely associated with this group but had some features which differentiated it.

Not all the causes of facial pain can be covered in this chapter but Table 12.1 provides a list of possible

diagnoses that need to be considered when dealing with a patient with orofacial pain. For updates, a paper in *Current Opinion in Supportive and Palliative Care* summarizes evidence-based publications published

Table 12.1 Differential diagnosis for orofacial pain

Musculoligamentous/ soft tissue causes	Temporomandibular disorder (myofascial face pain) Internal derangements of TMJ Persistent idiopathic orofacial pain/ atypical facial pain, facial neuralgia Salivary gland disease Oral lesions such as lichen planus, oral ulcers, candidiasis Cancer
Dentoalveolar causes	Dentinal Periodontal Pulpal Cracked tooth syndrome – often chronic and difficult to diagnose Maxillary sinusitis Thermal sensitivities Atypical odontalgia which may be trigeminal neuropathic pain/phantom tooth pain Post-traumatic nerve injuries including chemical
Neurologic/vascular causes	Trigeminal neuralgia Glossopharyngeal Cluster headache Postherpetic neuralgia Burning mouth syndrome, oral dysesthesia, glossodynia Cranial arteritis Pre-trigeminal neuralgia Ramsay Hunt SUNCT/SUNA Paroxysmal hemicrania

Evidence-Based Chronic Pain Management. Edited by C. Stannard, E. Kalso and J. Ballantyne. © 2010 Blackwell Publishing.

between 2007–2009 and highlights studies of special interest [4]. Further details on the characteristics and management of these pains can be found in textbooks such as *Assessment and Management of Orofacial Pain* [5] and *Orofacial Pain* [6].

Chronic idiopathic facial pain/ persistent facial pain/atypical facial pain

Background

This is currently the most controversial condition as it is likely to be a very heterogeneous group. This diagnosis was often made when all other causes of facial pain had been excluded and in those patients who do not report pain round the temporomandibular joint (TMJ). In 2002 a study conducted among dental and medical specialties showed that the majority preferred the term "atypical facial pain" but there was a wide range of terminologies. The management of these cases, however, suggested much more unity [7].

Pathophysiology

This remains largely unknown but several proposals have been put forward:
• an orofacial form of migraine
• medically unexplained symptoms
• psychogenic origin.
Psychologic factors are implicated in all pain conditions, irrespective of etiology or duration, and this group of patients are probably no different from other chronic pain sufferers. It is probable that some of these patients do have neuropathic pain related to previous trauma, infection or dental treatment.

Epidemiology

Given the difficulty in diagnosis and the lack of clear diagnostic criteria that could be used in epidemiologic studies, little is known about the incidence and prevalence of this condition [8]. Data from the secondary care sector show that 80% of sufferers are women and the highest prevalence is in the age group 40–50 years. A recent community-based study (2299 subjects) found that 7% suffered from chronic orofacial pain. Of this group, 27% reported one or more of these conditions: chronic facial pain, irritable bowel syndrome, chronic fatigue and chronic widespread pain, and 18% reported one pain, 6% reported another chronic pain in a distant part of the body and 2% reported three different pain syndromes. The common factors to these four conditions were female gender, high levels of health anxiety, reassurance-seeking behaviors, other somatic symptoms and recent adverse events [9]. There are few data on prognosis although Feinmann showed that 70% can be rendered pain free in the long term but may require medication and counseling [10].

Clinical features

The International Headache Society (IHS) criteria of 2004 introduced the term "persistent idiopathic facial pain" and provided specific criteria [11]. These were used by Zebenholzer *et al.* [12] to test their sensitivity, specificity and positive and negative predictive value in 97 patients referred to a neurologic service with facial pain. They provided the following criteria (italics are their additions to changes to the IHS criteria).

A Pain in the face, present daily *for at least 1 month* and persisting for all or most of the day, *with a least four characteristics from group B* (fulfilling criteria B and C)

B 1. Pain is confined at onset to a limited area on one side of the face
   2. Pain is deep and poorly localized
   3. *Intensity is moderate or severe but not unbearable*
   4. *Pain paroxysms do not occur*
   5. *Pain is not precipitated from trigger areas or by daily activities*

C Both of the following:
   1. No autonomic symptoms
   2. No sensory loss or other physical signs *but dysesthesia may occur*

D Investigations negative *including X-ray of the face and jaws does not demonstrate relevant abnormality.*

It is important to add that the symptoms and signs cannot be attributed to any other disorder. Zebenholzer *et al.* [12] suggest that there should be a category of "probable" which means that not all the symptoms need to be present to make the diagnosis. Using these criteria, the authors suggest that most patients could be classified with accuracy which would thus make comparisons of management easier.

Box 12.1 Interventions supported by evidence

Drug/therapy	Daily dose range	Efficacy	Side effects	Level of evidence
Persistent facial pain				
Amitriptyline	10–150 mg	Good	None reported but known to cause drowsiness, dry mouth	RCT*
Dothiepin (dosulepin) included biteguard	25–150 mg	Likely to be effective Insufficient evidence for biteguard	Drowsiness, dry mouth, dizziness	SR, RCT*
Fluoxetine	20 mg	Good	None reported but known to cause postural hypotension, sleep disturbance	RCT*
Phenelzine	45 mg	Improved both pain and associated depression	None reported but known to cause postural hypotension, dizziness, insomnia, dry mouth	RCT
TMD				
Amitriptyline	10–150 mg	Good	None reported but known to cause drowsiness, dry mouth	RCT*
Dothiepin (dosulepin) included biteguard	25–75 mg	Likely to be effective Insufficient evidence for biteguard	Drowsiness, dry mouth, dizziness	RCT*
Ibuprofen and diazepam	Ibuprofen 400 mg, diazepam 10–20 mg	Diazepam on its own or in combination with ibuprofen effective but ibuprofen on its own not effective	Nil stated but dependency is high with diazepam, gastrointestinal problems with ibuprofen	RCT
Piroxicam	20 mg	Good	None reported but as with other NSAIDs	RCT
Mersyndol, analgesic and antihistamine	450 mg paracetamol, 9.75 mg codeine and 5 mg doxylamine up to two	Effective	Drowsiness	RCT

Treatment	Dose/regimen	Efficacy	Side effects	Evidence
Occlusal splints	Night-time use mainly	Weak but effective in adolescents	None reported	2 SR, several RCT
CBT	6–12 sessions** over 4 months	Effective but not maintained after conclusion of therapy in some studies	None reported	Several RCT
CBT, biofeedback or combination of both	12 sessions**	All showed improvement but combined was highest effect and maintained at 1 year	None reported	2 RCT
Trigeminal neuralgia				
Baclofen	50–80 mg	Good	Ataxia, lethargy, fatigue, nausea, vomiting, beware rapid withdrawal	SR, RCT
Carbamazepine	300–1000 mg	Excellent	Drowsiness, ataxia, headaches, nausea, vomiting, constipation, blurred vision, rash, introduce slowly, drug interactions	SR, RCT
Lamotrigine	200–400 mg	Good when added to other antiepileptic drug	Dizziness, drowsiness, constipation, ataxia, diplopia, irritability, rapid dose escalation leads to rashes	SR, RCT
Oxcarbazepine	300–1200 mg	Excellent	Vertigo, fatigue, dizziness, nausea, hyponatremia in high doses, no major drug interactions	SR, RCT
Gabapentin and ropivicain	300–600 mg gabapentin, 5 injections into trigger points	NNT 2.4 at 4 weeks, improved quality of life	None reported	RCT

* Same trial had a mix of patients. ** A session is normally a period of 1–2 hours spent with a clinical psychologist.
CBT, cognitive behavioral therapy; NNT, number needed to treat; RCT, randomized controlled trial; SR, systematic review; TMD, temporomandibular disorders.

Based on this and previous work by others, the clinical features of persistent idiopathic facial pain are as folllows.
- Character: nagging, dull, throbbing, sharp, aching
- Severity: varies, mild to severe but not unbearable
- Site: radiation, unilateral, bilateral, no anatomic area, deep, poorly localized
- Duration periodicity: intermittent/constant, may be periods of pain relief
- Provoking factors: chewing, stress, fatigue but not touch provoked
- Relieving factors: rest, relaxation
- Associated factors: pain in other areas, personality changes, life events, no autonomic symptoms

Management

As with all other chronic pain, the approach must be biopsychosocial with active patient involvement. Patients need to feel that they are understood and clinicians must acknowledge the patient's experience of pain without attempting to validate its source. It is crucial that medical management includes challenging maladaptive beliefs and behaviors regarding health and illness and this may need a multidisciplinary approach with active participation by the patient.

Searching the literature shows that there have been systematic reviews on medical management of chronic idiopathic facial pain as there are several randomized controlled trials (RCT). However, it is important to remember that the diagnostic criteria used in these trials may have been different and so the results need to be interpreted with care. In some trials the patients also had TMD pain or even neuropathic pain.

Interventions supported by evidence

There are two systematic reviews [13, 14] on the use of antidepressants which used data from three RCT to suggest that they may be effective in atypical facial pain [14–17]. There is also a systematic review that looks at all types of pharmacologic treatments for this condition [18]. Only the larger studies will be included here.

Lascelles [17] used phenelzine in 40 atypical facial pain patients in a cross-over study and found it to be effective. The study by Feinmann & Harris [15] involving 93 patients with mixed chronic facial pain assessed the effect of dothiepin (dosulepin) versus placebo using a dose titration. At 9 weeks, 71% were pain free but withdrawal of drug at 6 months led to

relapse in some patients. There was a high drop-out rate and it is not possible to separate out the patients with different types of pain. The largest study was by Harrison et al. [16] which included 178 patients with mixed chronic facial pain who were divided into four groups: fluoxetine, placebo, cognitive behavioral treatment (CBT) with placebo, CBT with fluoxetine, and followed up for 3 months. Fluoxetine reduced pain at 3 months compared to placebo. CBT on its own was not effective in reducing pain but did improve patients' control of their lives. These improvements were maintained when drug therapy ceased.

Sharav et al. [19] showed the effectiveness of low- or high-dose amitriptyline 25 mg or 100 mg but their patients had a mixture of chronic idiopathic facial pain, TMD pain and even neuropathic pain.

Forsell et al. [20] used venlafaxine versus placebo in 30 patients in a double-blind cross-over RCT. Ten patients did not complete – eight due to adverse side effects and two due to noncompliance. There was no difference between placebo and active drug in terms of pain intensity although there was more significant improvement in pain relief scores in the active treatment group. There were no differences in terms of anxiety and depression. Efficacy of this drug was only modest but this could be due to small sample size as the study itself was of high quality.

Interventions refuted by evidence

In a double-blind placebo-controlled cross-over trial, al Balawi et al. [21] injected subcutaneous sumatriptan (6 mg) in 19 patients on one occasion. Some relief was noted in comparison to placebo but the effect was not sustained. All patients experienced one or more adverse event but these were all mild.

Commonly used interventions currently unproven

Cognitive behavioral therapy has been shown to be effective in chronic pain but there is only one study of its use in chronic idiopathic facial pain which showed that it did not relieve pain but affected patients' ability to control their pain [16]. The program included education about gate control theory, pain-coping strategies, relaxation, assertiveness, communication training, maintenance of gains and coping with acute exacerbations. This treatment is often used in combination with tricyclic antidepressants.

Box 12.2   Interventions refuted by evidence or insufficient evidence

Drug/therapy	Daily dose range	Efficacy	Side effects	Level of evidence
Persistent facial pain				
Sumatriptan	6 mg sc	Limited		RCT
Venlafaxine	75 mg	Limited	Most common are fatigue, loss of appetite, nausea, dry mouth	RCT
TMD				
Biofeedback only		None		1 SR
Acupuncture		None		2 SR
TENS		None		1 SR
Occlusal adjustments		Not effective	Irreversible changes	2 SR
Botulinum toxin	150 MU	Not effective	Injection pain, paralysis, asymmetric smile	RCT
Clonazepam	0.25–1 mg	Weak	Sedation	RCT
Triazolam	0.25–0.5 mg	Improves sleep but not pain	Impaired memory, confusion	RCT
Trigeminal neuralgia				
Dextromethorphan	120–920 mg	Worse	Mild cognitive impairment, dizziness and ataxia	RCT
Clomipramine	20–75 mg	Unknown	None stated	RCT
Pimozide	4–12gm	Excellent	Severe side effects limit its use: extrapyramidal, tremor, rigidity, memory loss	SR, RCT
Proparacaine hydrochloride	2 drops of 0.5% solution for 20 min	Ineffective		RCT
Tocainide	60 mg/kg	Ineffective	Rash, nausea, paresthesia, aplastic anemia	SR, RCT
Topiramate	25–250 mg	May be effective	Irritability, cognitive impairment, gastrointestinal, fatigue	SR, RCT
Tizanidine	6–18 mg	Ineffective	Drowsiness, dizziness, alters liver enzymes	SR,RCT

RCT, randomized controlled trial; SR, systematic review; TENS, transcutaneous electrical nerve stimulation; TMD, temporomandibular disorders.

Discussion of evidence

All the studies are small and may contain a very heterogeneous group of patients. Given the prevalence of orofacial pain, it is surprising that there are so few high-quality studies. Although there is some evidence for the success of antidepressants, some patients do not have a good response and this could be due to certain patient characteristics: nonanxious somatizers, dysfunctional health beliefs, history of unsuccessful surgery, no life event before pain onset. Treatment needs to be continued for a long time and relapses are common. As in other chronic pain, CBT is helpful in improving quality of life but may not directly result in a decrease in pain intensity.

Cost and feasibility of treatment/ cost benefit

If the diagnostic criteria were clearer and more generally recognized then many unnecessary investigations and dental treatments could be avoided. However, there is a group of patients who need long-term care to prevent relapse and take up a large amount of resources.

Box 12.3 Commonly used interventions currently unproven

Drug/therapy	Daily dose range	Efficacy	Side effects
Persistent facial pain			
CBT with or without tricyclic antidepressants	6–12 sessions	High	If drugs used: drowsiness, dryness
Information and reassurance		High	
TMD			
Ultrasound		Unknown	
Heat		Unknown	
Exercises		May be effective	
Information and reassurance		High	
Trigeminal neuralgia			
Clonazepam	4–8 mg	Low	Severe drowsiness
Pregabalin	150–600 mg	Good	Neurologic side effects
Phenytoin	200–300 mg	Good	Neurologic side effects, easy to overdose
Valproic acid	600–1200 mg	Poor	Neurologic side effects
Microvascular decompression		High; 70% pain free 10 years	0.5% mortality, hearing loss
Radiofrequency thermocoagulation		Good; 50% pain free 5 years	High % sensory loss
Percutaneous glycerol rhizotomy		Good; 50% pain free at 4 years	Sensory loss
Balloon decompression		Good; 50% pain free at 4 years	Masticatory problems
Gamma knife		Good; 50% pain free at 4 years	10% sensory loss

CBT, cognitive behavioral therapy; TMD, temporomandibular disorders.

The role of primary healthcare providers may be very important in continuing to provide support.

Future directions

Once the diagnostic criteria have been clarified, larger multicentered long-term RCT need to be done. Education of primary and secondary care providers is essential if this group of patients is to be recognized early and managed appropriately to prevent chronicity.

Cognitive behavioral therapy is often used after all other types of interventions have failed. This is in part related to the patients' expectations, which are usually to find relief of pain and not better ways of coping with it [22]. Williams [22] argues that this may not be the correct approach and that CBT should be offered earlier as it aims to provide maximum freedom from the negative impact of pain by changing the individual's relationship to it. It needs to be offered to patients with orofacial pain especially if they have risk factors.

Author's recommendations

Patients with chronic idiopathic pain need to be carefully assessed which includes eliciting their treatment goals and beliefs about treatments. In line with other chronic pain, unnecessary investigations and treatments make pain intractable and results in depressed patients. Clinicians often feel less optimistic about their ability to successfully manage these patients. A biopsychosocial approach to treatment is needed and CBT should be used alongside drug therapy in those who are found to have a high index of disability. The selective serotonin reuptake inhibitors (SSRI), especially fluoxetine and escitalopram or others such as venlafaxine, are often used as they cause fewer side effects than tricyclics, they do not interact with alcohol, do not result in weight gain and are safe in overdose but they may be less effective in pain relief. Written information is important and some patients may find it useful to talk to other patients with similar problems.

Temporomandibular disorders (TMD)

Myofascial pain, mandibular dysfunction, facial arthromyalgia, and masticatory myalgia are other terms used to describe pain related to the masticatory muscles, the temporomandibular joint (TMJ) or both [23].

Background

Temporomandibular disorder pain is common and found mainly in young and middle-aged women. It has been estimated that up to 75% of the US population may suffer from this condition at some stage in their lives and that the prevalence in any given year is 10–12%. There are five diagnostic systems with varying degrees of reliability, accuracy and predictive ability and there are at present no objective investigations that can be done to confirm the diagnosis made on history and examination. The system that has been most extensively studied is the Research Diagnostic Criteria (RDC) for TMD developed by an international group in the 1990s [23]. This lack of consensus hampers epidemiologic data collection. Drangsholt & LeResche [24] did a systematic review on this topic and the following data are from their review.

There appears to be little change in numbers of people seeking treatment for TMD over the last 5–10 years. The natural history of the disorder is extremely variable with only a small group being persistent.

Depression and somatization are the best predictors of chronicity. About 25% of sufferers are likely to be disabled by the pain and more will take time off work than utilize healthcare facilities. Risk factors which may also be causative include: female gender, depression, and multiple pain conditions. This adds to the evidence that these patients belong to the generic group of patients who suffer chronic pain. Other risk factors for which the evidence is less robust may include bruxism, exogenous reproductive hormones, trauma and hypermobility. Primary prevention is still not possible but there is no doubt

that, as with other chronic facial pain, misdiagnosis, unnecessary investigations and irreversible dental therapies contribute to chronicity. Recent case reports have highlighted that patients with TMD are more likely to report migraines, back pain and fibromyalgia than none cases [4]. For more comprehensive coverage of this topic, the reader is directed to the recent text by Laskin et al. [25] which includes the surgical management of joint and disk disorders, which will not be covered here.

Etiology

Pain in and around the TMJ can be related to problems with the joint itself, e.g. congenital, traumatic, ankylosis, neoplastic or arthritides or with the muscle of mastication themselves. The latter are by far the most common. The causes of TMD remain controversial and range from a wide variety of occlusal and skeletal abnormalities, trauma, bruxism, parafunctional activity and psychologic, including vulnerability to chronic pain. A systematic review showed no association between malocclusion, functional occlusion and TMD in a community-based population [26]. There is now more emphasis on nondental causes and involvment of specific hormones as well as neurotropin nerve growth factor.

Clinical features

The main symptoms of TMD pain are as follows.
- Site: TMJ and associated musculature, unilateral or bilateral
- Radiation: associated muscles, temple, neck
- Character: dull, aching, throbbing, sometimes sharp
- Severity: mild to moderate
- Duration: weeks to years
- Periodicity: continuous, can be intermittent or worse on waking or at the end of the day
- Provoking factors: jaw movement, eating, stress
- Relieving factors: jaw rest, tricyclic drugs
- Associated factors: limited mouth opening, TMJ parafunction, bruxism, anxiety, other pain sites

The effect of TMD pain on quality of life has been assessed in large population-based studies using the Graded Chronic Pain Scale [27]. This scale yields four grades: Grades 3 and 4 are associated with increasing high levels of psychosocial disability whereas Grades 1 and 2 relate to high pain intensity but relatively little daily living disability. In these studies 15–18% had Grade

3 disability and 3–6% Grade 4. These patients score high on depression, are high users of healthcare services and are resistant to change with treatment. Turp [2] showed that 66% of a group of 278 TMD patients referred to a tertiary center had widespread pain and these patients scored significantly higher on the Pain Disability Index and the Beck Depression Inventory.

Examination involves the application of pressure to a variety of specific anatomic sites (trigger points) to see if the muscles are tender. The range of movement of the mandible is then evaluated in vertical opening, protrusive and lateral positions. These ranges of movements are measured in three positions: when pain free, with unassisted maximal opening and assisted maximal opening. The distance is measured between the incisive edge of the upper central incisor and the lower mandibular incisor in millimeters and there is reasonable agreement in these measurements. Although joint sounds and crepitus are listened for, they are not highly diagnostic. Crepitus may indicate an arthrosis.

Investigations

A wide variety of diagnostic investigations have been used, e.g. jaw tracking, thermograph, electromyography, sonography, but none has been validated and shown to be of diagnostic value. The main investigations are computed tomography (CT) and magnetic resonance imaging (MRI) scans principally to look for internal disk derangements. If autoimmune disorders are suspected then blood tests may be indicated.

Management

In 1995 Antczak-Bouckoms [28] reviewed the strength of evidence for management of TMD pain and found more than 4000 references to TMD, of which about 1200 related to management. However, the majority of these were reviews, with 15% being clinical studies and of these less than 5% (51) were RCT. Treatments used often reflect the healthcare professional's views as to the cause of the pain and vary from conservative, psychologic, and physical to medical and surgical.

Conservative management involves the provision of information and reassurance and psychologic management strategies range from simple behavioral changes through to full courses of CBT. A vast range of physical therapies has been used which include posture training, thermal applications, mechanical exercises, biofeedback and EMG, hypnosis, relaxation, imagery, ultrasound, phonophoresis and iontophoresis, acupuncture and TENS. It is thought that provision of an ideal occlusion will reduce abnormal muscle activity and so reduce pain. A variety of so-called stabilization splints have been used which are worn at night when it is thought most likely that patients clench and grind their teeth (parafunctional habit). The oral appliances predominantly cover one or other arch either completely or partially. Some attempt to realign the maxillomandibular relationship whereas others do not seek to change the relationship. They can be made of soft plastic but many are rigid and attached to the teeth by clasps. Evidence for their efficacy has not been proven.

Medical therapy involves a range of drugs from analgesics to antidepressants. Surgery, including injections into the joints, is mainly used for disk and joint disorders and will not be discussed here; details can be found in Laskin et al. [25].

Interventions supported by evidence

There are several high-quality trials showing that CBT is effective when used in patients with TMD although the majority of earlier studies are not methodologically sound and lack long-term follow-up. The use of the RDC classification enables more homogeneity between subjects and identification of those who have greater disability and poorer psychosocial adaptation to their TMD and it is probably these who benefit most from CBT. Dworkin et al. [29] identified 117 such patients and enrolled them in a RCT which compared usual TMD treatment with six sessions of CBT over a 4-month period together with usual TMD care. This intervention was effective but only during the time it was delivered and at 1 year it was no better than usual care [29]. This finding is in contrast to more recent studies which also involved short- and long-term outcomes (1 year) [30–32]. CBT sessions varied from 12 1- to 2-hour sessions [30, 31] to four sessions [32] and the shorter ones were still effective. Most of these trials relied on patients having workbooks to complete between sessions and on regular telephone contact. Gatchel et al. [33] have shown that early intervention using six 1-hour sessions for patients with acute TMD reduced pain levels, improved coping abilities and reduced stress at 1 year and so prevented chronicity.

Some of the studies have included groups having biofeedback either on its own or in combination with CBT [30, 31]. These were methodologically sound RCTs that used no treatment as a control and the Gardea *et al.* [30] study included a 1-year follow-up. Improvements were found not only in pain intensity but in a range of other outcomes, including mood.

A systematic review suggested that there is insufficient evidence either for or against the use of stabilization splint therapy over other active interventions for the treatment of TMD but there is some weak evidence that these splints can reduce pain severity, at rest and on palpation, when compared to no treatment [34, 35]. Further evidence-based guidelines have been published by the European Academy of Craniomandibular Disorders (EACD) [36].

In a cross-over trial of 30 patients comparing mersyndol with placebo, there was a statistically significant improvement, no adverse effects with two drop-outs (pain relief, did not want to do trial) [37].

Singer & Dionne [38] randomized 49 patients into four parallel groups: diazepam, ibuprofen, diazepam and ibuprofen, and placebo, and found ibuprofen was no better than diazepam or placebo but ibuprofen and diazepam or diazepam on its own were better than placebo for pain relief.

Amitriptyline 10–30 mg or 50–150 mg is effective in both TMD and chronic idiopathic pain irrespective of dose [19] but in an open labeled cohort study, Plesh [39] showed that its effectiveness is greatest at 6 weeks and tails off after 1 year.

The Feinmann & Harris [15] study described in the section above on the use of dothiepin (dosulepin) and splints also included patients with TMD. Although the dothiepin (dosulepin) decreased pain by 50%, only 38% wore the soft occlusal appliance to the end of the trial and so there is insufficient evidence to support the use of the splints.

Interventions refuted by evidence or insufficient evidence

Koh & Robinson [40], in their systematic review (identified 660 trials on TMD therapy but only six fulfilled the inclusion criteria), assessed the effectiveness of occlusal adjustment for treating TMD in adults and preventing TMD and found there was no evidence to support this therapy. This has also been confirmed by others.

Jedel & Carlsson's systematic review of seven controlled clinical trials to assess the efficacy of biofeedback, acupuncture and TENS in TMD once again showed poor methodology and no evidence for effectiveness of these therapies [41]. Another systematic review on acupuncture came to the same conclusions [42].

Of the pharmacologic therapies, clonazepam versus placebo in 20 patients decreased pain but the study was very small and the 25% drop-out rate makes these results difficult to interpret [43].

There are no trials of sufficient quality on the use of oral opioids.

Botulinum toxin has been used in a small trial of 15 patients with muscular TMD pain but no evidence for effectiveness was found and one-third of the patients were lost to follow-up [44].

Commonly used interventions currently unproven

A vast majority of patients will respond well to a clear explanation and reassurance, especially if given by an empathic clinician, but there are no trials to prove its effectiveness.

Mechanical exercises are often prescribed as it is thought that patients with pain are often reluctant to use the body part that is causing pain. Use of occlusal appliances is common as these are easy for dental surgeons to construct and they are more familiar with this method of treatment rather than systemic drugs. Patients with TMD pain can be divided into three treatment groups based on their response to the Graded Chronic Pain Scale: minimal contact approach (one or two sessions with or without the help of a psychologist), integrated approach (with appliances, biofeedback and stress management led by hygienist) and a structured behavioral programme (psychologist led for six sessions) [45].

Discussion of evidence

The fact that such a variety of treatments is still used provides some evidence that there is no one method of treating these patients. The majority of patients will improve with very little need for therapy but with directed education. There then remains a small cohort of patients who remain difficult to manage. These are the patients who visit a wide range of healthcare providers and are ultimately seen in the tertiary care sector. Turp [2] showed that the average number of providers seen by TMD patients referred to a tertiary care center was 4.9 and that over 60% had at least one nondental treatment and 28% were dissatisfied with the care they had received.

From the current evidence, it is clear that as with other chronic pain, a biopsychosocial approach is necessary as behavior and attitudes need to change and patients need to self-manage their condition. Turner et al. [32] and Gatchel et al. [33] have shown that changing TMD patients' beliefs and pain-coping strategies through the use of CBT can have a modest effect on future pain and functioning. Combining CBT with biofeedback may yield even better results as the latter has a more immediate effect and appears to be more physiologically orientated.

There is some evidence that NSAIDs may be of some benefit but the side effects of these medications need to be taken into account. Benzodiazepines may be useful but they should not be used except in the short term due to dependency. As with other chronic pain, there is some evidence that tricyclic antidepressants as well as the newer SSRI may be of benefit. It is highly likely that dental treatment is not the way forward and the American Dental Association has stated that all treatments that attempt to address a possible occlusal disharmony should be reversible. Occlusal appliances which do not attempt to alter occlusion and which are only worn at night may be useful in patients who do not have a stable occlusion or those who have marked parafunctional habits. The EACD stress the importance of providing adequate information [36]. However, as with all other chronic pain conditions, a biopysychosocial approach is crucial especially in those patients who have pain beyond the TMJ area.

Cost and feasibility of treatment/ cost benefit

There are a variety of studies that have looked at direct costs based mainly on the production of some form of appliances. In 1995 it was estimated that 2.9% of the US total expenditure on dental services was on production of occlusal appliances and it was estimated that the minimum cost of treating TMD sufferers is $400 per year. There are also indirect costs associated with time off work or decreased work efficiency and it is estimated that

these are similar to those of back pain and headache sufferers.

Future directions

There is a need to look again at the diagnostic criteria and classification of TMD pain and to reach consensus so that improved RCT are designed for many of the treatments in current use. Long-term cohort studies are needed to determine prognosis as well as risk factors. A holistic approach is required as many TMD patients are also chronic pain sufferers.

Author's recommendations

The majority of patients with TMD consult a dentist and they tend to provide physical treatments which in many cases appear to be effective. However, this is much more likely to be a reflection of the natural history of the condition. It is essential that TMD patients have a careful assessment which includes psychosocial factors and takes into account the presence of other chronic pain sites. The small minority of patients who cannot be managed by careful explanation and education need a course of CBT. The CBT should be delivered at the start of management, possibly in combination with an antidepressant, and not at the end when all other treatments have been tried.

Trigeminal neuralgia

Background

Trigeminal neuralgia is classified as a neuropathic pain but it has some very specific features that make it a fairly unique type of facial pain.

The International Association for the Study of Pain (IASP) defines trigeminal neuralgia as "a sudden and usually unilateral severe brief stabbing recurrent pain in the distribution of one or more branches of the fifth cranial nerve" [46]. Trigeminal neuralgia is classified broadly into idiopathic and secondary forms. Secondary trigeminal neuralgia includes that due to any form of tumor, benign or malignant, multiple sclerosis or arteriovenous malformations.

Trigeminal neuralgia is probably the only nondental facial pain that can be managed highly successfully with a variety of surgical procedures. It is therefore very important to be able to distinguish this pain from other forms of facial pain which do not respond to surgical management. Although it is a condition managed primarily by neurologists and neurosurgeons, many patients first see a dentist as they perceive their pain to be of dental origin. This leads to misdiagnosis, unnecessary dental extractions (in up to 60%) and delays in treatment.

Etiology

The exact etiology of trigeminal neuralgia is still unknown but considerable progress has been made in recent years to put forward a mechanism for this pain. Most researchers would agree that in the majority of patients with classic trigeminal neuralgia, the pain is generated due to compression of the trigeminal nerve in most instances by vascular structures but in a small proportion due to other causes. The compression is most likely to occur at the so-called root entry zone which is defined as the point at which the peripheral and central myelin of the Schwann cells and astrocytes meet. Compression of the nerve at this point results in plaques of demyelination. Nerve injury results in hyperexcitability of injured afferents which result in after-discharges large enough to result in a non-nociceptive signal being perceived as pain. This leads to wind-up and both peripheral and central sensitization.

This theory has been put forward by Devor *et al.* and is known as the ignition theory hypothesis [47]. It is supported by electron microscopy appearances of the trigeminal nerve taken from patients with trigeminal neuralgia [48] and they also showed evidence of remyelination which could result in the pain remissions that are so characteristic of this condition. However, not all patients are found to have compression of the trigeminal nerve and even if found, not all patients have 100% pain relief for the duration of their life. There are likely to be other factors involved, given the rarity of the disease, and there may be genetic causes.

Epidemiology

Trigeminal neuralgia is considered a rare condition and until recently its crude annual incidence was reported as 5.7 for women and 2.5 for men per 100,000. However, a community-based London study put it at 8 per 100,000. The peak incidence has been reported as being in the 50–60 age group and increases with age. A more recent study using general practice research databases in the UK suggested

a prevalence of 26.4 per 100,000 [49]. However, the diagnostic criteria were very broad and therefore may have included other patients with unilateral facial pain. The major risk factor for trigeminal neuralgia is multiple sclerosis.

Clinical features

Although on the face of it, classic trigeminal neuralgia is easily diagnosed, it has long been recognized that there are other forms of trigeminal neuralgia which most frequently have been called atypical trigeminal neuralgia. Neurosurgeons have suggested that these two forms should be called type 1 and type 2 [50]. The atypical forms are more difficult to differentiate from other forms of unilateral pain and may also be associated with some form of trigeminal neuropathy, as suggested by Nurmikko & Eldridge [51].

The major differentiator between classic and atypical trigeminal neuralgia is in the character and its timing. Patients with classic trigeminal neuralgia report just a sharp shooting electric shock-like pain that lasts for a few seconds and may be repeated many times a day. After weeks or months, a period of complete pain remission may result which may last weeks or months. The atypical trigeminal neuralgia patients also have a sharp shooting electric shock but they have a burning, dull, aching after-pain. In some patients this just lasts for several minutes to a few hours and then gradually disappears, leaving a completely pain-free period. Other patients, however, report that this after-pain is persistent and there is no completely pain-free interval. It is this latter type of pain that may not respond as effectively to surgical management. It is postulated that this pain may be a continuation of the original condition. However, it could have a different etiology and therefore represent another disease form. There is currently no evidence of sufficient quality to support these theories. It has been suggested that many patients with trigeminal neuralgia will report a memorable onset and neurosurgeons have gone so far as to suggest that this could be a prognostic factor for improved outcomes.

The following clinical features are consistent with those published by the IHS [11] and IASP [46].

- Site: along one or more divisions of the trigeminal nerve, unilateral only, 3% bilateral
- Radiation: within trigeminal nerve

- Character: shooting, sharp, stabbing, electric shock-like, may be some burning
- Severity: usually severe but can be mild
- Duration: each attack lasts for seconds to maximum 2 minutes but attacks can follow in rapid succession
- Periodicity: paroxysmal with periods of complete pain remission which gradually get shorter
- Provoking factors: daily activities such as eating, talking, washing the face or cleaning the teeth but can be spontaneous
- Relieving factors: avoiding trigger factors, drugs
- Associated factors: stereotype attacks in the individual patient

Trigeminal neuralgia is relatively rare in only the first division and if it is reported as being present only in the first division then other causes should be carefully ascertained such as paroxysmal hemicrania, SUNCT (short-lasting unilateral neuralgiform headaches with conjunctival tearing) or SUNA (short-lasting neuralgiform pain with autonomic symptoms). It is important to note whether the pain is evoked by light touch activities and/or whether it occurs spontaneously as drugs may be more effective in reducing the number of spontaneous attacks. This is of considerable significance, as it is these spontaneous attacks that are more likely to reduce quality of life and make patients live in fear of having an attack at a time when they are away from their usual sources of support. Although the pain can be mild, there are reports of patients committing suicide due to the severity of this pain. Many patients with trigeminal neuralgia report the severity of their pain being worse during the day and only a third of patients will report experiencing pain at night resulting in awakening. There is evidence to suggest that trigeminal neuralgia patients will develop depression which will lift once the pain is successfully managed [52].

On examination, many patients will exhibit no neurologic deficit. However, this may be very subtle and may change with time. Sensory testing is essential as this will potentially differentiate between symptomatic and idiopathic trigeminal neuralgia. Patients will exhibit trigger areas from which pain is initiated and this could be classified as a form of allodynia.

Investigations

Currently there are no objective investigations that can be used to validate the clinical findings.

Radiologic investigations are important to differentiate between symptomatic and idiopathic trigeminal neuralgia. MRI is used to identify neurovascular compressions and needs to be of high quality in order to identify them. There are only a few studies that are of high enough quality to provide evidence for its use.

Sensory testing is not done routinely but there is evidence to suggest that qualitative sensory testing (QST) and evoked potentials may play an important role in differentiating between symptomatic and idiopathic trigeminal neuralgia [53, 54].

Management

Evidence-based guidelines have now been published on diagnosis and management [53, 54]. All patients will initially be treated medically but many will proceed to surgical management. There is currently insufficient evidence to suggest at which time point patients should be transferred from medical to surgical treatments or which is the most successful surgical treatment. There are no RCT of the major forms of surgical management that are in current use. Trials in trigeminal neuralgia are difficult to conduct due to a variety of factors including the rarity of the condition, its paroxysmal nature and the difficulty of using a placebo as opposed to an active form of control.

Intervention supported by evidence

There are Cochrane systematic reviews on the use of anticonvulsant drugs in neuropathic pain which include trials of patients with trigeminal neuralgia and there is a separate Cochrane review on nonepileptic drugs in the use of trigeminal neuralgia [55-57] as well as a regularly updated online entry in *Clinical Evidence* [58]. Many of these trials are small, conducted in the era when RCT had less rigorous quality controls. The largest number of RCT have been done on carbamazepine and there is good evidence to show that this drug is highly effective in patients with classic trigeminal neuralgia.

Oxcarbazepine, which is a daughter drug of carbamazepine, has been evaluated in RCT and a small systematic review (all abstracts) comparing it to carbamazepine. It has some improved efficacy over carbamazepine and much better tolerability. Oxcarbazepine has a much lower potential for drug interactions as it does not rely on the liver cytochrome system. A small RCT using gabapentin in combination with five ropivicaine injections on a weekly basis showed this drug to be highly effective [59].

There are no high-quality studies on the use of polypharmacy, as often done in epilepsy.

Interventions refuted by evidence

A number of drugs used in RCT are ineffective or their side effect profile is severe enough to exclude their use: tocainide, tizanidine and pimozide [55]. There are two RCT of the use of streptomycin injections at trigger points which were shown to be ineffective [60].

Commonly used interventions currently unproven

Pregabalin, which has been licensed for use in neuropathic pain, has been shown to be effective in a cohort study [62].

A systematic review of the literature on surgical management has been carried out and only those studies which have used independent observers to assess outcomes have been used to provide evidence [53, 54, 61].

Surgical management can be carried out at three different levels. Peripheral treatments are carried out at trigger points and have included a range of treatments such as cryotherapy, laser therapy, alcohol injections and neurectomies. All provide only short-term pain relief, mostly under 1 year.

There is a range of other ablative procedures, the majority at the level of the Gasserian ganglion, which aim to reduce sensory transmission and hence pain. A needle is passed through the foramen ovale under radiographic control. Once within the ganglion, one of three procedures can be carried out. The nerve can be subjected to radiofrequency thermocoagulation using temperatures between 60° and 90°C, it can be bathed in glycerol or compressed by a Foley catheter balloon. The results are fairly similar and the median pain relief period is 4–5 years. All will result in varying degrees of sensory deficit and other trigeminal nerve injuries are also reported. Aseptic meningitis and temporary diplopia are reported as well as arrhythmias when performing balloon compressions. The results are summarized in Table 12.3.

Posterior fossa procedures are either ablative or nondestructive. The ablative procedure is that of gamma knife radiation which is the least invasive of all the procedures. A recent study by Regis *et al.* [63], which is a cohort study with independent observers, suggested that the results are similar to those of other ablative procedures with similar pain relief periods but only 10% of patients report some form of sensory loss.

The currently most favored procedure is microvascular decompression. This is a major neurosurgical procedure that involves entry into the posterior fossa, identification of the vascular compression and dislodging the vessel/s from the trigeminal nerve. This can be achieved either by the use of Teflon or by making vascular slings to keep the offending vessels away from the nerve. At 10 years 70% of patients may still remain pain free but most recurrences occur within the first 2 years. As this is a major surgical procedure, it can result in the usual complications such as pulmonary emboli and gastrointestinal bleeds. It is associated with 0.4–0.5% mortality and a very small number of patients may suffer cerebral infarcts and hemorrhage, resulting in strokes. Immediate postoperative complications include meningitis, both bacterial and aseptic, and CSF leaks. The major neurologic deficit is ipsilateral hearing loss due to either damage to the mastoid air cells or trauma to the eighth nerve itself. The satisfaction of patients undergoing this procedure is high and up to 75% will report complete satisfaction after a mean of 5 years follow-up [64]. Patients in whom no nerve compression is found may have a partial sensory rhizotomy performed and this will then result in sensory loss. Pain recurrence rates appear to be similar but patients are highly likely to have sensory loss which reduces their quality of life [64].

There are now several national support groups, e.g. in the US, UK and Australia, which provide patients with information through a variety of means – books [65, 66], internet, email, phone lines and conferences – and there is anecdotal evidence that they are effective not only in providing information but in putting sufferers in touch with each other and so lessening their fears and loneliness [66].

Discussion of evidence

There is relatively good evidence to support the use of a variety of drugs.

Carbamazepine is the gold standard despite its high level of side effects and potential for drug interactions.

All patients are likely to suffer side effects when on high doses of carbamazepine and therefore it needs to be used at the lowest level possible to achieve pain control. Oxcarbazepine is therefore a very useful alternative [53, 54].

A decision analysis study using 156 patients with trigeminal neuralgia showed that they preferred surgical management to medical but the stage at which this change should be done has not been determined. Of the surgical procedures, there is a very slight preference for microvascular decompression. However, many patients fear this operation and therefore may not choose it until their pain becomes unbearable. From independent case series reports, there is some evidence to suggest that microvascular decompression is a successful form of treatment for trigeminal neuralgia. In those patients who do not want to undergo major surgery or are not fit for it then the ablative procedures at the Gasserian ganglion level can lead to acceptable pain relief and freedom from the need to use drugs.

Cost and feasibility of treatment/ cost benefit

There is very little evidence for this, although there has been one study comparing cost feasibility between gamma knife surgery and other neurosurgical procedures. The long-term use of drug therapy and the need for regular monitoring need to be taken into account when compared to surgical procedures which may initially be more costly but do not require such intensive patient follow-up.

Future directions

It is essential to clarify the diagnostic criteria of the different forms of trigeminal neuralgia and perform long-term cohort studies to see how the clinical features change over time. More epidemiologic studies are needed to define the prevalence and potential risk factors and risk groups as this could help to determine preventive procedures and to provide details on prognosis. Newer anticonvulsant drugs or drugs which address the mechanisms of neuropathic pain need to be evaluated in RCT, taking into account the severity and paroxysmal nature of this condition. There is also an urgent need to address the surgical management of trigeminal neuralgia by innovative ways of looking at RCT, given that there is no current evidence to suggest one technique as being superior to others. More basic science research, including genetic studies, is urgently needed. Some of the research needs in this field are summarized in *Insights* [66].

Author's recommendations

Care needs to be taken in eliciting and recording the clinical features of trigeminal neuralgia so the correct treatment is offered. The first-line drug should be carbamazepine but as soon as it loses efficacy or becomes poorly tolerated, other drugs such as oxcarbazepine should be used. Patients should be investigated with MRI and referred for an early surgical opinion so they have time to think through the variety of treatment options available. In patients who are medically fit and have a identifiable compression on MRI, microvascular decompression is the most satisfactory procedure when performed by a skilled neurosurgeon.

Whenever possible, patients should be provided with information about patient support groups and the range of literature that is available to them. A well-informed patient is likely to achieve better pain control and be more satisfied with outcomes.

References

1. Macfarlane TV, Kincey J, Worthington HV. The association between psychological factors and oro-facial pain: a community-based study. *Eur J Pain* 2002; **6**: 427–434.
2. Turp JC. *Temporomandibular Pain - Clinical Presentation and Impact.* Quintessenz Verlags-GmbH, Berlin, 2000.
3. Woda A, Tubert-Jeannin S, Bouhassira D, *et al.* Towards a new taxonomy of idiopathic orofacial pain. *Pain* 2005; **116**: 396–406.
4. Zakrzewska JM. Facial pain: an update. *Curr Opin Support Palliat Care* 2009; **3**: 125–130.
5. Zakrzewska JM, Harrison SD *Assessment and Management of Orofacial Pain.* Elsevier Science, Amsterdam, 2002.
6. Zakrzewska JM. *Orofacial Pain.* Oxford, Oxford University Press, 2009.
7. Elrasheed AA, Worthington HV, Ariyaratnam S, Duxbury AJ. Opinions of UK specialists about terminology, diagnosis, and treatment of atypical facial pain: a survey. *Br J Oral Maxillofac Surg* 2004; **42**: 566–571.
8. Zakrzewska JM, Hamlyn PJ. Facial pain. In: Crombie I, Linton SJ, LeResche L, von Korff M (eds) *Epidemiology of Pain.* IASP Press, Seattle, 1999: 171–202.

9. Aggarwal VR, Lunt M, Zakrzewska JM, Macfarlane GJ, Macfarlane TV. Development and validation of the Manchester orofacial pain disability scale. *Community Dent Oral Epidemiol* 2005; **33**: 141–149.

10. Feinmann C. The long-term outcome of facial pain treatment. *J Psychosom Res* 1993; **37**: 381–387.

11. International Headache Society. The International Classification of Headache Disorders. *Cephalalgia* 2004; **2**(suppl 1): 9–160.

12. Zebenholzer K, Wober C, Vigl M, Wessely P, Wober-Bingol C. Facial pain in a neurological tertiary care centre – evaluation of the International Classification of Headache Disorders. *Cephalalgia* 2005; **25**: 689–699.

13. McQuay HJ, Tramer M, Nye BA, Carroll D, Wiffen PJ, Moore RA. A systematic review of antidepressants in neuropathic pain. *Pain* 1996; **68**: 217–227.

14. Saarto T, Wiffen PJ. Antidepressants for neuropathic pain. Cochrane Database of Systematic Reviews 2007, Issue 4. Art. No.: CD005454. DOI: 10.1002/14651858.CD005454.pub2.

15. Feinmann C, Harris M. Psychogenic facial pain. Part 2: Management and prognosis. *Br Dent J* 1984; **156**: 205–208.

16. Harrison SD, Glover L, Feinmann C, Pearce SA, Harris M. A comparison of antidepressant medication alone and in conjunction with cognitive behavioural therapy for chronic idiopathic facial pain. In: Jensen TS, Turner JA, Wiesenfeld-Hallin Z. *Proceedings of the 8th World Congress on Pain. Progress in Pain Research and Management.* IASP Press, Seattle, 1997: 663–672.

17. Lascelles RG. Atypical facial pain and depression. *Br J Psychiatry* 1966; **112**: 651–659.

18. List T, Axelsson S, Leijon G. Pharmacologic interventions in the treatment of temporomandibular disorders, atypical facial pain, and burning mouth syndrome. A qualitative systematic review. *J Orofac Pain* 2003; **17**: 301–310.

19. Sharav Y, Singer E, Schmidt E, Dionne RA, Dubner R. The analgesic effect of amitriptyline on chronic facial pain. *Pain* 1987; **31**: 199–209.

20. Forsell H, Tasmuth T, Tenovuo O, Hampf G, Kalso E. Venlafaxine in the treatment of atypical facial pain: a randomized controlled trial. *J Orofac Pain* 2004; **18**: 131–137.

21. al Balawi S, Tariq M, Feinmann C. A double-blind, placebo-controlled, crossover, study to evaluate the efficacy of subcutaneous sumatriptan in the treatment of atypical facial pain. *Int J Neurosci* 1996; **86**: 301–309.

22. Williams AC. Cognitive behavioral treatment.In: Dostrovsky JO, Carr DB, Koltzenburg M (eds) *Proceedings of the 10th World Congress on Pain.* IASP Press, Seattle, 2003: 825–837.

23. Dworkin SF, LeResche L. Research diagnostic criteria for temporomandibular disorders: review, criteria, examinations and specifications, critique. *J Craniomandib Disord* 1992; **6**: 301–355.

24. Drangsholt M, LeResche L. Temporomandibular disorder pain. In: Crombie I, Linton SJ, LeResche L, von Korff M (eds) *Epidemiology of Pain.* IASP Press, Seattle, 1999: 203–233.

25. Laskin DM, Greene CS, Hylander WL. *TMDs: An Evidence-Based Approach to Diagnosis and Treatment.* Quintessence, New Malden, Surrey, 2006.

26. Gesch D, Bernhardt O, Kirbschus A. Association of malocclusion and functional occlusion with temporomandibular disorders (TMD) in adults: a systematic review of population-based studies. *Quintessence Int* 2004; **35**: 211–221.

27. von Korff M, Dworkin SF, LeResche L. Graded chronic pain status: an epidemiologic evaluation. *Pain* 1990; **40**: 279–291.

28. Antczak-Bouckoms AA. Epidemiology of research for temporomandibular disorders. *J Orofac Pain* 1995; **9**: 226–234.

29. Dworkin SF, Turner JA, Mancl L, et al. A randomized clinical trial of a tailored comprehensive care treatment program for temporomandibular disorders. *J Orofac Pain* 2002; **16**: 259–276.

30. Gardea MA, Gatchel RJ, Mishra KD. Long-term efficacy of biobehavioral treatment of temporomandibular disorders. *J Behav Med* 2001; **24**: 341–359.

31. Mishra KD, Gatchel RJ, Gardea MA. The relative efficacy of three cognitive-behavioral treatment approaches to temporomandibular disorders. *J Behav Med* 2000; **23**: 293–309.

32. Turner JA, Mancl L, Aaron LA. Short- and long-term efficacy of brief cognitive-behavioral therapy for patients with chronic temporomandibular disorder pain: a randomized, controlled trial. *Pain* 2006; **121**: 181–194.

33. Gatchel RJ, Stowell AW, Wildenstein L, Riggs R, Ellis E III. Efficacy of an early intervention for patients with acute temporomandibular disorder-related pain: a one-year outcome study. *J Am Dent Assoc* 2006; **137**: 339–347.

34. Al-Ani MZ, Davies SJ, Gray RJM, Sloan P, Glenny AM. Stabilisation splint therapy for temporomandibular pain dysfunction syndrome. Cochrane Database of Systematic Reviews 2004, Issue 1. Art. No.: CD002778. DOI: 10.1002/14651858.CD002778.pub2.

35. Forsell H, Kalso E, Koskela P, Vehmanen R, Puukka P, Alanen P. Occlusal treatments in temporomandibular disorders: a qualitative systematic review of randomized controlled trials. *Pain* 1999; **83**: 549–560.

36. De Boever JA, Nilner M, Orthlieb JD et al. Recommendations by the EACD for examination, diagnosis, and management of patients with temporomandibular disorders and orofacial pain by the general dental practitioner. *J Orofac Pain* 2008; **22**: 268–278.

37. Gerschman JA, Reade PD, Burrows GD. Evaluation of a proprietary analgesic/antihistamine in the management of pain associated with temporomandibular joint pain dysfunction syndrome. *Aust Dent J* 1984; **29**: 300–304.

38. Singer E, Dionne R. A controlled evaluation of ibuprofen and diazepam for chronic orofacial muscle pain. *J Orofac Pain* 1997; **11**: 139–146.

39. Plesh O, Curtis D, Levine J, McCall WD Jr. Amitriptyline treatment of chronic pain in patients with temporomandibular disorders. *J Oral Rehabil* 2000; **27**: 834–841.

40. Koh H, Robinson P. Occlusal adjustment for treating and preventing temporomandibular joint disorders. Cochrane Database of Systematic Reviews 2003, Issue 1. Art. No.: CD003812. DOI: 10.1002/14651858.CD003812.

41. Jedel E, Carlsson J. Biofeedback, acupuncture and transcutaneous electric nerve stimulation in the management of temperomandibular disorders: a systematic review. *Phys Ther Rev* 2003; **8**: 217–223.

42. Ernst E, White AR. Acupuncture as a treatment for temporomandibular joint dysfunction: a systematic review of randomized trials. *Arch Otolaryngol Head Neck Surg* 1999; **125**: 269–272.

43. Harkins S, Linford J, Cohen J, Kramer T, Cueva L. Administration of clonazepam in the treatment of TMD and associated myofascial pain: a double-blind pilot study. *J Craniomandib Disord* 1991; **5**: 179–186.

44. Nixdorf DR, Heo G, Major PW. Randomized controlled trial of botulinum toxin A for chronic myogenous orofacial pain. *Pain* 2002; **99**: 465–473.

45. Ohrbach R, Sherman J. Temporomandibular disorders. In: Dworkin RH, Breitbart WS (eds) *Psychosocial Aspects of Pain: A Handbook for Health Care Providers.* IASP Press, Seattle, 2004: 405–425.

46. Merskey H, Bogduk N. *Classification of Chronic Pain. Descriptors of Chronic Pain Syndromes and Definitions of Pain Terms*, 2nd edn. IASP Press, Seattle, 1994.

47. Devor M, Amir R, Rappaport ZH. Pathophysiology of trigeminal neuralgia: the ignition hypothesis. *Clin J Pain* 2002; **18**: 4–13.

48. Love S, Coakham HB. Trigeminal neuralgia: pathology and pathogenesis. *Brain* 2001; **124**: 2347–2360.

49. Hall GC, Carroll D, Parry D, McQuay HJ. Epidemiology and treatment of neuropathic pain: the UK primary care perspective. *Pain* 2006; **122**: 156–162.

50. Eller JL, Raslan AM, Burchiel KJ. Trigeminal neuralgia: definition and classification. *Neurosurg Focus* 2005; **18**: E3.

51. Nurmikko TJ, Eldridge PR. Trigeminal neuralgia – pathophysiology, diagnosis and current treatment. *Br J Anaesth* 2001; **87**: 117–132.

52. Zakrzewska JM, Sawsan J, Bulman JS. A prospective, longitudinal study on patients with trigeminal neuralgia who underwent radiofrequency thermocoagulation of the Gasserian ganglion. *Pain* 1999; **79**: 51–58.

53. Cruccu G, Gronseth G, Alksne J *et al.* AAN-EFNS guidelines on trigeminal neuralgia management. *Eur J Neurol* 2008; **15**: 1013–1028.

54. Gronseth G, Cruccu G, Alksne J *et al.* Practice parameter: the diagnostic evaluation and treatment of trigeminal neuralgia (an evidence-based review): report of the Quality Standards Subcommittee of the American Academy of Neurology and the European Federation of Neurological Societies. *Neurology* 2008; **71**: 1183–1190.

55. Wiffen PJ, Collins S, McQuay HJ, Carroll D, Jadad A, Moore RA. Anticonvulsant drugs for acute and chronic pain. Cochrane Database of Systematic Reviews 2005, Issue 3. Art. No.: CD001133. DOI: 10.1002/14651858.CD001133.pub2.

56. Wiffen PJ, McQuay HJ, Moore RA. Carbamazepine for acute and chronic pain in adults. Cochrane Database of Systematic Reviews 2005, Issue 3. Art. No.: CD005451. DOI: 10.1002/14651858.CD005451.

57. He L, Wu B, Zhou M. Non-antiepileptic drugs for trigeminal neuralgia. Cochrane Database of Systematic Reviews 2006, Issue 3. Art. No.: CD004029. DOI: 10.1002/14651858. CD004029.pub2.

58. Zakrzewska JM, Linskey ME. Trigeminal neuralgia. *Clin Evid (Online)* 2009; pii, 1207.

59. Lemos L, Flores S, Oliveira P *et al.* Gabapentin supplemented with ropivacain block of trigger points improves pain control and quality of life in trigeminal neuralgia patients when compared with gabapentin alone. *Clin J Pain* 2008; **24**: 64–75.

60. Zakrzewska JM. Trigeminal neuralgia. In: Zakrzewska JM, Harrison SD (eds) *Assessment and Management of Orofacial Pain.* Elsevier Sciences, Amsterdam, 2002: 267–370.

61. Zakrzewska JM, Lopez BC. Quality of reporting in evaluations of surgical treatment of trigeminal neuralgia: recommendations for future reports. *Neurosurgery* 2003; **53**: 110–122.

62. Obermann M, Yoon MS, Sensen K *et al.* Efficacy of pregabalin in the treatment of trigeminal neuralgia. *Cephalalgia* 2008; **28**: 174–181.

63. Regis J, Metellus P, Hayashi M, Roussel P, Donnet A, Bille-Turc F. Prospective controlled trial of gamma knife surgery for essential trigeminal neuralgia. *J Neurosurg* 2006; **104**: 913–924.

64. Zakrzewska JM, Lopez BC, Kim SE, Coakham HB. Patient reports of satisfaction after microvascular decompression and partial sensory rhizotomy for trigeminal neuralgia. *Neurosurgery* 2005; **56**: 1304–1311.

65. Weigel G, Casey KF. *Striking Back. The Trigeminal Neuralgia Handbook.* Trigeminal Neuralgia Association, Gainesville, FL, 2000.

66. Zakrzewska JM. *Insights: Facts and Stories Behind Trigeminal Neuralgia.* Trigeminal Neuralgia Association, Gainesville, FL, 2006.

CHAPTER 13

Pelvic and perineal pain in women

William Stones[1] and Beverly Collett[2]

[1] Department of Obstetrics and Gynaecology, Aga Khan University Hospital, Nairobi, Kenya
[2] Pain Management Service, University Hospitals of Leicester, Leicester, UK

Pathophysiology of chronic pelvic and perineal pain in women

A classic clinical observation in women presenting with chronic pelvic pain is the poor correlation between identifiable pathologic processes, the chronicity and severity of pain and the impact of symptoms on quality of life.

This is exemplified by endometriosis, a condition affecting women predominantly in the reproductive age group and characterized by the presence of endometrial glands and stroma outside the endometrial cavity. The condition is thought to arise mainly by implantation of endometrial tissue following retrograde menstruation via the fallopian tubes [1]. It presents a clinical spectrum, with endometriotic deposits sometimes observed at laparoscopy in the absence of symptoms or tissue damage, through subfertility apparently associated with endometriosis but in the absence of pain, to chronic pain associated with disabling pain symptoms and often gross damage to the pelvic organs through abnormal invasion of endometriotic deposits into the pelvic tissues, neovascularization and adhesion formation. In a series of asymptomatic multiparous patients undergoing sterilization, the prevalence was 26/3384 (3.7%) [2]. There is a relationship between the depth of invasion of endometriosis and the intensity of pain symptoms,

established with some difficulty through small but detailed histopathologic studies [3]. In this study nerve fibers could usually be identified in specimens of deeply invading endometriosis. Pain was present in 17% of those with deposits invading <2 mm, 53% of those with 2–4 mm deposits, 37% of those with 5–10 mm deposits and all six women with very deep deposits of >10 mm. No wholly reliable predictive set of criteria has emerged from studies of symptom profiles. Only the severity of dysmenorrhea was useful in predicting the diagnosis of endometriosis at laparoscopy [4].

Based on a study of uterine specimens removed at hysterectomy for endometriosis, other forms of chronic pelvic pain and for nonpain indications, Atwal *et al.* proposed a concept of reinnervation and microneuroma formation as a mechanism for uterine pain and tenderness, with these features being seen in specimens from patients with painful conditions but not in those from patients without pelvic pain [5]. The study did not proceed to characterize the neurotransmitter profile of the nerves which may have given further information about the sensory processes and pathways involved. The neurotransmitter expression of nerves growing into experimental implants in a rat model mimicking endometriosis did indicate the presence of both autonomic and sensory components [6].

Some of the above may be explained by the extent to which pathologic processes are associated with the release of inflammatory mediators, which again may reflect biologic variations in the response to tissue damage. Immune hypotheses have been proposed in relation to endometriosis, but there are

Evidence-Based Chronic Pain Management. Edited by C. Stannard, E. Kalso and J. Ballantyne. © 2010 Blackwell Publishing.

no data to link specific patterns of host response with symptoms. Although mechanisms of visceral nociception have been clarified through animal experimental studies of the feline bladder [7], and processes such as activation of silent afferents following inflammation have been demonstrated, there is a dearth of evidence as to the place of such mechanisms in the pathophysiology of abnormal visceral sensation in women. Nevertheless, in the clinical setting, it is a frequent observation that chronic pain can develop following infection that has apparently resolved, which may point to processes such as the activation of silent afferents. Chlamydial infection, in particular, is often associated with tissue damage in the absence of acute symptoms and may account for visceral sensitization. Adhesions may form after inflammation due to sepsis, following surgery and may be associated with endometriosis. Innervation of adhesion tissue has been described [8]. However, any causal relationship with pain symptoms is unclear.

Vulvodynia is a chronic disorder in women, characterized by provoked or constant vulvar pain of varying intensity without obvious concomitant clinical pathology. Two subsets of vulvodynia are recognized: generalized and localized pain subtypes, the latter currently referred to as vestibulodynia or vestibulitis.

With regard to vulval or perineal pain, trauma is often suspected as a causal factor in the pathogenesis, whether during childbirth or through injury to the pelvis. Again, such episodes may be coincidental. Nerve conduction studies to assess damage to the pudendal innervation have proved of marginal value in clinical practice. A syndrome of entrapment of the pudendal nerve in Alcock's canal has been described [9]. It is not clear whether neuropathic processes are involved in this proposed mechanism, what the impact of surgical intervention is on the conduction properties of afferent fibers and whether central sensitization is a feature of the clinical presentation.

Immune and inflammatory mediators have been considered in the pathogenesis of endometriosis and have also received much attention in the case of vulval vestibulitis or vestibulodynia.

As with endometriosis, it is unclear whether the primary problem is inflammation or the associated nociceptive processes. Evidence for the latter is the observation in a functional MRI study of increased cerebral neuronal activity during painful vulval vestibular stimulation among patients with vulval vestibulitis syndrome compared with that seen among controls [10]. At the tissue level there is evidence for neuronal proliferation [11] but no excess of cyclo-oxygenase or inducible nitric oxide activity [12]. Previous causative hypotheses around human papillomavirus or herpes genitalis infection have been discounted in molecular studies of clinical biopsy specimens.

Pelvic muscle spasm may be a feature of chronic pelvic pain [13] and it is often difficult to establish whether this is the primary problem or is a natural response to the presence of pelvic tenderness arising from another condition such as endometriosis. Spasm of the levators certainly contributes to additional distressing symptoms such as urinary retention, constipation and dyspareunia.

A vascular pain mechanism, pelvic venous congestion, has been proposed as a cause of chronic pelvic pain and relevant endothelially mediated vascular pain mechanisms have been demonstrated in human studies. There are questions about the association between pain symptoms and particular radiologic or ultrasound appearances that have become somewhat more difficult to interpret with the advent of interest among interventional radiologists in embolization of "pelvic varices" [14].

Hormonal factors are important mediators of nociception in both animal and human experimental models. Variations of pain threshold and behavior were demonstrated in relation to sex hormone exposure in rats at different stages of the estrus cycle. Responses to distension of the uterus and vagina and pain behaviors overall showed heightened responsiveness during metestrus and diestrous compared to proestrus and estrus [15]. Meta-analysis of studies of women undergoing experimental exposure to different pain modalities at different stages of the menstrual cycle indicated an effect size of 0.40 for variation in pain sensitivity between the most and least sensitive phase [16].

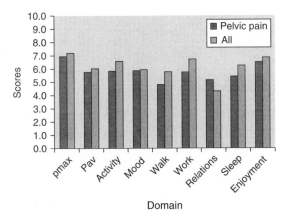

Figure 13.1 Pain intensity among UK pain clinic patients with chronic pain (all causes) and women with chronic pelvic pain [19].

As with chronic pain in general, genetic factors may give rise to susceptibility to pelvic pain. In clinical genetic epidemiologic studies, it is difficult to distinguish between genetic susceptibility to a condition such as endometriosis, that may give rise to pain, and susceptibility to pain *per se*. In an Australian cohort of female twins who were questioned on two occasions 8 years apart, the longitudinally stable variance attributable to genetic and environmental factors could be calculated. Whereas 39% of the variance in reported menstrual flow was accounted for by genetic factors, the corresponding figure for dysmenorrhea was 55%, and for functional limitation from menstrual symptoms was 77% [17]. Using the same twin cohort, the genetic contributions to endometriosis and somatic distress (as a proxy for nociception) were 38% and 15% respectively [18].

Once patients with chronic pelvic and vulval pain reach the stage of assessment in a pain clinic, it appears that the pattern of symptom impact is similar to that seen in other chronic painful conditions in terms of severity and lifestyle impact (Fig. 13.1). It remains a clinical challenge to individualize assessment and treatment either to focus on "specific" pathologies such as endometriosis or to emphasize pain management and understanding of the pathophysiology as discussed above. Best clinical practice suggests an approach that recognizes both dimensions.

Table 13.1 Classification of causes of chronic pelvic pain. Reproduced from Stones [20].

Inflammatory, infective
Chronic salpingitis

Inflammatory, noninfective
Endometriosis
Vulvodynia with dermatosis

Mechanical
Uterine retroversion
Adhesions

Functional
Pelvic congestion
Irritable bowel syndrome

Neuropathic
Postsurgical
Dysesthetic vulvodynia
Vulval vestibulodynia

Musculoskeletal
Pelvic floor myalgia
Abdominal and pelvic trigger points
Postural muscle strain

Classification of the causes of pelvic pain

Table 13.1 shows the classification of the causes of chronic pelvic pain.

Epidemiology of chronic pelvic and vulval/perineal pain in women

Population data on pain prevalence in women are available. A US-based telephone survey interviewed respondents aged 18–50 years [21]; 17,927 households were contacted, 5325 women agreed to participate, and of these 925 reported pelvic pain of at least 6 months' duration, including pain within the past 3 months. Having excluded those pregnant or postmenopausal and those with only cycle-related pain, 773/5263 (14.7%) were identified as suffering from chronic pelvic pain. A British population survey used a postal sample of 2016 women randomly selected from the Oxfordshire Health Authority register of 141,400 women aged 18–49 years [22]. Chronic pelvic pain was defined as recurrent pain of at least

6 months' duration, unrelated to periods, intercourse or pregnancy. For the survey, a "case" was defined as a woman with chronic pelvic pain in the previous 3 months, and on this basis the prevalence was 483/2016 (24.0%). There were significant associations between chronic pelvic pain and the specific symptoms of dysmenorrhea and dyspareunia.

In the setting of UK primary care consultations, data from 284,162 women aged 12–70 years who had a general practice contact in 1991 were analyzed to identify subsequent contacts over the following 5 years [23]. The monthly prevalence rate was 21.5/1000 and the monthly incidence rate was 1.58/1000. The authors highlighted the burden of disease represented by these data, pointing out the comparability with migraine, back pain and asthma in primary care. Older women had higher monthly prevalence rates: for example, the rate was 18.2/1000 in the 15–20 year age group and 27.6/1000 in women over 60 years of age. This association was thought to be due to persistence of symptoms in older women, the median duration of symptoms being 13.7 months in 13–20 year olds and 20.2 months in women over 60 years [24].

The presence of symptoms does not necessarily reflect healthcare seeking. This was highlighted in the UK population survey described above: of 483 women with chronic pelvic pain, 195 (40.4%) had not sought a medical consultation, 127 (26.3%) reported a past consultation and 139 (28.8%) reported a recent consultation for pain [25]. The US telephone survey discussed above also drew attention to the large numbers of women with symptoms who do not seek medical attention. Seventy-five percent of this sample had not seen a healthcare provider in the previous 3 months.

With regard to vulval pain, the single available population-based sample survey was undertaken in Boston, USA [26]. Census records were used to sample 4915 women aged 18–64 years using a self-administered questionnaire. Approximately 16% of respondents reported histories of chronic burning, knife-like pain or pain on contact that lasted for at least 3 months or longer. These symptoms were present in nearly 7% at the time of the survey. As with the pelvic pain surveys discussed above, a substantial proportion of women reported that they had not sought treatment. Of those who did seek healthcare,

60% saw three or more doctors but a positive diagnosis was frequently absent.

Risk factors

Consideration of risk factors for chronic pelvic and perineal pain necessitates a recognition of the complex interplay of pathophysiologic processes discussed above, reproductive history and status, the psychologic mediators of the impact of adverse life experiences, and co-morbidity such as depression. Typically, in the literature the direction of causality is difficult to establish. As an example, depression may be a risk factor for chronic pain, or at least for greater symptom impact, while chronic pain may naturally give rise to mood disturbance. In the early literature, an attempt was made to separate physical from psychologic processes. In more recent studies, the similar prevalence of mood disturbance in those with and without a specific cause for pelvic pain has been established [27].

Abuse as a child, whether sexual or physical, may predispose to chronic pelvic pain. Direct causality cannot be inferred as many individuals who have suffered such abuse do not suffer from chronic pain in later life. The research literature is beset with the problem of appropriate comparison groups. A comparison of adverse experiences was made with three groups of 30 patients each, two of patients from a tertiary referral multidisciplinary clinic and a group without pain [28]. The two groups of pain patients were those with pelvic pain, and those with other types of pain. Among the pelvic pain group, 12 (40%) reported sexual abuse compared to five (17%) in each of the two comparison groups. Experience of physical abuse was the same in all groups although women with pelvic pain had a higher score for somatization, i.e. the experience and communication of somatic distress and symptoms.

The role of infection is sometimes overstated with regard to chronic pelvic pain, notwithstanding the proposed mechanism of visceral sensitization by agents such as chlamydia discussed above. In vulval vestibulitis syndrome (VVS), researchers have undertaken numerous studies attempting to elucidate the significance of infection as a risk factor for vestibular pain. The role of candidiasis has not been confirmed, with conflicting data reporting an association with recurrent candida in 80% of VVS cases [29] or no difference in the prevalence compared with controls [30]. The diagnosis of candidiasis in the afore-mentioned studies was often presumptive; hence, early misdiagnosis of VVS as candidiasis could have contributed to the observed statistical linkage. More recent investigations, which corroborated referring physician statements or prior laboratory results with patient reports, found VVS risk to be associated with a history of bacterial vaginosis, *Candida albicans*, pelvic inflammatory disease, trichomoniasis, and vulvar dysplasia [31]. Case–control studies from North America suggest that VVS is more common in white compared to African-American women [32], but this was not confirmed in the population-based survey of Harlow & Stewart [26].

Latthe & colleagues [33] undertook a systematic review of 48 factors predisposing women to chronic pelvic pain, dyspareunia and dysmenorrhea. Factors associated in the analysis with noncyclical pelvic pain were drug or alcohol abuse, miscarriage, prolonged menstrual flow, pelvic inflammatory disease, previous cesarean section, pelvic pathology, abuse (sexual and physical), and psychologic co-morbidity. Odds ratios and confidence intervals for some of these associations are shown in Table 13.2. While the review establishes associations of interest, one needs to bear in mind that the assembled data are drawn from very diverse settings ranging from population surveys to tertiary medical facilities. Furthermore, some of the associations may be self-fulfilling: the diagnosis of "pelvic inflammatory disease" is often given to women

presenting with pain despite the absence of objective features of infection, and patients with recurrent or "unexplained" pain may be given a psychologic or psychiatric label by default.

Treatment of pelvic pain

Interventions supported by RCT evidence

Laparoscopic surgery for endometriosis

Discussion of the role of hysterectomy is beyond the scope of this chapter.

An early randomized comparison of laparoscopic surgery for mild or moderate endometriosis showed evidence of benefit. Sixty-three patients were randomized to laser ablation of endometriotic deposits and laparoscopic uterine nerve ablation, or expectant management (diagnostic laparoscopy alone). At 6 months, 62.5% of those in the laser laparoscopy group reported improvement or resolution of symptoms compared with 22.6% in the expectant group [34]. With regard to severe endometriosis treated by laparoscopic excision or delayed for 6 months, symptom relief was obtained by 16/20 (80%) of those operated on versus versus 6/19 (32%) of those in whom treatment was delayed [35].

Surgery versus cognitive therapy and biofeedback for pelvic muscle relaxation for vulval vestibulitis syndrome (vestibulodynia)

A 12-week trial of either cognitive behavior therapy or biofeedback for pelvic muscle relaxation using electromyography was compared with

Table 13.2 Odds ratios and 95% confidence intervals for factors associated with chronic noncyclical pelvic pain in women. Adapted from Latthe *et al.* [33] with permission from BMJ Publishing Group Ltd.

Factor	Odds ratio and 95% confidence intervals
Drug/alcohol abuse	4.61 (1.09 to 19.38)
Miscarriage	3.00 (1.27 to 7.09)
Duration of menstrual flow	3.13 (1.62 to 6.05)
History of pelvic inflammatory disease	6.35 (2.66 to 15.16)
Previous cesarean section	3.18 (1.91 to 5.30)
"Pelvic pathology"	2.45 (1.30 to 4.61)
Abuse	2.45 (1.47 to 4.06)
Psychosomatic symptoms	8.01 (5.16 to 12.44)

vestibulectomy in 78 women. Post-treatment and 6-month follow-up results were superior in the vestibulectomy group, although scores improved in all the groups [36].

Surgery versus conservative management for pudendal nerve entrapment

Sixteen women were randomized to each of two groups, either a group who underwent surgery to decompress the pudendal nerve or a group treated by conservative management. On an intention-to-treat basis, 50% of the intervention group were improved compared to 6.2% of the control group at 3 months. Analyzing by actual treatment, 71.4% of the surgery group were improved at 12 months compared to 13.3% of the control group. At 4 years, eight of those randomized to surgery were still improved (50%). The authors conclude that while the intervention is worthwhile, other modalities of treatment are likely to be needed in addition [37].

Multidisciplinary management

The use of a multidisciplinary approach in the treatment of women with chronic pelvic pain led to a positive outcome in a self-rating scale (odds ratio (OR) 4.15, 95% confidence interval (CI) 1.91–8.99, n = 106) and in daily activity but not in pain scores, by comparison with those receiving "conventional care" [38].

Counseling supported by ultrasound scanning

Often patients with pelvic pain are anxious about the potential for disease. A randomized comparison of expectant management versus counseling supported by ultrasound scanning to demonstrate normal anatomy showed benefit for the intervention both in terms of pain scores (OR 6.77, 95% CI 2.83–16.19, n = 90) and mood [39].

Hormonal therapy for ovarian suppression

Progestogen (medroxyprogesterone acetate) was effective in reducing chronic pelvic pain after 4 months' treatment as reflected in pain scores (OR 2.64, 95% CI 1.33–5.25, n = 146) and a self-rating scale (OR 6.81, 95% CI 1.83–25.3, n = 44), but benefit was not sustained 9 months post treatment [40, 41]. Medroxyprogesterone acetate plus psychotherapy was effective in terms of pain scores (OR 3.94, 95% CI 1.2–12.96, n = 43) but not in the self-rating scale at the

end of treatment. Benefit was not sustained post treatment. Venography scores for pelvic congestion, symptom and examination scores, mood and sexual function were improved to a greater extent 1 year after treatment with goserelin compared to progestogen [42].

Treatments with conflicting evidence from randomized studies

Presacral neurectomy and laparoscopic uterine nerve ablation

Presacral neurectomy (PSN) and laparoscopic uterine nerve ablation (LUNA) are both surgical procedures that involve the disruption of sensory nerve afferents that carry pain stimuli from the pelvis. In LUNA, the uterosacral ligaments are transsected close to their insertion at the cervix, thus interrupting part of the Lee-Frankenhauser nerve plexus. In PSN, the presacral nerve plexus is isolated and cut proximally and distally. Complications associated with LUNA are rare; there have been isolated cases of uterine prolapse and bladder dysfunction. PSN has been associated with more serious complications such as hematoma formation, major vessel injury, constipation and bladder dysfunction, though these are rare in experienced hands. A number of studies have suggested benefit from LUNA and PSN for primary and secondary dysmenorrhea, including randomized trials [43, 44]. However, a large multicenter study examining the effectiveness of LUNA in pelvic pain (n = 487) has recently finished, with indications of negative findings with respect to pain relief (KS Khan, personal communication).

Short-term results for PSN and LUNA for dysmenorrhea seem to be similar, although PSN has better results in the long term as suggested by the single trial comparing the two procedures [45]. This showed no difference in the treatment groups up to 6 months (OR 0.7, 95% CI 2.9–82.7), although when responses were assessed at 12 months, PSN appeared to be more effective.

Treatments supported by nonrandomized studies but shown to be noneffective in RCT

Adhesiolysis

A number of nonrandomized studies have reported that division of adhesions is useful in the treatment of pelvic pain [46–48]. Overall, a meta-analysis showed that out of over 600 patients with pelvic pain, 76% would obtain relief from adhesiolysis. However, the two available RCT are not supportive. The outcome in women undergoing adhesiolysis via laparotomy was not different to that in women who did not undergo surgery on any outcome measure (OR 1.54, 95% CI 0.81–2.93, n = 148). However, the small subgroup with dense vascularized adhesions did show a significant benefit for surgery (OR for self-rating scale 16.59, 95% CI 2.16–127.2, n = 15) [49]. Using a laparoscopic approach, 29/52 patients reported improvement following adhesiolysis compared to 20/48 controls (OR 1.75 for improvement, 95% CI 0.8–3.82) [50].

Treatments supported by nonrandomized studies

Lidocaine for vulval vestibulitis syndrome (vestibulodynia)

Topical 5% lidocaine ointment applied overnight resulted in significant improvement in a group of 61 participants observed over a mean of 7 weeks. Seventy-six percent reported being able to have intercourse at the end of the study, compared to 36% before treatment; 57% achieved a 50% or greater improvement in symptoms [51].

Tricyclic and SNRI antidepressants

Tricyclic antidepressants and serotonin and noradrenaline reuptake inhibitor (SNRI) antidepressants have been shown to be helpful in neuropathic pain [52, 53]. The question remains as to whether these drugs relieve pelvic pain and vulvodynia. Although there have been anecdoctal reports of benefit in small groups of patients with vulvodynia [54, 55], there are no published randomized controlled studies to clarify the position.

Anticonvulsants

Gabapentin blocks the $\alpha 2\delta$ subunit of the calcium channel and has been shown to be effective for the treatment of neuropathic pain [52]. A small series of patients with vulvodynia reported a favorable response to gabapentin, but no controlled trials have been published [56]. One small trial has suggested a synergistic effect between amitriptyline and gabapentin.

Biofeedback

Twenty-nine patients with moderate to severe vulvar vestibulitis were given electromyographic assessment of the pelvic floor muscles. The patients were then given a portable home trainer biofeedback device and instructions to perform biofeedback-assisted pelvic floor muscle rehabilitation exercises. Patients were evaluated on a monthly basis for vestibulodynia and dyspareunia; 51.7% demonstrated markedly reduced introital tenderness and 93.3% were able to resume sexual activity without discomfort [57].

Treatments not shown to be effective: evidence of no benefit

Photographic reinforcement

A randomized comparison of pain outcomes following laparoscopy was undertaken to assess the potential benefit of showing laparoscopic images to patients as a method of "photographic reinforcement" of the explanation of normal findings at surgery [58]. Two hundred and thirty-five women undergoing diagnostic laparoscopy for the investigation of pelvic pain were randomized. Pain scores at 6 months were reported in 45 and 57 women in the intervention and control groups respectively. Pain scores and other measures were not significantly different but there was a trend towards less favorable outcomes in the photographic reinforcement group.

Treatments not shown to be effective: no evidence of benefit

SSRI antidepressants

No improvement in pain scores was seen in a small study of women with pelvic pain taking sertraline compared to placebo. The SF-36 subscale "Health perception" showed a small improvement in the sertraline arm, while the "Role functioning-emotional" subscale showed a large fall in the sertraline arm [59].

Writing therapy

The aim of this intervention was to allow patients to identify and express the thoughts and feelings associated with their pain as a means of reducing their impact. The main effects of writing about the stress of pelvic pain were limited [60]. Weighted mean differences (95% CI) on the various subcategories of McGill Pain Questionnaire were: sensory pain 0.07 (−0.31 to −0.45), affective pain −0.12 (−0.42 to −0.18) and evaluation pain −1.16 (−1.96 to −0.36). Women with higher baseline ambivalence about emotional expression appear to respond more positively to this intervention, thus showing a subgroup who may benefit specifically from this type of psychologic approach.

Static magnetic therapy

The effects of wearing small magnets as therapy for chronic pelvic pain versus placebo were assessed [61]. No difference was seen following 2 weeks' treatment but some significant differences appeared at 4 weeks as assessed by the Pain Disability Index and the Clinical Global Impression Scale but not the McGill Pain Questionnaire. Analyzed in terms of weighted mean differences, the differences were nonsignificant and there was a substantial drop-out rate. The putative mechanism of action of this modality is unclear but some data from other settings have indicated benefit, such as therapy for diabetic neuropathic foot pain. It is suggested that magnetic fields modify the abnormal discharge of damaged C-fiber afferents [62].

Issues of cost-effectiveness

The costs and benefits of different forms of endometriosis treatment have been reviewed [63]. In this condition there are choices to be made between hormonal therapy and surgery. Costs associated with surgery are heavily dependent on the capacity to undertake "one-stop" diagnostic and therapeutic laparoscopy. While appropriate for minimal to moderate disease, this approach is not feasible for complex late-stage endometriosis surgery, which requires careful planning, including bowel preparation. In recent years, the costs of medical treatments have reduced, but there is still a lack of long-term safety data relating to the use of gonadotrophin-releasing hormone (GnRH) agonists with "add-back" estrogen. Therefore, laparoscopic surgery remains the preferred option in many cases. Other forms of treatment for pelvic and vulval pain have not been analyzed systematically for cost-effectiveness.

Box 13.1   Treatment options

Interventions supported by RCT evidence

Laparoscopic surgery for endometriosis
Vestibulectomy
Pudendal nerve release
Multidisciplinary management
Counseling with ultrasound scanning
Hormonal therapy for ovarian suppression

Interventions with conflicting evidence from RCTs

PSN and LUNA

Treatments supported by nonrandomized studies but shown to be noneffective in RCT

Adhesiolysis

Treatments supported by nonrandomized studies

Lignocaine ointment for vulvar vestibulitis
Tricyclic antidepressants
Gabapentin
Biofeedback

The future: strategies to improve the evidence base for the treatment of pelvic and vulval/perineal pain in women

In the clinical setting it is usually unrealistic to try to collect patients with a definitive pathologic diagnosis for treatment trials in pelvic and vulval/perineal pain. Moreover, the case mix seen in particular clinics is highly influenced by referral patterns and the specialist interest of the practitioner. Inevitably, there will be heterogeneity between units both in patients' clinical presentation and in the chronicity and severity of pain and associated functional impairment.

A practical approach to generating informative studies might involve the following elements.

• Definition of entry criteria based on pain intensity, duration and symptom impact using validated measures such as the Brief Pain Inventory.

• Grouping of participants on the basis of related constellations of symptoms. For example, it makes clinical sense to group those with mainly focal vulval vestibular symptoms separately from those with more generalized pelvic pain secondary to endometriosis. But patients often have symptoms referable to other pelvic organs, especially the bowel and bladder, and it is unrealistic to exclude them from studies of "pelvic pain." Moreover, such symptom overlap is consistent with current concepts of viscerovisceral and viscerosomatic convergence in sensory innervation.

- Where feasible, identification of a neuropathic element through sensory testing may help to strengthen understanding of treatment mechanisms as well as providing repeatable outcome measures within the same individual.
- Defining "packages" of interventions for comparison, in recognition that chronic pain management almost always involves (and indeed should involve) more than one treatment modality.

Authors' recommendations

This chapter has identified treatments for which evidence is stronger, and those that are at the less robust end of the spectrum. It has not been possible satisfactorily to review the full range of "general" chronic pain treatment modalities that are offered to patients with chronic pelvic, vulval or perineal pain. For example, opioids have an important place for many patients but tend to be conceptualized as a treatment for chronic pain rather than for a specific subgroup of chronic pain patients. Thus, while they are very important in practice, it is unlikely that a substantial body of RCT evidence on their use in this specific patient group will emerge.

It is interesting to reflect on the presence of a number of surgical interventions in the list of effective treatments. The evidence suggests that these are valuable and their presence in a review of pain treatments perhaps extends the conceptual boundaries of the multidisciplinary approach. As emphasized by the French group who have pioneered surgery for pudendal neuralgia, surgery needs to be undertaken along with other pain management interventions and not as a single modality. Again, women with endometriosis have often not received multidisciplinary pain interventions because they have been considered to have a gynaecologic condition amenable to surgery. In reality, they benefit substantially from the combination of appropriate surgery with other pain management modalities.

A significant barrier to research and service development in this area is that it has a relatively low priority for the pharmaceutical industry. In addition, funding combinations of interventions is especially unattractive to industrial sponsors because of regulatory requirements. Therefore, the reality is that substantial clinical trial activity is likely to be dependent on competitive grant funding. For research funding bodies, formal comparisons of treatment packages have not been seen as sufficiently novel or original. To generate a climate where such studies are given appropriate priority by funding bodies requires considerable effort from health service researchers, patient organizations and professional societies.

References

1. Sampson JA. Perforating hemorrhagic (chocolate) cysts of the ovary. Their importance and especially their relation to pelvic adenomas of the endometrial type ('adenomyoma' of the uterus, rectovaginal septum, sigmoid etc). *Arch Surg Chicago* 1921; **3**: 245–323.
2. Sangi-Haghpeykar H, Poindexter AN III. Epidemiology of endometriosis among parous women. *Obstet Gynecol* 1995; **85**: 983–992.
3. Cornillie FJ, Oosterlynck D, Lauweryns JM, Koninckx PR. Deeply infiltrating pelvic endometriosis: histology and clinical significance. *Fertil Steril* 1990; **53**: 978–983.
4. Forman RG, Robinson JN, Mehta Z, Barlow DH. Patient history as a simple predictor of pelvic pathology in subfertile women. *Hum Reprod* 1993; **8**: 53–55.
5. Atwal G, du Plessis D, Armstrong G, Slade R, Quinn M. Uterine innervation after hysterectomy for chronic pelvic pain with, and without, endometriosis. *Am J Obstet Gynecol* 2005; **193**: 1650–1655.
6. Berkley KJ, Dmitrieva N, Curtis KS, Papka RE. Innervation of ectopic endometrium in a rat model of endometriosis. *Proc Natl Acad Sci USA* 2004; **101**: 11094–11098.
7. McMahon SB. Are there fundamental differences in the peripheral mechanisms of visceral and somatic pain? *Behav Brain Sci* 1997; **20**: 381–391.
8. Tulandi T, Chen M, Al-Took S, Watkin K. A study of nerve fibers and histopathology of postsurgical, postinfectious, and endometriosis-related adhesions. *Obstet Gynecol* 1998; **92**: 766–768.
9. Labat JJ, Robert R, Bensignor M, Buzelin JM. Neuralgia of the pudendal nerve – anatomoclinical considerations and therapeutic approach. *J d'Urologie* 1990; **96**: 239–244.
10. Pukall CF, Strigo IA, Binik YM, Amsel R, Khalife S, Bushnell MC. Neural correlates of painful genital touch in women with vulvar vestibulitis syndrome *Pain* 2005; **115**: 118–127.
11. Bornstein J, Goldschmid N, Sabo E. Hyperinnervation and mast cell activation may be used as histopathologic

diagnostic criteria for vulvar vestibulitis. *Gynecol Obstet Invest* 2004; **58**: 171–178.

12. Bohm-Starke N, Falconer C, Rylander E, Hilliges M. The expression of cyclooxygenase 2 and inducible nitric oxide synthase indicates no active inflammation in vulvar vestibulitis. *Acta Obstet Gynaecol Scand* 2001; **80**: 638–644.

13. Abbott JA, Jarvis SK, Lyons SD, Thomson A, Vancaille TG. Botulinum toxin type A for chronic pain and pelvic floor spasm in women: a randomized controlled trial. *Obstet Gynecol* 2006; **108**: 915–923.

14. Stones RW. Pelvic vascular congestion: half a century later. *Clin Obstet Gynecol* 2003; **46**: 831–836.

15. Bradshaw HB, Temple JL, Wood E, Berkley KJ. Estrous variations in behavioral responses to vaginal and uterine distention in the rat. *Pain* 1999; **82**: 187–197.

16. Riley J L, Robinson ME, Wise EA, Price DD. A meta-analytic review of pain perception across the menstrual cycle. *Pain* 1999; **81**: 225–235.

17. Treloar SA, Martin NG, Heath AC. Longitudinal genetic analysis of menstrual flow, pain, and limitation in a sample of Australian twins. *Behav Genet* 1998; **28**: 107–116.

18. Zondervan KT, Cardon LR, Kennedy SH, Martin NG, Treloar SA. Multivariate genetic analysis of chronic pelvic pain and associated phenotypes. *Behav Genet* 2005; **35**: 177–188.

19. Stones RW, Price C. Health services for women with chronic pelvic pain. *J Roy Soc Med* 2002; **95**: 531–535.

20. Stones RW. Chronic pelvic pain. In: Edmonds K (ed) *Dewhurst's Textbook of Obstetrics and Gynaecology*, 7th edn. Blackwell Publishing, Oxford, 2007: 423–429.

21. Mathias, SD, Kuppermann M, Liberman RF, *et al.* Chronic pelvic pain: prevalence, health-related quality of life, and economic correlates. *Obstet Gynecol* 1996, **87**: 321–327.

22. Zondervan KT, Yudkin PL, Vessey MP, *et al.* Chronic pelvic pain in the community – symptoms, investigations, and diagnoses. *Am J Obstet Gynecol* 2001; **184**: 1149–1155.

23. Zondervan KT, Yudkin PL, Vessey MP, *et al.* Patterns of diagnosis and referral in women consulting for chronic pelvic pain in UK primary care. *Br J Obstet Gynaecol* 1999; **106**: 1156–1161.

24. Zondervan KT, Yudkin PL, Vessey MP et al.Prevalence and incidence of chronic pelvic pain in primary care: evidence from a national general practice database. *British Journal of Obstetrics and Gynaecology* 1999b; **106**:1149–1155.

25. Zondervan KT, Yudkin PL, Vessey MP, *et al.* The community prevalence of chronic pelvic pain in women and associated illness behaviour. *Br J Gen Pract* 2001; **51**: 541–547.

26. Harlow BL, Stewart EG. A population-based assessment of chronic unexplained vulvar pain: have we underestimated the prevalence of vulvodynia? *J Am Med Women's Assoc* 2003; **58**(2): 82–88.

27. Waller KG, Shaw RW. Endometriosis, pelvic pain, and psychological functioning. *Fertil Steril* 1995; **63**: 796–800.

28. Collett BJ, Cordle CJ, Stewart CR, Jagger C. A comparative study of women with chronic pelvic pain, chronic nonpelvic pain and those with no history of pain attending general practitioners. *Br J Obstet Gynaecol* 1998; **105**: 87–92.

29. Mann MS, Kaufman RH, Brown D Jr, Adam E. Vulvar vestibulitis: significant clinical variables and treatment outcome. *Obstet Gynecol* 1992; **79**: 122–125.

30. Bazin S, Bouchard C, Brisson J, Morin C, Meisels A, Fortier M. Vulvar vestibulitis syndrome: an exploratory case–control study. *Obstet Gynecol* 1994; **83**: 47–50.

31. Smith EM, Ritchie JM, Galask R, Pugh EE, Jia J, Ricks-McGillan J. Case–control study of vulvar vestibulitis risk associated with genital infections. *Infect Dis Obstet Gynecol* 2002; **10**: 193–202.

32. Foster DC, Woodruff JD. Case-control study of vulvar vestibulitis syndrome. *J Women's Health* 1995; **4**: 677–680.

33. Latthe P, Mignini L, Gray R, Hills R, Khan, K. Factors predisposing women to chronic pelvic pain:systematic review. *BMJ* 2006; **332**: 749–755.

34. Sutton CJG, Ewen SP, Whitelaw N, Haines P. Prospective, randomized, double-blind, controlled trial of laser laparoscopy in the treatment of pelvic pain associated with minimal, mild, and moderate endometriosis. *Fertil Steril* 1994; **62**(4): 696–700.

35. Abbott J, Hawe J, Hunter D, Holmes M, Finn P, Garry R. Laparoscopic excision of endometriosis: a randomized, placebo-controlled trial. *Fertil Steril* 2004; **82**: 878–884.

36. Bergeron S, Binik YM, Khalife S, *et al.* A randomized comparison of group cognitive behavioral therapy, surface electromyographic biofeedback, and vestibulectomy in the treatment of dyspareunia resulting from vulvar vestibulitis. *Pain* 2001; **91**: 297–306.

37. Robert R, Labat JJ, Bensignor M, *et al.* Decompression and transposition of the pudendal nerve in pudendal neuralgia: a randomized controlled trial and long-term evaluation. *Eur Urol* 2005; **47**(3): 403–408.

38. Peters AA, van Dorst E, Jellis B, van Zuuren E, Hermans J, Trimbos JB. A randomized clinical trial to compare two different approaches in women with chronic pelvic pain. *Obstet Gynecol* 1991; **77**: 740–744.

39. Ghaly AFF. The psychological and physical benefits of pelvic ultrasonography in patients with chronic pelvic pain and negative laparoscopy. A random allocation trial. *J Obstet Gynaecol* 1994; **14**: 269–271.

40. Farquhar CM, Rogers V, Franks S, Pearce S, Wadsworth J, Beard RW. A randomized controlled trial of medroxyprogesterone acetate and psychotherapy for the treatment of pelvic congestion. *Br J Obstet Gynaecol* 1989; **96**: 1153–1162.

41. Walton SM, Batra HK. The use of medroxyprogesterone acetate 50mg in the treatment of painful pelvic conditions: preliminary results from a multicentre trial. *J Obstet Gynaecol* 1992; **12** (suppl 2): s50–53.

42. Soysal ME, Soysal S, Vicdan K, Ozer S. A randomized controlled trial of goserelin and medroxyprogesterone acetate in the treatment of pelvic congestion. *Hum Reprod* 2001; **16**: 931–939.

43. Johnson NP, Farquhar CM, Crossley Y, *et al.* A double–blind randomised controlled trial of laparoscopic uterine nerve

ablation for women with chronic pelvic pain. *Br J Obstet Gynaecol* 2004; **111**: 950–959.

44. Perez J. Laparoscopic presacral neurectomy. Results of the first 25 cases. *J Reprod Med* 1990; **35**: 625–630.

45. Chen F, Chang S, Chu K, Soong Y. Comparison of laparoscopic presacral neurectomy and laparoscopic uterine nerve ablation for primary dysmenorrhea. *J Reprod Med* 1996; **41**: 463–466.

46. Mueller M, Tshudi J, Herrmann U, Klaiber C. An evaluation of laparosocpic adhesiolysis in patients with chronic abdominal pain. *Surg Endosc* 1995; **9(7)**: 802–804.

47. Saravelos H, Li T, Cooke I. An analysis of the outcome of microsurgical and laparosocpic adhesiolysis for chronic pelvic pain. *Hum Reprod* 1995; **10**(11): 2895–2901.

48. Steege J, Stout A. Resolution of chronic pelvic pain after laparoscopic lysis of adhesions. *Am J Obstet Gynecol* 1991; **165**: 278–281.

49. Peters AAW, Trimbos-Kemper GCM, Admiraal C, Trimbos JB. A randomized clinical trial on the benefit of adhesiolysis in patients with intraperitoneal adhesions and chronic pelvic pain. *Br J Obstet Gynaecol* 1992; **99**: 59–62.

50. Swank DJ, Hop WC, van Erp WF, Jenssen IM, Bonjier HJ, Jeekel J. Laparoscopic adhesiolysis in patients with chronic abdominal pain: a blinded randomised controlled multicentre trial. *Lancet* 2003; **361**: 1247–1251.

51. Zolnoun DA, Hartmann KE, Steege JF. Overnight 5% lidocaine ointment for treatment of vulvar vestibulitis. *Obstet Gynecol* 2003; **102**: 84–87.

52. Finnerup NR, Otto M, McQuay HJ, Jensen TS, Sindrup SH. Algorithm for neuropathic pain treatment: an evidence based proposal. *Pain* 2005; **118**: 289–305.

53. Goldstein DJ, Lu Y, Detke MJ, Lee TC, Iyengar S. Duloxetine vs placebo in patient with painful diabetic neuropathy. *Pain* 2005; **116**: 109–118.

54. McKay M. Dysaesthetic ('essential ') vulvodynia: treatment with amitriptyline. *J Reprod Med* 1993; 38: 9–13.

55. Munday PE. Response to treatment in dysaesthetic vulvodynia. *J Obstet Gynaecol* 2001; **21**: 610–613.

56. Ben-David B, Friedman M. Gabapentin therapy for vulvodynia. *Anesth Analg* 1999; **89**: 1459–1460.

57. Mckay E, Kaufman RH, Docotr U, Berkova Z, Glazer H, Redko V. Treating vulvar vestibulitis with electromyographic biofeedback of pelvic floor musculature. *J Reprod Med* 2001; **46**: 337–342.

58. Onwude L, Thornton J, Morley S, Lilleyman J, Currie I, Lilford R. A randomised trial of photographic reinforcement during postoperative counselling after diagnostic laparoscopy for pelvic pain. *Eur J Obstet Gynecol Reprod Biol* 2004; **112**: 89–94.

59. Engel CC, Walker EA, Engel AL, Bullis J, Armstrong A. A randomized, double-blind crossover trial of sertraline in women with chronic pelvic pain. *J Psychosom Res* 1998; **44**: 203–207.

60. Norman S, Lumley M, Dooley J, Diamond M. For whom does it work? Moderators of the effects of written emotional disclosure in a randomised trial among women with chronic pelvic pain. *Psychosom Med* 2004; **66**: 174–183.

61. Brown C, Pharm D, Ling F, Wan J, Pills A. Efficacy of static magnetic field therapy in chronic pelvic pain: a double-blind study. *Am J Obstet Gynecol* 2002; **187**: 1581–1587.

62. Weintraub MI, Wolfe GI, Barohn RA, *et al*. Static magnetic field therapy for symptomatic diabetic neuropathy: a randomized, double-blind, placebo-controlled trial. *Arch Phys Med Rehab* 2003; **84**: 736–746.

63. Stones RW, Thomas EJ. Cost-effective medical treatment of endometriosis. In: Bonnar J (ed) *Recent Advances in Obstetrics and Gynaecology, no.19*. Churchill Livingstone, Edinburgh, 1995: 139–152.

CHAPTER 14

Perineal pain in males

Andrew P. Baranowski

Pain Management Centre, National Hospital for Neurology and Neurosurgery, University College London Hospitals, London, UK

Introduction

For the purpose of this chapter, the pelvis will be regarded as the area below a transverse section through the body taken at the level of the iliac crest and above a transverse section drawn just below the external genitalia. This is not the true anatomic pelvis but has been defined in this way to include those pain syndromes that may be referred to the true anatomic pelvis.

Background to perineal/pelvic pain syndromes in males

Perineal/pelvic pain in the male relates to either a well-defined pathology or one of the pain syndromes. Well-defined pathologies would include the cancers and infectious diseases that may produce pain; the management of such pathologic process will not be discussed in this chapter as treatment of the primary cause is described in numerous texts and is the treatment of choice when possible.

The pain syndromes, by definition, are poorly defined in terms of classical pathology; in particular, there is no evidence of tumor, infection or inflammation as a cause of pain. Over the past few years a number of mechanisms have been suggested that would explain some of the features of these conditions. In certain cases, most notably the pelvic neuralgias and myalgias, "classical pathological processes"

Evidence-Based Chronic Pain Management. Edited by
C. Stannard, E. Kalso and J. Ballantyne. © 2010 Blackwell
Publishing.

are being used to explain the mechanisms for the pain syndrome; in other cases "chronic pain mechanisms" are being invoked. Some of the pain syndromes will thus be recategorized, with time, into the well-defined pathology group.

Historically the perineal/pelvic pain syndromes were classified by a terminology that implied a pathologic process that could not be confirmed. For instance, testicular pain was referred to as "chronic orchitis" despite there being no evidence of infection or even inflammation. Other spurious terms used include "chronic prostatitis" for pain perceived to arise from the "prostate" and "interstitial cystitis" for pain perceived in the "bladder." The European Association for Urology (EAU) modified the axial taxonomy of the International Association for the Study of Pain in 2003, publishing a pain syndrome classification based on perceived site of pain. Pain perceived to be in the prostate, from the clinical history and examination, according to that taxonomy is to be known as prostate pain syndrome, pain perceived in the testis as testicular pain syndrome and in the bladder as bladder pain syndrome. This classification does not imply any pathologic process; in particular, it is not meant to imply a pain source in the organ, only that the perceived sensation appears associated with that organ. There may be associated symptoms such as swelling, urinary frequency or urgency and the mechanisms for these are beginning to be understood.

Most of the recent emphasis on classification has been in the fields of prostate pain and bladder pain. The NIH in 1990 included chronic prostate pain under its classification of "prostatitis." This is now considered by many to have been a mistake. However, it did allow clinicians to divide the chronic prostate pains into those with inflammation on examination of the prostatic secretions and those without evidence of inflammation (in both of these groups, by definition, there was no evidence of infection). Recent experience suggests that the mechanisms in both groups may be similar and that the presence of inflammatory cells has no therapeutic implications and does not affect prognosis. Recently, the European Association for the Study of Interstitial Cystitis (ESSIC) agreed that the term "interstitial cystitis" should be abandoned for the term bladder pain syndrome. It further subdivided the condition according to changes in the bladder seen on cystoscopy and biopsy.

The new taxonomy has had a number of consequences. First, patient groups and some clinicians have raised concerns about the implications of the name changes for "the sake of name change." These groups raise concerns about costs, particularly in those countries where a specific named diagnosis is necessary to obtain treatment. Second, there is a move away from an organ-based taxonomy and towards a mechanism-based approach. For the purpose of this chapter, we shall discuss evidence-based treatments as appropriate for both mechanism-based and organ-specific diagnoses.

Current understanding of relevant pathophysiology for perineal/pelvic pain syndromes

Visceral chronic pain mechanisms

There are differences between the nociceptive processes involved in visceral pain compared to those in somatic pain. However, it is well established that central hypersensitivity changes can occur in both types of pain. The implications are that normal sensory stimuli can be perceived in a magnified form with the result that innocuous sensations may be perceived as pain or that normally unperceived sensory stimuli become perceived. The latter dysaesthesias may be the cause of urinary frequency and urgency in the bladder pain syndromes, the urge to defecate in bowel hypersensitivities and sensory changes associated with ejaculation in the prostate pain syndromes. These central changes may occur as a result of an acute painful insult such as associated with infection. The insult to the organ results in activation of normally silent,

"sleeping" afferents and in changes in the receptive fields of second-order neuronal pathways within the central nervous system.

Multiple chemical changes may be implicated in these changes. N-methyl-D-aspartic acid (NMDA) is implicated in central neuromodulation as NMDA blockade can reduce the visceral hyperalgesia response in both psychophysical and electrophysiologic investigations. Nerve growth factor (NGF) has direct and indirect effects upon primary afferents with the result that the primary afferents are more sensitive to stimuli; that is, more activity is generated in them per unit of stimulus. The tachykinins may be involved in sensitization of the micturition reflex following bladder inflammation and may have a significant role in the production of neurogenic edema, such as may be seen in certain subgroups of bladder pain syndrome. Adenosine triphosphate (ATP) acting upon the P2X1 receptors and agents acting on the sodium channel receptors have also been implicated. As well as chemical changes, structural and local cell genetic changes occur and as a result the changes of sensory perception associated with the organ may persist for many months or even years after the original insult.

Recent evidence points to the existence of both visceral-visceral hyperalgesias and dysesthesias as well as visceral-muscular hyperalgesias. Central changes throughout the neuraxis may occur as a result of an insult such as acute distension or inflammation of an organ. These central changes may alter the neuroprocessing of signals from organs not involved in the primary pathology so that those organs become hypersensitive (visceral-visceral hyperalgesia) or affecting muscles (visceral-muscular hyperalgesia). Visceral-visceral hyperalgesia and hypersensitivity may explain why many patients have pain and sensory abnormalities associated with multiple organs.

A number of chronic perineal/pelvic pain syndromes may involve chronic infection or inflammation that cannot be identified. The evidence that such pathologies cause chronic pain is hotly debated and there is a general trend away from diagnoses which imply undected infection or inflammation.

Muscle hyperalgesia

The mechanisms involved in visceral-visceral hyperalgesia may be responsible for sensory perception abnormalities perceived in the muscles. Muscle hyperalgesia may arise as a result of a visceral insult (visceral-muscle hyperalgesia), primary muscle insult (e.g. trauma to the muscle itself) or secondary to other musculoskeletal abnormalities (e.g. mechanical back pain producing a referred pelvic muscle hyperalgesia). Additionally, primary muscle dysfunction with pain may result in visceral hyperalgesia, visceral sensitivity and visceral dysfunction. Muscles are closely approximated to the viscera and nerves and in consequence, the muscles may physically interact with those structures. For instance, irritable pelvic floor muscles may affect bladder function, producing urinary frequency and a sensation of urgency associated with poor urinary flow, intermittent urinary flow, hesitancy and *pis en deux*. Similarly, changes in the structure (e.g. lax pelvic floor muscles) or function (e.g. spasm of the pelvic floor muscles) may affect adjacent nerves. Such mechanisms have been proposed as possible causes of pudendal neuralgia.

Peripheral nerve injury

The innervation of the pelvis and perineum is complex and is well described. The pathophysiology of nerve injury and the pain associated with this are also well described. There are a number of classic nerve injury syndromes which may present as pelvic/perineal pain.

Central nerve injuries

- Sacral roots (perineal and leg pain), e.g. cauda equina syndrome, arachnoiditis, presacral tumor.

Intra-abdominal/pelvic nerve injury

- Injury to pelvic plexus, superior and inferior hypogastric plexus, presacral sympathetic nerves and ganglion impar, prostatic plexus (deep pelvic pain), e.g. pelvic surgery and tumors.

Nerve injury affecting nerves anterior to the pelvis

- Pain from the thoracolumbar nerve (posterior branch – pelvic lumbago, lateral branch – lateral pelvic pain, anterior branch – inguinal and testicular pain), e.g. 12th rib syndrome, nerve root irritation due to canal stenosis or disk.
- Ilio-inguinal and iliohypogastric nerve injury (inguinal canal, suprapubic and scrotal/testicular pain), e.g following lumbar spinal surgery, incisions in the iliac abdominal region, Pfannenstiel incisions, inguinal surgery.
- Genitofemoral nerve injury (scrotal/testicular pain and inner thigh pain), e.g. abdominal aortic aneurism surgery, ureteric surgery, iliac surgery, inguinal surgery.
- Obturator nerve (pelvic and inner thigh pain), e.g. obturator canal entrapment, pelvic cancer.

Nerve injury to those nerves that enter the pelvis posteriorly

- Pudendal nerve (anal, perineal/vulvar, penis/clitoris, scrotal/testicular pain), e.g. nerve entrapment syndromes, pelvic floor muscle dysfunction, direct trauma.
- Inferior cluneal nerve (buttock pain extending to inner thighs/perineum), e.g. direct trauma, sitting for prolonged times, nerve entrapment.
- Perineal branches of the posterior femoral cutaneous nerve (perineal pain), e.g. direct trauma, sitting for prolonged times, nerve entrapment.
- Posterior femoral cutaneous nerve (posterior thigh pain), e.g. direct trauma, sitting for prolonged times, nerve entrapment.

The pain syndromes associated with injury of the posterior nerves in the region of the piriformis, superior gemellus, obturator internus and inferior gemellus muscles (the "posterior triangle") merit special mention as they have not been well described to date. Injury and disease processes in this area may involve one or more of these nerves with associated neuropathic symptoms. The sensory abnormalities that occur may be a result of involvement of the following nerves: sciatic, inferior cluneal, pudendal, posterior femoral cutaneous and the perineal branches of the posterior femoral cutaneous nerve.

Many perineal pains are now categorized as pudendal neuralgia. However, making such a diagnosis is not easy as many mechanisms may be involved, including damage to other nerves (as listed above) and the muscle hyperalgesias. For true pudendal neuralgia, the pain should be perceived in the distribution of the pudendal nerve or one of its branches. Other sensory/motor abnormalities may support the diagnosis such as numbness or paresthesia in an appropriate distribution or the absence of a bulbocavernosal reflex. Pudendal nerve conduction tests in the absence of hypoesthesia rarely help with the diagnosis. It has been suggested that bulbocavernosal electromyographs may be more helpful. Classically the pain is said to be worse with sitting and relieved by standing (or sitting on a toilet seat). However, such variations in pain may be associated with other "posterior triangle" nerves and the muscle hyperalgesias. The more pronounced the nerve damage, the less likely that there will be a variation in the pain with direct pressure over the nerves as the pain will be more constant. Thorough clinical examination by an experienced practitioner may help to distinguish the different types of pain. Selective nerve blocks of the pudendal nerve at the ischeal spine, under X-ray guidance and with neurotracing recognition of the nerves, is an essential part of making the diagnosis, but may also be therapeutic. Deeper injections under CT guidance may also help localize the source of the pain.

Psychology and psychiatry in male perineal/pelvic pain syndromes

Illusory pain associated with frank psychiatric disturbance is extremely uncommon. Other neurologic syndromes may produce pain in the pelvis/perineum but these are not well described in the absence of lesions demonstrated within the nervous system on scanning.

There is little evidence that negative sexual events (NSE) produce imaginary pain. Negative sexual events and other major life events may result in a state of emotional and physical tension. Such states may be associated with a number of physiologic changes, including muscle tension, with associated pain. Such changes may result in muscle hyperalgesia, nerve entrapment and the initiation of a persistent pain syndrome.

Chronic pelvic/perineal pain is associated with psychologic distress and sexual dysfunction in men. There is a complex interaction between the psychology, sexology, relationships and sociology of chronic pelvic pain. Patients who exhibit catastrophizing and who have poor pain-contingent resting and poor social support have poor outcomes from therapy.

Prevalence figures/epidemiology

Chronic perineal/pelvic pain in men is common. It is probably the most common reason for attendance at a urology clinic in males under 40.

Prostate pain/prostate pain syndrome

Worldwide prevalence of prostate pain is said to be 2–10% [1]; however, other pelvic pains may be included in this figure as diagnosis may be difficult. In a postal survey of 3000 Canadian men the majority of sufferers were aged 20–49 or over 70 [2], with 50% of men given the diagnosis of prostatitis symptoms at some point during their lives [3].

In the USA 8% of urology clinic patients and 1% of patients in general clinics are given the diagnosis of "prostatitis" [4].

Nickel and his group reviewed the National Institutes of Health (NIH) chronic prostatitis symptom index data [5]. This represents a cross-sectional postal survey of 2987 men aged 20–74 years in Canada (response rate of 29%). It identified 9.7% of subjects as having chronic prostatitis-like symptoms according to the NIH chronic prostatitis symptom index. In this group the average age of the prostatitis population was 50 years and the prevalence was 11.5% in men younger than 50, and 8.5% in the older men. The relatively low response rate raises the issue of nonresponder bias. Also, in this survey younger men were under-represented and the older age group over-represented. In a later study by this group [6], a prospective study of 8712 patients seen in a urology outpatient practice, prostatitis-type symptoms were identified in only 2.7% of the men.

Scrotal pain/scrotal pain syndrome (including testicular and epididymal pain syndromes)

The incidence of testicular pain not related to surgery is considered to be 1% [7]. Nickel *et al.* in 2005 diagnosed epididymitis in 0.9% of men presenting to a urology clinic [6].

Postsurgical pain is well described with the incidence of postvasectomy pain said to be 15–19% [8].

Bladder pain/bladder pain syndrome

There is disagreement over the terminology for pain perceived to be associated with the bladder. In the 1980s a conference of the National Institute of Diabetes and Digestive and Kidney Diseases (NIDDK) agreed criteria to ensure that the groups of patients enrolled in research studies would be relatively similar [9]. These criteria defined interstitial cystitis (IC) by exclusion with bladder pain, urgency and the finding of submucosal hemorrhages, called glomerulations, as the only positive elements and circumscribed lesions known as Hunner's lesions as an automatic inclusion criterion. The NIDDK criteria were accepted for research but were considered too restrictive for clinical use [10].

The International Continence Society defined a painful bladder syndrome in 2002 [11] and the European Association of Urology defined the bladder pain syndrome [12]. In a recent response (2007) to patient support groups, the ESSIC stated "The name Interstitial Cystitis (IC) has been under debate for several years. Originally, IC was synonymous with Hunner's lesion of the bladder, but has subsequently expanded to be used in an undefinable population of patients with bladder pain." The ESSIC went on to emphasize: "The International Continence Society (ICS) published a report of definitions in 2002, defining painful bladder syndrome (PBS) as – suprapubic pain related to bladder filling, accompanied by other symptoms such as increased daytime and night-time frequency in the absence of infection or other pathology – and IC as the above with "typical cystoscopic and histological features"." To be consistent with other pain terminology, the term painful bladder syndrome is likely to change to bladder pain syndrome and during the transition, bladder pain syndrome/interstitial cystitis (BPS/IC) is likely to be used to describe both conditions. This change in terminology, although scientifically rational, has caused much concern amongst patient support groups.

A study indicating that BPS/IC is underdiagnosed in both men and women was carried out from a mailing of the O'Leary-Sant interstitial cystitis questionnaire, sent to 10,000 subjects in the North Pacific. The prevalence of BPS/IC symptoms was between 6.2% and 11.2% for women and 2.3% and 4.6% for men. In a previous study in the same population, the prevalence of a physician diagnosis of BPS/IC was 0.2% in women and 0.04% in men. Therefore the prevalence of BPS/IC symptoms was 30–50-fold higher in women and 60–100-fold higher in men compared with the physician diagnosis of BPS/IC. The symptoms were of long standing (duration greater than 1 year) in 80% and bothersome (severity score 5 or greater) in 50%. The response rate was 35% and so the results of this study may reflect significant nonresponder bias [13].

There may be genetic influences on the development of BPS/IC as first-degree relatives of sufferers have a higher prevalence than the general population. It has been demonstrated that there is a particularly high proportion in the American Indians of Cherokee descent, approximately 17% [14]. BPS/IC is also reported to be associated with inflammatory bowel disease, systemic lupus erythematosus, irritable bowel syndrome and fibromyalgia [15].

Penile/perineal pain/penile pain syndrome

Not much is known about the incidence of these conditions. Pain referral to the penis from the pelvic floor muscles, base of the bladder and prostate appears not to be unusual. Similarly, as part of a picture of pelvic muscle hyperalgesia, trigger points within the ischiocavernosus and bulbospongiosus muscles may be detected and penile pain may arise as a result of pudendal neuralgia. Pure and idiopathic penile pain appears to be less common.

Risk factors

Very little information exists as to what may predispose to chronic perineal/pelvic pain in men.

It is generally accepted that in general a NSE does not predispose to chronic perineal/pelvic pain. However, such an experience will affect the way that a patient views his condition and how he manages it. Knowledge of the NSE may also affect in a negative way how those trusted with the care of the patient respond. There is no doubt that the care provided to victims of a NSE will have to be tailored to take the event into account. The relevance of this for male patients has been reviewed [16].

In the case of victims of torture, trauma to the perineal region may predispose to chronic pain. Very few data have been collected in relation to this. Similarly, very few data on the role of psychology have been correlated.

It is generally accepted that direct trauma may produce long-term damage and pain. Such trauma may be due to surgery or an accident or be wilfully inflicted. The incidence of chronic pain following surgery may be as high as 10 or 15%. In men, the classic nerve compression related to cycling does not appear to be as common as compression due to sitting at a computer/workstation for long periods.

Trip *et al.* [17, 18] have illustrated the importance of psychologic factors for the prognosis of men with chronic perineal/pelvic pain. Those who catastrophize or have poor coping strategies do poorly and one may assume are more prone to persistent chronic pain. In a recent review of patients with such pain in the author's institution, distress was high, with pain being only one cause. Problems with work, relationships, sexual relationships and loss of meaning of life appeared to be equally important stressors.

Management of perineal pain

Interventions supported by evidence

Chronic perineal/pelvic pain in men covers a diverse group of poorly understood conditions. In many cases the recommendations about treatments will arise from drawing parallels with the management of other conditions. The evidence presented below will primarily be for the pain syndromes (see above) as other well-described conditions have recognized clinical approaches for their management. To reach the diagnosis of a pain syndrome, organ-specific investigations by appropriate specialists (e.g. urologists) will have been undertaken to exclude the well-defined pathologies.

There are several summaries of evidence-based treatment for male perineal/pelvic pain and the following will draw upon these [12]. In all probability there are significant overlaps in the various perineal/pelvic pain syndromes and as a consequence, in addition to review of the evidence for specific treatment options in defined pain syndromes, the evidence for generic treatments based on putative underlying mechanisms is considered.

Drugs

Prostate pain syndrome

As the exact nature of this condition is poorly understood, specific drug treatment options do not exist. Drug use is primarily aimed at reducing spasm in the bladder outflow system (smooth and/or striated muscles) or the use of analgesics [19, 20].

Striated muscle relaxants are thought to be of help if there is pelvic floor muscle spasm or the presence of pelvic floor muscle trigger points. However, there are no prospective trials [21].

α Receptors are found in the bladder neck and prostate and **α blockers** are well recognized as medications that improve flow in the presence of lower urinary tract obstructive symptoms. Some studies do exist that suggest an improvement in the symptoms of patients with "NIH III a/b prostatitis" [22–25]. Whether this is due to improving outflow performance by blocking the α receptors of the bladder neck and prostate is not known.

The use of **antibiotics** remains controversial in the prostate pain syndrome (i.e. no proven infection). However, the current EAU guidelines indicate that "because some patients have been observed to improve with antimicrobial therapy"[26], "a trial treatment with antibiotics is recommended" [21, 24]. They go on to say: "Patients responding to antibiotics should be maintained on the medication for 4–6 weeks or even longer. If relapse occurs after discontinuation, continuous low-dose antimicrobial therapy should be reintroduced and sustained if effective" [27]. Long-term results with trimethoprim-sulfamethoxazole have remained poor [28–30]. Results of therapy with quinolones, including norfloxacin [31], ciprofloxacin [32, 33] and ofloxacin [34–36], seem to be more encouraging.

Analgesics are often a mainstay treatment but few studies on their long-term efficacy have been undertaken. Simple analgesics based on paracetamol should be considered initially. The use of nonsteroidal anti-inflammatory medications is widespread, but their use in the absence of inflammation is debatable. **Opioids** should only be considered if one or other of the national guidelines have been followed (e.g. British Pain Society guidelines). An intravenous opioid drug trial could be considered to help in the decision making for the long-term prescription of opioids. **Neuropathic analgesics** may have a role (see below).

Several small studies of hormone manipulation with the 5- α -reductase inhibitor **finasteride** support the view that it may favorably influence voiding and pain in a small percentage of patients [21, 37, 38]. **Anticholinergics** may be beneficial in reducing urgency urinary symptoms in some patients [39].

Positive effects of **phytotherapy** and **pentosanpolysulfate** (PPS) [40] have been reported, but these options need to be explored in prospective studies before any recommendations can be made.

There is little evidence for immune modulation using **cytokine inhibitors** [41, 42].

Scrotal pain syndrome

The research on the use of drugs in the management of scrotal pain, and testicular pain in particular, is limited [12]. There have been advocates for the use of **antibiotics** but as with the prostate pain syndrome, there appears to be no hard evidence for their use in the absence of a well-defined infection.

If urinary symptoms are present then, as with the prostate pain syndrome, it makes sense to manage these (see above). Similarly, the use of **NSAID** may have a role if inflammation is suspected. Otherwise, analgesics including **opioids** and therapies for neuropathic pain (see below) are often considered.

Bladder pain syndrome

A significant amount of research has been undertaken in this field and this has been summarized on a number of occasions [12]. Difficulties persist in agreeing diagnostic criteria; however, the following drugs have been suggested as being useful when the NIDDK classification for interstitial cystitis is used.

- Grade A recommendation (clinical studies of good quality and consistency including at least one randomized trial): **cimetidine, sodium pentosanpolysulfate** (**antibiotics**, but a limited role and only when infection documented).
- Grade B recommendations (well-conducted clinical studies without randomized trials): h**ydroxyzine, amitriptyline.**
- Grade C recommendation (absence of directly applicable clinical studies of good quality): **analgesics, corticosteroids, prostaglandins, immunosuppressants, oxybutynin, tolterodine, gabapentin** (preliminary data to date).

Penile pain syndrome

When there is no obvious known cause for penile pain, neuropathic pain medications may be considered.

Physical interventions

Prostate pain syndrome

Therapies, such as biofeedback, relaxation exercises, lifestyle changes (e.g. diet, discontinuing bike riding, changing a workstation), acupuncture, massage therapy, chiropractic therapy and meditation have all been suggested to improve symptoms [19, 21].

It is sometimes difficult to identify which component(s) of multidisciplinary therapy are the most effective. Hetrick *et al.* have suggested that biofeedback pelvic floor training, independent of other influences, may benefit this group of patients [43]. It is the author's clinical impression that treatment needs to be intensive and personalized and the role of the therapist is very important. Much has been written about trigger point therapy within the pelvis but there are few formal studies [44]. Individual patients appear to benefit providing they are managed as "a whole" with attention to posture, exercise and stretches as well as the trigger point release treatments.

Heat therapy, such as transrectal hyperthermia [45–48] and transurethral thermotherapy [49–52], have been reported to produce favorable results in some patients [20]. These treatment options are rarely used.

Scrotal pain syndrome

It has been suggested that there may be a role for surgery if an identifiable lesion can be demonstrated. Success rates of 50% or higher have been described [53–55]. However, in the absence of such a lesion, the role of surgery is debatable and may even be detrimental [12].

Microsurgical testicular denervation for scrotal pain syndrome has been descibed, but case series are small [56, 57]. Epidymectomy and orchidectomy are probably less successful (though 20% and 60% success rates, respectively, have been suggested) [55, 58] but are frequently undertaken.

Nerve blocks (L1 dorsal root renal/sympathectomy, groin blocks and pudendal/perineal (posterior triangle) blocks) may have a role in the management of scrotal pain syndrome as well as aiding differential diagnosis. However, there are no specific published data.

Bladder pain syndrome/IC

The following recommendations are the views from Fall *et al.* [12] with comments from Hanno *et al.* [59] inserted in square brackets when there is a difference in the recommendation.

- Grade A recommendation (clinical studies of good quality and consistency including at least one randomized trial): intravesical pentosanpolysulfate, intravesical dimethyl sulfoxide [Grade B recommendation in the Hanno reference], intravesical resinifaratoxin (consider as a research tool), transurethal coagulation of bladder lesions (e.g. Hunner's ulcers) if present, major surgery (cystectomy, diversionary surgery, bladder augmentation) if shrunken scarred bladder.

- Grade B recommendations (well-conducted clinical studies without randomized trials): electromotive drug administration (EMDA) with lidocaine, sacral neuromodulation [should be considered investigational], bladder training/physiotherapy/biofeedback].
- Grade C recommendation (sbsence of directly applicable clinical studies of good quality): intravesical anesthetics, intravesical heparin, intravesical hyaluronic acid, bladder distension, nerve blocks/epidural, diet, acupuncture.

Hanno *et al.* stated that cystolysis (denervation of the nerves from around the bladder), sympathetic and parasympathetic neurolysis are not indicated.

Penile pain syndrome

There is no specific evidence available for physical interventions for the management of penile pain with no obvious cause. However, if the penis is considered as a somatic structure, nerve blocks may have a role as in any other somatic structure, especially if there is a suggestion of a central process.

Psychology

Prostate pain syndrome

The role of psychologic intervention in prostate pain syndrome has been studied and further research is ongoing [17, 18, 60].

As might be expected, the severity of urinary symptoms is linked to pain. However, psychologic factors such as depression, pain-contingent resting and helplessness catastrophizing are stronger predictors of pain severity. Pain-contingent resting is the strongest predictor, with helplessness and catastrophizing also being predictive.

Presenters at a recent Société Internationale d'Urologie meeting (Cape Town, 2006) have stated that: "Taken together, these data suggest a biopsychosocial intervention in CP/CPPS is warranted and that cognitive/behavioral variables are targets for change because of their significant impact CP/CPPS patient adjustment."

Bladder pain syndrome

The EAU recommendations suggested that little research had been undertaken in this area but that psychologic tools should be considered.

Generic treatment options

Because many urogenital pain syndromes are poorly understood, generic treatment options may be considered. These will be most effective for neuropathic conditions with or without central sensitization and muscle spasm, trigger points or hyperalgesia.

Neuropathic pain therapy

Chong & Hester [61] have summarized the current knowledge in relation to the role of neuropathic analgesics in urogenital pain.

Tricyclic and tetracyclic antidepressant drugs may have a role if the clinical presentation suggests pain of neuropathic origin. The best evidence is for amitriptyline. SSRIs and SNRIs may have a role. The best evidence in neuropathic pain is for venlafaxine (but this has cardiac side effects) and duloxetine (which may also reduce stress incontinence).

Antiepileptic drugs have become very popular and several studies have suggested that gabapentin and pregabalin may have a role in urogenital pain. Other antiepileptics may be considered.

Opioids should be considered providing appropriate precautions are undertaken – see above.

Differential nerve blocks

Very little has been published on the therapeutic role of differential nerve blocks in urogenital pain [62]. However, it is clear that they may have a diagnostic role [63] as well as a possible therapeutic role. The evidence for a therapeutic role is often indirect and draws upon the evidence from pain perceived at other sites.

A comprehensive understanding of the anatomy is essential to be able to diagnose specific nerve involvement and access the nerves in a safe manner. The sympathetic, parasympathetic and somatic nerves can be blocked separately. Using appropriate imaging and neurotracing techniques allows nerves to be identified sequentially. For instance, in the region of the piriformis, the sciatic nerve, posterior femoral cutaneous nerve and its perineal nerve, inferior gluteal nerve, the nerve to obturator internus and the pudendal nerve can be separated out. A lot of attention has been paid to blocking these posterior nerves recently as well as the anterior nerves such as the ilio-inguinal, iliohypogastric and genitofemoral nerves. In our clinic, we now have to assess many more patients with nerve compression in the groin, buttock region and perineum than was done a few years ago. Some patients do gain long-term benefit from injections occasionally combined with pulsed radiofrequency neuromodulation while others are referred on for peripheral nerve surgery.

Trigger point treatments
There is no doubt that the muscles of the pelvis can develop trigger points similar to striated muscles at other sites with referred pain. The conditions seen may manifest as one or two trigger points with referred pain or as a more complex regional condition with central changes resulting in widespread muscle hyperalgesia and visceral dysfunction.

As with any other trigger point pathology, the patient needs to be considered as a whole. In particular,

Box 14.1 Treatment options

Condition	Intervention
Interventions supported by evidence	
Prostate pain syndrome	α Blockers
	NSAIDs
	Biofeedback and muscle-based therapies
Bladder pain syndrome	Hydroxyzine
	Amitriptyline
	PPS oral/intravesicular
	Intravesicular dimethyl sulfoxide
	Intravesicular vallinoids (contradictory results and side effects result in this treatment not having a high recommendation)
	Transurethral resection of Hunner's lesion
	Psychology
Muscle hyperalgesia	Relaxation+/−biofeedback+/−physical therapy (mainly male pelvic pain)
	Multidisciplinary pain management (for well-being/quality of life)
Commonly used interventions currently unproven	
Prostate pain syndrome	Muscle relaxants
	Antimicrobial therapy (in certain cases where response to trial occurs, quinolones probably best)
	Opioids (as part of multimodal therapy for treatment-refractory pain in collaboration with pain clinics)
	5-α-Reductase inhibitors (if benign prostatic hyperplasia is present)
Bladder pain syndrome	Analgesics
	Intravesicular hyaluronic acid
	Intravesicular chondroitin sulfate
	Nerve blockade
	Bladder training
	Physiotherapy
	Acupuncture
	Bladder resection and other surgery (for small-volume bladders, recurrent infection, reflux)
Peripheral neuralgia in pelvic pain	Nerve blocks
	Tricyclic antidepressants
	Anticonvulsants
General treatments	Paracetamol
	NSAIDs
	Tricyclic antidepressants
	Anticonvulsants
Interventions refuted by evidence	
Prostate pain syndrome	Antimicrobial therapy (in certain cases where no response to trial occurs)
Bladder pain syndrome	Bladder distension

the core muscles external to the pelvis may need addressing, e.g., paraspinal, gluteal and anterior abdominal wall muscles. The adductors and iliopsoas also need to be assessed and managed. Within the pelvis muscles such as coccygeus, iliococcygeus and pubococcygeus/rectalis may have trigger points, as may the piriformis and obturator internus muscles which span from the pelvis to the hip. The ischiocavernosus and bulbocavernosus may also be involved.

All these muscles can be reached for injection with appropriate imaging. Once more, the research in this field is minimal. However, evidence from other areas suggests that injecting, particularly if combined with postural work, stretching and pacing, may benefit these patients. We have a number of patients in whom botulinium toxin injections into some of these deeper pelvic muscles under CT guidance has given a significant response where other treatments have failed.

Author's recommendations

It is important that "well-defined" pathologies are identified and treated appropriately. With this in mind, the patient may be referred to a specialty clinician (e.g. urologist, gynecologist, urogynecologist). The symptoms and signs will usually define which is the most appropriate specialty and in some cases several specialties may be involved. Once "well-defined" pathologies, such as tumors and infections, have been excluded, these complex pain syndrome patients will require management in a multidisciplinary environment with the involvement of pain management physicians/ psychologists and physiotherapists. Close links will need to be maintained with the specialty clinicians (for specialty functional symptomatic treatments) and the family doctor.

In certain conditions the roles of functional/symptomatic treatments are fairly well defined, such as in the bladder pain syndromes. In others there is very little information. The priority has to be to obtain a balance between risk and proven benefit. In many cases there is little evidence for surgery; indications for surgery include severe incontinence, prolapse and recurrent proven infections. Nonsurgical interventions should be employed initially, including evaluation by an experienced urogenital pain management psychologist.

The pain management physician/anesthetist may use the tools of medications and injections as for any other chronic pain condition. For injection treatments, the pain management physician/anesthetist should be very familiar with the anatomy and the range of tools available to identify the targets appropriately. Experience with neurotracing and CT imaging is essential. In the future, ultrasound may also become important. Neuromodulation appears to have a role. However, the technique chosen usually depends upon the specialist performing the technique. We aim to provide both sacral root and retrograde spinal cord stimulation depending on the symptoms, with a trial of both if appropriate. Further research in relation to neuromodulation needs to be undertaken and until then both options should be available. Peripheral nerve (groin nerves and pudendal) neuromodulation is at an even earlier stage.

No patient with urogenital pain should be managed unless there is access to an experienced urogenital pain management clinical psychologist. However, such psychologists are a rare breed.

More centers of urogenital pain medicine with involvement of pain management physicians/anesthetists, psychologists and physiotherapists need to be set up with the aim of managing these complex patients within a multidisciplinary environment closely linked to specialty services.

References

1. Krieger JN, Ross SO, Riley DE, et al. Chronic prostatitis: epidemiology and role of infection. *Urology* 2002; **60**(6, suppl.A): 8–13.
2. Roberts RO, Lieber MM, Rhodes, T, et al. Prevalence of a physician-assigned diagnosis of prostatitis: the Olmsted County study of urinary symptoms and health status among men. *Urology* 1998; **51**(4): 578–584.
3. Stamley TA. *Pathogenesis and Treatment of Urinary Tract Infections.* Williams and Wilkins, Baltimore, 1980: 342–429.
4. McNaughton Collins M, Stafford RS, O'Leary MP, et al. How common is prostatitis? A national survey of physician visits. *J Urol* 1998; **159**: 1224–1248.
5. Nickel JC, Downey J, Hunter D, et al. Prevalence of prostatitis-like symptoms in a population based study using the National Institutes of Health chronic prostatitis symptom index. *J Urol* 2001; **165**: 842–845.
6. Nickel J, Teichman J, Gregoire M, et al. Prevalence, diagnosis, characterization, and treatment of prostatitis, interstitial cystitis, and epididymitis in outpatient urological practice: the Canadian PIE Study. *Urology* 2005; **66**(5): 935–940.
7. Bowsher D. Neurogenic pain syndromes and their management. *Br Med Bull* 1991; **47**(3): 644–666.

8. Granitsiotis P, Kirk D. Chronic testicular pain: an overview. *Eur Urol* 2004; **45**(4): 430–436.

9. Gillenwater JY, Wein AJ. Summary of the National Institute of Arthritis, Diabetes, Digestive and Kidney Diseases Workshop on Interstitial Cystitis, National Institutes of Health, Bethesda, Maryland, August 28–29, 1987. *J Urol* 1988; **140**: 203–206.

10. Peeker R, Fall M. Toward a precise definition of interstitial cystitis: further evidence of differences in classic and nonulcer disease. *J Urol* 2002; **167**: 2470–2472.

11. Abrams PH, Cardozo L, Fall M, *et al*. The standardisation of terminology of lower urinary tract function: report from the standardisation sub-committee of the international continence society. Neuro*urol Urodynam* 2002; **21**: 167.

12. Fall M, Baranowski AP, Fowler CJ, *et al*. *Guidelines on Chronic Pelvic Pain*. European Association of Urology, Arnhem, The Netherlands, 2003.

13. Clemens JQ, Meenan RT, Richard T, *et al*. Prevalence of interstitial cystitis symptoms in a managed care population. *J Urol* 2005; **174**(2): 576–580.

14. Forrest JB, Schmidt S. Interstitial cystitis, chronic nonbacterial prostatitis and chronic pelvic pain syndrome in men: a common and frequently identical. clinical entity. *J Urol* 2004; **172**(6): 2561–2562.

15. Fall M, Baranowski A, Fowler C, *et al*. European Association of Urology guidelines on chronic pelvic pain. *Eur Urol* 2004; **46**(6): 681–689.

16. Baranowski A. Complex Chronic pelvic pain in men. In: Baranowski A, Abrams P, Fall M (eds) *Urogenital Pain in Clinical Practice*. Marcel Dekker, New York, 2008.

17. Tripp A, Nickel JC, Wang Y, *et al.*, and the National Institutes of Health-Chronic Prostatitis Collaborative Research Network (NIH-CPCRN) Study Group. Catastrophizing and pain-contingent rest predict patient adjustment in men with chronic prostatitis/chronic pelvic pain syndrome. *J Pain* 2006; **7**(10): 697–708.

18. Nickel JC, Tripp DA, Wang Y, *et al.*, and the NIH-CPCRN Study Group. Biopsychosocial factors in quality of life in CP/CPPS. Category III chronic prostatitis/chronic pelvic pain syndrome: Insights from the National Institutes of Health Chronic Prostatitis Collaborative Research Network Studies. *Curr Prostate Rep* 2007; **5**: 141–148.

19. Nickel JC, Weidner W. Chronic prostatitis: current concepts and antimicrobial therapy. *Infect Urol* 2000; **13**: 22.

20. Nickel JC. Prostatitis: evolving management strategies. *Urol Clin North Am* 1999; **26**: 737–751.

21. Olavi L, Make L, Imo M. Effects of finasteride in patients with chronic idiopathic prostatitis: a double-blind, placebo-controlled, pilot study. *Eur Urol* 1998; **33**: 24.

22. Barbalias GA, Meares EM Jr, Sant GR. Prostatodynia: clinical and urodynamic characteristics. *J Urol* 1983; **130**: 514–517.

23. Osborn DE, George NJ, Rao PN, *et al*. Prostatodynia – physiological characteristics and rational management with muscle relaxants. *Br J Urol* 1981; **53**: 621–623.

24. de la Rosette JJ, Karthaus HF, van Kerrebroeck PE, de Boo T, Debruyne FM. Research in 'prostatitis syndromes': the use

25. of alfuzosin (a new alpha 1-receptor-blocking agent) in patients mainly presenting with micturition complaints of an irritative nature and confirmed urodynamic abnormalities. *Eur Urol* 1992; **22**: 222–227.

25. Neal DE Jr, Moon TD. Use of terazosin in prostatodynia and validation of a symptom score questionnaire. *Urology* 1994; **43**: 460–465.

26. Brunner H, Weidner W, Schiefer HG. Studies on the role of Ureaplasma urealyticum and Mycoplasma hominis in prostatitis. *J Infect Dis* 1983; **147**: 807–813.

27. de la Rosette JJ, Debruyne FM. Nonbacterial prostatitis: a comprehensive review. *Urol Int* 1991; **46**: 121–125.

28. Drach GW. Trimethoprim sulfamethoxazole therapy of chronic bacterial prostatitis. *J Urol* 1974; **111**: 637–639.

29. McGuire EJ, Lytton B. Bacterial prostatitis: treatment with trimethoprim-sulfamethoxazole. *Urology* 1976; **7**: 499–500.

30. Meares EM. Long-term therapy of chronic bacterial prostatitis with trimethoprim- sulfamethoxazole. *Can Med Assoc J* 1975; **112**: 22–25.

31. Schaeffer AJ, Darras FS. The efficacy of norfloxacin in the treatment of chronic bacterial prostatitis refractory to trimethoprim-sulfamethoxazole and/or carbenicillin. *J Urol* 1990; **144**: 690–693.

32. Childs SJ. Ciprofloxacin in treatment of chronic bacterial prostatitis. *Urology* 1990; **35**: 15–18.

33. Weidner W, Schiefer HG, Brahler E. Refractory chronic bacterial prostatitis: a re-evaluation of ciprofloxacin treatment after a median follow up of 30 months. *J Urol* 1991; **146**: 350–352.

34. Cox CE. Ofloxacin in the management of complicated urinary tract infections, including prostatitis. *Am J Med* 1989; **87**: 61S–68S.

35. Pust RA, Ackenheil-Koppe HR, Gilbert P. Clinical efficacy of ofloxacin (Tarivid) in patients with chronic bacterial prostatitis: preliminary results. *J Chemother* 1989; **1**(suppl 4): 471.

36. Remy G, Rouger C, Chavanet P. Use of ofloxacin for prostatitis. *Rev Infect Dis* 1988; **10**(suppl 1): 173.

37. Golio G. The use of finasteride in the treatment to chronic nonbacterial prostatitis. In: Abstracts of the 49th Annual Meeting of the Northeastern Section of the American Urological Association, Phoenix, AZ, 1997; 128.

38. Holm M, Meyhoff HH. Chronic prostatic pain. A new treatment option with finasteride? *Scand J Urol Nephrol* 1997; **31**: 213–215.

39. Meares EJ. Prostatitis and related disorders. In: Walsh PC, Retik AB, Stamey TA, Vaughan EDJ, (eds) *Campbell's Urology*. WB Saunders, Philadelphia, 1992: 807.

40. Wedren H. Effects of sodium pentosanpolysulphate on symptoms related to chronic non-bacterial prostatitis. A double-blind randomized study. *Scand J Urol Nephrol* 1987; **21**: 81–88.

41. Canale D, Scaricabarozzi I, Giorgi P, Turchi P, Ducci M, Menchini-Fabris GF. Use of a novel non-steroidal anti-inflammatory drug, nimesulide, in the treatment of abacterial prostatovesiculitis. *Andrologia* 1993; **25**: 163–166.

42. Canale D, Turchi P, Giorgi PM, Scaricabarozzi I, Menchini-Fabris GF. Treatment of abacterial prostato-vesiculitis with nimesulide. *Drugs* 1993; **46**(suppl 1): 147–150.

43. Hetrick DC, Glazer H, Liu YW, *et al*. Pelvic floor electromyography in men with chronic pelvic pain syndrome: a case-control study. *Neurol Urodynam* 2006; **25**(1): 46–49.

44. Wise D, Anderson R. *A Headache in the Pelvis: A New Understanding and Treatment for Prostatitis and Chronic Pelvic Pain Syndromes*, 5th edn. National Centre for Pelvic Pain Research, Occidental, CA, 2008.

45. Kamihira O, Sahashi M, Yamada S, Ono Y, Ohshima S. Transrectal hyperthermia for chronic prostatitis. *Nippon Hinyokika Gakkai Zasshi* 1993; **84**: 1095–1098.

46. Kumon H, Ono N, Uno S, *et al*. Transrectal hyperthermia for the treatment of chronic prostatitis. *Nippon Hinyokika Gakkai Zasshi* 1993; **84**: 265–271.

47. Montorsi F, Guazzoni G, Bergamaschi F, *et al*. Is there a role for transrectal microwave hyperthermia of the prostate in the treatment of abacterial prostatitis and prostatodynia? *Prostate* 1993; **22**: 139–146.

48. Shaw TK, Watson GM, Barnes DG. Microwave hyperthermia in the treatment of chronic abacterial prostatitis and prostatodynia: results of a double-blind placebo controlled trial. *J Urol* 1993; **149**: 405A.

49. Choi NG, Soh SH, Yoon TH, Song MH. Clinical experience with transurethral microwave thermotherapy for chronic nonbacterial prostatitis and prostatodynia. *J Endourol* 1994; **8**: 61–64.

50. Michielsen D, van Camp K, Wyndaele JJ, Verheyden B. Transurethral microwave thermotherapy in the treatment of chronic abacterial prostatitis: a 2 years follow-up. *Acta Urol Belg* 1995; **63**: 1–4.

51. Nickel JC, Sorenson R. Transurethral microwave thermotherapy of nonbacterial prostatitis and prostatodynia: initial experience. *Urology* 1994; **44**: 458–460.

52. Nickel JC, Sorensen R. Transurethral microwave thermotherapy for nonbacterial prostatitis: a randomized double-blind sham controlled study using new prostatitis specific assessment questionnaires. *J Urol* 1996; **155**: 1950195-4; discussion 1954–1955.

53. Gray CL, Powell CR, Amling CL. Outcomes for surgical management of orchalgia in patients with identifiable intrascrotal lesions. *Eur Urol* 2001; **39**: 455–459.

54. Yaman O, Ozdiler E, Anafarta K, Gogus O. Effect of microsurgical subinguinal varicocele ligation to treat pain. *Urology* 2000; **55**: 107–108.

55. Padmore DE, Norman RW, Millard OH. Analyses of indications for and outcomes of epididymectomy. *J Urol* 1996; **156**: 95–96.

56. Heidenreich A, Olbert P, Engelmann UH. Management of chronic testalgia by microsurgical testicular denervation. *Eur Urol* 2002; **41**: 392–397.

57. Choa RG, Swami KS. Testicular denervation. A new surgical procedure for intractable testicular pain. *Br J Urol* 1992; **70**: 417–419.

58. Sweeney P, Tan J, Butler MR, McDermott TE, Grainger R, Thornhill JA. Epididymectomy in the management of intrascrotal disease: a critical reappraisal. *Br J Urol* 1998; **81**: 753–755.

59. Hanno P, Baranowski AP, Rosamilia A, *et al. International Continence Society Guidelines on chronic pelvic pain.* International Consultation on Incontinence (ICI), 2005.

60. McNaughton-Collins M. The impact of chronic prostatitis/chronic pelvic pain syndrome on patients. *World J Urol* 2003: **21**(2): 86–89.

61. Chong MS, Hester J. Pharmacotherapy for neuropathic pain with special reference to urogenital pain. In: Baranowski AP, Abrams P, Fall M (eds) *Urogenital Pain in Clinical Practice*. Marcel Dekker, New York, 2008.

62. Naja MZ, Al-Tannir MA, Maaliki H, El-Rajab M, Ziade MF, Zeidan A. Nerve-stimulator-guided repeated pudendal nerve block for treatment of pudendal neuralgia. *Eur J Anaesthesiol* 2006; **23**(5): 442–444.

63. Robert R, Labat JJ, Bensignor M, *et al*. Decompression and transposition of the pudendal nerve in pudendal neuralgia: a randomized controlled trial and long-term evaluation. *Eur Urol* 2005; **47**(3): 403–408.

CHAPTER 15

Pain from abdominal organs

Timothy J. Ness[1] *and L. Vandy Black*[2]

[1]Department of Anesthesiology, University of Alabama at Birmingham, Birmingham, AL, USA
[2]Department of Pediatric Hematology-Oncology, University of Alabama at Birmingham, Birmingham, AL, USA

Sources of abdominal pain

Pain localized to the abdomen can have multiple etiologies, a subset of which have their sites of origin in viscera within or immediately adjacent to the peritoneal cavity such as the gastrointestinal tract, hepatobiliary structures/pancreas, urologic structures, and reproductive organs. Etiologies include focal processes secondary to infection, cancer, other sources of inflammation or obstruction, idiopathic systemic diseases, and functional alterations. The substrates of sensory processing from these viscera are diffusely organized so that sensations from these structures can be perceived as similarly diffuse and may be localized to general body regions or be perceived as located within nonvisceral structures. Organ-specific localization may require technologic extensions of the physical exam (e.g. endoscopy) that allow for direct stimulation or examination of abdominal organs. Often diagnoses are descriptive in nature with only indirect evidence for an organ's involvement due to an association of the pain with a bodily function such as swallowing, micturition or defecation.

Evaluation of abdominal symptoms

Abdominal pain is a common presenting symptom in emergency rooms and primary care clinics. When coupled with chest symptoms, it is the number 1 cited reason for patients seeking urgent care evaluations. Initial approaches include a basic history and physical exam that assesses the acute versus chronic nature of the complaints, exacerbating and ameliorating factors, and definition of co-existing disease. A key consideration is potential signs and symptoms associated with neoplastic and infectious processes (e.g. weight loss, fevers, night sweats, and chills) since a failure to initiate timely therapy can have significant consequences related to the progression of life-threatening disease processes. The use of medications which alter bowel motility or bladder function, even when prescribed for other uses (e.g. antidepressants), must be considered. Palpation and auscultation of the abdomen can identify abdominal wall rigidity or localized tenderness suggesting a peritoneal process or an underlying mass suggestive of a neoplastic, infectious or obstructive process. Rectal and pelvic exams may give additional information related to local pathology. Neurologic examination may demonstrate evidence of nerve entrapment, neuropathy or localized radiculopathy. Testing for fecal blood, urinalysis, blood cell count with white cell differential, serum amylase/lipase levels, electrolytes and liver function tests all are considered routine. Radiographic evaluations, endoscopic evaluations, ultrasonography, and other advanced imaging or tissue/fluid sampling studies have become routine, but should ideally be dependent upon the persistence or progression of complaints.

Visceral pain arising from cancer

Pathophysiology

The diagnosis of cancer should be considered when evaluating presumably "chronic" disorders. This topic is the subject of an entire chapter in this text, so only

Evidence-Based Chronic Pain Management. Edited by C. Stannard, E. Kalso and J. Ballantyne. © 2010 Blackwell Publishing.

brief mention will be given here, but cancer-related pain is illustrative of all other visceral pains.

Neoplasms can arise in all visceral structures and dull constant pain is often an early symptom. Some neoplasms occur more commonly in the presence of recurrent inflammatory processes such as chronic pancreatitis and ulcerative colitis, so establishment of a "benign" diagnosis does not preclude development of a malignant process [1]. Pain can be induced by stimulation of abdominal viscera in three ways: chemical stimulation that occurs secondary to local inflammatory or tissue-damaging processes; chemical stimulation that occurs secondary to ischemia; or high-intensity mechanical stimulation that is secondary to compressive/obstructive processes (which may be modified by inflammation or ischemia). Cancer can obviously be the etiology of all three of these types of stimuli. It can infiltrate a primary viscus or extend into a neighboring organ. It can cause bowel obstruction with secondary distension. There can be liver metastases that produce capsular or diaphragmatic irritation, portal vascular distension, ascites, and obstruction of the biliary tree. There can be ischemia and necrosis of viscera due to mesenteric vessel involvement. Extension of the disease process into retroperitoneal, parietal peritoneal, abdominal wall or bony structures can produce nonvisceral pain that is equal to or greater than that due to the visceral process. In addition, neuropathic pain can result from lumbosacral plexus invasion or spinal cord compression. Sequelae of antineoplastic treatments can outlive the primary process in the form of postoperative pain syndromes, stent-related complications, and chemotherapy- or radiation therapy-induced neuropathies. Cancer serves as an "all-of-the-above" answer for possible pain mechanisms and so requires due consideration.

Evaluation and treatment

Cancer involving the upper gastrointestinal tract and organs located in the upper abdomen generally produces chest or upper abdominal symptoms. Lower gastrointestinal tract lesions and pelvic organ cancers generally result in symptoms localized to the lower abdomen, pelvis or perineum. Unfortunately, due to the potential presence of metastatic extension prior to diagnosis, no symptomatology or location is pathognomonic for any specific disease site. Visceral cancers may be asymptomatic until obstruction or invasion of

other structures occurs. Anorexia, weight loss, fatigue, nausea and other nonspecific symptoms are common. Further investigation is prompted by the presence of anemia, hematemesis, melena, hematuria, and palpable masses on physical exam. Referral to an oncologist for a definitive diagnostic work-up and possible surgical exploration/biopsy is always appropriate though initial diagnostic imaging may need to be performed so that referral can be facilitated.

Treatment of the cancer (surgery, chemotherapy, radiotherapy) is considered the primary treatment for pain whether it is curative or palliative. Temporizing medical treatments are the first line of palliative therapy with the aggressive use of opioids, anti-inflammatories, antiemetics, antispasmodics, stimulants, and other indicated adjuvants. Neurolytic procedures including cordotomy are considered options in some cases with the particular site of treatment determined by the site of the cancer. Further discussion related to the evaluation and treatment of cancer pain will be deferred to the chapter on that topic.

Visceral pain arising from the gastrointestinal tract

General issues

An early distinction that must be determined when evaluating pain arising in the gastrointestinal (GI) tract is whether the suspected pathophysiology is potentially tissue and/or life threatening or whether it represents a condition in which quality of life is the main endpoint of therapy. Infectious, inflammatory, and ischemic processes may require urgent treatment, whereas other disorders with lesser potential for global physiologic disruption may be evaluated and treated at a slower pace.

Chronic mesenteric ischemia – ischemic colitis

Pathophysiology/epidemiology

Mesenteric ischemia, when recognized, prompts immediate treatment in a way similar to the treatment of cardiac angina with focused attempts to either reduce the metabolic demand or to improve blood and oxygen delivery. Acute mesenteric ischemia is not common but due to the severity of consequences, accounts for 0.1% of hospital admissions [2]. Severe abdominal pain may be precipitated by the ingestion of a meal which increases the metabolic demands on the GI tract. As a consequence, weight loss and poor nutritional status due to a fear of eating may compromise patients already in ill health due to vascular disease. End-stage phenomena associated with mesenteric ischemia include necrosis of the gut wall with subsequent perforation and peritonitis. A compromised mucosal barrier can also result in the release of gram-negative bacterial endotoxin, leading to systemic manifestations.

Evaluation and treatment

Abdominal bruits, poor peripheral pulses, and arteriographic evidence of stenosis or occlusion in the three main mesenteric arteries are all consistent with the diagnosis of *abdominal* angina. Embolic events, arterial thrombosis, venous occlusion, and low flow states due to poor cardiac output all produce similar results. Approximately half of the cases of morbidity due to mesenteric vascular disease present as ischemic colitis which is usually diagnosed by colonoscopy. It is notable that approximately 20% of patients with ischemic colitis develop evidence of peritonitis requiring surgical treatment. These patients may present with persistent diarrhea, rectal bleeding or weight loss. The gold standard for the diagnostic work-up of mesenteric ischemia is angiography, which has both a sensitivity and specificity close to 100% [3]. However, less invasive methods such as magnetic resonance angiography (MRA) and computed tomography (CT) also have diagnostic value [2].

Treatments for mesenteric vasculopathy are highly dependent upon whether the patient has peritoneal signs. When such signs are present, a patient must undergo an exploratory laparotomy. In this setting, potential treatment options are surgical in nature and include resection of necrotic and perforated bowel with thromboembolectomy, patch angioplasty, endarterectomy, and bypass procedures, depending on the individual vascular anatomy and the cause of the occlusion (i.e. embolus or thrombus). "Second-look" surgeries may also be necessary [3]. Percutaneous transluminal angioplasty has been successful in one case report of a patient with a thrombosis of the superior mesenteric artery [4], but this approach is generally not advocated given the significant risk of rethrombosis [2].

In patients without suspected peritonitis, thrombolytics such as tissue plasminogen activator (t-PA), urokinase, and streptokinase have been used successfully in some patients [2] but to date, there are no studies which compare these agents to each other or other therapies. The use of vasodilators has been supported by both animal and human studies [2]. However, these are rarely used as monotherapy, unless a patient is felt to be a poor surgical candidate. Clinically, Boley *et al.* demonstrated a decreased mortality rate of 54% (compared to a traditional 70–80%) when utilizing early angiography and papaverine in the management of patients with suspected acute mesenteric ischemia [5]. This has led to the frequent perioperative use of papaverine to reduce splanchnic vasoconstriction; however, there are no randomized controlled trials to support its efficacy. Finally, animal studies suggest the potential role of angiotensin-converting enzyme (ACE) inhibitors, gastric inhibitory peptide, iloprost (a synthetic derivative of prostacyclin), and similar compounds to increase mesenteric flow, but these await full translation [2].

Inflammatory bowel disease

Pathophysiology/epidemiology

Inflammatory bowel disease (IBD) consists of two recurrent gastrointestinal inflammatory disorders (ulcerative colitis (UC) and Crohn's disease (CD)) which have many similarities in symptomatology and histopathology. Where they differ is in the extent of the disease process, incidence of relapse, and associated complications such as fistula formation. In UC, the gastrointestinal component of the disease process is restricted to the colon, whereas in CD, there can be involvement in any portion of the gastrointestinal tract. These are highly disruptive disorders that can become emergently severe due to local spread of infection and alterations in nutrient, fluid, and electrolyte levels. Based on epidemiologic data, it is suspected that IBD has some genetic basis to its etiology. It is 3–6 times more common in Jews than non-Jews and more common in whites than blacks or Asians. UC is 3–5 times more common than CD, but has less impact on the healthcare system since recurrent exacerbations are less frequent and severe.

Evaluation and treatment

The diagnosis of inflammatory bowel disease is based on biopsy, colonoscopic/endoscopic appearance, and/or surgical evaluation prompted by abdominal pain, fever, and altered bowel habits (e.g. bloody diarrhea).

Table 15.1 Levels of evidence

Level	Type of evidence
I	Evidence obtained from meta-analysis of multiple, well-designed, controlled studies. Randomized trials with low false-positive and false-negative errors (high power).
II	Evidence obtained from at least one well-designed, experimental study. Randomized trials with high false-positive or false-negative errors (low power).
III	Evidence obtained from well-designed, quasi-experimental studies such as nonrandomized, controlled single-group, pre/post, cohort, and time or matched case–control series.
IV	Evidence from well-designed, nonexperimental studies such as comparative and correlational descriptive and case studies.
V	Evidence from case reports and clinical examples.

Grade	
A	There is evidence of type I or consistent findings from multiple studies of type II, III or IV
B	There is evidence of type II, III or IV and findings are generally consistent
C	There is evidence of type II, III or IV and findings are inconsistent
D	There is little or no systematic empiric evidence

Box 15.1 Pain treatment options: inflammatory bowel disease (and associated arthropathies) [8–15]

Treatments with Grade B evidence

Immunosuppressants (azothioprine, corticosteroids – Level II)

Salicylates (sulfasalazine, olsalazine – Level II and III)

COX-2 inhibitors (Level III)

TNF-α blockade (infliximab but not etanercept – Level II) [14]

Granulocyte macrophage-colony stimulating factor (Level II)

Probiotics (Level III)

Oral antibiotics (rifaximin, metronidazole "-azines" (Level II and III)

Treatments with Grade C evidence

Enema/suppositories (mesalazine, nicotine – Level III)

Opioids (Level IV)

Radiation enteritis or local infection by organisms such as shigella, salmonella, amoebiasis or *Clostridium difficile* excludes the diagnosis. The formation of fistulas, abscesses, strictures, perforation and toxic dilation can all occur as local complications of IBD. All are more common in CD than UC. IBD may also be associated with arthritis, skin changes and evidence of liver disease.

Treatment of IBD is a rapidly evolving field, with many new agents under investigation [6], and a full discussion of such treatments is beyond the scope of this chapter. In general, UC can be "cured" by colectomy since by definition, one cannot have colitis without a colon. However, CD is a life-long illness with the goals of therapy generally revolving around symptom relief. The mainstays of pharmacologic therapy include corticosteroids, aminosalicylates, and immune modulators such as the thiopurines [7]. A brief summary of options for pain relief and levels of evidence (Table 15.1) is outlined in Box 15.1.

One pharmacologic approach which has been recently debated in the literature includes the use of tumor necrosis factor-α (TNF-α) inhibitors [9]. Infliximab is one of the most well-studied agents in this class and has been proven effective for induction and maintenance therapies by multiple clinical trials and a recent Cochrane review [10]. In one study, a clinical response was observed at 4 weeks in 65% of patients with CD who received a single dose of infliximab (5 mg/kg, 10 mg/kg or 20 mg/kg), compared with 17% of patients who received placebo [11]. In the ACCENT I study (A Crohn's Disease Clinical Trial Evaluating Infliximab in a New Long Term Treatment Regimen), patients who received maintenance therapy with infliximab had higher rates of remission at 30 weeks than those patients treated with placebo [12]. Additional studies, including ACCENT II, have also found infliximab effective in treating draining fistulas in CD as compared to placebo, with a complete resolution in 36% of patients at 54 weeks versus 19% of control patients [13]. With regard to UC, two large trials, referred to as ACT (Active Ulcerative Colitis) I and II, evaluated the effects of infliximab. In ACT I, patients refractory to steroids and immune modulators were treated with infliximab at a dose of 5 mg/kg or 10 mg/kg versus placebo. Patients treated with infliximab had response rates of around 50% versus 30% in the placebo group. ACT II, which also included patients refractory to 5-amino-salicylic acid, reported remission rates of 26% and 36% in patients treated with infliximab 5 mg/kg or 10 mg/kg, respectively, as compared to remission rates of 11% in patients treated with a placebo [14].

Despite the promising results of infliximab, some of the other TNF-α blockers have not been as efficacious. One study treated 43 patients with CD with either etanercept 25 mg or placebo and found no difference in response or remission rates at weeks 2, 4 or 8 [15]. Potential limitations of the TNF-α antagonists include infections, infusion reactions, autoimmune phenomenon, and immunogenicity [7].

Diverticular disease

Pathophysiology/epidemiology
Diverticuli, sacs or pouch openings off the main lumen of the gut, occur most commonly in the colon but can also occur at any other GI tract site. They typically arise at the site of penetrating blood vessels which represent "weak" sites in the colon wall. Colonic diverticuli are generally pain free but severe abdominal pain and infection may result if their mouth (opening to the lumen) becomes inflamed and/or obstructed. The disorder is then termed diverticulitis and is associated with pain, altered bowel habits, abscess formation, obstruction, colonic distension, and bleeding. In the absence of infection or inflammatory changes, diverticuli may present with recurrent, episodic left lower quadrant colicky pain and the disorder is termed diverticulosis.

Evaluation/treatment
Diverticuli are identified on colonoscopy or via radiographic imaging of the colon. If diverticulitis is present, then evidence of infection coupled with physical exam or radiographic findings of a mass adjacent to the colon forms the diagnosis [16]. Investigative studies that identify diverticuli are often prompted by GI bleeding since colonic diverticuli are the most common source of lower gastrointestinal tract bleeding. Treatment of diverticulitis may be medical with antibiotics or surgical with resection and drainage. Roughly 1% of all patients with colonic diverticula require surgical management. An estimated 15–30%

of patients requiring hospital admission are treated surgically. Follow-up studies of postoperative patients reveal that between 2% and 10% will continue to have major symptoms that they find troublesome, and up to 25% of patients will have minor symptoms [16,17]. Therefore, even though segmental colonic resection may be required for some patients to control bleeding, consensus panels have been unable to definitively recommend surgery for pain control [18].

Preventive treatments for diverticular disease have revolved around fiber and other dietary modifications. Food items such as seeds or corn are discouraged due to the potential for blocking of the mouths of existent diverticuli, but fiber is encouraged because high colonic bulk content decreases the intracolonic pressure that leads to the development of the diverticuli [17]. The prophylactic use of antibiotics can also prevent complications from diverticular disease [19–21]. In a study of 307 patients, rifaximin with fiber supplementation was found to be more effective than fiber supplementation alone in reducing symptoms of uncomplicated diverticular disease [19]. Another study compared different doses of both mesalazine and rifaximin and found mesalazine 800 mg twice a day for 10 days out of the month to be the most effective at reducing symptoms [20].

Irritable bowel syndrome (functional bowel disorders)

Pathophysiology/epidemiology
Irritable bowel syndrome (IBS) is one of several functional bowel disorders, including noncardiac chest pain, functional dyspepsia, epigastric pain syndrome, postprandial distress syndrome and chronic proctalgia, which represent diagnoses of exclusion that are based on symptomatology [22]. IBS has been demonstrated to be associated with abnormalities of motility and/or sensation in different subpopulations. The diagnosis of IBS is given to 40–70% of referrals to gastroenterologists.

IBS typically presents in the third or fourth decades of life and has a female to male ratio of 2:1. In general populations, up to 20% of women and 10% of men experience symptomatology consistent with IBS, but most people with these symptoms do not seek medical care. Of those who do seek care, 50–60% have significant symptomatology consistent with depression and/or an anxiety disorder [23, 24]. IBS symptomatology is present in many cultures, with similar prevalences noted in Britain, China, India, Japan, New Zealand, the United States and South America. Other disorders without identifiable histopathology such as fibromyalgia and mixed headaches are common co-morbidities [24].

There exist many diverse hypotheses related to the etiology of IBS, ranging from the purely psychosocial to neuropathic processes producing visceral hypersensitivity (the equivalent of somatic hyperalgesia/allodynia). Peripheral sensitizing substances such as cytokines released by mast cells have been hypothesized as mechanistic agents of hypersensitivity [25].

Evaluation and treatment

The diagnosis of IBS requires the positive findings of disturbed bowel habits and a history of pain/discomfort coupled with negative findings for neoplastic, infectious or inflammatory causes. It is defined by the Rome criteria, now in their third form [26], as 3 months of continuous or recurrent symptoms of abdominal pain or discomfort associated with two of the following: an improvement with defecation and/or a change in stool consistency (appearance) and/or a change in stool frequency. At least three different clinical presentations are given the diagnosis of IBS, two of which have pain/discomfort as a minor component (watery diarrhea group and alternating constipation/diarrhea group respectively). There is a third subgroup of IBS patients who have abdominal pain as their primary symptom and altered bowel movements as a secondary or exacerbating complaint. In this group, pain is typically in the left lower quadrant or in the suprapubic region and may be precipitated by food ingestion and a need to defecate. Bloating, mucus in the stools and flatulence are often prominent, and anxiety may exacerbate these symptoms. Although there is great variation between patients, the particular symptom complex for a given patient generally remains constant. Generalized abdominal tenderness to palpation is common. The classic physical finding is a tender, palpable sigmoid colon in the left lower quadrant.

As a diagnosis of exclusion, imaging and laboratory findings should be negative for neoplasm, inflammatory bowel disease, infection, diverticulosis or other intra-abdominal processes. Colonoscopy and/or barium enema radiography should be negative for any focal lesions. Stool samples should not have occult blood or infectious agents present. It is generally agreed that the colons of most patients with IBS are exceptionally reactive to physiologic stimuli such as eating [27]. Unfortunately, this finding is only supportive evidence for the diagnosis. Motility studies and sensation evocation with a distending balloon in the rectum or sigmoid colon may prove valuable in the stratification of patients into different subgroups.

Irritable bowel syndrome has frequent exacerbations and may have spontaneous resolution. As a consequence, open trials are of limited value due to high placebo rates. Interventional treatments are not a major component of therapy because, by definition of the disease, there is no structural pathology to treat. Life-threatening pathology can be ruled out without an exhaustive investigation. However, the patient needs to be assured that their symptoms are believed. There are no universally accepted treatments for IBS [26-28] but some therapeutic options are listed in Box 15.2. Due to the typically stable nature of a patient's symptom complex, once significant pathology has been ruled out, additional or repeat investigation is not necessary unless the symptom complex changes.

Box 15.2 Pain treatment options: irritable bowel syndrome [28–35]

Treatments with Grade B evidence

Dietary modification (Level III)
  Food avoidance (caffeine, milk products, legumes)
  Addition of fiber/bran/bulking agents
Behavioral therapies (Level II–IV)
Antidepressants (SSRIs – Level II, tricyclics – Level II and III)
5HT-3 antagonists (diarrhea predominant; safety issues – Level I subset)
5HT-4 agonists (constipation predominant; safety issues – Level I subset)
Probiotics/antibiotics (Level II and III)
Acupuncture (Level III)
TENS (Level III)

Treatments with Grade C evidence

Anticholinergics/antispasmodics (Level II–IV dependent on drug)

Drugs acting via serotonin receptors as either 5HT-3 antagonists (alosetron) or 5HT-4 agonists (tegaserod) have been utilized in clinical practice for certain subgroups of patients. In large, randomized, double-blind, placebo-controlled trials involving patients with diarrhea-predominant IBS, alosetron decreased stool frequency and bowel urgency, relieved abdominal pain and discomfort, and improved health-related quality of life measures [27]. Tegaserod has been shown in randomized clinical trials to be moderately effective for the global relief of symptoms in patients with IBS. In an analysis of eight randomized trials, patients assigned to tegaserod were 20% more likely than those assigned to placebo to have a global relief of their symptoms, with a number needed to treat of 17 to achieve a clinically significant benefit. However, marketing of tegaserod was suspended in March 2007, when analysis of the data from clinical trials identified a significant increase in the number of cardiovascular ischemic events (myocardial infarction, stroke, and unstable angina) in patients taking the drug (13 events in 11, 614 patients) as compared with those receiving placebo (one event in 7031 patients), but all these events occurred in patients with known cardiovascular disease, cardiovascular risk factors or both [29]. In July 2007, the Food and Drug Administration (FDA) approved an investigational new-drug program for tegaserod with access restricted to women younger than 55 years of age who have constipation-predominant IBS without known cardiovascular problems [27].

Cognitive behavioral therapy (CBT) (a combination of cognitive and behavioral techniques) is the best studied psychologic treatment for IBS [30]. Cognitive techniques are aimed at changing catastrophic or maladaptive thinking patterns underlying the perception of somatic symptoms [31]. Behavioral techniques aim to modify dysfunctional behaviors through relaxation techniques, contingency management (rewarding healthy behaviors) or assertion training. Some randomized controlled trials have also shown reductions in IBS symptoms with the use of gut-directed hypnosis (aimed at improving gut function), which involves relaxation, changes in beliefs, and self-management [30–32]. Data from head-to-head comparisons of psychotherapy with pharmacotherapy for IBS are lacking. The magnitude of improvement that has been reported with psychologic treatments seems to be

similar to or greater than that reported with medications studied specifically for bowel symptoms in IBS, although comparisons are limited by, among other things, the lack of a true placebo control in trials of psychotherapies. In a meta-analysis of 17 randomized trials of cognitive treatments, behavioral treatments or both for IBS (including hypnosis), as compared with control treatments (including waiting list, symptom monitoring, and usual medical treatment), those patients who were randomly assigned to CBT were significantly more likely to have a reduction in gastrointestinal symptoms of at least 50% (OR 12; 95% CI 6–260), and the estimated number needed to treat with CBT or hypnotherapy for one patient to have improvement was estimated to be two [30].

Proctalgia fugax

Pathophysiology/treatment

Defined as episodic spasms of pain localized to the rectum and anus occurring at irregular intervals and without an identifiable cause, proctalgia fugax is highly prevalent, occurring in 14–19% of healthy subjects [36]. Episodes are normally brief (seconds to minutes) and infrequent (usually <6/year). Proctalgia fugax is not the same as chronic proctalgia, which is pain that is more continuous in nature and typically of lower intensity. Spasms of the sigmoid colon, levator ani, and/or pelvic floor musculature have been postulated as sources of the pain. Local anorectal pathology (fissures, abscesses) needs to be ruled out as alternative treatable sources of pain and spasm. Various activities may precipitate episodes such as bowel movements, sexual activity, stress, and temperature changes. As a consequence, avoidance behaviors may occur, with obvious consequences for quality of life.

No etiology or method of treating/preventing proctalgia fugax has been universally accepted. The brief nature of most episodes makes most reactive pharmacologic treatments inadequate since the episode resolves spontaneously prior to the onset of treatment effects. Inhaled salbutamol, clonidine, nitroglycerine, antispasmodics, botulinum A toxin, and calcium channel blockers have all been reported as effective in either reactive or preventive fashions, but none in controlled trials. Heat or pressure applied to the perineum, food/drink consumption, dilation of the anal sphincter, assumption of a knee-to-chest position, and assumption of other postures have also been anecdotally reported as beneficial.

Visceral pain arising from the hepatobiliary system and pancreas

Chronic pancreatitis

Pathophysiology/epidemiology

The symptoms of pancreatitis can be associated with pancreatic cell death and/or with ductal fibrosis and calcification and are generally grouped into acute (isolated episodes with serum amylase and lipase elevations) and chronic (identical symptoms that may lack measurable laboratory abnormalities) forms [37–39]. Whereas acute pancreatitis generally resolves without permanent structural abnormalities, most forms of chronic pancreatitis are associated with permanent abnormalities. Acute-on-chronic episodes may occur in a patient with known chronic changes that become coupled to an acute necrotic episode. Alcohol abuse is the primary etiology in 70–80% of cases of chronic pancreatitis in nontropical regions. Only 5–10% of heavy drinkers develop symptomatic chronic pancreatitis, implying that other etiologic factors (e.g. genetic, infectious, nutritional) also contribute to its development. Other potential causes include a pancreas divisum, genetic causes (hereditary type), previous trauma, previous obstructive episodes, hyperparathyroidism, hyperlipidemia, and α_1-antitrypsin deficiency. Like many chronic pain disorders, the magnitude of identifiable pathology does not correlate with reports of pain.

Experimentally, chronic pancreatitis may be induced in animals by the administration of toxins, but attempts to form epidemiologic links in humans to specific toxins, other than alcohol and cigarette smoking [38], have not been successful. However, diets with too much or too little fat and/or protein have also been implicated. In fact, it has been proposed that increases in oxidative stress underlie the pathophysiology of chronic pancreatitis. In this scenario, there would exist periodic bursts of free radical formation producing subsequent injury. A co-morbidity of chronic pancreatitis is cirrhosis of the liver which complements the "cirrhosis" of the pancreas.

Pancreatic fluids have been noted to have altered protein content and to form "sludge" or intraductal "plugs" that calcify into stones with secondary inflammatory and fibrotic reactions. A common consequence of stone formation/fibrosis is intraductal hypertension, which may contribute to the continuous pain that develops in some chronic pancreatitis patients. Unfortunately, relief of ductal obstruction does not invariably result in pain relief.

Evaluation/treatment

The pain of chronic pancreatitis is pain that is typically described as deep, boring and epigastric in location with radiation through to the back. The pain may be episodic in nature but may advance until it is continuous. Exacerbations of pain may be produced by eating, particularly fatty foods. Sitting upright or leaning forward may decrease the pain. It is normally coupled with nausea and vomiting, so dehydration and malnutrition may be the formal indications for medical intervention. It may be possible to palpate an inflammatory mass on physical exam, but abdominal guarding usually precludes such findings. Subjects with alcoholic chronic pancreatitis often have stigmata associated with extensive alcohol use and associated liver failure.

In advanced disease, laboratory tests of pancreatic insufficiency (e.g. steatorrhea) or islet cell loss (e.g. glucose intolerance) may manifest. Elevated serum amylase and lipase levels change unreliably in chronic stages of the disease. Diagnostic imaging (radiographs, ultrasound, computed tomography) demonstrating diffuse intraductal calcium deposition will support the diagnosis in 30–90% of cases, depending upon the modality employed. ERCP (endoscopic retrograde cholangiopancreatography) is the "gold standard" for chronic pancreatitis. Stratification into severity of disease is based on a grading of ductal abnormalities. An incidental finding that is not uncommon during surgical treatment of chronic pancreatitis is evidence of pancreatic cancer.

Some practice guidelines do exist for the treatment of pain due to chronic pancreatitis [39]. Unfortunately, most published treatment options are only validated mainly by case reports and retrospective series. Few studies of chronic pancreatitis pain have employed rigorously controlled methodologies and even fewer have demonstrated robust effects of the studied treatment. A list of potential treatment options is given in Box 15.3. Based on epidemiologic data, abstinence from alcohol is an absolute behavioral alteration that must occur when the etiology of the pancreatitis is alcohol related. An individual who continues to abuse

Box 15.3 Pain treatment options: chronic pancreatitis [37–45]

Treatments with Grade B evidence
Abstinence from alcohol (Level III)
Antioxidants and micronutrients (Level II)
Cholecystokinin receptor antagonists (Level II)

Treatments with Grade C evidence
Opioids (including K-ORAs; Level II and III)
Anti-inflammatory drugs (Level III)
Endoscopic management (stents, sphincterotomy, stone removal) (Level III evidence – inferior to surgical intervention) [44, 45]
Oral pancreatic enzyme treatment (Level II)
Octreotide (prevents complications of pancreatic procedures – Level II)
Neurolysis (Level IV)
Intraceliac local anesthetic and/or steroid injections (Level IV)
Surgical diversion or resection (Level III)
Pseudocystic drainage (percutaneous, endoscopic, surgical) (Level IV)
Shock-wave lithotripsy of pancreatic stones (Level III)

steroid injections provided pain relief in 4/16 patients [41]. However, 11 of the 12 patients who did not obtain relief were narcotic dependent, whereas none of the four who obtained relief were narcotic dependent. This finding emphasizes the complexity of treating pain in a population of patients with chemical dependencies and other abnormal psychologic and psychosomatic behaviors.

In another report [42] which investigated the mode of delivering the nerve blocks, 25% of patients with CT-guided celiac plexus blocks experienced pain relief compared to 43% of patients who were treated by endoscopic ultrasound-guided celiac plexus blocks. The benefit from endoscopic ultrasound-guided celiac plexus also persisted for longer than that of the CT-guided blocks. More importantly, paraplegia has not been described after endoscopic ultrasound-guided celiac plexus block. The same group of investigators more recently published their prospective experience with endoscopic ultrasound-guided celiac plexus blocks with steroids in 90 patients with pain resulting from chronic pancreatitis [43]. A significant improvement in pain scores occurred in 55% of these patients. The benefit persisted beyond 12 weeks in 26% of the patients and beyond 24 weeks in 10%. Younger patients (<45 years) and patients with previous pancreatic surgery for chronic pancreatitis did not appear to benefit from the blocks.

The current evidence indicates that endoscopic ultrasound-guided celiac plexus blocks are safe and well tolerated with excellent temporary results in some patients. Unfortunately, reliable predictors of success are lacking. In the absence of long-term studies in patients with chronic pancreatitis, the role of endoscopic ultrasound-guided celiac plexus blocks should be limited to treating flares of chronic pain in patients with otherwise limited therapeutic options.

Surgical diversion or resection is often viewed as the definitive treatment of chronic pancreatitis despite the absence of prospective randomized studies. The endoscopic placement of stents, sphincterotomy, dilation and/or stone removal are well-established alternatives to surgery in the treatment of biliary tract diseases, and similar techniques for the relief of chronic pancreatic pain have been developed. However, recent randomized comparisons of endoscopic versus surgical management of ductal obstruction have suggested the superiority of surgical interventions. In one study [44], patients with

alcohol despite the diagnosis of chronic pancreatitis has a 50% mortality rate at 5-year follow-up. If they abstain from drinking, it takes more than 25 years to have a similar mortality rate. It has been commonly reported that total abstinence from alcohol achieves pain relief in up to 50% of patients, particularly those with mild to moderate disease [39].

Celiac plexus blocks with local anesthetics have been used for diagnostic purposes as well as a primary therapy for pain in association with chronic pancreatitis. Although widely used, there have been relatively few formally reported experiences with nerve blocks for the long-term treatment of chronic pancreatitis. Leung et al. [40] studied the use of celiac plexus blocks in 23 patients with chronic pancreatitis. Twelve of the 23 had complete analgesia, whereas six had partial relief. There was no effect in five patients. The mean pain-free period was 2 months. There was less of an effect in patients with previous pancreatic surgery, and repeat blocks were unhelpful. Because of concerns about potential irreversible nerve injury, the injection of steroids as opposed to alcohol has been recommended when using celiac plexus blocks for the treatment of chronic pancreatitis. In one study, chronic pancreatitis and a distal obstruction of the pancreatic duct without an inflammatory mass were randomized to undergo endoscopic transampullary drainage of the pancreatic duct (n = 19) or operative pancreaticojejunostomy (n = 20). At 24 months of follow-up, patients treated surgically had lower pain scores and required fewer procedures. Complete or partial pain relief was achieved in 32% of patients who underwent endoscopic drainage as compared with 75% of patients assigned to surgical drainage. Another study of 72 patients found surgery superior to endoscopic sphincterotomy with stenting and/or stone removal [45].

Opioids are the primary pharmacologic analgesic therapy for advanced chronic pancreatitis, although some have suggested the use of "adjuvants" such as antidepressants. There is the unfortunate but common experience of clinicians that patients who have alcoholic pancreatitis may exchange their alcohol addiction for an opioid addiction. Patients with substance abuse histories develop painful diseases and ethically require treatment, but clinicians still experience significant angst in association with symptom-based treatment rather than etiology-based treatment.

Postcholecystectomy syndrome

Pathophysiology/treatment
One in four patients who undergo cholecystectomy for uncomplicated gallstone disease or acute cholecystitis continues to have persistent abdominal pain 5 years after their surgery [46]. This postcholecystectomy syndrome consists of pain which is typically in the right upper quadrant of the abdomen and is similar to that of cholecystitis. It is exacerbated by eating, may be associated with nausea, and is often described as dull and colicky. An appropriate work-up can rule out a definable pathology such as a retained bile duct stone or secondary pancreatitis. Endoscopic retrograde cholangiopancreatography/manometry may identify abnormal pressures or motility within the biliary duct and if observed, elevated sphincter of Oddi pressures suggest sphincter dysfunction as the cause of the syndrome [47]. Treatments include sphincterotomy or stenting when elevated pressures are noted. Nifedipine has been reported to help with sphincter dysfunction, but there is no high-level evidence for any treatment option. Often there is no objective identification of the pain's etiology, so treatment is empiric.

Visceral pain arising from urologic organs

Urolithiasis

Pathophysiology/treatment
Irritative effects of stones moving within the urinary system (renal pelvis/calices, ureters, bladder, urethra) can lead to severe pain (renal colic) and if sufficiently obstructive to urine flow, can destroy kidney function. It may be recurrent in "stone-formers" and may be continuous when numerous or large renal pelvic (staghorn) calculi are present. It occurs in 15% of white men and 6% of all women in industrialized countries [48]. Diagnosis is based on history of stone formation and/or imaging studies (intravenous pyelogram or CT). The primary treatment for the disorder is the removal of the stone by spontaneous passage, which may be assisted by fragmentation using lithotripsy, or it may require surgical removal.

Drugs which relax the ureters include nonsteroidal anti-inflammatory drugs (NSAIDs), nifedipine, and tamsulosin, all of which have been demonstrated to facilitate stone passage. Otherwise, pain treatments employed are intended to be "temporizing" with the goal of relieving pain and ureteral spasming until stone removal occurs. These treatments are listed in Box 15.4. The two principal classes of agents used to treat pain from renal colic are NSAIDs and opioids. NSAIDs are often considered the first-line therapy because they directly address the underlying etiology of the pain by inhibiting prostaglandin synthesis and subsequently reducing vasodilation, intrarenal pressure, and urinary tract inflammation. In fact, some studies have shown NSAIDs to be superior to opioids in reducing pain scores and the need for further analgesic therapies [49]. Therapies to reduce stone formation include alkalinization of the urine, avoidance of certain drugs, use of thiazide diuretics, and dietary alterations.

Polycystic kidney disease

Pathophysiology/treatment
This autosomal dominant genetic disease is associated with cyst formation, rupture, infection and secondary compression or traction of neighboring structures which can produce low back pain, abdominal pain, headache, chest pain, flank pain and/or leg pain

Box 15.4 Pain treatment options: urolithiasis [48–51]

Treatments with Grade A or B evidence

Agents to assist stone passage [51]

NSAIDs (Level I)

Calcium channel blockers (nifedipine) (Level I)

α-Adrenoceptor antagonists (tamsulosin, terazocin, doxazocine) (Level II)

Nitroglycerine and other nitrates (Level IV)

Lithotripsy (Level I)

Analgesics, antispasmodics

Opioids including tramadol (Level II or III)

Antimuscurinics (Level III or IV)

Phosphodiesterase IV inhibitors (Level II)

Surgical procedures for stone removal (Level III)

Acupuncture (Level III)

TENS (Level II)

Drug and dietary modification to prevent stone formation

[52, 53]. Eventually the disorder leads to kidney failure. Renal stone formation and liver cyst formation are both common co-morbidities. Therapeutic regimens have been proposed which suggest a general progression from nonpharmacologic methods to non-narcotic analgesics and minimally invasive procedures to progressively more invasive procedures and the use of opioids [54]. Procedures unique to polycystic kidney disease include surgical or percutaneous drainage of the cysts to decompress the lesions, sometimes followed by marsupialization to avoid fluid reaccumulation. In a study by Brown *et al.* [55], 50% of patients were pain free 12–28 months after laparoscopic marsupialization. More recently, Casale and colleagues [56] reported treating 12 patients aged 8–19 years (mean age 12.4) with laparoscopic renal denervation and nephropexy. All these patients had autosomal dominant polycystic kidney disease with chronic pain that was refractory to narcotic use. All patients were reportedly pain free following surgery with a mean follow-up period of 25.5 months.

Loin pain-hematuria syndrome

Pathophysiology/treatment

This is a descriptive diagnosis of obscure etiology with the primary symptom of severe flank pain and the laboratory finding of hematuria. It may be secondary to an immunoglobulin A nephritis, but its existence as a clinicopathologic entity has been questioned [57] since in most cases, it is a diagnosis of exclusion. In a research setting, renal biopsies of subjects with the diagnosis of loin-pain hematuria suggest a glomerular source of the hematuria [58]. Treatments by some have been aggressive, utilizing interventions such as intraureteric capsaicin, nephrectomy, extensive surgical sympathectomy of the kidney, and renal autotransplantation. However, recurrence of pain following these procedures is common. Meticulous screening of patients for other urologic, nephrologic or psychiatric etiologies of pain prior to surgical intervention is recommended. Results of injection therapies are usually viewed as short-lived. There is no high-level evidence for any of these treatment options.

Painful bladder syndrome – interstitial cystitis

Pathophysiology/epidemiology

Painful bladder syndrome (PBS; alternatively known as bladder pain syndrome) is a descriptive diagnosis that has been recently advocated for use on an international level as descriptive of a complex of urologic complaints including pain [59]. Thought to be an early form of the disorder interstitial cystitis (IC), there is an expectation that a majority of patients with PBS might have a common etiology. Notably, IC has no agreed etiology, pathophysiology or treatment and nor does the less defined PBS. The prevalence of IC is estimated to be 2 in 10,000 with a female to male ratio of 10:1. Patients with IC are 10–12 times more likely to report childhood bladder problems than the general population [60]. IC is frequently associated with other chronic disorders such as inflammatory bowel disease, systemic lupus erythematosus, irritable bowel syndrome, "sensitive" skin, fibromyalgia and allergies [61].

Interstitial cystitis does have a defining pathology in that the diagnosis, as defined by a study group of the United States National Institute of Diabetes, Digestive and Kidney Diseases, requires the presence of mucosal ulcers (a Hunner's patch) or "glomerulations." The latter are small submucosal petechial hemorrhages viewed cystoscopically after sustained distension of the bladder (hydrodistension). Glomerulations are not unique to IC but occur in other forms of cystitis (e.g. radiation cystitis) and may even be a normal variant. As a consequence, the formal diagnosis of IC also requires exclusion of known disorders which produce pain and/or glomerulations (e.g. viral infection, chemotherapy exposure).

There is good evidence that there is a disruption of the normal urothelial barrier in most if not all IC patients. The etiology of the breakdown in the urothelial barrier and the consequences of this breakdown in IC are, as yet, unknown. One theory proposes that the breakdown of the urothelial barrier results from a failure to maintain adequate formation of glycosaminoglycans, the protective coating of the urothelium. Another theory proposes that IC is a systemic autoimmune disease presenting as a local manifestation with associated immunologic dysfunction, including possible abnormal mast cell activity. The most mechanistic theory to date relates the breakdown of the urothelial barrier to the presence of a specific peptide present within the urine of IC patients that impairs urothelial regrowth. Named the antiproliferative factor (APF), this low molecular weight peptide is a member of the Frizzled 8 protein family [62]. APF has been identified in over 90% of rigorously diagnosed IC patients and, at present, is the best laboratory diagnostic test for IC. Unfortunately, it is currently only available as a research tool. Whether APF is present due to developmental, immunologic, infectious, genetic or neurologic causes has not been determined. It has been demonstrated to produce a downregulation of genes which stimulate epithelial proliferation and an upregulation of genes that inhibit cell growth. Independent of the specific reason for urothelial disruption, the simplest explanation of the consequences of this breakdown is that it allows an exposure of urinary constituents, bacterial products and cell death products to bladder sensory nerves that normally are protected by an intact urothelial barrier. "Toxic" urine exposure may then produce either direct activation or sensitization of peripheral and/or central nervous system structures. It is likely that all these theories are correct for subsets of patients and that multiple different pathophysiologies are being grouped together under one diagnosis.

Evaluation/treatment

Pain, nocturia, urgency and frequency are the primary symptoms of IC. Pain may be localized to the lower abdomen, pelvis, groin and/or perineum [60]. The onset of the disease may follow an "event" but is notable for a rapid progression of symptomatology. Depression and anxiety are frequent co-morbidities. In one analysis, Clemens and associates reported that 25% of patients with IC also carried an *International Statistical Classification of Diseases* (ICD)-9 diagnosis of depressive disorder and 19% carried a diagnosis of anxiety. In this study, compared to controls, patients with IC were also more likely to suffer from fibromyalgia, gastritis, headaches, esophageal reflux and back pain, and were more likely to have a history of child abuse [63]. Suprapubic tenderness to palpation may accompany a diagnosis of IC. Although a history of frequent urinary tract infections is twice as common in IC patients as in non-IC patients, most report infrequent urinary tract infections (<1/year) prior to the onset of their symptoms, and they typically have sterile urine on laboratory exam. A cystoscopic examination of the bladder wall is necessary to meet the research definition of IC (Hunner's patch or glomerulations needed). The intravesical potassium sensitivity test has been employed as an alternative diagnostic procedure with good sensitivity (70–90%) for subjects meeting formal research criteria, but it lacks specificity [64].

The ultimate goal of therapy is to neutralize the factor or factors responsible for a disease process. In the absence of any known causative factors, the treatments for IC have been guided by theory and/or prudence. A given patient's therapy typically progresses from the least invasive treatments to the more invasive. A list of potential treatments for IC is given in Box 15.5. While there are no universally accepted treatments, most patients are initially treated with oral medications such as NSAIDs, antihistamines, antidepressants or cyclosporine, among others [65]. These are based on varying degrees of evidence as outlined in the box. A comparison of cyclosporine to pentosan polysulfate has found cyclosporine to be more effective in reducing urinary frequency with a response rate of 75% for cyclosporine versus 19% for pentosan polysulfate [66, 67]. More invasive treatments such as electrical nerve stimulation, nerve blocks or surgical resection may be required in some patients [65, 68].

Epidemiologically, IC is most prevalent in young to middle-aged women, implying there may be a

Box 15.5 Pain treatment options: interstitial cystitis [59–68]

Treatments with Grade B evidence

Antidepressants (Level I subset)
Cyclosporine (Level III)

Treatments with Grade C evidence

Dietary modification (Level IV)

Hydrodistension (with or without intravesical treatments – Level IV)

Components: dimethyl sulfoxide, heparin, corticosteroids, bicarbonate, hyaluronic acid, clorpactin, intravesical Bacillus Calmette-Guerin (Level III – subsets respond)

Systemic medications

Antihistamines/mast cell stabilizers (Level III)

Opioids/B&O suppositories (Level III)

Nonsteroidal anti-inflammatories (Level III – may worsen some)

Pentosan polysulfate (Level II – subsets respond)

Pyridium (Level IV)

TENS (Level IV)

S3 nerve root stimulation (Level II and III for urinary frequency – not pain)

Local anesthetic nerve blocks (Level IV)

Surgical resection/diversion (Level III)

Behavioral therapies (Level IV)

Hyperbaric oxygen therapy (Level III)

resolution of symptomatology that occurs with time. It has been reported that up to 50% of patients diagnosed with IC have spontaneous remissions with durations of 1–80 months. All clinical trials related to IC have been hampered by the likely inclusion of a heterogeneous clinical population. This may become less problematic in the future with the advent of a diagnostic test for APF, which would allow for the objective enrollment of study participants into clinical trials.

Visceral pain arising from reproductive organs

General statements

Approximately half of the world's population has experienced a monthly recurrence of abdominal pain associated with the menstrual cycle. The degree of distress and disruption of activities of daily living produced by this cycling phenomenon varies widely in the population. Menstrual cramps in the perimenstrual period and *Mittelschmerz* (pain at the time of ovulation) are viewed as "normal" but when they become noncyclic or when they lead to a severe disruption of activity, then investigations and interventions may be performed. Gynecologic pains can be divided into two sites of pain localization: the abdomen/pelvis and the perineum (vulvodynia). The latter disorder is discussed in a separate chapter of this text along with nonspecific pelvic pains of several types. The types of pain discussed here will be attributed to specific intra-abdominal female reproductive organs. Brief mention will also be made of orchialgia, a male correlate to ovarian pain.

Dysmenorrhea

Pathophysiology/epidemiology

A painful monthly "flow" can occur either secondary to underlying endocrine/pelvic pathology or it may be "primary," in which case, there is no other identifiable pathology. It is thought that dysmenorrhea is due to contractions (cramping) of the uterus when it expels menstrual constituents. This cramping produces high-intensity mechanical stimuli and focal uterine ischemia. In addition to the mechanical stimulation and ischemia, the uterine afferents and central neuronal processing may be sensitized due to hormonal alterations since this has been noted in other species. Various products of inflammation (prostaglandins, leukotrienes) are produced by the sloughing, necrotic uterine lining which can also produce a sensitization/activation of uterine afferent neurones. It should not be surprising that there could be a significant generation of pain at the time of menses.

Evaluation/treatment

The initial clinical evaluation of dysmenorrhea requires simple history taking to assess the cyclic nature of the pain and a physical exam to evaluate the secondary forms of dysmenorrhea (imperforate hymen, uterine/tubal abnormalities, adenomyosis or leiomyoma (fibroids)). Treatment of such secondary forms is the primary etiologic therapy. Other potential options are listed in Box 15.6. Due to its common occurrence, most

Box 15.6 Pain treatment options: dysmenorrhea [69–73]

Treat sources of secondary dysmenorrhea
Endometriosis (see Box 15.7)
Hysterectomy – bilateral salpingo-oophorectomy
Other endocrine/metabolic disorders

Treatments with Grade A or B evidence for primary dysmenorrhea

Oral contraceptives/progesterones (Level I)
Nonsteroidal anti-inflammatories (Level I)

Treatments with Grade C evidence for primary dysmenorrhea

Medical treatments
  Opioids (Level III)
  Transdermal nitroglycerine (Level III)
  Guaifenesin (Level III)
Denervation [72]
Uterosacral nerve ablation (Level II and III)
Presacral neurectomy (Level I–III)
Complementary and alternative treatments
  TENS (Level II)
  Acupuncture/acupressure (Level III)
  Aromatherapy (Level III)
  Magnet therapy (Level III)

---

cases of dysmenorrhea are presumed to be primary, and cyclo-oxygenase inhibitors such as the NSAIDs are considered the first-line reactive treatment [69]. Multiple studies have confirmed that NSAIDs are more effective than placebo in relieving menstrual pain. However, when compared with each other, no specific NSAID has been shown to be superior. Ideally, these medications should be administered on a scheduled basis and begun 1–2 days before the expected onset of menstruation [70]. Oral contraceptives may also be used as a preventive measure. These have also been shown to be more effective than placebo in reducing menstrual symptoms and the need for additional pain medications in a double-blinded, randomized controlled trial [71]. In fact, the combination of NSAIDs and oral contraceptives is able to alleviate pain in 75–80% of women suffering from primary dysmenorrhea [70].

Typically when conservative pharmacologic management of presumed primary dysmenorrhea has failed, a laparoscopy is performed in an attempt to identify potentially treatable sources of secondary dysmenorrhea. If no pelvic pathology is identified, then surgical/neuroablative treatment may be considered. Other potential options with varying degrees of supportive evidence include long-acting hormonal therapies and nontraditional remedies such as vitamin E and B1 supplementation, magnesium supplementation, various other dietary and herbal remedies, acupuncture, and transcutaneous electrical nerve stimulation (TENS). A Cochrane review of high-frequency TENS for the treatment of dysmenorrhea found it to be more effective than placebo in relieving menstrual-related pain. However, the TENS group did experience a higher rate of muscle vibration, skin tightness, headache, and skin irritation [70–73].

Endometriosis

Pathophysiology/epidemiology

When endometrial glands and stroma are found outside the uterine cavity, the term "endometriosis" is employed. It is estimated to be present in 1–2% of the general female population and in approximately half of women who undergo laparoscopy for pelvic pain. Common sites where endometriosis is found include the ovaries, the peritoneum coating (both visceral and somatic), and the cul-de-sac. It can be found in any part of the abdominal cavity and may "erode" into other structures such as the GI tract. Its severity is graded on a I–IV staging scale. The leading theory related to the development of endometriosis suggests that retrograde menses extrude out of the fallopian tubes and onto pelvic/abdominal structures, with subsequent implantation of viable endometrial tissue. Although a source of secondary dysmenorrhea, it can be associated with pain in all parts of the menstrual cycle.

Evaluation/treatment

There are many variants of presentation for endometriosis including dyspareunia, urinary urgency, increased frequency, bladder pain, back pain, rectal pain, and pain radiating to the thighs, perineum or vagina. It may produce hormonal alterations causing abnormal uterine bleeding or infertility. Hematuria and bowel or ureteral obstruction can occur from the erosion of endometrial tissue into neighboring viscera or compression of tubular structures. A pelvic exam may demonstrate multiple, focal sites

Box 15.7 Pain treatment options: endometriosis [74–76]

Treatments with Grade A or B evidence
Medical treatments
Hormonal–metabolic
Oral contraceptives/progesterones (Level I)
Danazol (Level II)
GnRH agonists (Level I)
Gestrione (Level II)
Aromatase inhibitors (Level I and II)
Analgesic
Nonsteroidal anti-inflammatories (Level I)

Treatments with Grade C evidence
Opioids (Level III)
Surgical ablation (Level II)
Hysterectomy/bilateral salpingo-oophorectomy (Level II)
Denervation
Uterosacral nerve ablation (Level III)
Presacral neurectomy (Level I–III)

Note: recommendations may differ for adolescent and adult patients [76].

of tenderness or sites of fibrosis within the pelvis. A definitive diagnosis requires histologic confirmation via a laparoscopic examination.

Pain treatment options echo those put forward for dysmenorrhea, with analgesic and neuroablative procedures viewed as temporizing or palliative (Box 15.7). In general, the medical management of endometriosis typically starts with hormonal treatments. Surgical treatment, often performed at the time of diagnostic laparoscopy, may consist of resection, fulguration or the laser ablation of identified sites of endometriosis. More severe disease may prompt more radical interventions which can include hysterectomy, bilateral salpingo-oophorectomy, appendectomy, and extensive resection of any suspicious lesions [74–76].

Ovarian pain

Pathophysiology/treatment
Ovaries can be painful when cystic structures form as part of the polycystic ovarian syndrome or if torsion of the ovary or compression of neighboring structures occurs due to dermoid cyst enlargement. An iatrogenic

chronic pain disorder that relates to the ovary is the ovarian remnant syndrome where a previous surgical resection of an ovary was incomplete. Characterized by pelvic and/or flank pain that normally does not arise until several years after the original surgery, the pain may be cyclic in nature. It has been speculated that ovarian remnant syndrome may become more common due to techniques of laparoscopic surgery that increase the risk of leaving small portions of ovarian tissue *in situ* [77]. Work-up is similar to that for any painful adnexal mass, and treatment is typically surgical, with complete resection of remaining tissues. Therapies similar to those employed for dysmenorrhea and endometriosis may have some benefit.

Orchialgia

Pathophysiology/treatment
Pain originating from the testes may be felt within the abdomen or may be localized within the scrotum [78]. Pains from such areas have a wide differential diagnosis, including local processes such as tumor, infection (e.g. epididymitis), varicocele/hydrocele/spermatocele, and testicular torsion. Previous surgeries such as inguinal hernia repair and vasectomy as well as noniatrogenic trauma can all lead to chronic inflammatory processes as well as altered sensation and associated chronic pain. Neuropathic etiologies ranging from diabetic neuropathy and entrapment neuropathies to spinal disk disease to the use of statin drugs may all present with testicular pain. Scrotal pain should be differentiated from testicular pain since the nerve supplies differ and may represent differing sites of pathology along sacral versus thoracolumbar pathways. Due to the "personal" nature of the site of pain, concerns related to psychologic etiologies or sequelae of this chronic pain are maintained.

Treatment of chronic orchialgia has traditionally started with anti-inflammatories and/or antibiotics, but often proceeds to surgical procedures including epididymectomy, orchiectomy or denervation procedures. Long-term outcomes are unknown and retrospective series have suggested limited benefit, particularly in subsets of patients with other pain disorders. There may be benefit from the use of antidepressants, anticonvulsants, membrane-stabilizing agents, opiates and, in some patients, sympatholytic treatments. However, because of the wide differential diagnosis of testicular pain, no specific treatment has high-level evidence for its use [79].

Other disorders with abdominal pain as a symptom

Familial Mediterranean fever

Pathophysiology/treatment

This is an autosomal recessive genetic disease linked to chromosome 16 which usually manifests between ages 5 and 15 years [80, 81]. Known gene mutations have been found in substantial numbers of people from various Mediterranean populations. It has been linked to alterations in the innate immune system involving the protein pyrin. The disease is characterized by periodic febrile episodes without an identifiable triggering event, serous peritonitis, pleuritis, synovitis, and a rash that may resemble erysipelas. Abdominal pain episodes of varying intensity may occur anywhere from twice per week to once per year, but most commonly occur at 2–4 week intervals with acute episodes lasting 1–3 days. Chest pain and arthralgias occur in 75% of episodes. Renal failure due to amyloidosis is a potential sequel. Laboratory evaluation may indicate an elevated white blood count or an elevated sedimentation rate, but these are not necessary criteria for diagnosis.

Systemic analgesics are the primary treatment, though various case reports have advocated for more aggressive measures. Colchicine is the treatment recommendation of a European consensus conference based on Level I evidence [82] as daily colchicine has been demonstrated to decrease the frequency of attacks and the risks of amyloidosis. Prophylactic antibiotics, hormones, antipyretics, immunotherapy, psychotherapy, thalidomide, interferon-α, infliximab, dietary alterations, chloroquine, and phenylbutazone have all been tried with limited success (Level III and IV evidence).

Porphyria

Pathophysiology/treatment

There are several related genetic disorders which are associated with the increased formation of porphyrins or their precursors. These disorders are collectively termed porphyria [83, 84]. The most frequently encountered of these is intermittent acute porphyria (IAP) which is associated with colicky abdominal pain that is intermittent, may be associated with environmental exposures, and which can last for days to months. Since it is transmitted as an autosomal dominant disorder with incomplete penetrance, family history may or may not be helpful in the diagnosis. Certain drugs such as barbiturates, benzodiazepines, alcohol, phenytoin, ketamine, etomidate, meprobamate, and corticosteroids have been implicated as "triggers" of a crisis, so are generally avoided. Other gastrointestinal signs and symptoms such as vomiting, constipation, and abdominal distension are common and may complicate the initial diagnosis. Neural demyelination can occur, resulting in various neurologic and psychiatric symptoms. The urine and blood tests which are useful for the diagnosis of porphyria may only be valid during crises, though increased urinary porphobilinogen secretion confirms the diagnosis. Genetic testing of asymptomatic members in IAP families is now routine.

Treatment is based on avoiding known triggers and treating crises with intravenous fluids and/or an increased carbohydrate intake. The key treatment of porphyria involves stopping heme synthesis. Intravenous hematin (4 mg/kg of body weight) provides negative feedback to the heme synthetic pathway and shuts down the productions of porphyrins and porphyrin precursors. Aggressive treatments including liver transplant have been suggested. Nontriggering analgesics include most opioids with the exception of pentazocine.

Adhesions

Pathophysiology/treatment

The laparoscopic demonstration of intra-abdominal adhesions in patients with abdominal/pelvic pain is common (16–51% of patients). Two separate randomized trials [85, 86] suggest that unless adhesions are very dense and producing bowel obstruction, adhesiolysis appears unlikely to produce a reliable benefit. Attempts to control or prevent adhesions with the use of anti-inflammatory agents, peritoneal instillates or surgical barriers have not affected pain-related outcomes [87]. Medical treatments are otherwise empiric and supportive in nature with no clear evidence guiding the best practice.

Future research priorities

As is apparent from the sparse amount of high-grade evidence for most therapies related to pain arising from abdominal organs, there are many lines of investigation available for researchers that are of high clinical significance. Despite the clinical importance of visceral pain disorders, their treatment continues to be a matter of debate rather than implementation of evidence-based therapies. Those disorders with high-grade evidence are of the shorter, time- and event-limited variety such as the passage of kidney stones. It is the chronic disorders that have clinicians and researchers alike scratching their heads. This, in part, may relate to the seemingly contradictory needs for both "lumping" and "splitting" in relation to the disorders. It is clear that not all painful disorders have the same mechanisms, as the local environments, adequate stimuli and evoked responses may be radically different for adjacent organ systems. For example, the presence of the bacterium *E. coli* will lead to massive physiologic and sensory responses when invading the lumen of the normally sterile urinary bladder, but lives unobtrusively in the lumen of the neighboring sewage-filled colon.

To understand the mechanisms of inflammation, primary afferent neuronal responses and reflex activation that are unique to each organ system is vital to an understanding of the painful disorders associated with those organs. Despite the need for that *splitting* approach to research, it must also be recognized that there is need for *lumping* when considering the responses evoked by stimuli arising from different organ systems. Commonalities of sensation type, quality, affective impact, physiologic response and even referred localization (which may be identical for different organs) are present for all visceral systems. Hence, therapies may need to focus to a greater degree on these higher order response elements associated with painful disorders. One of the failures of research related to therapies is that studies generally have either too great a focus on a specific organ-based mechanism, with an ignoring of total body effects, or the opposite, too great a focus on response factors with too little emphasis on what is evoking these responses. It is unlikely that a single pill or a single behavioral therapy will abolish all the reactions evoked in a chronically painful disorder. Our research needs to reflect the therapeutic need for multilevel, multimodal therapy.

General recommendations related to therapeutics

Just as there is a need for research related to multimodal therapy, there is also a need to deliver multimodal therapy. Physicians want a "cookbook" related to the treatment of medical disorders where a specific label for a disorder is associated with a defined treatment sequence. At present, we do not have such a cookbook related to chronically painful disorders and so individual assessment, personal judgment and the "art" of medicine all factor into treatment plans. When faced with the evaluation and treatment of a painful disorder, it is necessary to undertake basic evaluations that assess the potential for reversible or time-important disorders such as infection, ischemia or cancer. After that, there may be a need for additional organ-specific assessment but there may be an even greater need for global response-related treatments such as behavioral interventions that may not be as dependent upon the particular organ evoking the responses. Too often, treatment strategies turn to such response-related therapeutics as monotherapy only after extensive organ-based procedures and treatments have failed. For the sake of patients suffering from painful disorders, let us avoid monotherapy and search for the best combination of therapeutics. Evidence-based medicine will hopefully carry us to a fully defined list of combination therapeutics that are most effective, but until that day the clinician must systemically determine for themselves the optimal combinations.

Conclusion

Chronic abdominal pain arising from visceral structures is a common clinical entity with multiple etiologies both known and unknown. The pain is often poorly localized with referral of pain to somatic sites. Pain arising in the viscera can signal life- or tissue-threatening disorders with grave consequences. It may also be a sensation out of proportion to the identifiable pathology. Evidence-based medicine related to various painful disorders is limited; therefore, a systematic approach to the reported symptom is prudent and utilization of multimodal therapeutics is recommended.

References

1. Andren-Sandberg A, Dervenis C, Lowenfels B. Etiologic links between chronic pancreatitis and pancreatic cancer. *Scand J Gastroenterol* 1997; **32**: 97–103.

2. Kozuch PL, Brandt LJ. Review article: diagnosis and management of mesenteric ischaemia with an emphasis on pharmacotherapy. *Aliment Pharmacol Ther* 2005; **21**: 201–215.

3. Brandt LJ, Boley SJ. AGA technical review on intestinal ischaemia. *Gastroenterology* 2000; **118**: 954–968.

4. van Deinse WH, Zawacki JK, Phillips D. Treatment of acute mesenteric ischaemia by percutaneous transluminal angioplasty. *Gastroenterology* 1986; **91**: 475–478.

5. Boley SJ, Sprayregan S, Siegelmann SS, et al. Initial results from an aggressive roentgenological and surgical approach to acute mesenteric ischemia. *Surgery* 1977; **82**: 848–855.

6. Kaser A, Tilg H. Novel therapeutic agents in the treatment of IBD. *Expert Opin Ther Targets* 2008; **12**(5): 553–563.

7. Carter MJ, Lobo AJ, Travis SPL. Guidelines for the management of inflammatory bowel disease in adults. *Gut* 2004. **53**(suppl V): v1–16.

8. Gerson LB, Triadafilopoulos G. Palliative care in inflammatory bowel disease: an evidence-based approach. *Inflamm Bowel Dis* 2000; **6**: 228–243.

9. Rahimi R, Nikfar S, Abdollahi M. Do anti-tumor necrosis factors induce response and remission in patients with acute refractory Crohn's disease? A systemic meta-analysis of controlled clinical trials. *Biomed Pharmacother* 2007; **61**: 75–80.

10. Behm BW, Bickston SJ. Tumor necrosis factor-alpha antibody for maintenance of remission in Crohn's disease. Cochrane Database of Systematic Reviews 2008; Issue 1, Art. No. CD006893. DOI: 10.1002/14651858.CD006893.

11. Targan SR, Hanaver SB, van Deventer SJ, et al. A short term study of chimeric monoclonal antibody cA2 to tumor necrosis factor alpha for Crohn's disease. *N Engl J Med* 1997; **337**: 1029–1035.

12. Hanauer SB, Feagan BG, Lichtenstein GR, et al. Maintenance infliximab for Crohn's disease: the ACCENT I randomized trial. Lancet 2002; **359**: 1541–1549.

13. Sands BE, Anderson FH, Bernstein CN, et al. Infliximab maintenance therapy for fistulizing Crohn's disease. *N Engl J Med* 2004; **350**: 876–885.

14. Chang JT, Lichtenstein GR. Drug insight: antagonists of tumor-necrosis factor-alpha in the treatment of inflammatory bowel disease. *Nat Clin Pract Gastroenterol Hepatol* 2006; **3**: 220–228.

15. Sandborn WJ, Hanauer SB, Katz S, et al. Etanercept for active Crohn's disease: a randomized, double-blind, placebo controlled trial. *Gastroenterology* 2001; **121**: 1088–1094.

16. Frattini J, Longo WE. Diagnosis and treatment of chronic and recurrent diverticulitis. *J Clin Gastroenterol* 2006. **40**(suppl 3): S145–S149.

17. Place RJ, Simmang CL. Diverticular disease. *Best Pract Res Clin Gastroenterol* 2002; **16**: 135–148.

18. Kohler L, Sauerland S, Neugebauer E. Diagnosis and treatment of diverticular disease: results of a consensus development conference. The Scientific Committee of the European Association for Endoscopic Surgery. *Surg Endosc* 1999; **13**: 430–436.

19. Colecchia A, Vestito A, Pasqui F, et al. Efficacy of long-term cyclic administration of the poorly absorbed antibiotic Rifaximin in symptomatic, uncomplicated colonic diverticular disease. *World J Gastroenterol* 2007; **13**(2): 264–269.

20. Comparato G, Fanigliulo L, Cavallaro LG, et al. Prevention of complications and symptomatic recurrences in diverticular disease with mesalazine: a 12-month follow-up. *Dig Dis Sci* 2007; **52**: 2934–2941.

21. Petruzziello L, Iacopini F, Bulajic M. Review article: uncomplicated diverticular disease of the colon. *Aliment Pharmacol Ther* 2006; **23**: 1379–1391.

22. Cremoni F, Talley NJ. Irritable bowel syndrome: epidemiology, natural history, health care seeking and emerging risks. *Gastroenterol Clin North Am* 2005; **34**: 189–204.

23. Roy-Byrne PP, Davidson KW, Kessler RC, et al. Anxiety disorders and comorbid medical illness. *Gen Hosp Psychiatr* 2008; **30**: 208–225.

24. Riedl A, Schmidtmann M, Stengel A, et al. Somatic comorbidities of irritable bowel syndrome: a systemic analysis. *J Psychosom Res* 2008; **64**: 573–582.

25. Tobin MC, Moparty B, Farhadi A, et al. Atopic irritable bowel syndrome: a novel subgroup of irritable bowel syndrome with allergic manifestations. *Ann Allergy Asthma Immunol* 2008; **100**(1): 49–53.

26. Spiller R. Clinical update: irritable bowel syndrome. *Lancet* 2007; **369**: 1586–1588.

27. Mayer EA. Irritable bowel syndrome. *N Engl J Med* 2008; **358**: 1692–1699.

28. Farthing MJG. Treatment options in irritable bowel syndrome. *Best Pract Res Clin Gastroenterol* 2004; **18**: 773–786.

29. Pasricha PJ. Desperately seeking serotonin … a commentary on the withdrawal of tegaserod and the state of drug development for functional and motility disorders. *Gastroenterology* 2007; **132**: 2287–2290.

30. Lackner JM, Mesmer C, Morley S, et al. Psychologic treatments for irritable bowel syndrome: a systemic review and meta-analysis. *J Consult Clin Psychol* 2004; **72**: 1100–1113.

31. Lackner JM, Jaccard J, Krasner SS, et al. Self-administered cognitive behavioral therapy for moderate to severe IBS: clinical efficacy, tolerability, feasibility. *Clin Gastroenterol Hepatol* 2008; **6**(8): 899–906.

32. Whorwell PJ. The history of hypnotherapy and its role in the irritable bowel syndrome. *Aliment Pharmacol Ther* 2005; **22**: 1061–1067.

33. Quartero AO, Meiniche-Schmidt V, Muris J, Rubin G, de Wit N. Bulking agents, antispasmodic and antidepressant medication for the treatment of irritable bowel syndrome. Cochrane Database of Systematic Reviews 2005, Issue 2. Art. No.: CD003460. DOI: 10.1002/14651858.CD003460.pub2.

34. Bijkerk CJ, Muris JW, Knottnerus JA, Hoes AW, de Wit NJ. Systematic review: the role of different types of fiber in the treatment of irritable bowel syndrome. *Aliment Pharmacol Ther* 2004; **19**: 245–251.

35. Hayee B, Forgacs I. Psychological approach to managing irritable bowel syndrome. *BMJ* 2007; **334**: 1105–1109.

36. Bharucha AE, Wald A, Enck P, Rao, S. Functional anorectal disorders. *Gastroenterology* 2006; **130**: 1510–1518.

37. Gupta V, Toskes PP. Diagnosis and management of chronic pancreatitis. *Post Grad Med* 2005; **81**: 491–497.

38. Witt H, Apte MV, Keim V, Wilson JS. Chronic pancreatitis: challenges and advances in pathogenesis, genetics, diagnosis and therapy. *Gastroenterology* 2007; **132**: 1557–1573.

39. Warshaw AL, Banks PA, Fernandez-Del Castillo C. AGA Technical Review: treatment of pain in chronic pancreatitis. *Gastroenterology* 1998; **115**: 765–776.

40. Leung JW, Bowen-Wright M, Aveling W, *et al.* Coeliac plexus block for pain in pancreatic cancer and chronic pancreatitis. *Br J Surg* 1983; **70**: 730–732.

41. Busch EH, Atchison SR. Steroid celiac plexus block for chronic pancreatitis: results in 16 cases. *J Clin Anesth* 1989; **1**: 431–433.

42. Gress F, Schmitt C, Sherman S, *et al.* A prospective randomized comparison of endoscopic ultrasound and computed tomography-guided celiac plexus block for managing chronic pancreatitis pain. *Am J Gastroenterol* 1999; **94**: 900–905.

43. Gress F, Schmitt C, Sherman S, *et al.* Endoscopic ultrasound-guided celiac plexus block for managing abdominal pain associated with chronic pancreatitis: a prospective single center experience. *Am J Gastroenterol* 2001; **96**: 409–416.

44. Cahen DL, Gouma DJ, Nio Y, *et al.* Endoscopic versus surgical drainage of the pancreatic duct in chronic pancreatitis. *N Engl J Med* 2007; **356**: 727–729.

45. Dite P, Ruzicka M, Zboril V, Novoty I. A prospective, randomized trial comparing endoscopic and surgical therapy for chronic pancreatitis. *Endoscopy* 2003; **35**: 553–558.

46. Vetrhus M, Berhane T, Soreide O, Sondenaa K. Pain persists in many patients five years after removal of the gallbladder: observations from two randomized controlled trials of symptomatic, noncomplicated gallstone disease and acute cholecystitis. *J Gastroint Surg* 2005; **9**: 826–831.

47. Behar J, Corazziari E, Guelrud M, Hogan W, Sherman S, Toouli J. Functional gallbladder and sphincter of Oddi disorders. *Gastroenterology* 2006; **130**: 1498–1509.

48. Micali S, Grande M, Sighinolfi MC, de Carne C, de Stefani S, Bianchi G. Medical therapy of urolithiasis. *J Endourol* 2006; **20**: 841–847.

49. Micali S, Grande M, Sighinolfi MC, *et al.* Medical therapy for urolithiasis. *J Endourol* 2006; **20**(11): 841–847.

50. Davenport K, Timoney AG, Keeley FX. Conventional and alternative methods for providing analgesia in renal colic. *Br J Urol Int* 2005; **95**: 297–300.

51. Beach MA, Mauro LS. Pharmacologic expulsion treatment of ureteral calculi. *Ann Pharmacother* 2006; **40**: 1361–1368.

52. Torres VE, Harris PC, Pirson Y. Autosomal dominant polycystic kidney disease. *Lancet* 2007; **369**: 1287–1301.

53. Bajwa ZH, Sial KA, Malik AB, Steinman TI. Pain patterns in patients with polycystic kidney disease. *Kidney Int* 2004; **66**: 1561–1569

54. Bajwa ZH, Gupta S, Warfield CA, Steinman TI. Pain management in polycystic kidney disease. *Kidney Int* 2001; **60**: 1631–1644.

55. Brown JA, Torres VE, King BF, Segura JW. Laparoscopic marsupialization of symptomatic polycystic kidney disease. *J Urol* 1996; **156**: 22–27.

56. Casale P, Meyers K, Kaplan B. Follow-up for laparoscopic renal denervation and nephropexy for autosomal dominant polycystic kidney disease-related pain in Pediatrics. *J Endourol* 2008; **22**(5): 991–993.

57. Lall R, Mailis A, Rapoport A. Hematuria-loin pain syndrome: its existence as a discrete clinicopathological entity cannot be supported. *Clin J Pain* 1997; **13**: 171–177.

58. Spetie DN, Nadasdy T, Nadasdy G, *et al.* Proposed pathogenesis of idiopathic loin-pain-hematuria syndrome. *Am J Kidney Dis* 2006; **47**: 419–427.

59. Payne CK, Joyce GF, Wise M, Clemens JQ, Urologic Diseases in America Project. Interstitial cystitis and painful bladder syndrome. *J Urol* 2007; **177**: 2042–2049.

60. Bogart LM, Berry SH, Clemens JQ. Symptoms of interstitial cystitis, painful bladder syndrome and similar diseases in women: a systematic review. *J Urol* 2007; **177**: 450–456.

61. Alagiri M, Chottiner S, Ratner V, Slade D, Hanno PM. Interstitial cystitis: unexplained associations with other chronic disease and pain syndromes. *Urology* 1997; **49**(suppl 5A): 52–57.

62. Keay SK, Szekely Z, Conrads TP, *et al.* An antiproliferative factor from interstitial cystitis patients is a frizzled 8 protein-related sialoglycopeptide. *Proc Natl Acad Sci USA* 2004; **101**: 11803–11808.

63. Clemens JQ, Meenan RT, O'Keefe Rosetti MC, *et al.* Case-control study of medical comorbidites in women with interstitial cystitis. *J Urol* 2008; **179**; 2222–2225.

64. Stanford EJ, Dell JR, Parsons CL. The emerging presence of interstitial cystitis in gynecologic patients with chronic pelvic pain. *Urology* 2006; **69**(suppl 4A): 53–59.

65. Phatak S, Foster HE Jr. The management of interstitial cystitis: an update. *Nat Clin Pract Urol* 2006; **3**: 45–53.

66. Sairanen J, Tammela TL, Leppilahti M, *et al.* Cyclosporine A and pentosan polysulfate sodium for the treatment of interstitial cystitis: a randomized comparative study. *J Urol* 2005; **174**: 2235–2238.

67. Buffington CA. Cyclosporine A and pentosan polysulfate sodium for the treatment of interstitial cystitis: a randomized comparative study. *J Urol* 2006; **176**(2): 838.

68. Chancellor MB, Yoshimura N. Treatment of interstitial cystitis. *Urology* 2004; **63**(suppl 1): 85–92.

69. Marjoribanks J, Proctor M, Farquhar C, Sangkomkamhang US, Derks RS. Nonsteroidal anti-inflammatory drugs for primary dysmenorrhoea. Cochrane Database of Systematic Reviews 2003, Issue 4. Art. No.: CD001751. DOI: 10.1002/14651858. CD001751.

70. Sanfilippo J, Erb T. Evaluation and management of dysmenorrhea in adolescents. *Clin Obstet Gynecol* 2008; **51**(2): 257–267.

71. Davis A, Westhoff C, O'Connell K, *et al*. Oral contraceptives for dysmenorrhea in adolescent girls. *J Obstet Gynecol* 2005; **106**: 97–104.

72. Proctor M, Latthe P, Farquhar CM, Khan KS, Johnson N. Surgical interruption of pelvic nerve pathways for primary and secondary dysmenorrhoea. Cochrane Database of Systematic Reviews 2005, Issue 4. Art. No.: CD001896. DOI: 10.1002/14651858.CD001896.pub2.

73. Lefebvre G, Pinsonneault O, Antao V, *et al*. Primary dysmenorrheal consensus guideline. *J Obstet Gynaecol Can* 2005; **27**: 1117–1146.

74. American College of Obstetricians and Gynecologists. Medical management of endometriosis. ACOG Practice Bulletin No. 11. *Int J Gynaecol Obstet* 2000; **71**: 183–196.

75. Practice Committee of American Society of Reproductive Medicine. Treatment of pelvic pain associated with endometriosis. *Fertil Steril* 2006; **86**(suppl 4): S18–S27.

76. American College of Obstetricians and Gynecologists Committee on Adolescent Health Care. Endometriosis in adolescents. Committee Opinion 310. *Obstet Gynecol* 2005; **105**: 921–927.

77. Nezhat CH, Seidman DS, Nezhat FR, Mirmalek SA, Nezhat CR. Ovarian remnant syndrome after laparoscopic oophorectomy. *Fertil Steril* 2000; **74**: 1024–1028.

78. Granitsiotis P, Kirk D. Chronic testicular pain; an overview. *Eur Urol* 2004; **45**: 430–436.

79. Wesselmann U, Burnett AL, Heinberg LJ. The urogenital and rectal pain syndromes. *Pain* 1997; **73**: 269–294.

80. Simon A, van der Meer JWM. Pathogenesis of familial periodic fever syndromes or hereditary autoinflammatory syndromes. *Am J Physiol Integr Comp Physiol* 2007; **292**: R86–R98.

81. Simon A, van der Meer JWM, Drenth JPH. Familial Mediterranean fever – a not so unusual cause of abdominal pain. *Best Pract Res Clin Gastroenterol* 2005; **19**: 199–213.

82. Kallinich T, Haffner D, Niehues T, *et al*. Colchicine use in children and adolescents with familial Mediterranean fever: literature review and consensus statement. *Pediatrics* 2007; **119**: 474–483.

83. Sassa S. Modern diagnosis and management of the porphyrias. *Br J Haematol* 2006; **135**: 281–292.

84. Anderson KE, Bloomer JR, Bonkovsky HL, *et al*. Recommendations for the diagnosis and treatment of the acute porphyrias. *Ann Intern Med* 2005; **142**: 439–450.

85. Swank DJ, Swank-Bordewijk SC, Hop WC, *et al*. Laparoscopic adhesiolysis in patients with chronic abdominal pain: a blinded randomized controlled multi-centre trial. *Lancet* 2003; **361**: 1247–1251.

86. Peters AA, Trimbos-Kemper GC, Admiraal C, Trimbos JB, Hermans J. A randomized clinical trial on the benefits of adhesiolysis in patients with intraperitoneal adhesions and chronic pelvic pain. *Br J Obstet Gynaecol* 1992; **99**: 59–62.

87. Practice Committee of the American Society for Reproductive Medicine. Control and prevention of peritoneal adhesions in gynecologic surgery. *Fertil Steril* 2006; **86**(suppl 4): S1–S5.

CHAPTER 16

Postsurgical pain syndromes

Fred Perkins and Jane Ballantyne

National Anesthesia Service, United States Department of Veteran Affairs, White River Junction, VT, USA

Background

As surgery becomes safer and appropriate to increasing numbers of individuals, and as the population ages, surgery is less feared and more widely undertaken. This trend is accompanied by an increasing awareness of the problem of persistent postsurgical pain. Whereas once one felt lucky to survive surgery, and not surprised by long-term sequelae, now one can reasonably expect a full recovery. Persistent pain can considerably alter risk:benefit assessments in surgical decision making, and it follows that progress in surgical management must include efforts to understand and avoid persistent postsurgical pain. This is an area of research that has received much attention, especially over the last decade. A number of comprehensive reviews can be found in the literature [1–3] and evidence is beginning to accrue that helps quantify the problem as well as understand its basis. This chapter provides an overview of that evidence.

Prevalence

Given the fragmented nature of postsurgical follow-up, it is perhaps not surprising that rates of persistent postsurgical pain were largely unknown until attention was drawn to the problem. Table 16.1 summarizes data from recent studies attempting to quantify the problem of persistent postsurgical pain. These

Evidence-Based Chronic Pain Management. Edited by
C. Stannard, E. Kalso and J. Ballantyne. © 2010 Blackwell
Publishing.

summary prevalence data do not help in determining the severity, duration or tolerability of the pain, or its true burden, but do provide a measure of the proportion of individuals affected. The table draws a distinction between persistent pain arising when there was no pre-existent pain or pre-existent pain was unrelated, versus persistent pain occurring as unresolved pain after surgery that attempts to improve pain. The former – postsurgical chronic pain syndromes – are predominantly neuropathic pain syndromes, whereas the latter – persistent postsurgical pain conditions – are multifactorial and often associated with the original condition. What has surprised the medical community is how commonly persistent postsurgical pain occurs in both circumstances.

Definition and timing of postsurgical pain

Pain is nearly universal following any surgical procedure, and this postoperative pain is assumed to resolve over a relatively short period measured in days or weeks. It is usually assumed that acute postoperative pain is primarily the result of nociceptive and inflammatory input from the surgical injury, although in some surgical models, nerve injury may be a significant component even during the acute phase. It is also reasonable to assume, on the basis of clinical presentation as well as investigational data, that most persistent postsurgical pain, at least after nonpain-related surgery, is predominantly neuropathic [3, 4]. Chronic pain has traditionally been defined as pain lasting more than 3 or 6 months [5] yet given the complexity of mechanisms of persistent postinjury pain, and the variations in recovery times for each component,

Table 16.1 Prevalence of postoperative pain by procedure

Surgical procedure	Prevalence of chronic pain	Prevalence of preoperative pain
Pain new in location or character*		
Lower extremity amputation [2]	Stump pain 62% Phantom pain 70%	Very common if ischemic disease
Breast surgery:		
Augmentation mammoplasty [41]	20%	Rare
Simple mastectomy [2]	30%	Rare
Mastectomy + axillary node dissection [2]	50%	Rare
Thoracotomy:		
Posterolateral approach [2]	50%	Rare
VATS [2]	31%	Rare
Radical prostatectomy [73]	32%	Rare
Hysterectomy [70]	32%	62%, associated with uterine pathology
Sternotomy:		
CABG [74]	30%	Angina common
Valve replacement [75]	32%	Rare
Colectomy [68]	28%	Rare
Laparoscopic cholecystectomy [67]	23%	Common and usually associated with cholelithiasis
Vasectomy [76]	15%	Rare
Inguinal hernia repair [62]	12%	Incident pain common
Cesarean section [66]	6%	(Labor pain)
Lens implantation [65]	<1%	Rare
Persistence of pre-existing pain˜		
Pelvic fracture open fixation [72]	48%	Almost universal and associated with fracture
Lumbar discectomy [71]	44%	Common and associated with nerve root impingement
Hip replacement [64]	20%	Almost universal and associated with joint disease
Root canal [69]	12%	Common and associated with tooth decay

* Most common syndromes of persistent or chronic pain, surgery was not undertaken for pain relief, pain is usually neuropathic

˜ Pain severe and present longer than expected, surgery was for pain relief, pain multifactorial and often associated with original condition (e.g. continued inflammation)

CABG, coronary artery bypass graft; VATS, video-assisted thoracoscopic surgery.

this type of definition does not help distinguish acute from long-lived processes. More satisfactorily in the present context, and perhaps in all cases of acute progressing to chronic pain, chronic pain can be defined as "pain that extends beyond the period of tissue healing and/or with low levels of identified pathology that are insufficient to explain the presence and/or extent of pain" [6]. This definition allows that aberrancy in the pain process can arise at different times, depending on a number of surgical and patient factors. Callesen *et al.* [7] presented data from a large case series of hernia repairs and found that the prevalence of groin pain decreased from 3 months to 6 months to 12 months and then stabilized. Similar data for

persistent pain following thoracotomy have been presented by Gottschalk's group [8] and the same is true for breast surgery [9]. For lower extremity amputation, Jensen *et al.* documented a relatively constant prevalence of pain between 1 and 2 years [10]. Thus the first year after surgery may be a critical time for intervention when pain processes may be amenable to modification before they have stabilized.

Risk factors

There have been a number of risk factors identified for the development of chronic pain following surgery (Table 16.2). Some of these factors are surgery specific while others are more general.

Table 16.2 Risk factors for persistent postoperative pain

Surgical nerve injury
Continued inflammatory response (e.g. mesh hernia repair)
Pre-existing pain
Severity of postoperative pain
Radiation or chemotherapy postoperatively
Increased baseline pain sensitivity
Genetic predisposition
Psychologic vulnerability
Female gender
Younger age

Surgical factors

Some studies have indicated that nerve damage during surgery is associated with an increased prevalence of chronic pain [11–13]. Yet the prevalence of nerve damage in surgical models typically associated with persistent pain (thoracotomy, breast surgery and inguinal hernia repair) is much higher than the prevalence of pain [2]. Either the persistence of pain varies with the type of nerve damage or there are other factors, including patient factors, that produce the difference. Data are lacking regarding the specific type(s) of nerve damage that may be associated with an increased incidence of chronic pain, but it is interesting that S. Weir Mitchell [14] noted over 100 years ago that nerve damage from contusion or incomplete transection was more likely to result in long-term pain (in particular, causalgia) than nerve transection. Preliminary observations suggest that preserving the intercostal brachial nerve during mastectomy may decrease risk of persistent pain [4, 15]. Several newer thoracotomy techniques may produce less nerve injury, and early results suggest better pain outcomes. These include use of thoracoscopy in preference to fully open procedures with rib retractors, and the practice of muscle-sparing thoracotomy in preference to the conventional posterolateral approach [12, 16]. A number of other minimally invasive procedures are likely to be associated with less nerve injury and better pain outcomes, and early data support this assumption [3]. High rates of persistent postherniorrhaphy pain may be associated with an inflammatory process induced by the use of mesh in the repair, and preliminary results suggest that the use of lightweight mesh may reduce chronic inflammatory pain [17].

Pre-existing pain

Convincing correlations between pain before surgery and persistent postsurgical pain have been demonstrated. For example, phantom limb pain has been correlated with duration and severity of preamputation pain, typically in patients requiring amputation for vascular disease [10, 18]. Similar associations have been demonstrated for other surgeries including breast, inguinal hernia and gallbladder, but with less consistency [2].

Increase in early postoperative pain and postoperative opioid consumption

Increased intensity of acute pain (and as a surrogate, the amount of opioid consumed in the immediate postoperative period) has been a robust predictor of chronic pain. This raises the question as to whether acute pain in some way causes chronic pain, and if so whether effective early postoperative analgesia is a method of decreasing chronic pain. Another possibility is that more severe acute pain is a marker for more intense nociceptive stimulation, or possibly increased individual sensitivity to pain, and in those cases improved acute pain control would be less likely to affect pain persistence. Although the exact mechanisms for the association between acute pain severity and pain persistence are unclear, the use of early and aggressive postoperative pain therapy seems logical and should be investigated.

Postoperative radiation and chemotherapy

Administration of chemotherapy increases the incidence of phantom limb pain, and may affect chronic pain in other surgical models [2, 19]. In the case of breast surgery, both radiation and chemotherapy during postoperative recovery have been shown to increase the likelihood of postmastectomy pain in the breast and arm [2].

Pain sensitivity

Patients may differ considerably in their sensitivity to pain. It has been demonstrated that pain sensitivity as measured by pain rating during a first-degree burn can predict the extent of pain following anterior cruciate ligament reconstruction [20]. Thermal pain sensitivity as measured by the heat pain unpleasantness was a significant predictor of pain intensity following cesarean section [21]. Other patient factors have not been predictive of postoperative pain, such as pain sensitivity as measured by pressure algometry [22] or tolerance to ice water immersion. Variations in pain sensitivity are increasingly attributed to genetic differences in both the generation and experiencing of pain. For example, functional polymorphisms of catecholamine-O-methyltransferase (COMT) have been associated with changes in pain sensitivity, and the melanocortin-1 receptor gene that produces red hair and freckles has been shown to alter κ-opioid analgesia [3].

Patient characteristics

There are individual factors that appear to be of importance. Women experience more acute and chronic pain following thoracic surgery than men [23]. After herniorrhaphy, older patients are less likely to develop persistent pain [24, 25]. Psychosocial factors may also play an important role in the development of chronic pain, which is amply documented in chronic pain of nonsurgical origin, though less so in persistent postsurgical pain. It might be surmised, however, that stress, anxiety, fear of pain and the natural tendency to associate pain with poor outcome or death might have a negative impact on the pain experience, if not on pain progression. In one study, persistent functional abdominal pain was associated with stress, vulnerability and symptoms of psychologic stress after cholecystectomy [26]. In another study of lower extremity amputees, psychosocial variables predicted phantom pain up to 2 years after amputation [27].

Common postsurgical pain syndromes

Lower extremity amputation

Phantom and stump pain after lower extremity amputation is well described in both the historic and recent literature, making this the best described and recognized of the persistent postsurgical pain syndromes. The reported incidence in the literature varies from 30% to 81% [2]. Incidence data are, of course, determined by the time point at which they are measured, and postamputation pain does tend to decrease over the course of the first year after surgery, although it may stabilize and persist after this [10, 28].

The presence of intense preoperative pain in the extremity increases the likelihood of developing phantom limb pain, according to some studies [18, 29]. Probably related to this, postamputation pain seems to be more common in amputation for cancer rather than trauma [19]. A great deal of excitement was engendered when Bach *et al.* reported a significant decrease in the incidence of phantom limb pain attributable to the use of 72 hours dense epidural blockade prior to amputation in a quasi-randomized but small trial [30]. This study strongly suggested that "pre-emptive" analgesia worked, at least in the case of limb amputation. However, this study has been reproduced only once in another small quasi-randomized study [31] and in a newer, large, truly randomized trial, this observation was not confirmed [32]. However, the larger study used preoperative epidural treatment for only 18 hours, and used less dense blockade. Whether or not dense and prolonged neural blockade prior to amputation can reduce phantom limb pain remains an open question. Little study has been made of the role of anesthetic choice (regional versus general) or surgical technique on the prevalence of postamputation pain, so no conclusions can be made in this respect.

In addition to preamputation limb pain being a strong predictor of postamputation pain prevalence and severity, there is also evidence that early postoperative limb pain predicts long-term phantom limb pain. Stump pain at 1 week is significantly associated with phantom pain at 1 week, and persistent stump and phantom pain are also closely associated [2]. Chemotherapy administration during recovery after amputation has been shown to increase the likelihood of phantom limb pain [19]. Nerve sheath infusion of local anesthetic was shown to decrease the incidence of phantom limb pain in one small case series [33] but a later small randomized trial failed to confirm this finding [34]. Uncertainty about the benefit of nerve sheath infusion remains. Although conceptually, it would seem that early treatment of postamputation pain with adjuncts such as anticonvulsants and antidepressants might reduce pain persistence, there are virtually no published data to support this.

Breast surgery

The majority of studies of chronic pain following breast surgery involve women with cancer. There are also some reports of reasonable quality following augmentation mammoplasty or reduction mammoplasty. Studies of both cancer surgery and augmentation mammoplasty document a significant prevalence of chronic pain following breast surgery (see Table 16.1). For women undergoing cancer surgery, there are also problems with persistent arm pain following axillary dissection. Radiation therapy and chemotherapy following breast surgery will further increase the prevalence of persistent pain [2]. At least one group of researchers has noted a decrease in the incidence of arm pain and symptoms as surgeons have become more careful in the handling of the nerves in the axilla [35]. There are now a number of studies demonstrating that axillary sentinel node biopsy is associated with less persistent pain than a primary axillary dissection. One of these is a randomized controlled study in which women were randomized to a sentinel node study arm or an axillary dissection study arm [36]. Women in the sentinel node arm where cancer was found in a sentinel node also underwent an axillary dissection. Women who did not have cancer in the sentinel node were less likely to receive adjuvant cancer therapy and were significantly less likely to develop persistent axillary pain (8% at 24 months) compared to those who had a primary axillary dissection and adjuvant therapy (39% at 24 months). In Table 16.3 the Odds ratios of this study and two prospective case series [37, 38] studies are summarized. Women with negative nodes on a sentinel node biopsy are significantly less likely to develop arm pain and other arm symptoms. Women who underwent a secondary axillary node dissection were as likely or more likely to develop chronic pain as those who underwent a primary axillary node dissection [37].

Breast-conserving surgery has been associated with a higher prevalence of chronic pain than simple mastectomy [2] but only in studies where persistent pain

was assessed as a tertiary, not a primary or secondary outcome, and the association has not been found consistently. There are no randomized studies here.

Recently there have been two randomized controlled studies that looked at the influence of perioperative paravertebral blockade on persistent pain following breast surgery. Both found a significantly lower prevalence of chronic pain in women who had the block. One [35] was a follow-up study of 60 women who had participated in an acute perioperative pain study [39]. In this study the prevalence of pain at both 6 months and 12 months was significantly lower among the women who had received a block (17% versus 40% at 6 months, and 7% versus 33% at 12 months). The second study [40] was smaller (29 subjects) and involved the placement of a paravertebral catheter preoperatively in the patients in the treatment arm. This was dosed with 10 ml of 0.25% bupivacaine prior to surgery and reinjected every 12 hours for 48 hours with the same dose. A telephone follow-up inquired about pain 3 months following surgery ("Do you have chronic pain as a result of your breast surgery?"). The paravertebral block group had significantly lower pain prevalence at 3 months (0% versus 80%). If the 6-month data from the first study are combined with the 3-month data from the second study then the calculated odds ratio of persistent pain in the paravertebral block groups is 0.05 (0.02–0.11).

There are a number of randomized controlled studies that have looked at perioperative interventions to decrease the prevalence of persistent pain after breast surgery. Romundstad et al. [41] compared a single dose of methylprednisolone (125 mg) to a single dose of parecoxib (40 mg) to placebo in women undergoing augmentation mammoplasty. At 12 months the prevalence of rest pain in the three groups was 16%, 7%, and 16% respectively, with no significant differences. Evoked pain was found in 16%, 14%, and 29% respectively, again with no significant differences (P = 0.085). The calculated odds ratio and 95% confidence intervals for methylprednisolone compared to placebo were 0.49 (0.30–0.74), and for parecoxib 0.40 (0.25–0.64).

Fassoulaki and colleagues published two randomized controlled studies of perioperative gabapentin [42, 43]. In the first [42], women received gabapentin 1200 mg per day (400 mg three times a day), starting the evening before surgery, or mexiletine 600 mg per day (200 mg three times per day) or placebo three

Table 16.3 Sentinel node compared to primary axillary dissection

Sentinel (only)	Axillary dissection	Odds ratio	95% CI	Quality	Ref
8%	31%	0.14	0.09–0.21	RCT	36
16%	50%	0.19	0.15–0.24	CS	37,38

RCT, randomized controlled study; CS, case series.

times per day. There were no significant differences in pain prevalence or intensity, or in analgesic requirement at 3 months follow-up, although the character of the pain in the control group tended to be burning rather than throbbing, aching or stabbing. In the second study [43], women undergoing breast cancer surgery received a combination of gabapentin 1600 mg per day (400 mg four times a day) for 10 days starting the evening before surgery, plus EMLA cream (20 g) for 3 days starting the day of surgery, plus intraoperative irrigation of the brachial plexus with 10 ml of 0.75% ropivacaine. The control group underwent placebo administration of each of the interventions. This study found significantly decreased pain prevalence at both 3-month and 6-month follow-up in the intervention group (30% versus 57% at 6 months). The calculated odds ratio for pain at 6 months is 0.32 (0.18–0.62). Whether gabapentin can alter long-term pain following breast surgery is not clear, and follow-up at 12 months and longer is needed.

Thoracotomy

Persistent pain following thoracotomy may have a prevalence as high as 50% [2] and anecdotal reports suggest the syndrome is extremely troublesome to both patients and surgeons. The prevalence of preoperative pain is low (12%), but chronic pain is more likely to develop if preoperative pain is present [23].

The use of thoracic epidural analgesia with local anesthetics has been strongly advocated [44] although the data may seem conflicting. There are three randomized controlled trials that look at the effect of adding intraoperative epidural analgesia to postoperative epidural analgesia [23, 45, 46] Obata et al. [45] and Senturk et al. [46] both found a decreased prevalence of pain at 6 months when patients received a continuous infusion of local anesthetic starting before skin incision in patients undergoing posterolateral thoracotomy (see Table 16.4). In contrast,

Table 16.4 Pain prevalence at 6 months following thoracotomy, effect of intraoperative local anesthetic

Intra-op + post-op	Post-op only	Odds ratio	95% CI	Quality	Ref
38%	65%	0.33	0.22–0.50	RCT	45,46

Ochroch et al. [23] did not find a significant effect of intra- and postoperative epidural local anesthetic versus postoperative only on a mixed surgical population (32% posterolateral thoracotomy and 68% muscle-sparing thoracotomy) followed for 48 weeks. However, Ochroch's study was powered to look for a 10 mm decrease in average pain intensity (using a 0–100 mm VAS) rather than looking at persistent pain prevalence. In addition, this study was a multifactorial analysis and as such was significantly underpowered for showing an overall significant effect on persistent postsurgical pain. The three trials also differed in the local anesthetic used, and in the concentration of local anesthetic as well as the amount of epidural opioid.

There has been little effort to assess the role of paravertebral blockade on persistent pain after thoracotomy, so it is difficult to reach conclusions on this intervention. Studies show decreased acute pain intensity using perioperative paravertebral blockade [47] but with no long-term follow-up. A meta-analysis concluded that paravertebral blockade and thoracic epidural analgesia provided equivalent analgesia, but paravertebral blockade had a better side effect profile [48]. A randomized controlled trial comparing preincision local anesthetic infiltration with saline infiltration in patients undergoing posterolateral thoracotomy found no difference in acute or chronic pain intensity [49]. Pain prevalence data were not reported.

A subsequent report from Ochroch et al. [50] using data from their 2002 study [23] looked at the effect of surgical incision type and found that patients who underwent posterolateral thoracotomy were more limited in their physical activity than those who had muscle-sparing incisions, despite no significant differences in pain prevalence or pain intensity between the groups. Previous studies [2] have suggested that incision type is of importance regarding the prevalence of chronic pain, and this is an area that needs further investigation.

There are reports that handling of intercostal nerves at closure following posterolateral thoracotomy can alter the prevalence of persistent pain. When patients were randomized (n = 114) to having the intercostal nerves protected by an intercostal muscle harvest, the average intensity of postoperative pain decreased acutely and for the 12 weeks of follow-up [51]. Total pain prevalence at 12 weeks was not reported, but the prevalence of moderate to severe pain at 12 weeks was 22% for the nerve-protected group and 28% for the control group (not significant). In a case series (n = 280) closure with sutures placed through the lower rib rather than under it (where the intercostal nerve could be compressed) resulted in significantly less intense pain through 3 months follow-up, and patients from the control group were more likely to use neuropathic pain descriptors on the short form of the McGill Pain Questionnaire [52]. Pain prevalence data were not reported.

Inguinal hernia repair

There are a number of excellent reviews on postherniorrhaphy pain [24, 25, 53]. To date, no differences in persistent pain have been found between different anesthetic techniques or different postoperative analgesic methods [54]. However, a number of studies have looked at the effect of different surgical techniques, and found differences. These studies include comparison of open hernia repair with mesh to laparoscopic repair with mesh; the identification and sectioning of major nerves compared to preservation of these nerves; the use of lightweight mesh compared to regular mesh; and the comparison of open mesh repairs to open nonmesh repairs.

Table 16.5 is a summary of the effects of different surgical interventions on the probability of persistent pain. These data are presented as odds ratios and their 95% confidence intervals. A systematic review of nerve preservation compared to sectioning found three randomized controlled trials and four cohort

Table 16.5 Surgical options and persistent pain, hernia repair

Experimental	Control	Odds ratio	95% CI	Quality	Ref
Laparoscopic repair	Open repair	0.56	0.44–0.70	M	57, 58
Lightweight mesh	Standard mesh	0.67	0.49–0.91	RCT, 2	17, 61
Open mesh	Open nonmesh	0.63	0.42–0.96	M	77
Nerve sectioning	Nerve identification	1.10	0.76–1.15	M	55

M, meta-analysis; RCT, randomized controlled study.

trials [55]. Intentional sectioning of the ilio-inguinal and iliohypogastric nerves did not alter the probability of persistent pain following hernia repair at 6 months (21% prevalence of pain for nerve sectioning and 23% prevalence for nerve preservation). An early systematic review comparing open hernia repair to laparoscopic repair [56] noted that few studies reported the prevalence of chronic pain, and there were no significant differences. Two more recent reviews of the same topic [57, 58] found a significant decrease in risk of chronic pain with laparoscopic repair (8% prevalence) compared to open mesh repair (13% prevalence). A review of open hernia repair using mesh versus not using mesh found a lower prevalence of persistent pain and a lower hernia recurrence rate with mesh repairs [59]. These findings are similar to the findings from a Cochrane Database Review [60] in which cumulative data revealed a prevalence of 6% for chronic pain following mesh repairs and 10% for open repairs. There have been a number of recent randomized controlled studies comparing lightweight mesh to standard mesh [17, 61] but there has not been a rigorous meta-analysis or systematic review. The combined prevalence of chronic pain with lightweight mesh was 27%, while with standard mesh it was 33%.

Surgical treatment of chronic pain following hernia repair has been reviewed recently [62]. Neurectomy of the ilio-inguinal, iliohypogastric, genitofemoral or lateral femoral cutaneous nerve was described in 14 papers, mostly reporting good outcomes. However, the reviewers questioned the quality of these studies in terms of methodology, pre- and intraoperative diagnostic criteria and follow-up. They also found insufficient data on the effect of removal of mesh or staples to make a recommendation on this. Medical management of persistent postherniorrhaphy pain is limited to a few case reports.

Summary of present evidence and its limitations

Now that it is becoming clear that chronic postsurgical pain is more prevalent and troublesome than was once thought, it becomes incumbent on those involved in surgical care to make efforts to understand, prevent and treat the phenomenon. Patient factors, surgical factors, and anesthesia/analgesia factors all appear to influence the development and degree of postsurgical pain.

With regard to surgical technique, current evidence suggests that technique can alter the likelihood of developing persistent pain following inguinal hernia repair and axillary dissection. For thoracotomy, the data are less clear, but early evidence suggests that less traumatic surgery and closures that minimize damage to intercostal nerves may reduce pain intensity and prevalence. There is no evidence to suggest that surgical technique makes a difference to postamputation pain. It is interesting that how the major nerves are handled has not been formally addressed. Ligatures are frequently used around major nerves to control bleeding, and this has a striking similarity to at least one of the animal models of neuropathic pain [63].

Anesthetic and analgesic interventions have not been shown to alter persistent pain following inguinal hernia surgery, but the number and quality of studies are poor. There are good data that paravertebral blockade can alter the prevalence of persistent pain following breast surgery. Likewise, the data are moderately good regarding the use of intraoperative and postoperative epidural analgesia for posterolateral thoracotomy. There is still uncertainty about the role of anesthetic and analgesic interventions for reducing postamputation pain.

The addition of adjuvant analgesics holds promise to decrease the prevalence of persistent pain following breast surgery (gabapentin, methylprednisolone, parecoxib), but the majority of the studies were for only 3–6 months. Evidence is not sufficient to make a strong recommendation for use of these agents, but trials should now be focused on high-risk populations, including amputees and patients with severe immediate postsurgical pain. Longer term follow-up is also needed.

Author's recommendations

Current evidence suggests that surgical technique has an important role in minimizing persistent pain after surgery, but that specific modifications, such as use of minimally invasive and muscle- or nerve-sparing techniques and lightweight mesh (for hernia repairs), are needed, not simply careful technique. Conduction blockade (paravertebral and epidural) is helpful for reducing persistent pain in the case of breast surgery and thoracotomy. Postoperative adjuvant analgesia should be considered for patients in high-risk surgical groups.

References

1. Macrae WA, Davies HTO. Chronic postsurgical pain. In: Crombie IK, Croft PR, Linton SJ, LeResche L, von Korff M (eds) *Epidemiology of Pain*. IASP Press, Seattle, 1999: 125–142.
2. Perkins FM, Kehlet H. Chronic pain as an outcome of surgery. *Anesthesiology* 2000; **93**: 1123–1133.
3. Kehlet H, Jensen TS, Woolf CJ. Persistent postsurgical pain: risk factors and prevention. *Lancet* 2006; **367**: 1618–1625.
4. Jung BF, Ahrendt GM, Oaklander AL, Dworkin RH. Neuropathic pain following breast cancer surgery: proposed classification and research update. *Pain* 2003; **104**: 1–13.
5. Merskey H, Bogduk N. *Classification of Chronic Pain. Descriptions of Chronic Pain Syndromes and Definitions of Pain Terms*, 2nd edn. IASP Press, Seattle, WA, 1994.
6. Jacobson L, Mariano AJ. General considerations of chronic pain. In: Loeser JD, Butler SH, Chapman CR, Turk DC (eds) *Bonica's Management of Pain*, 3rd edn. Lippincott Williams and Wilkins, Baltimore, MD, 2001: 241–254.
7. Callesen T, Bech K, Kehlet H. Chronic pain after inguinal hernia repair – a prospective study after 500 operations. *Br J Surg* 1999; **86**: 1528–1531.
8. Landreneau RJ, Mack MJ, Hazelrigg SR, Naunheim K, Dowling RD, Ritter P, *et al.* Prevalence of chronic pain after pulmonary resection by thoracotomy or video-assisted thoracic surgery. *J Thorac Cardiovasc Surg* 1994; **107**: 1079–1085.
9. Tasmuth T, Kataja M, Blomqvist C, von Smitten K, Kalso E. Treatment-related factors predisposing to chronic pain in patients with breast cancer – a multivariate approach. *Acta Oncol* 1997; **36**: 625–630.
10. Jensen TS, Krebs B, Nielsen J, Rasmussen P. Immediate and long-term phantom limb pain in amputees: incidence, clinical characteristics and relationship to pre-amputation limb pain. *Pain* 1985; **21**: 267–278.
11. Benedetti F, Amanzio M, Casadio C, Filosso PL, Molinatti M, Oliaro A, *et al.* Postoperative pain and superficial abdominal reflexes after posterolateral thoracotomy. *Ann Thorac Surg* 1997; **64**: 207–210.
12. Benedetti F, Vighetti S, Ricco C, Amanzio M, Bergamasco L, Casadio C, *et al.* Neurophysiologic assessment of nerve impairment in posterolateral and muscle-sparing thoracotomy. *J Thorac Cardiovasc Surg* 1998; **115**: 841–847.
13. Bratschi HU, Haller U. Significance of the intercostobrachial nerve in axillary lymph node excision. *Geburtshilfe und Frauenheilkunde* 1990; **50**: 689–693.
14. Mitchell SW. *Injuries of Nerves*. J. B. Lippincott, Philadelphia, 1872.
15. Macrae WA. Chronic pain after surgery. *Br J Anaesth* 2001; **87**: 88–98.
16. Rogers ML, Henderson L, Mahajan RP, Duffy JP. Preliminary findings in the neurophysiological assessment of intercostal nerve injury during thoracotomy. *Eur J Cardiothorac Surg* 2002; **21**: 298–301.
17. O'Dwyer PJ, Kingsnorth AN, Molloy RG, Small PK, Lammers B, Horeyseck G. Randomized clinical trial assessing

impact of a lightweight or heavyweight mesh on chronic pain after inguinal hernia repair. *Br J Surg* 2005; **92**: 166–170.

18. Nikolajsen L, Ilkjaer S, Krøner K, Christensen JH, Jensen TS. The influence of preamputation pain on postamputation stump and phantom pain. *Pain* 1997; **72**: 393–405.

19. Smith J, Thompson JM. Phantom limb pain and chemotherapy in pediatric amputees. *Mayo Clin Proc* 1995; **70**: 357–364.

20. Werner MU, Duun P, Kehlet H. Prediction of postoperative pain by preoperative nociceptive responses to heat stimuli. *Anesthesiology* 2004; **100**: 115–119.

21. Pan PH, Coghill R, Houle TT, Seid MH, Lindel WM, Parker RL, et al. Multifactorial preoperative predictors of postcesarean section pain and analgesic requirements. *Anesthesiology* 2006; **104**: 417–425.

22. Katz J, Jackson M, Kavanagh BP, Sandler AN. Acute pain after thoracic surgery predicts long-term post- thoracotomy pain. *Clin J Pain* 1996; **12**: 50–55.

23. Ochroch EA, Gottschalk A, Augostides J, Carson KA, Kent L, Malayaman N, et al. Long-term pain and activity during recovery from major thoracotomy using thoracic epidural analgesia. *Anesthesiology* 2002; **97**: 1234–1244.

24. Aasvang E, Kehlet H. Chronic postoperative pain: the case of inguinal herniorrhaphy. *Br J Anaesth* 2005; **95**: 69–76.

25. Poobalan AS, Bruce J, Cairns W, Smith S, King PM, Krukowski ZH, et al. A review of chronic pain after inguinal herniorrhaphy. *Clin J Pain* 2003; **19**: 48–54.

26. Jørgensen LS, Christiansen PM, Raundahl U, Østgaard SE. Long-lasting functional abdominal pain and duodenal ulcer are associated with stress, vulnerability and symptoms of psychological stress. *Dan Med Bull* 1996; **43**: 359–363.

27. Hanley MA, Jensen MP, Ehde DM, Hoffman AJ, Patterson DR, Robinson LR. Psychosocial predictors of long-term adjustment to lower-limb amputation and phantom limb pain. *Disabil Rehabil* 2004; **26**: 882–893.

28. Sherman R, Sherman C. Prevalence and characteristics of chronic phantom limb pain among American veterans. *Am J Phys Med Rehabil* 1983; **62**: 227–238.

29. Krane EJ, Heller LB. The prevalence of phantom limb sensation and pain in pediatric amputees. *J Pain Symptom Manage* 1995; **10**: 21–29.

30. Bach S, Noreng MF, Tjellden NU. Phantom limb pain in amputees during the first 12 months following limb amputation, after preoperative lumbar epidural blockade. *Pain* 1988; **33**: 297–301.

31. Jahangiri M, Bradley JWP, Jayatunga AP, Dark CH. Prevention of phantom pain after major lower limb amputation by epidural infusion of diamorphine, clonidine and bupivacaine. *Ann Roy Coll Surg Engl* 1994; **76**: 324–326.

32. Nikolajsen L, Ilkjaer S, Christensen JH, Krøner K, Jensen TS. Randomised trial of epidural bupivacaine and morphine in prevention of stump and phantom pain in lower-limb amputation. *Lancet* 1997; **350**: 1353–1357.

33. Fisher A, Meller Y. Continuous postoperative regional analgesia by nerve sheath block for amputation surgery – a pilot study. *Anesth Analges* 1991; **72**: 300–303.

34. Pinzur MS, Gupta P, Pluth T, Vrbos L. Continuous postoperative infusion of a regional anesthetic after an amputation of the lower extremity. *J Bone Joint Surg* 1996; **78-A**: 1501–1505.

35. Kairaluoma PM, Bachman MS, Rosenberg PH, Pere PJ. Preincisional paravertebral block reduces the prevalence of chronic pain after breast surgery. *Anesth Analges* 2006; **103**: 703–708.

36. Veronesi U, Paganelli G, Viale G, Luini A, Zurrida S, Galimberti V, et al. A randomized comparison of sentinel-node biopsy with routine axillary dissection in breast cancer. *N Engl J Med* 2003; **349**: 546–553.

37. Husen M, Paaschburg B, Flyger HL. Two-step axillary operation increases risks of arm morbidity in breast cancer patients. *Breast* 2006; **15**: 620–628.

38. Schulze T, Mucke J, Markwardt J, Schlag PM, Bembenek A. Long-term morbidity of patients with early breast cancer after sentinel lymph node biopsy compared to axillary lymph node dissection. *J Surg Oncol* 2006; **93**: 109–119.

39. Kairaluoma PM, Bachman MS, Korpinen AK, Rosenberg PH, Pere PJ. Single-injection paravertebral block before general anesthesia enhances analgesia after breast cancer surgery with and without associated lymph node biopsy. *Anesth Analges* 2004; **99**: 1837–1843.

40. Iohom G, Abdalla H, O'Brien J, Szarvas S, Buckley E, Butler M, et al. The associations between severity of early postoperative pain, chronic postsurgical pain and plasma concentration of stable nitric oxide products after breast surgery. *Anesth Analges* 2006; **103**: 995–1000.

41. Romundstad L, Breivik H, Roald H, Romundstad PR, Stubhaug A. Chronic pain and sensory changes after augmentation mammoplasty: long term effects of preincisional administration of methylprednisolone. *Pain* 2006; **124**: 92–99.

42. Fassoulaki A, Patris K, Sarantopoulos C, Hogan Q. The analgesic effect of gabapentin and mexiletine after breast surgery. *Anesth Analges* 2002; **95**: 985–991.

43. Fassoulaki A, Triga A, Melemeni A, Sarantopoulos C. Multimodal analgesia with gabapentin and local anesthetics prevents acute and chronic pain after breast surgery for cancer. *Anesth Analges* 2005; **101**: 1427–1432.

44. Gottschalk A, Cohen SP, Yang S, Ochroch EA. Preventing and treating pain after thoracic surgery. *Anesthesiology* 2006; **104**: 594–600.

45. Obata H, Saito S, Fujita N, Fuse Y, Ishizaki K, Goto F. Epidural block with mepivacaine before surgery reduces long-term post-thoracotomy pain. *Can J Anaesth* 1999; **46**: 1127–1132.

46. Senturk M, Ozcan PE, Talu GK, Kiyan E, Camci E, Ozyalin S, et al. The effects of three different analgesia techniques on long-term postthoracotomy pain. *Anesth Analges* 2002; **94**: 11–15.

47. Richardson J, Sabanathan S, Jones J, Shah RD, Cheema S, Mearns AJ. A prospective, randomized comparison of preoperative and continuous epidural or paravertebral bupivacaine on post-thoracotomy pain, pulmonary function and stress response. *Br J Anaesth* 1999; **83**: 387–392.

48. Davies RG, Myles PS, Graham JM. A comparison of the analgesic efficacy and side-effects of paravertebral vs epidural

blockade for thoracotomy – a systematic review and meta-analysis of randomized trials. *Br J Anaesth* 2006; **96**: 418–426.

49. Cerfolio RJ, Bryant AS, Bass CS, Bartolucci AA. A prospective, double-blind, randomized trial evaluating the use of preemptive analgesia of the skin before thoracotomy. *Ann Thorac Surg* 2003; **76**: 1055–1058.

50. Ochroch EA, Gottschalk A, Augoustides JG, Aukburg SJ, Kaiser LR, Shrager JB. Pain and physical function are similar following axillary, muscle-sparing vs posterolateral thoracotomy. *Chest* 2005; **128**: 2664–2670.

51. Cerfolio RJ, Bryant AS, Patel B, Bartolucci AA. Intercostal muscle flap reduces the pain of thoracotomy: a prospective randomized trial. *J Thorac Cardiovasc Surg* 2005; **130**: 987–993.

52. Cerfolio RJ, Price TN, Bryant AS, Bass CS, Bartolucci AA. Intracosal sutures decrease the pain of thoracotomy. *Ann Thorac Surg* 2003; **76**: 407–412.

53. Callesen T. Inguinal hernia repair: anesthesia, pain and convalescence. *Dan Med Bull* 2003; **50**: 203–218.

54. Bay-Nielsen M, Perkins FM, Kehlet H. Pain and functional impairment 1 year after inguinal herniorrhaphy: a nationwide questionnaire study. *Ann Surg* 2001; **233**: 1–7.

55. Wijsmuller AR, van Veen RN, Bosch JL, Lange JF, Kleinrensink GJ, Lange JF. Nerve management during open hernia review. *Br J Surg* 2007; **94**: 17–22.

56. Collaboration EH. Laparoscopic compared with open methods of groin hernia repair: systematic review of randomised controlled trials. *Br J Surg* 2000; **87**: 860–867.

57. Schmedt CG, Sauerland S, Bittner R. Comparison of endoscopic procedures vs Lichtenstein and other open mesh techniques for inguinal hernia repair: a meta-analysis of randomized trials. *Surg Endosc* 2005; **19**: 188–199.

58. McCormack K, Wake B, Perez J, Fraser C, Cook J, McIntosh E, *et al.* Laparoscopic surgery for inguinal hernia repair; systematic review of effectiveness and economic evaluation. *Health Technol Assess* 2005; **9**: 1–203.

59. Grant AM. Open mesh versus non-mesh repair of groin hernia: meta-analysis of randomised trials based on individual patient data. *Hernia* 2002; **6**: 130–136.

60. McCormack K, Scott NW, Go PMNYH, Grant AM, EU Hernia Trialists. Laparoscopic techniques versus open techniques for inguinal hernia repair. Cochrane Database of Systematic Reviews 2005 Aug 12; 4.

61. Bringman S, Wollert S, Osterberg J, Smedberg S, Granlund H, Heikkinen T-J. Three-year results of a randomized clinical trial of lightweight or standard polypropylene mesh in Lichtenstein repair of primary inguinal hernia. *Br J Surg* 2006; **93**: 1056–1059.

62. Aasvang E, Kehlet H. Surgical management of chronic pain after inguinal hernia repair. *Br J Surg* 2005; **92**: 795–801.

63. Bennett GJ, Xie Y-K. A peripheral mononeuropathy in rat that produces disorders of pain sensation like those seen in man. *Pain* 1988; **33**: 87–107.

64. Nikolajsen L, Brandsborg B, Jensen TS, Kehlet H. Chronic pain following total hip arthroplasty: a nationwide questionnaire study. *Acta Anaesthesiol Scand* 2006; **50**: 495–500.

65. Snellingen T, Evans JR, Ravilla T, Foster A. Surgical interventions for age-related cataract. Cochrane Database of Systematic Reviews 2006; 1: 1–28.

66. Nikolajsen L, Sorensen HC, Jensen TS, Kehlet H. Chronic pain following Caesaran section. *Acta Anaesthesiol Scand* 2004; **48**: 111–116.

67. Bisgaard T, Rosenberg J, Kehlet H. From acute to chronic pain after laparoscopic cholecystectomy: a prospective follow-up analysis. *Scand J Gastroenterol* 2005; **40**: 1358–1364.

68. Lavand'homme P, de Kock M, Waterloos H. Intraoperative epidural analgesia combined with ketamine provides effective preventive analgesia in patients undergoing major digestive surgery. *Anesthesiology* 2005; **103**: 813–820.

69. Polycarpou N, Ng YL, Canavan D, Moles DR, Gulabivala K. Prevalence of persistent pain after endodontic treatment and factors affecting its occurrence in cases with complete radiographic healing. *Int Endodont J* 2005; **38**: 169–178.

70. Brandsborg B, Nikolajsen L, Hansen CT, Kehlet H, Jensen TS. Risk factors for chronic pain after hysterectomy. *Anesthesiology* 2007; **106**: 1003–1012.

71. Atlas SJ, Keller RB, Wu YA, Deyo RA, Singer DE. Long-term outcomes of surgical and nonsurgical management of sciatica seconday to a lumbar disc herniation: 10 year results from the Maine lumbar spine study. *Spine* 2005; **30**: 927–935.

72. Meyhoff CS, Thomsen CH, Rasmussen LS, Nielsen PR. High incidence of chronic pain following surgery for pelvic fracture. *Clin J Pain* 2006; **22**: 167–172.

73. Gottschalk A, Smith DS, Jobes DR, Kennedy SK, Lally SE, Noble VE, *et al.* Preemptive epidural analgesia and recovery from radical prostatectomy. *JAMA* 1998; **279**: 1076–1082.

74. Bruce J, Drury N, Poobalan AS, Jeffrey RR, Smith WC, Chambers WA. The prevalence of chronic chest and leg pain following cardiac surgery: a historical cohort study. *Pain* 2003; **104**: 265–273.

75. Jensen MK, Andersen C. Can chronic poststernotomy pain after cardiac valve replacement be reduced using thoracic epidural analgesia? *Acta Anaesthesiol Scand* 2004; **48**: 871–874.

76. Awsare NS, Krishnan J, Boustead GB, Hanbury DC, McNicholas TA. Complications of vasectomy. *Ann Roy Coll Surg Engl* 2005; **87**: 406–410.

77. Grant AM. Open mesh versus non-mesh repair of groin hernia: meta-analysis of randomised trials based on individual patient data. *Hernia* 2002; **6**: 130–136.

CHAPTER 17

Painful diabetic neuropathy

Christina Daousi[1] and Turo J. Nurmikko[2]

[1]University Hospital Aintree, Clinical Sciences Center, Liverpool, UK
[2]Division of Neurological Science, School of Clinical Sciences, University of Liverpool, Clinical Sciences Center, Liverpool, UK

Introduction

Worldwide, 120 million people are estimated to have diabetes and this figure is predicted to rise to 221 million by the year 2010. The total number of people with diabetes is projected to rise to 366 million by 2030, as a result of population growth, urbanization, aging, increasing prevalence of obesity and adoption of sedentary lifestyles. These figures highlight the growing public health burden of diabetes across the world, which will inevitably lead to increased morbidity and mortality as a consequence of the rise in the complications associated with diabetes.

Diabetic neuropathy is one of the most common complications of diabetes and potentially one of the most debilitating. The total annual cost of diabetic neuropathy and its complications in the USA was estimated in 2003 to be around 12 billion US dollars, and up to a third of the direct medical costs of diabetes were attributed to diabetic peripheral neuropathy [1].

The enormous human and economic costs associated with this complication of diabetes make the study of the size of the problem, its underlying pathophysiologic mechanisms and the application of evidence-based therapeutic approaches of paramount importance and a healthcare priority.

Diabetic neuropathy is not a single entity but a heterogeneous group of disorders that encompasses a wide range of abnormalities. One common classification scheme is based on the anatomic distribution and it includes two main types: diffuse neuropathy and focal neuropathies. The most common diffuse neuropathy in patients with diabetes is chronic distal symmetric sensorimotor polyneuropathy, affecting predominantly the feet and lower legs, but progressively becoming more proximal with time and duration of diabetes, evolving in a symmetric pattern from the most distal extremities to more proximal areas, in a "glove and stocking" distribution. This type of neuropathy can predispose to the development of neuropathic foot ulceration, can cause neuropathic pain or can be associated with both.

Sensorimotor neuropathy affects large and small afferent nerve fibers to varying degrees, resulting in mixed symptoms and sensory loss. Its onset is usually insidious and can sometimes be one of the presenting features in patients with type 2 diabetes mellitus. It may be asymptomatic and discovered incidentally on routine clinical examination or it may manifest with a variety of sensory symptoms mainly in the lower limbs and, in more severe cases, in the fingers and hands.

The character of pain in diabetic neuropathy can be highly diverse with patients tending to have a variety of symptoms (Table 17.1), which can also vary in nature over time. Pain is often worse at night or may be exacerbated when tired or stressed. Many patients with neuropathic pain exhibit persistent or paroxysmal pain that is independent of a stimulus, and can be shooting, lancinating or burning. On the other hand, patients may experience stimulus-evoked pain which has two key features: hyperlagesia (increased pain response to a suprathreshold noxious stimulus, far beyond that of a normal response) and allodynia (pain elicited by a non-noxious stimulus).

Evidence-Based Chronic Pain Management. Edited by C. Stannard, E. Kalso and J. Ballantyne. © 2010 Blackwell Publishing.

Table 17.1 Symptoms commonly reported by patients with painful diabetic neuropathy

Burning
Shooting, lancinating
Pins and needles, tingling
Hot or cold sensations in the feet
Aching, cramping
Itching, numbness
"Walking on marbles"
Irritation of feet by bedclothes

Epidemiology and natural history of chronic painful diabetic neuropathy

Estimates of the prevalence of chronic painful diabetic neuropathy (CPDN) vary substantially. In a hospital diabetic clinic population, 8% of patients had typical lower limb neuropathic symptoms, over twice that of a control group [2]. One study found that 11% of insulin-treated patients aged 15–59 years had painful symptoms [3] while another reported that 20% of patients with type 2 diabetes had neuropathic pain after 10 years of diabetes [4], although details of pain duration and severity were not given.

In a community-based study of patients with type 1 and 2 diabetes attending primary or secondary care clinics [5], using a structured questionnaire and examination, 350 people with diabetes were assessed and compared with 344 age- and sex-matched controls from the same locality. This is the largest study to date in which well-defined criteria of painful diabetic neuropathy and validated measures of pain severity and quality have been used, giving a better representation of the extent of the problem in the population with diabetes in the community. The estimated prevalence of chronic (>1 year's duration) painful diabetic neuropathy was 16.2% compared with 4.9% in the control sample. Pain was present across all age ranges and was equally common in those attending either hospital or community clinics. It was also revealed that CPDN was severe, frequently under-reported and undertreated in people with diabetes [5].

There is limited information regarding the natural history of painful neuropathy. Some longitudinal studies have shown a general tendency for painful neuropathic symptoms to improve [6–10] but others have found no change [11–13]. These conflicting results can be explained by the inclusion of patients with short duration of pain and with varying neuropathic syndromes which are known to have different prognoses [14]. Only three previous studies have concentrated on patients with neuropathic pain for over 6 months [9–11].

Pathogenesis of neuropathic pain in chronic pain diabetic neuropathy

Data from basic research indicate that multiple pathophysiologic mechanisms may underlie neuropathic pain and that different mechanisms may co-exist in a single patient and perhaps change over time [15]. There is considerable agreement that both peripheral and central processes contribute to the chronic neuropathic pain in CPDN, and that these different mechanisms may explain the qualitatively different symptoms and signs that patients experience [16].

There is now mounting evidence that not only the damaged neurones but also the altered properties of the nondamaged sensory neurones projecting into damaged neurons play a crucial role in the generation of neuropathic pain. However, the precise nature of the mechanisms underlying these changes remains to be fully elucidated [17].

At the molecular level, some of the important changes that occur and may contribute to the generation and maintenance of chronic neuropathic pain can be summarized as follows [18]:
- abnormal expression of sodium channels in the periphery
- increased activity at glutamate receptor sites
- reduction of GABA inhibition
- alteration of calcium influx into cells [19].

Therapies for painful diabetic neuropathy

Drug treatments currently used in the management of painful diabetic neuropathy are not neuroprotective and neither do they restore nerve damage but are aimed simply at relieving the patients' symptoms and improving their functioning and quality of life. There is no single therapy that will benefit all patients with painful neuropathy, and there are few data comparing drug classes or examining combinations of drugs and most trials are of short duration.

Glycemic control

An abundance of evidence supports the importance of tight glycemic control in the prevention of diabetic complications, including diabetic neuropathy [20, 21]. It is possible that maintenance of stable blood glucose control is also important [22] so optimal glycemic control should always be the goal when managing the patient with CPDN.

Antidepressants

Tricyclic antidepressants (TCAs)

Tricyclic antidepressants remain the best studied class of drugs used in the management of neuropathic pain in general and for the management of painful diabetic neuropathy in particular [23, 24]. A number of randomized, double-blinded, placebo-controlled trials have demonstrated their efficacy and relatively good safety profile. Their main mode of action appears to involve inhibition of norepinephrine and serotonin reuptake at the neuronal synapse, therefore inhibiting transmission of pain.

Of the tricyclic agents, amitriptyline and imipramine remain the mainstay of treatment in CPDN. The main side effects of TCAs are mainly anticholinergic and include dry mouth, blurred vision, sedation, constipation, urinary hesitancy, postural dizziness, and prolongation of electrocardiographic QT interval. Their use requires caution in patients with glaucoma, elderly male patients with possible underlying prostate hypertrophy and patients with underlying cardiac disease and cardiac arrhythmias.

In a randomized, double-blind cross-over study, 29 patients with painful diabetic neuropathy received 6 weeks of amitriptyline and 6 weeks of an "active" placebo [25]. Amitriptyline was superior to placebo in relieving pain from week 3 through to week 6. Patients who were able to tolerate higher amitriptyline doses reported greater relief, through the maximum dose of 150 mg at night. The analgesic effect of amitriptyline was independent of its antidepressant effects [25].

Twelve patients with severe, painful diabetic neuropathy were treated with imipramine and placebo in a fixed-dose, double-blind, cross-over study of 5 plus 5 weeks [26]. Seven patients experienced notable improvement while receiving imipramine and none while receiving placebo. The rating of specific symptoms at the end of each treatment period showed a beneficial effect of imipramine on pain, paresthesia, dysesthesia, numbness and nocturnal exacerbation [26].

Desipramine, a selective noradrenaline reuptake inhibitor and a metabolite of imipramine, has been shown to be effective as an alternative therapy [27–29], having fewer anticholinergic side effects with fewer sedative effects than amitriptyline or imipramine but is now no longer available in the UK.

Two randomized, double-blind, cross-over studies in patients with painful diabetic neuropathy were carried out comparing amitriptyline with the relatively selective norepinephrine reuptake inhibitor desipramine in 38 patients, and comparing the selective blocker of serotonin reuptake fluoxetine with placebo in 46 patients [29]. Fifty-seven patients were randomly assigned to a study as well as to the order of treatment, permitting comparison among all three drugs and placebo as the first treatment. Both amitriptyline and desipramine were superior to placebo. Fluoxetine was effective only in depressed patients, unlike amitriptyline and desipramine that were effective in both depressed and nondepressed patients [29].

A double-blind, cross-over controlled clinical trial on the efficacy of a nortriptyline-fluphenazine combination was carried out in patients with painful diabetic polyneuropathy [30]. Significant relief of both pain and paresthesia was obtained with this combination. The differences were statistically significant. Side effects were frequent but not usually severe enough to lead to cessation of these medications [30].

In another systematic review of antidepressant usage in painful diabetic neuropathy, number needed to treat (NNT) to achieve at least 50% pain relief for TCAs was reported as 3.5 [23] and 2.6 by another group, although this did include one nondiabetic neuropathic trial [31].

In order to evaluate which antidepressant is more effective and what role the newer antidepressants can play in treating neuropathic pain, a Cochrane Collaborative systematic review was carried out of randomized trials of antidepressants in neuropathic pain [32]. Fifty trials of 19 antidepressants were considered eligible (2515 patients) for inclusion, including five trials for diabetic neuropathy. The NNT for effectiveness of antidepressants in CPDN was 1.3 (95% confidence interval (CI) 1.2−1.5), relative risk (RR) 12.4 (95% CI 5.2−29.2). The best evidence available was for amitriptyline. There were only limited data for the effectiveness of SSRI, therefore it was not possible to identify the most effective antidepressant; this question will probably be answered only after more studies of SSRIs in CPDN are conducted [32].

Selective serotonin reuptake inhibitors (SSRIs)
Overall, there is limited evidence for the efficacy of these drugs in clinical trials [23]. The effect of the SSRI paroxetine at a fixed dose of 40 mg daily on diabetic neuropathy symptoms was examined in comparison to imipramine and placebo in one randomized, double-blind, cross-over study [33]. Paroxetine significantly reduced the symptoms of neuropathy but was somewhat less effective than imipramine. No patients on paroxetine dropped out due to side effects and no withdrawal symptoms were reported, unlike the imipramine-treated group in which five patients discontinued the study because of intolerable side effects and 4/19 patients completing the study reported withdrawal symptoms after discontinuing imipramine [33].

The effect of the SSRI citalopram at a fixed dose of 40 mg daily on diabetic neuropathy symptoms was examined in a double-blind, placebo-controlled, cross-over study for two 3-week periods [34]. Citalopram significantly relieved the symptoms of neuropathy in comparison with placebo. Two of 17 patients in the study, both receiving citalopram, had to drop out because of side effects. Side effect ratings were significantly higher during administration of citalopram than placebo, but citalopram was generally well tolerated.

Another SSRI, fluoxetine, has not been shown to be superior to placebo in one study [29].

Serotonin-norepinephrine reuptake inhibitors (SNRIs)
Venlafaxine extended release
Venlafaxine extended release (ER) is a SNRI which has recently been investigated in CPDN. One multicenter, double-blind, randomized, placebo-controlled study included 244 patients with painful diabetic neuropathy and examined the efficacy and safety of 6 weeks of venlafaxine ER (75 mg and 150–225 mg)

treatment [35]. Baseline pain intensity was 68.7 mm (moderately severe). At week 6, the percentage reduction from baseline in VAS pain intensity was 27% (placebo), 32% (75 mg), and 50% (150−225 mg; P < 0.001 versus placebo). Mean VAS pain relief scores in the 150−225 mg group were significantly greater than placebo at week 6 (44 versus 60 mm; P < 0.001). The NNT for 50% pain intensity reduction with venlafaxine ER 150−225 mg was 4.5 at week 6. Nausea and somnolence were the most commonly reported adverse events. Seven patients on venlafaxine had clinically important ECG changes during treatment. The NNT value for higher dose venlafaxine ER was comparable to those of tricyclic antidepressants and the anticonvulsant gabapentin [35].

In another randomized, double-blind, placebo-controlled, three-way cross-over study, the efficacy of venlafaxine over placebo was examined and compared to imipramine [36]. Forty patients were assigned to one of the treatment sequences each of 4 weeks duration, and 29 completed all three studies, 15 of whom had CPDN. The daily doses were venlafaxine 225 mg and imipramine 150 mg. The sum of the individual pain scores during treatment week 4 was lower on venlafaxine (80% of baseline score; P = 0.006) and imipramine (77%; P = 0.001) than on placebo (100%) and did not show any statistical difference between venlafaxine and imipramine (P = 0.44). NNT to obtain one patient with moderate or better pain relief were 5.2 for venlafaxine and 2.7 for imipramine [36].

Although venlafaxine appears to be effective in the relief of symptoms associated with CPDN and has a relatively safe side effect profile, its use can only be supported in cases where other first-line treatments have failed to produce clinically significant improvements at maximally tolerated doses, at least until further studies with larger numbers of patients with CPDN are conducted. One of its main benefits is certainly the once-daily dosing schedule of its ER preparation.

Duloxetine
Duloxetine is a balanced and potent dual SNRI; it lacks other significant receptor or channel activities and neuroprotective properties [37]. Serotonin and norepinephrine are thought to inhibit pain by interfering with descending pain inhibition pathways of the brainstem and spinal cord [37].

In a 12-week, multicenter, double-blind study, 457 patients experiencing pain due to diabetic polyneuropathy were randomly assigned to treatment with duloxetine 20, 60, 120 mg daily or placebo [38]. Duloxetine 60 and 120 mg daily demonstrated statistically significant greater improvement compared with placebo on the 24-h average pain score, beginning 1 week after randomization and continuing through the 12-week trial. Duloxetine treatment was considered to be safe and well tolerated with less than 20% discontinuation due to adverse events [38].

In another multicenter, parallel, double-blind, randomized, placebo-controlled trial, 348 patients with pain due to diabetic peripheral neuropathy without co-morbid depression were randomly assigned to receive duloxetine 60 mg once daily, duloxetine 60 mg twice daily or placebo, for 12 weeks [39]. Compared with placebo-treated patients, both duloxetine-treated groups improved significantly more (P < 0.001) on the 24-h average pain score. Duloxetine demonstrated superiority to placebo in all secondary analyses of the primary efficacy measure and in most secondary measures for pain. Discontinuations due to adverse events were more frequent in the duloxetine 60 mg bd (12.1%) than the placebo-treated (2.6%) group. Duloxetine showed no adverse effects on diabetic control, and both doses were safely administered and well tolerated [39].

Similar findings were reported in an independent confirmatory study conducted to assess the efficacy and safety of duloxetine in CPDN [40]. Duloxetine 60 mg od and 60 mg bd demonstrated improvement in the management of CPDN and showed rapid onset of action, with separation from placebo beginning at week 1 on the 24-h average pain severity score. For all secondary measures for pain (except allodynia), mean changes showed an advantage of duloxetine over placebo, with no significant difference between 60 mg od and 60 mg bd. Clinical Global Impression of Severity and Patient's Global Impression of Improvement evaluation demonstrated greater improvement in duloxetine- than placebo-treated patients. Duloxetine showed no notable interference with diabetic control, and both doses were safely administered [40].

Comparison of antidepressants and antiepileptic drugs

In a systematic review of randomized controlled trials to evaluate the effectiveness and safety of antidepressants,

21 placebo-controlled treatments in 17 randomized controlled trials were included, involving 10 antidepressants used for a variety of neuropathic pain syndromes including CPDN [41]. The main outcomes were global judgments, pain relief or reduction in pain intensity of more than 50% from baseline, and information about minor and major adverse effects. In six of 13 diabetic neuropathy studies the odds ratios showed significant benefit compared with placebo. The combined odds ratio was 3.6 (95% CI 2.5–5.2), with a NNT for benefit of 3 (2.4–4). There were fewer than 200 patients in total with CPDN included in these studies, and no single study had enrolled more than 50 patients. Across all pain syndromes included in the review, comparisons of TCAs did not show any significant difference between them; they were significantly more effective than benzodiazepines in the three comparisons available. Paroxetine and mianserin were less effective than imipramine. Overall, antidepressants were effective in relieving neuropathic pain compared with placebo.

In a systematic review to determine the relative efficacy and adverse effects of antidepressants and anticonvulsants in the treatment of diabetic neuroapathy and postherpetic neuralgia, 16 reports on painful diabetic neuropathy compared antidepressants with placebo (491 patient episodes) and three compared anticonvulsants with placebo (321) [23]. The NNT for at least 50% pain relief with antidepressants was 3.4 (95% CI 2.6–4.7) and with antiepileptic drugs 2.7 (2.2–3.8). Antidepressants and antiepileptic drugs had the same efficacy and incidence of minor adverse effects in these two neuropathic pain conditions. There was no evidence that SSRIs were better than older antidepressants, and no evidence that gabapentin was better than older antiepileptic drugs. In these trials patients were more likely to stop taking antidepressants than antiepileptic drugs because of adverse effects [23].

Antiepileptic drugs

Gabapentin

Gabapentin, a second-generation antiepileptic agent licensed for use in the management of partial seizures, has found over the last decade application in the management of neuropathic pain, including chronic pain associated with CPDN. Gabapentin is one of the few drugs licensed in the UK with an indication specifically for treatment of neuropathic pain.

Gabapentin is structurally related to γ-aminobutyric acid (GABA) but does not appear to bind to its receptors. Its proposed mechanism of action involves binding to the α2δ-1 subunit of voltage-gated calcium channels and modulation of the release of excitatory neurotransmitters.

In an 8-week, randomized, double-blind, placebo-controlled trial, involving 165 patients with CPDN, gabapentin-treated patients had significantly lower mean daily pain scores compared with placebo [42]. Improvement was also shown in a number of secondary measures such as sleep interference scores, the Short-Form McGill Pain Questionnaire scores, Patient Global Impression of Change and Clinical Global Impression of Change, the Short-Form 36 Quality of Life Questionnaire scores, and the Profile of Mood States. These results were achieved by titrating gabapentin from 900 to 3600 mg daily or to the maximum tolerated dosage. The main side effects experienced by patients included dizziness, somnolence and confusion. The NNT for 50% pain relief in this study was 3.7 [31]. Another small-scale RCT study with gabapentin titrated only to a maximum dose of 900 mg daily failed to demonstrate superiority over placebo [43].

In a randomized, double-blinded, double-dummy, cross-over study comparing the efficacy of gabapentin (900–1800 mg daily) with amitriptyline (25–75 mg daily), no advantage of gabapentin over amitriptyline was shown [44]. The total number of patients experiencing any adverse event was similar in both groups, but the frequency with which weight gain was encountered as a side effect was higher in the amitriptyline group.

In another small 12-week, open-label, prospective, randomized trial comparing the efficacy and tolerability of gabapentin and amitriptyline monotherapy in CPDN, 25 patients were randomized to receive either gabapentin, titrated from 1200 mg/day to a maximum of 2400 mg/day, or amitriptyline, titrated from 30 mg/day to a maximum of 90 mg/day [45]. Both drugs were titrated over a 4-week period and maintained at the maximum tolerated dose for 8 weeks. Gabapentin produced greater improvements than amitriptyline in pain and paresthesia [45]. Additionally, gabapentin was better tolerated than amitriptyline. Adverse events were more frequent in the amitriptyline group than in the gabapentin group. Side effects were the main limiting factor preventing dose escalation [45].

A systematic review of the literature involving both controlled and uncontrolled studies of gabapentin used in a variety of neuropathic pain conditions, including CPDN, has suggested that effectiveness may be reduced if one limits administration of the drug to very low doses (<1800 mg daily), whereas rapid dose escalation may be associated with increased central nervous system side effects such as dizziness, somnolence, headache and confusion [46].

In a more recent and similar review of the evidence supporting the use of gabapentin in the treatment of adults with varying neuropathic pain syndromes including CPDN, titration to 1800 mg daily was recommended for greater efficacy and doses up to 3600 mg daily were found to be needed in many patients [47]. Therefore, although the maximum licensed dose (for pain) in the UK is 1800 mg per day, it may be necessary to use a higher dosage (providing it is tolerated) to improve efficacy.

Pregabalin

Pregabalin is another second-generation antiepileptic drug that has recently been licensed in the UK for the treatment of neuropathic pain conditions, including CPDN. Pregabalin, like gabapentin, is an analog of the neurotransmitter GABA but it does not appear to exert its action through binding of the GABA receptors. Its proposed mechanism of action involves binding with high affinity to the α2δ subunit of voltage-gated calcium channels, thereby reducing the release of excitatory neurotransmitters.

A number of studies have explored the efficacy of pregabalin in CPDN. One hundred and forty-six (146) patients were randomized to receive placebo (n = 70) or pregabalin at a fixed dose of 300 mg/day (n = 76) for 8 weeks [48]. Pain relief and improved sleep began during week 1 and remained significant throughout the study (P < 0.01). A total of 40% of the pregabalin-treated patients reported at least 50% reduction in pain scores compared with only 14.5% in the placebo group. Pregabalin was well tolerated despite a greater incidence of dizziness and somnolence than placebo. Most adverse events were mild to moderate and did not result in withdrawal [48].

In another study, 338 patients with a 1–5-year history of CPDN and average weekly pain scores ≤4 on an 11-point numeric pain-rating scale were enrolled in a 5-week, double-blind, multicenter, placebo-controlled study [49]. Patients were randomized to receive one of three doses of pregabalin or placebo three times daily. Patients in the 300 mg and 600 mg/day pregabalin groups showed improvements in endpoint mean pain score (primary efficacy measure) versus placebo (P = 0.0001), but no effect at 75 mg daily. Improvements were also seen in weekly pain scores, Sleep Interference Score, Patient Global Impression of Change, Clinical Global Impression of Change, SF McGill Pain Questionnaire, and multiple domains of the SF-36 Health Survey. Improvements in pain and sleep were seen as early as week 1 and were sustained throughout the 5 weeks [49].

Another relatively short-duration (6 weeks), randomized, double-blind, multicenter study enrolled 246 men and women with painful diabetic neuropathy who received pregabalin (150 or 600 mg/day) or placebo [50]. Pregabalin 600 mg/day significantly decreased mean pain score to 4.3 (versus 5.6 for placebo, P = 0.0002) and increased the proportion of patients who had a greater than 50% decrease in pain from baseline (39% versus 15% for placebo, P = 0.002). Pregabalin also significantly reduced sleep interference, past week and present pain intensity, sensory and affective pain scores. More patients receiving pregabalin 600 mg/day than placebo showed improvement, as rated on the Clinical and Patient Global Impression of Change scales. Pregabalin 150 mg/day was essentially no different from placebo. Dizziness was the most commonly reported side effect [50].

Another 12-week randomized, double-blind, multicenter, placebo-controlled, parallel-group study evaluated the efficacy and safety of pregabalin in patients with chronic postherpetic neuralgia or CPDN [51]. Patients were randomized to placebo (n = 65) or to one of two pregabalin regimes: a flexible schedule of 150, 300, 450, and 600 mg/day with weekly dose escalation based on patients' individual responses and tolerability (n = 141) or a fixed schedule of 300 mg/day for 1 week followed by 600 mg/day for 11 weeks (n = 132). Both regimes significantly reduced mean pain scores versus placebo (P = 0.002, P < 0.001) and were superior to placebo in improving pain-related sleep interference (P < 0.001). The most commonly reported adverse events for pregabalin-treated patients were dizziness, peripheral edema, weight gain and somnolence, and appeared to be dose dependent [51].

From the above studies, it has become apparent that pregabalin is effective for the treatment of neuropathic pain associated with diabetic neuropathy but not at all doses. Pregabalin administered at a dosage of 75 mg or 150 mg daily does not produce significant clinical improvement in patients with CPDN compared with placebo. Higher doses (300–600 mg/day) can show clinical efficacy even within 1 week of initiation of treatment. The dosing schedule used in three of the trials described above was three times daily and only in one of the major trials was a twice-daily regime chosen [51]. Moreover, pregabalin similarly to gabapentin, has demonstrated efficacy in improvement of a number of secondary endpoints such as sleep interference SF-McGill pain scores and SF-36 Health Survey scores. In view of the relatively short duration of the trials conducted so far, there are no long-term data that show durability of the effects of pregabalin over a longer period of time.

Like gabapentin, pregabalin is also renally excreted and dose reduction is required in patients with renal impairment. Otherwise, there are limited clinically significant interactions with other classes of drugs and there is no evidence of hepatic metabolism or interference with the P450 cytochrome system.

Topiramate

This is another newer generation antiepileptic drug that has also been investigated in CPDN. It may exert its analgesic actions via several potential mechanisms; it has been proposed that this agent blocks α-amino-3-hydroxy-5-methylisoxazole-4-propionic acid (AMPA) glutamate receptors, and interferes with depolarization of voltage-activated sodium channels and with calcium influx into cells [52].

In order to evaluate the efficacy and tolerability of topiramate in painful diabetic neuropathy, patients with moderate to extreme pain were randomized to placebo or topiramate (100, 200 or 400 mg/day) in three similar double-blind trials involving a total of 1259 patients [53]. The primary efficacy endpoint was pain reduction from final visit to baseline on the 100 mm VAS for the intention-to-treat populations. After 18–22 weeks of double-blind treatment, although reductions in pain scores were numerically greater with topiramate in two studies, the differences between topiramate and placebo in VAS scores or in the secondary efficacy endpoints did not reach statistical significance in any of the three studies. Across all tudies, 24% of topiramate-treated patients and 8% of placebo-treated patients discontinued due to adverse events with no difference in the occurrence of serious adverse experiences [53].

Another independent placebo-controlled trial used different methodology to assess the efficacy and tolerability of topiramate in CPDN [54]. This was a 12-week, multicenter, randomized, double-blinded trial that included 323 subjects with CPDN and pain VAS score of at least 40 on a scale from 0 (no pain) to 100 (worst possible pain). Topiramate (n = 214) or placebo (n = 109) was titrated to 400 mg daily or to the maximum tolerated dose. Twelve weeks of topiramate treatment reduced pain VAS score more effectively than placebo (P = 0.038). Fifty percent of topiramate-treated subjects and 34% of placebo-treated subjects responded to treatment, defined as >30% reduction in pain VAS score (P = 0.004). Topiramate monotherapy also reduced worst pain intensity and sleep disruption. Diarrhea, loss of appetite, and somnolence were the most commonly reported adverse events in the topiramate group. Overall, 48% of patients withdrew in the active group, nearly half being due to adverse events including gastrointestinal symptoms and somnolence but also some due to cognitive dysfunction.

It was also noted that the topiramate-treated group experienced a more significant reduction in body weight than the placebo group (-2.6 versus $+0.2$ kg weight loss for placebo; $P < 0.001$), an effect believed to be mediated through the carbonic anhydrase properties of topiramate.

Because the bulk of evidence suggests no benefit from topiramate at better tolerated doses of 100 mg/d and 200 mg/d, and evidence regarding higher doses is conflicting, topiramate is unlikely to have a useful role in the management of CDPN.

Lamotrigine

Lamotrigine, another newer antiepileptic agent, is believed to exert its antiallodynic effects by blocking sodium channels in a use-dependent manner, thereby limiting spontaneous firing, and by inhibiting the release of glutamate and aspartate, well-characterized excitatory neurotransmitters [55].

In one small study a total of 59 patients were randomly assigned to receive either lamotrigine (titrated from 25 to 400 mg/day) or placebo over a 6-week period [56]. The primary outcome measure was reduction in pain intensity. Eighty-three percent of patients receiving lamotrigine and 73% receiving placebo completed the study. Daily pain score in the lamotrigine-treated group was reduced from $6.4 +/- 0.1$ to $4.2 +/- 0.1$ and in the control group from $6.5 +/- 0.1$ to $5.3 +/- 0.1$ ($P < 0.001$ for lamotrigine doses of 200, 300, and 400 mg). Secondary efficacy measures remained unchanged. The global assessment of efficacy favored lamotrigine treatment over placebo, and the adverse events profile was similar in both groups [56].

In two other relatively large replicate, randomized, double-blind, placebo-controlled studies, lamotrigine was inconsistently effective for pain associated with diabetic neuropathy but was generally safe and well tolerated [57]. Patients (n = 360 per study) with painful diabetic neuropathy were randomized to receive lamotrigine 200, 300 or 400 mg daily or placebo during the 19-week treatment phase, including a dose escalation and fixed-dose maintenance phase. The mean reduction in pain intensity score from baseline to week 19 (primary endpoint) was greater in patients receiving lamotrigine 400 mg than placebo in only one of the two studies. Lamotrigine 200 and 300 mg did not significantly differ from placebo at week 19 in either study. Lamotrigine 300 and 400 mg were only occasionally more effective than placebo for secondary efficacy endpoints. Adverse events were reported more frequently in the lamotrigine-treated patients compared with placebo. The most common adverse events with lamotrigine were headache and rash.

Given the limited efficacy and the need for very slow dose escalation and potential for severe, life-threatening side effects, lamotrigine cannot be recommended for CPDN except in exceptional circumstances. The manufacturer has reached the same conclusion and announced it will not pursue further development and study of the drug in CDPN [57].

Carbamazepine

Carbamazepine use is nowadays limited in the management of painful diabetic neuropathy in the UK. Older studies [58–61] found that carbamazepine was beneficial in one study, although the patients had a variety of neuropathic syndromes [58], two were not RCT [60, 61] and the fourth was very brief [59]. The NNT for the positive study [58] was 3.3.[62].

Oxcarbazepine

More recently oxcarbazepine, another novel antiepileptic agent, has been evaluated in the management of neuropathic pain [63, 64]. Oxcarbazepine has been developed through structural modification of the carbamazepine molecule with the intention of avoiding metabolites causing side effects, and significant differences have emerged between the two drugs. The mechanism of action of oxcarbazepine involves mainly blockade of sodium currents but differs from carbamazepine by modulating different types of calcium channels [65]. Its potential advantages include a better safety profile with apparently fewer adverse events.

In one multicenter, placebo-controlled trial involving 146 patients, oxcarbazepine was initiated at a dose of 300 mg/day and titrated to a maximum dose of 1800 mg/day (66). After 16 weeks, oxcarbazepine-treated patients experienced a significantly larger decrease in the average change in VAS score from baseline compared with placebo (p = 0.01). A reduction in mean VAS score occurred as early as week 2 of the study. Global assessment of therapeutic effect rating was improved in more oxcarbazepine patients than placebo and patients on oxcarbazepine experienced better quality of sleep. Most adverse events were mild to moderate in severity and transient (66).

In another multicenter, double-blind, placebo-controlled, 16-week study, a total of 141 patients with CPDN were randomized to oxcarbazepine (1200 mg/day) (n = 71) or placebo (n = 70) [67]. The reduction in mean VAS score from baseline to the last study week (primary efficacy point) was similar between the oxcarbazepine and placebo groups. The majority of adverse events were mild to moderate in severity and resolved over the course of the study [67].

As part of a multicenter, double-blind, placebo-controlled, dose-ranging 16-week study, a total of 347 patients were randomized to oxcarbazepine 600 mg/day (n = 83), 1200 mg/day (n = 87), 1800 mg/day (n = 88) or placebo (n = 89) [68]. No difference between any oxcarbazepine group and the placebo group was noted for the primary efficacy variable (change in mean VAS score from baseline to the last week of the study). Statistically significant differences were found between the oxcarbazepine 1200 mg/day (P = 0.038) and 1800 mg/day (P = 0.005) groups and placebo in the overall mean weekly VAS scores for the entire double-blind treatment phase. Although the primary efficacy variable did not reach statistical significance, patients taking oxcarbazepine 1200 and 1800 mg/day did show improvements in VAS scores compared with placebo.

Lacosamide

Lacosamide is a novel antiepileptic drug known to produce a reduction in neuronal discharge and synaptic excitability in experimental models of epilepsy through an unknown mechanism. In the first Phase II randomized, placebo-controlled, parallel-group study, in 119 patients with CPDN of a mean duration of over 3 years, pain reduction was reported as significantly greater by patients on the active drug when compared to placebo [69]. The stable maintenance period on 400 mg/day was limited to 4 weeks, with a 3-week uptitration and 1 week tapering phase. Due to the relatively small number of patients entered into the study, the primary intention-to-treat efficacy analysis was based on last observation carried forward (LOCF) population. Progressive reduction of the VAS scores from 6.6 (1.6) to 3.7 (2.6) in patients on active medication versus reduction of 6.5 (1.7) to 4.5 (2.6) in patients on placebo provided a treatment difference of 0.9 (P = 0.039). Treatment emergent adverse effects were mostly mild or moderate with some central nervous system related (dizziness, nausea and anxiety) more common during lacosamide. Despite borderline efficacy, its relative tolerability associated with probably a novel mode of action, different from those of other antiepileptic drugs, suggests larger trials are warranted [69].

Other antiepileptic drugs

Older studies in CPDN of phenytoin, clonazepam and sodium valproate have been reported, but only two have been randomized placebo-controlled trials, with conflicting results [24]. A NNT of 2.1 has been reported for phenytoin [62]. A more recent, 4-week, relatively small randomized, placebo-controlled study of sodium valproate found it was more effective than placebo at reducing pain [70]. Similar results were found by the same group in a separate 3-month study of equivalent size [71].

There are few data directly comparing antidepressants and antiepileptic agents [72] although separate reviews suggest that there are few differences in analgesic efficacy or side effects [41, 62]. This has been confirmed more recently [23].

Antiarrhythmic agents

Lidocaine and mexiletine

Intravenous lidocaine has been shown to be beneficial in the relief of neuropathic pain in a few studies [73, 74]. In a randomized, double-blind, cross-over study of patients with painful diabetic neuropathy of more than 6 months duration, intravenous lidocaine was shown to have a significant beneficial effect 1 and 8 days after infusion compared with after saline infusion ($P < 0.05$ and $P < 0.02$, respectively) [73]. The duration of the individual effect ranged from 3 to 21 days, and it did not affect the objective measurements of neuropathy.

The analgesic effect of intravenous lidocaine was also evaluated in a small study of patients with neuropathic pain of varying etiology [74]. The response was compared with that of ischemic pain. Disorders manifesting as deafferentation or central neuralgias appeared in that study to be affected favorably by lidocaine IV whereas pain of peripheral origin remained unaffected [74]. The lack of an oral agent and the need for ECG monitoring during the infusion along with its associated adverse effects render intravenous lidocaine an unpopular treatment choice.

The efficacy of an oral antiarrhythmic agent, mexiletine, a type 1b antiarrhythmic drug, has been demonstrated to be variable in a small number of studies [24] with little evidence of efficacy superior to placebo [75]. It requires regular electrocardiographic monitoring and is contraindicated in patients with underlying cardiovascular disease, therefore it is now rarely used in the management of painful diabetic neuropathy.

Lidocaine patch

The treatment of painful diabetic polyneuropathy is often inadequate and frequently limited by the systemic adverse effects of medications or the inadequate clinical response of the patients, therefore necessitating the evaluation of novel treatments. One such treatment is the 5% lidocaine patch which can be useful in patients suffering from touch-evoked allodynia, hyperalgesia or pain paroxysms [76].

Forty patients with peripheral neuropathic pain syndromes of varying etiology completed a prospective, randomized, placebo-controlled, two-way, cross-over study [76]. Patients suffering from pain in a localized skin area with intensity above 40 mm on the

VAS were included. At the discretion of the patients, up to four patches (covering a maximum of 560 cm^2) were applied onto the maximally painful area for 12 consecutive hours daily, always either by day or at night. Throughout the study, ongoing pain, allodynia, quality of neuropathic symptoms, quality of sleep, and adverse events were assessed. As an add-on therapy, the lidocaine patch 5% was effective in reducing ongoing pain ($P = 0.017$) and allodynia ($P = 0.023$) during the first 8 hours after application [76].

In another study patients with CPDN, postherpetic neuralgia and low back pain, who had partial response to gabapentin-containing analgesic regimens, were enrolled [77]. Eligible patients were included in this open-label, nonrandomized, prospective, 2-week study in which the lidocaine patch 5% was applied to the area of maximal pain, using no more than a total of four patches changed every 24 hours whilst patients were maintained on their other analgesic regimens. In the combined patient population (n = 77), 2 weeks of treatment with the lidocaine patch 5% significantly improved all four composite measures on the Neuropathic Pain Scale ($P < 0.01$). Overall, eight patients (10%) experienced mild to moderate treatment-related adverse effects [77].

In another open-label, flexible-dosing, 3-week study with a 5-week extension period, 56 patients with painful diabetic polyneuropathy of longer than 3 months duration were treated with the 5% lidocaine patch, a maximum of four patches daily for 18 hours [78]. Patients showed significant improvements in pain and quality-of-life outcome measures during the 3-week treatment period. These benefits were maintained in a subgroup of patients treated for an additional 5 weeks, during which taper of concomitant analgesic therapy was possible. Adverse events were minimal, and systemic accumulation of lidocaine did not occur [78].

The findings from the last two studies described above [77, 78], in view of their open-label nature, will have to be replicated and confirmed in larger, placebo-controlled studies in the future.

Opioids

Controversy surrounds the role of opioids in the management of neuropathic pain but they can be of use when other therapies have been ineffective [24, 79–81]. There are concerns not only about the responsiveness of neuropathic pain to opioid treatment [82] but also the possibilities of dependency, tolerance or addiction, along with the frequency of associated side effects and the lack of long-term trial evidence [24].

Controlled-release (CR) oxycodone has reported to be effective in two randomized double-blind placebo-controlled studies [83, 84]. One multicenter, randomized, double-blind, placebo-controlled, parallel-group study included 159 subjects with moderate to severe pain due to diabetic neuropathy [83]. Treatment began with either one 10 mg tablet of CR oxycodone (n = 82) or identical placebo (n = 77) every 12 hours. Treatment lasted up to 6 weeks. At an average dose of 37 mg per day, CR oxycodone provided more analgesia than placebo (P = 0.002) in the intention-to-treat cohort. Overall, 80 (96%) of 82 subjects given CR oxycodone and 52 (68%) of 77 subjects who received placebo reported adverse events. The most common adverse events in the CR oxycodone group were opioid related [83].

Fifty-six patients with diabetic neuropathy with moderate or greater pain for at least 3 months underwent washout from all opioids 2–7 days before randomization to 10 mg CR oxycodone or active placebo every 12 hours [84]. The dose was increased, approximately weekly, to a maximum of 40 mg twice a day CR oxycodone, with cross-over to the alternative treatment after a maximum of 4 weeks. CR oxycodone resulted in significantly lower pain scores and disability. Scores from six of the eight SF-36 domains (a quality of life assessment tool) were significantly better during CR oxycodone treatment. The NNT to obtain one patient with at least 50% pain relief was 2.6 and clinical effectiveness scores favored treatment with CR oxycodone over placebo (P = 0.0001) [84].

In these two studies, CR oxycodone was used both as sole agent and in combination with other adjuvant pain medications and side effects were very common in both studies and included nausea, headaches, constipation and drowsiness.

Tramadol

Tramadol is a synthetic, opioid-like analgesic which is known to be a weak inhibitor of serotonin and noradrenaline reuptake and shows very low affinity for the μ-opioid receptors [85]. It has been found to be effective in the treatment of pain in diabetic neuropathy in two double-blind, placebo-controlled, randomized trials and its long-term pain-relieving properties were shown in a 6-month open-label extension study [86–88].

A multicenter randomized, double-blind, placebo-controlled, parallel-group study to evaluate the efficacy of tramadol in CPDN consisted of a wash-out/screening phase, during which all analgesics were discontinued, and a 42-day double-blind treatment phase [86]. A total of 131 patients with CPDN were treated with tramadol four times daily (n = 65) or placebo (n = 66). The primary efficacy analysis compared the mean pain intensity scores in the tramadol and placebo groups obtained at day 42 of the study or at the time of discontinuation. Tramadol, at an average dosage of 210 mg/day, was significantly (P < 0.001) more effective than placebo for treating the pain of diabetic neuropathy [86]. Patients in the tramadol group scored significantly better in physical (P = 0.02) and social functioning (P = 0.04) ratings than patients in the placebo group. The most frequently occurring adverse events with tramadol were nausea, constipation, headache, and somnolence [86].

In another randomized, double-blind, placebo-controlled and cross-over study, 45 patients (15 of whom had CPDN) were assigned to one of the two treatment sequences [88]. The dose of tramadol slow-release tablets was titrated to at least 200 mg/day and at the highest 400 mg/day. Thirty-four patients completed the study. Their ratings for pain (P = 0.001), paraesthesia (P = 0.001) and touch-evoked pain (P < 0.001) were lower on tramadol than on placebo, as were their ratings of allodynia (P = 0.012) [88].

A NNT of 3.1 has been calculated for the use of tramadol in the setting of CPDN [31].

If opioids are used as adjunctive therapy for neuropathic pain, they should be administered when other more established therapies such as antidepressants or antiepileptic drugs have been tried. Other partially effective treatments should be continued [79, 89, 90]. Regular review, use of opioids for a trial period and a definitive treatment plan are vital to increase the chances of success. Sustained-release opioids are recommended although immediate-release opioids can be used for breakthrough pain [89, 90].

Antioxidants

Evidence suggests that oxidative stress resulting from enhanced free radical formation and/or deficits in antioxidant defense may play a major role among the putative pathogenic mechanisms of diabetic neuropathy [91–93]. A meta-analysis of four trials (ALADIN I, ALADIN III, SYDNEY and NATHAN II) comprising a total of 1258 diabetic patients with positive sensory symptoms of polyneuropathy showed that treatment over 3 weeks with intravenous α-lipoic acid (ALA) was safe and significantly improved both positive neuropathic symptoms and neuropathic deficits to a clinically meaningful degree [92]. A recent randomized, double-blind, placebo-controlled, dose–response trial over 5 weeks (ALADIN II) showed that oral treatment with ALA at a dose of 600 mg per day improved neuropathic symptoms and deficits in patients with distal diabetic polyneuropathy [94]. Detailed results of longer duration trials recently completed are awaited.

Topical nitrates

Considerable evidence implicates impaired nitric oxide (NO) generation in the pathogenesis of diabetic neuropathic pain through defects in local vasodilation [95].

The role of isosorbide dinitrate (ISDN) spray has recently been explored in a double-blind, randomized, placebo-controlled, cross-over study [96]. ISDN spray reduced overall neuropathic pain (P = 0.02) and burning sensation (P = 0.006). No treatment difference was observed with other sensory modalities (hot/cold sensation, tingling, numbness, hyperesthesia, and jabbing-like sensation). At study completion, 11 patients (50%) reported benefit and wished to continue using the ISDN spray, four (18%) preferred the placebo spray, and the remaining seven (32%) were undecided.

More recently, glyceryl trinitrate patches have been shown to be promising as an alternative to ISDN spray in the alleviation of burning pain in diabetic neuropathy [95] but their role remains to be confirmed in larger, double-blind, placebo-controlled clinical trials.

Other topical therapies

Capsaicin, the main ingredient of the red chilli pepper, acts by depleting the nociceptive C-fibers of substance P. A meta-analysis of four randomized, double-blind, placebo-controlled trials in painful diabetic neuropathy found capsaicin overall to be more effective than placebo [97]. However, it is not possible to totally blind either participants or investigators

to the potential irritant side effects of capsaicin, and it may therefore be that the studies were not in fact "blind." Long-term follow-up data are also limited. The release of large amounts of substance P following the application of the cream results in a transient worsening of the symptoms during the first week or two of capsaicin use. The burning sensation, time to achieve pain reduction, and the need to apply it four times daily to the affected areas limit its usefulness.

Op-site® film has been found to be helpful in reducing pain in some patients in an open study, but application can be problematic and it is probably only useful for allodynia.

Other drugs

A variety of drugs have been tried with varying degrees of scientific proof of their efficacy which on the whole cannot be recommended for routine usage. Most trials had methodologic flaws, were very small or are only published so far in abstract form.

Oral dextromethorpan and memantine, N-methyl-D-aspartate receptor antagonists, have shown variable efficacy in pain reduction in very small randomized, placebo-controlled trials. Levodopa has also led to pain reduction in a small randomized controlled trial. Good evidence for the effectiveness of drugs such as aspirin or NSAID is lacking [24].

Stimulation therapies

Transcutaneous electrical nerve stimulation (TENS) was used in a 4-week, single-blind study that randomized 31 patients with type 2 diabetes and symptoms and signs of peripheral neuropathy, to receive either active electrotherapy or sham therapy [98]. Patients in the active group had a 52% reduction in pain compared with 27% in controls. In another study, 54 patients with diabetes who were using a TENS device were identified, and the patients' symptoms prior to and following electrotherapy were assessed [99]. Forty-one (76%) patients reported a mean 44% subjective improvement in their neuropathic pain with TENS electrotherapy, which they had continued to use as an adjunct to their conventional analgesic drugs for a mean of 1.7 years. In another small (n = 26), single-blind study TENS was also shown to be a useful adjunctive modality when combined with a pharmacologic agent such as amitriptyline, to augment symptomatic pain relief [100].

The value of percutaneous electrical nerve stimulation (PENS) in painful diabetic neuropathy was assessed in one short-term sham-controlled cross-over study which randomized 50 patients to receive either active PENS or sham PENS (acupuncture only) [101]. Patients who received active therapy showed a significant reduction in pain scores.

The effects of traditional acupuncture in CPDN were studied in one uncontrolled trial [102]. Forty-six patients (of whom more than half were on standard medical treatment for painful neuropathy) received up to six courses of classic acupuncture analgesia over 10 weeks; over 75% noted an improvement in pain symptoms. The patients were followed up for a period that ranged from 18 to 52 weeks during which time only 8/34 needed further acupuncture.

Electrical spinal cord stimulation (ESCS) involves the delivery of a low-voltage electrical current to the dorsal structures of the spinal cord in order to reduce pain perception. In a small study, ESCS has been shown to be effective and safe in the treatment of severe, resistant, painful neuropathy, confirming its place in the contemporary management of chronic intractable pain when all other conventional treatment strategies have failed [103]; the beneficial effects can last many years [104] and the majority of complications are of a technical nature and tend to occur during the first 6 months of implantation.

The mechanisms behind the pain-relieving effects of ESCS are still obscure. Although these data do support a role for electrotherapy in the symptomatic treatment of CPDN, there are obvious deficiencies as it is not possible to perform conventional double-blind studies because of failure to "blind" the patients to the electrical sensation when active and sham therapies are applied. The studies also tend to be small and/or of short duration. However, the lack of significant reported or observed side effects from these electroanalgesic therapies appears encouraging. ESCS is an expensive procedure and is suitable only for selective cases of CPDN when managed in specialist centers where the necessary expertise and facilities are available.

Author's recommendations

Based on the number needed to treat (NNT) system, TCA have been shown to be most effective when dosed from 25 to 150 mg daily, with two systematic reviews reporting a NNT of 2.6 by one group [31] and 3.5 by another [23]. It is important to emphasize that the majority of the trials evaluating the efficacy and safety of TCA were of relatively small size that may have led to an overestimation of their benefits.

Because of the well-characterized side effects of TCA, they should not be chosen as the first-line treatment for patients with certain co-morbidities such as known cardiac arrhythmias, electrocardiographic abnormalities, postural hypotension, unexplained falls and balance problems, glaucoma and prostatic hypertophy. All these medical conditions can potentially be exacerbated by the use of TCA in view of their well-known anticholinergic properties. Because of the higher prevalence of these disorders among the elderly, alternative first-line medications frequently have to be chosen for this population. These recommendations are in line with those developed by the Diabetic Peripheral Neuropathic Pain Consensus Treatment Guidelines Advisory Board in 2006 [105] which were formulated to help guide treatment decisions so that an optimal balance between pain relief and side effects is achieved.

When the use of a TCA is contraindicated (quite frequently the case), the newer antiepileptic drugs gabapentin and pregabalin can be considered. The use of pregabalin is supported by greater clinical trial evidence compared with gabapentin. Pregabalin administered at a dosage of 75 mg or 150 mg daily does not produce significant clinical improvement in patients with CPDN compared with placebo. Higher doses (300–600 mg/day) have to be administered and these can show clinical efficacy even within 1 week of initiation of treatment. The dosing schedule should be three times or twice daily. Moreover, pregabalin, similarly to gabapentin, has demonstrated efficacy in improvement of a number of other clinically important parameters such as sleep interference. They are both renally excreted and dose reduction is required in patients with renal impairment but they do not interfere with the hepatic P450 cytochrome system. In view of the relatively short duration of the trials conducted so far, there are no long-term data as yet that show durability of the effects of pregabalin over a longer period of time.

The SNRI duloxetine has been licensed in the US and Europe with a specific indication for the treatment of neuropathic pain associated with CPDN. Although its superiority over placebo has been demonstrated in large, multicenter, randomized, double-blind studies, there has been no head-to-head comparison with the traditional TCA or the antiepileptic drugs, and given its cost and the existing data on its gastrointestinal, neuropsychologic and possible hepatic adverse effects and risk of interactions with other drugs, its place as a first-line agent in the management of pain associated with CPDN remains to be further elucidated.

Although the use of CR oxycodone in CPDN is supported by evidence from at least two large RCT, and the use of tramadol by one RCT in patients with CPDN and another RCT that included patients with painful neuropathy, a minority of whom were identified with CPDN, the concerns regarding dependency, tolerance or addiction when used on a long-term basis should make them second-line agents in the management of CPDN. In refractory cases of CPDN, opioids such as tramadol may prove useful in the suppression of breakthrough pain.

There is a dearth of studies on the use of combination pharmacotherapy in neuropathic pain. In one study involving 57 patients (35 with CDPN, 22 with postherpetic neuralgia), in which the patients were randomly allocated to four 5-week periods of maximum tolerated doses of placebo, gabapentin, morphine or gabapenin-morphine combination, the investigators showed better pain relief during the combination than either drug alone, despite lower doses [106]. While this type of combination therapy is not unusual in clinical practice, it is noteworthy that common combinations of antidepressants and antiepileptic drugs seem not to have been subjected to similar clinical trials. Yet combined use of a TCA with sedative effects as an adjunct to an antiepileptic drug may prove beneficial, especially in cases where sleep disturbance is a prominent feature.

Future research directions

Knowledge of the precise epidemiology and especially natural history of CPDN is of vital importance and will help to design and implement effective management strategies. With regard to pharmacologic agents currently available and licensed for treatment of CPDN, it is important to emphasize the need for a consensus on standard outcome measures to be evaluated in drug trials that would enable easier comparison of treatment efficacy.

There is also an urgent need for further well-designed trials of drug combinations and alternative therapies. These will provide the clinical evidence necessary to design effective and widely accepted treatment algorithms that will only improve pain relief.

Further research is also needed to understand and identify the underlying pathogenetic mechanisms contributing to the symptoms in an individual, The ultimate goal is to be able to safely bridge clinical findings with basic mechanisms and subsequently to apply mechanism-tailored treatment strategies that will increase the chances of successful pain relief.

Conclusion

Chronic painful diabetic neuropathy is a common complication of diabetes but is often under-reported and inadequately treated [24]. Management of this condition can be challenging but antidepressants and antiepileptic drugs remain the mainstays of treatment (Box 17.1).

Box 17.1 Pharmacologic and other treatments used in CPDN

Treatments supported by evidence
TCA
Pregabalin, gabapentin
Duloxetine
Oxycodone CR, tramadol
Venlafaxine ER
Carbamazepine

Treatments not consistently proven to be efficacious with current evidence
Topiramate, oxcarbazepine
Lamotrigine

Treatments with limited evidence
Capsaicin, 5% lidocaine patch
ISDN spray, GTN patch
Citalopram, paroxetine, fluoxetine
Phenytoin
Dextromethorphan, memantine
TENS, PENS, ESCS, acupuncture

Treatments refuted by evidence
Mexiletine
NSAIDs, aspirin

References

1. Gordois A, Scuffham P, Shearer A, Oglesby A, Tobian JA. The health care costs of diabetic peripheral neuropathy in the US. *Diabetes Care* 2003; **26**: 1790–1795.

2. Chan AW, MacFarlane IA, Bowsher DR, Wells JC, Bessex C, Griffiths K. Chronic pain in patients with diabetes mellitus; comparison with a non-diabetic population. *Pain Clinic* 1990; **3**: 147–159.

3. Boulton AJ, Knight G, Drury J, Ward JD. The prevalence of symptomatic, diabetic neuropathy in an insulin-treated population. *Diabetes Care* 1985; **8**: 125–128.

4. Partanen J, Niskanen L, Lehtinen J, Mervaala E, Siitonen O, Uusitupa M. Natural history of peripheral neuropathy in patients with non-insulin-dependent diabetes mellitus. *N Engl J Med* 1995; **333**: 89–94.

5. Daousi C, MacFarlane IA, Woodward A, Nurmikko TJ, Bundred PE, Benbow SJ. Chronic painful peripheral neuropathy in an urban community: a controlled comparison of people with and without diabetes. *Diabet Med* 2004; **21**: 976–982.

6. Archer AG, Watkins PJ, Thomas PK, Sharma AK, Payan J. The natural history of acute painful neuropathy in diabetes mellitus. *J Neurol Neurosurg Psychiatr* 1983; **46**: 491–499.

7. Mayne N. The short-term prognosis in diabetic neuropathy. *Diabetes* 1968; **17**: 270–273.

8. Young RJ, Ewing DJ, Clarke BF. Chronic and remitting painful diabetic polyneuropathy. Correlations with clinical features and subsequent changes in neurophysiology. *Diabetes Care* 1988; **11**: 34–40.

9. Benbow SJ, Chan AW, Bowsher D, MacFarlane IA, Williams G. A prospective study of painful symptoms, small-fibre function and peripheral vascular disease in chronic painful diabetic neuropathy. *Diabet Med* 1994; **11**: 17–21.

10. Daousi C, Benbow SJ, MacFarlane IA. The natural history of chronic painful peripheral neuropathy in a community diabetes population. *Diabet Med* 2006; **23**(9): 1021–1024.

11. Boulton AJ, Armstrong WD, Scarpello JH, Ward JD. The natural history of painful diabetic neuropathy – a 4-year study. *Postgrad Med J* 1983; **59**: 556–559.

12. Bischoff A. The natural course of diabetic neuropathy. A follow-up. *Horm Metab Res Suppl* 1980; **9**: 98–100.

13. Fry IK, Hardwick C, Scott G. Diabetic neuropathy: a survey and follow-up of 66 cases. *Guys Hosp Rep* 1962; **111**: 113–129.

14. Watkins PJ. Natural history of the diabetic neuropathies. *Q J Med* 1990; **77**: 1209–1218.

15. Hansson P. Neuropathic pain: clinical characteristics and diagnostic workup. *Eur J Pain* 2002; **6**(suppl A): 47–50.

16. Dworkin RH. An overview of neuropathic pain: syndromes, symptoms, signs, and several mechanisms. *Clin J Pain* 2002; **18**: 343–349.

17. Koltzenburg M, Scadding J. Neuropathic pain. *Curr Opin Neurol* 2001; **14**: 641–647.

18. Attal N, Bouhassira D. Mechanisms of pain in peripheral neuropathy. *Acta Neurol Scand Suppl* 1999; **173**: 12–24.

19. Jensen TS. Anticonvulsants in neuropathic pain: rationale and clinical evidence. *Eur J Pain* 2002; **6**(suppl A): 61–68.

20. Boulton AJ, Drury J, Clarke B, Ward JD. Continuous subcutaneous insulin infusion in the management of painful diabetic neuropathy. *Diabetes Care* 1982; **5**: 386–390.

21. Ziegler D, Dannehl K, Wiefels K, Gries FA. Differential effects of near-normoglycaemia for 4 years on somatic nerve dysfunction and heart rate variation in type 1 diabetic patients. *Diabet Med* 1992; **9**: 622–629.

22. Oyibo SO, Prasad YD, Jackson NJ, Jude EB, Boulton AJ. The relationship between blood glucose excursions and painful diabetic peripheral neuropathy: a pilot study. *Diabet Med* 2002; **19**: 870–873.

23. Collins SL, Moore RA, McQuay HJ, Wiffen P. Antidepressants and anticonvulsants for diabetic neuropathy and postherpetic neuralgia: a quantitative systematic review. *J Pain Symptom Manage* 2000; **20**: 449–458.

24. Benbow SJ, Daousi C, MacFarlane IA. Painful diabetic neuropathy. In: Barnett AH (ed) *Best Research and Practice Compendium: Diabetes*. Elsevier, Edinburgh, 2005.

25. Max MB, Culnane M, Schafer SC, *et al.* Amitriptyline relieves diabetic neuropathy pain in patients with normal or depressed mood. *Neurology* 1987; **37**: 589–596.

26. Kvinesdal B, Molin J, Froland A, Gram LF. Imipramine treatment of painful diabetic neuropathy. *JAMA* 1984; **251**: 1727–1730.

27. Max MB, Kishore-Kumar R, Schafer SC, *et al.* Efficacy of desipramine in painful diabetic neuropathy: a placebo-controlled trial. *Pain* 1991; **45**: 3–9.

28. Sindrup SH, Gram LF, Skjold T, Grodum E, Brosen K, Beck-Nielsen H. Clomipramine vs desipramine vs placebo in the treatment of diabetic neuropathy symptoms. A double-blind cross-over study. *Br J Clin Pharmacol* 1990; **30**: 683–691.

29. Max MB, Lynch SA, Muir J, Shoaf SE, Smoller B, Dubner R. Effects of desipramine, amitriptyline, and fluoxetine on pain in diabetic neuropathy. *N Engl J Med* 1992; **326**: 1250–1256.

30. Gomez-Perez FJ, Rull JA, Dies H, *et al.* Nortriptyline and fluphenazine in the symptomatic treatment of diabetic neuropathy. A double-blind cross-over study. *Pain* 1985; **23**: 395–400.

31. Sindrup SH, Jensen TS. Pharmacologic treatment of pain in polyneuropathy. *Neurology* 2000; **55**: 915–920.

32. Saarto T, Wiffen PJ. Antidepressants for neuropathic pain. Cochrane Database of Systematic Reviews 2007, Issue 4. Art. No.: CD005454. DOI: 10.1002/14651858.CD005454.pub2.

33. Sindrup SH, Gram LF, Brosen K, Eshoj O, Mogensen EF. The selective serotonin reuptake inhibitor paroxetine is effective in the treatment of diabetic neuropathy symptoms. *Pain* 1990; **42**: 135–144.

34. Sindrup SH, Bjerre U, Dejgaard A, Brosen K, aes-Jorgensen T, Gram LF. The selective serotonin reuptake inhibitor citalopram relieves the symptoms of diabetic neuropathy. *Clin Pharmacol Ther* 1992; **52**: 547–552.

35. Rowbotham MC, Goli V, Kunz NR, Lei D. Venlafaxine extended release in the treatment of painful diabetic neuropathy: a double-blind, placebo-controlled study. *Pain* 2004; **110**: 697–706.

36. Sindrup SH, Bach FW, Madsen C, Gram LF, Jensen TS. Venlafaxine versus imipramine in painful polyneuropathy: a randomized, controlled trial. *Neurology* 2003; **60**: 1284–1289.

37. Smith TR. Duloxetine in diabetic neuropathy. *Expert Opin Pharmacother* 2006; **7**: 215–223.

38. Goldstein DJ, Lu Y, Detke MJ, Lee TC, Iyengar S. Duloxetine vs. placebo in patients with painful diabetic neuropathy. *Pain* 2005; **116**: 109–118.

39. Raskin J, Pritchett YL, Wang F, *et al.* A double-blind, randomized multicenter trial comparing duloxetine with placebo in the management of diabetic peripheral neuropathic pain. *Pain Med* 2005; **6**: 346–356.

40. Wernicke JF, Pritchett YL, D'Souza DN, *et al.* A randomized controlled trial of duloxetine in diabetic peripheral neuropathic pain. *Neurology* 2006; **67**: 1411–1420.

41. McQuay HJ, Tramer M, Nye BA, Carroll D, Wiffen PJ, Moore RA. A systematic review of antidepressants in neuropathic pain. *Pain* 1996; **68**: 217–227.

42. Backonja M, Beydoun A, Edwards KR, *et al.* Gabapentin for the symptomatic treatment of painful neuropathy in patients with diabetes mellitus: a randomized controlled trial. *JAMA* 1998; **280**: 1831–1836.

43. Gorson KC, Schott C, Herman R, Ropper AH, Rand WM. Gabapentin in the treatment of painful diabetic neuropathy: a placebo controlled, double blind, crossover trial. *J Neurol Neurosurg Psychiatry* 1999; **66**: 251–252.

44. Morello CM, Leckband SG, Stoner CP, Moorhouse DF, Sahagian GA. Randomized double-blind study comparing the efficacy of gabapentin with amitriptyline on diabetic peripheral neuropathy pain. *Arch Intern Med* 1999; **159**: 1931–1937.

45. Dallocchio C, Buffa C, Mazzarello P, Chiroli S. Gabapentin vs. amitriptyline in painful diabetic neuropathy: an open-label pilot study. *J Pain Symptom Manage* 2000; **20**: 280–285.

46. Mellegers MA, Furlan AD, Mailis A. Gabapentin for neuropathic pain: systematic review of controlled and uncontrolled literature. *Clin J Pain* 2001; **17**: 284–295.

47. Backonja M, Glanzman RL. Gabapentin dosing for neuropathic pain: evidence from randomized, placebo-controlled clinical trials. *Clin Ther* 2003; **25**: 81–104.

48. Rosenstock J, Tuchman M, LaMoreaux L, Sharma U. Pregabalin for the treatment of painful diabetic peripheral neuropathy: a double-blind, placebo-controlled trial. *Pain* 2004; **110**: 628–638.

49. Lesser H, Sharma U, LaMoreaux L, Poole RM. Pregabalin relieves symptoms of painful diabetic neuropathy: a randomized controlled trial. *Neurology* 2004; **63**: 2104–2110.

50. Richter RW, Portenoy R, Sharma U, LaMoreaux L, Bockbrader H, Knapp LE. Relief of painful diabetic peripheral neuropathy with pregabalin: a randomized, placebo-controlled trial. *J Pain* 2005; **6**: 253–260.

51. Freynhagen R, Strojek K, Griesing T, Whalen E, Balkenohl M. Efficacy of pregabalin in neuropathic pain evaluated in a 12-week, randomized, double-blind, multicenter, placebo-controlled trial of flexible- and fixed-dose regimens. *Pain* 2005; **115**: 254–263.

52. Beydoun A, Backonja MM. Mechanistic stratification of antineuralgic agents. *J Pain Symptom Manage* 2003; **25**: S18–S30.

53. Thienel U, Neto W, Schwabe SK, Vijapurkar U. Topiramate in painful diabetic polyneuropathy: findings from three double-blind placebo-controlled trials. *Acta Neurol Scand* 2004; **110**: 221–231.

54. Raskin P, Donofrio PD, Rosenthal NR, *et al.* Topiramate vs. placebo in painful diabetic neuropathy: analgesic and metabolic effects. *Neurology* 2004; **63**: 865–873.

55. Dickenson AH, Matthews EA, Suzuki R. Neurobiology of neuropathic pain: mode of action of anticonvulsants. *Eur J Pain* 2002; **6**(suppl A): 51–60.

56. Eisenberg E, Lurie Y, Braker C, Daoud D, Ishay A. Lamotrigine reduces painful diabetic neuropathy: a randomized, controlled study. *Neurology* 2001; **57**: 505–509.

57. Vinik AI, Tuchman M, Safirstein B, *et al.* Lamotrigine for treatment of pain associated with diabetic neuropathy: results of two randomized, double-blind, placebo-controlled studies. *Pain* 2007; **128**: 169–179.

58. Rull JA, Quibrera R, Gonzalez-Millan H, Lozano CO. Symptomatic treatment of peripheral diabetic neuropathy with carbamazepine (Tegretol): double blind crossover trial. *Diabetologia* 1969; **5**: 215–218.

59. Wilton TD. Tegretol in the treatment of diabetic neuropathy. *S Afr Med J* 1974; **48**: 869–872.

60. Chakrabarti AK, Samantaray SK. Diabetic peripheral neuropathy: nerve conduction studies before, during and after carbamazepine therapy. *Aust N Z J Med* 1976; **6**: 565–568.

61. Badran AM, Aly MA, Sous ES. A clinical trial of carbamazepine in the symptomatic treatment of diabetic peripheral neuropathy. *J Egypt Med Assoc* 1975; **58**: 627–631.

62. McQuay H, Carroll D, Jadad AR, Wiffen P, Moore A. Anticonvulsant drugs for management of pain: a systematic review. *BMJ* 1995; **311**: 1047–1052.

63. Beydoun A, Kobetz SA, Carrazana EJ. Efficacy of oxcarbazepine in the treatment of painful diabetic neuropathy. *Clin J Pain* 2004; **20**: 174–178.

64. Carrazana E, Mikoshiba I. Rationale and evidence for the use of oxcarbazepine in neuropathic pain. *J Pain Symptom Manage* 2003; **25**: S31–S35.

65. Schmidt D, Elger CE. What is the evidence that oxcarbazepine and carbamazepine are distinctly different antiepileptic drugs? *Epilepsy Behav* 2004; **5**: 627–635.

66. Dogra S, Beydoun A, Mazzola J, Hopwood M, Wan Y. Oxcarbazepine in painful diabetic neuropathy: a randomized, placebo-controlled study. *Eur J Pain* 2005; **9**: 543–554.

67. Grosskopf J, Mazzola J, Wan Y, Hopwood M. A randomized, placebo-controlled study of oxcarbazepine in painful diabetic neuropathy. *Acta Neurol Scand* 2006; **114**: 177–180.

68. Beydoun A, Shaibani A, Hopwood M, Wan Y. Oxcarbazepine in painful diabetic neuropathy: results of a dose-ranging study. *Acta Neurol Scand* 2006; **113**: 395–404.

69. Rauck RL, Shaibani A, Biton V, Simpson J, Koch B. Lacosamide in painful diabetic peripheral neuropathy: a phase 2 double-blind placebo-controlled study. *Clin J Pain* 2007; **23**: 150–158.

70. Kochar DK, Jain N, Agarwal RP, Srivastava T, Agarwal P, Gupta S. Sodium valproate in the management of painful neuropathy in type 2 diabetes – a randomized placebo controlled study. *Acta Neurol Scand* 2002; **106**: 248–252.

71. Kochar DK, Rawat N, Agrawal RP, *et al.* Sodium valproate for painful diabetic neuropathy: a randomized double-blind placebo-controlled study. *QJM* 2004; **97**: 33–38.

72. Jose VM, Bhansali A, Hota D, Pandhi P. Randomized double-blind study comparing the efficacy and safety of lamotrigine and amitriptyline in painful diabetic neuropathy. *Diabet Med* 2007; **24**: 377–383.

73. Kastrup J, Petersen P, Dejgard A, Angelo HR, Hilsted J. Intravenous lidocaine infusion – a new treatment of chronic painful diabetic neuropathy? *Pain* 1987; **28**: 69–75.

74. Boas RA, Covino BG, Shahnarian A. Analgesic responses to i.v. lignocaine. *Br J Anaesth* 1982; **54**: 501–505.

75. Duby JJ, Campbell RK, Setter SM, White JR, Rasmussen KA. Diabetic neuropathy: an intensive review. *Am J Health Syst Pharm* 2004; **61**: 160–173.

76. Meier T, Wasner G, Faust M, *et al.* Efficacy of lidocaine patch 5% in the treatment of focal peripheral neuropathic pain syndromes: a randomized, double-blind, placebo-controlled study. *Pain* 2003; **106**: 151–158.

77. Argoff CE, Galer BS, Jensen MP, Oleka N, Gammaitoni AR. Effectiveness of the lidocaine patch 5% on pain qualities in three chronic pain states: assessment with the Neuropathic Pain Scale. *Curr Med Res Opin* 2004; **20**(suppl 2): 21–28.

78. Barbano RL, Herrmann DN, Hart-Gouleau S, Pennella-Vaughan J, Lodewick PA, Dworkin RH. Effectiveness, tolerability, and impact on quality of life of the 5% lidocaine patch in diabetic polyneuropathy. *Arch Neurol* 2004; **61**: 914–918.

79. Watson CP. The treatment of neuropathic pain: antidepressants and opioids. *Clin J Pain* 2000; **16**: S49–S55.

80. Sindrup SH, Jensen TS. Efficacy of pharmacological treatments of neuropathic pain: an update and effect related to mechanism of drug action. *Pain* 1999; **83**: 389–400.

81. Kalso E, Edwards JE, Moore RA, McQuay HJ. Opioids in chronic non-cancer pain: systematic review of efficacy and safety. *Pain* 2004; **112**: 372–380.

82. Arner S, Meyerson BA. Lack of analgesic effect of opioids on neuropathic and idiopathic forms of pain. *Pain* 1988; **33**: 11–23.

83. Gimbel JS, Richards P, Portenoy RK. Controlled-release oxycodone for pain in diabetic neuropathy: a randomized controlled trial. *Neurology* 2003; **60**: 927–934.

84. Watson CP, Moulin D, Watt-Watson J, Gordon A, Eisenhoffer J. Controlled-release oxycodone relieves neuropathic pain: a randomized controlled trial in painful diabetic neuropathy. *Pain* 2003; **105**: 71–78.

85. Lee CR, McTavish D, Sorkin EM. Tramadol. A preliminary review of its pharmacodynamic and pharmacokinetic properties, and therapeutic potential in acute and chronic pain states. *Drugs* 1993; **46**: 313–340.

86. Harati Y, Gooch C, Swenson M, *et al.* Double-blind randomized trial of tramadol for the treatment of the pain of diabetic neuropathy. *Neurology* 1998; **50**: 1842–1846.

87. Harati Y, Gooch C, Swenson M, *et al.* Maintenance of the long-term effectiveness of tramadol in treatment of the pain of diabetic neuropathy. *J Diabetes Complications* 2000; **14**: 65–70.

88. Sindrup SH, Andersen G, Madsen C, Smith T, Brosen K, Jensen TS. Tramadol relieves pain and allodynia in polyneuropathy: a randomized, double-blind, controlled trial. *Pain* 1999; **83**: 85–90.

89. Pain Society. Recommendations for the use of opioids for persistent non-cancer pain. A consensus statement prepared on behalf of the Pain Society, the Royal College of Anaesthetists, the Royal College of General Practitioners and the Royal College of Psychiatrists. 2004. Available from www.britishpainsociety.org/pdf/opioids_doc_2004.pdf.

90. Kalso E, Allan L, Dellemijn PL, *et al.* Recommendations for using opioids in chronic non-cancer pain. *Eur J Pain* 2003; **7**: 381–386.

91. Cameron NE, Eaton SE, Cotter MA, Tesfaye S. Vascular factors and metabolic interactions in the pathogenesis of diabetic neuropathy. *Diabetologia* 2001; **44**: 1973–1988.

92. Ziegler D, Nowak H, Kempler P, Vargha P, Low PA. Treatment of symptomatic diabetic polyneuropathy with the antioxidant alpha-lipoic acid: a meta-analysis. *Diabet Med* 2004; **21**: 114–121.

93. Ziegler D, Sohr CG, Nourooz-Zadeh J. Oxidative stress and antioxidant defense in relation to the severity of diabetic polyneuropathy and cardiovascular autonomic neuropathy. *Diabetes Care* 2004; **27**: 2178–2183.

94. Ziegler D, Ametov A, Barinov A, *et al.* Oral treatment with alpha-lipoic acid improves symptomatic diabetic polyneuropathy: the SYDNEY 2 trial. *Diabetes Care* 2006; **29**: 2365–2370.

95. Rayman G, Baker NR, Krishnan ST. Glyceryl trinitrate patches as an alternative to isosorbide dinitrate spray in the treatment of chronic painful diabetic neuropathy. *Diabetes Care* 2003; **26**: 2697–2698.

96. Yuen KC, Baker NR, Rayman G. Treatment of chronic painful diabetic neuropathy with isosorbide dinitrate spray: a double-blind placebo-controlled cross-over study. *Diabetes Care* 2002; **25**: 1699–1703.

97. Zhang WY, Li Wan PA. The effectiveness of topically applied capsaicin. A meta-analysis. *Eur J Clin Pharmacol* 1994; **46**: 517–522.

98. Kumar D, Marshall HJ. Diabetic peripheral neuropathy: amelioration of pain with transcutaneous electrostimulation. *Diabetes Care* 1997; **20**: 1702–1705.

99. Julka IS, Alvaro M, Kumar D. Beneficial effects of electrical stimulation on neuropathic symptoms in diabetes patients. *J Foot Ankle Surg* 1998; **37**: 191–194.

100. Kumar D, Alvaro MS, Julka IS, Marshall HJ. Diabetic peripheral neuropathy. Effectiveness of electrotherapy and amitriptyline for symptomatic relief. *Diabetes Care* 1998; **21**: 1322–1325.

101. Hamza MA, White PF, Craig WF, *et al.* Percutaneous electrical nerve stimulation: a novel analgesic therapy for diabetic neuropathic pain. *Diabetes Care* 2000; **23**: 365–370.

102. Abuaisha BB, Costanzi JB, Boulton AJ. Acupuncture for the treatment of chronic painful peripheral diabetic neuropathy: a long-term study. *Diabetes Res Clin Pract* 1998; **39**: 115–121.

103. Tesfaye S, Watt J, Benbow SJ, Pang KA, Miles J, MacFarlane IA. Electrical spinal cord stimulation for painful diabetic peripheral neuropathy. *Lancet* 1996; **348**: 1696–1701.

104. Daousi C, Benbow SJ, MacFarlane IA. Electrical spinal cord stimulation in the long-term treatment of chronic painful diabetic neuropathy. *Diabet Med* 2005; **22**: 393–398.

105. Argoff CE, Backonja MM, Belgrade MJ, *et al.* Consensus guidelines: treatment planning and options. Diabetic peripheral neuropathic pain. *Mayo Clin Proc* 2006; **81**: S12–S25.

106. Gilron I, Bailey JM, Tu D, Holden RR, Weaver DF, Houlden RL. Morphine, gabapentin or their combination for neuropathic pain. *N Engl J Med* 2005; **352**: 1324–1334.

CHAPTER 18

Postherpetic neuralgia

Turo J. Nurmikko

Division of Neurological Science, School of Clinical Sciences, University of Liverpool, Clinical Sciences Centre, Liverpool, UK

Introduction

Postherpetic neuralgia (PHN) is one of the best known neuropathic pain conditions and possibly the most investigated. Its unique and stereotypical clinical presentation with localized pain, allodynia, and sensory change has inspired a number of pathophysiologic studies. In the developing discipline of pain medicine in the latter part of the 20th century, PHN was seen as an archetype of neuropathic pain and its management was left to pain specialists who reported impressive case series with fascinating clinical details. The pain and sensory dysfunction and a seemingly stable natural course of PHN were also suitable for a multitude of clinical trials. Epidemiologic studies suggest, however, that PHN is usually mild and self-remitting and that most cases are managed in primary care [1, 2]. However, as the most common complication of the herpes zoster (HZ), which itself is the most common neurologic infection, PHN remains sufficiently prevalent to warrant special interest and to be recognized as a clinical problem, even if only a small unfortunate minority with shingles develop the most severe form of the disease.

Pathophysiology

Postherpetic neuralgia is the term used to describe the painful aftermath of HZ. At present no agreed criteria

exist for the definition of PHN definition, either relating to the time point of its development after the onset of HZ infection or the intensity and quality of discomfort required for the diagnosis. Many authors accept a time definition of pain for PHN of 3 or 4 months after the onset of rash, and some have adopted a concept of "clinically meaningful pain" rated at ≥ 3 out of 10 [3, 4]. Pain frequently precedes HZ (called preherpetic neuralgia), and usually outlasts the rash by some weeks.

Shingles, i.e. HZ, results from activation of the varicella zoster virus (VZV) which has remained latent in the dorsal root ganglia since the first infection (varicella). *In situ* hybridization has shown the latent VZV genome localized in 1–7% of sensory ganglion neurones. Latency seems to be established by cell-free virus [5]. Maintenance is associated with expression of six genes (ORF 4, ORF21, ORF29, ORF62, ORF 63, ORF 66) and the protein products from these genes. Cell-mediated immunity controls the transcriptional factors preventing viral transcription and a reduced T cell response results in viral replication taking place. The virus replicates in the ganglionic neurones, infects the neighboring cells and is then transmitted down the nerve axons to the skin where local infection results in blister formation [5, 6]. The virus also travels centrally, leading to inflammation of the meninges and spinal cord, albeit to a limited degree. Subclinical central nervous system inflammation is common, as shown in a study in which patients with HZ who were devoid of any central nervous system signs frequently had inflammatory changes in their cerebrospinal fluid and MRI [7].

Infected cells may undergo lysis. Histopathologic investigations of human spinal ganglia, obtained

---

Evidence-Based Chronic Pain Management. Edited by C. Stannard, E. Kalso and J. Ballantyne. © 2010 Blackwell Publishing.

at post mortem from patients with acute or subacute HZ, show neuronal loss and inflammatory infiltrates in ganglia, nerve and nerve root [8]. Most changes in the peripheral nerve appear to be the result of Wallerian degeneration of both large and small fibers. The inflammatory changes are then over time replaced by fibrous tissue. Some histopathologic studies of PHN report atrophy of the dorsal horn with limited but persistent inflammation with degeneration of sensory ganglia, sometimes extending contralaterally [9]. Epidermal nerve fiber density assessment from skin biopsies shows bilateral degeneration of terminal of peripheral fibers within the affected dermatome, possibly resulting from contralateral subclinical spread of the virus [10]. The combined data from these studies therefore demonstrate widespread neural damage that follows the primary inflammation. The association between neural pathology and pain is not clear, and neither is it known to what extent prompt use of antivirals or other interventions is capable of preventing the changes.

The clinical picture of PHN suggests several potential mechanisms for the generation and maintenance of pain. Patients frequently complain of a steady aching or burning pain and also sharp shooting pain and tactile allodynia [11]. Different pains may affect a distinct part of the affected dermatome. Sensory changes are equally varied, with severe loss of sensitivity reported approximately as commonly as preserved sensation, even in the same patient. Some 25–30% of patients with PHN appear to have reduced cutaneous thresholds for heat pain in the affected dermatome (heat hyperalgesia) [12, 13] while some are found to have almost complete deafferentation [13, 14]. In a minority of patients, introduction of capsaicin increases pain and causes local flare, best explained by peripheral sensitization [15]. In others, lack of small fiber-mediated nociceptive function is associated with preservation of large fiber-mediated functions [14, 16]. These patients may have mechanical allodynia, probably due to central sensitization. A unifying theory of pathophysiology suggests there are several subtypes of PHN which, at least in theory, can be distinguished on clinical and neurophysiologic grounds [17].

However, linking pathophysiologic mechanisms to specific treatments has so far eluded investigators. As novel specific receptor agonists and antagonists

are being developed, this may change in the future. By 2007 several Phase I and Phase II studies were under way to test a number of antagonists and agonists aimed at specific receptors and ion channels known to be associated with neuropathic pain (e.g. TRPV1, TPRM8, Nav1.8, Nav1.9, CB1, CB2).

Chronic PHN is commonly associated with psychiatric co-morbidity (sleep, low mood, tendency to social isolation) which together with pain may lead to significant disability [15].

Epidemiology of herpes zoster

Population-based epidemiologic data suggest an annual incidence of HZ between 1.3 and 4.1 per 1000 population [18–20]. Some longitudinal studies suggest an increase in incidence in the last two decades although the reason for this is not clear [5, 20]. The incidence is much higher in the elderly; a recent study suggests an incidence rate of 2.1 per 1000 person-years in those under 50 and 10.1 in those over 80, a fivefold difference [20]. Other large studies show a similar trend [1, 19]. These figures are generally accepted to reflect the natural decline in cell-mediated immunity with advancing age. All reported studies rely on the clinical presentation of HZ. Some studies suggest that 10% of the diagnoses of HZ made in primary care are in fact due to zosteriform herpes simplex. Other common misdiagnoses include common dermatologic diseases such as contact dermatitis, erysipelas and insect bites [5, 21]. By contrast, atypical forms of herpes zoster also exist, such as zoster sine herpete, in which rash does not develop.

Immunocompromised patients represent 8–10% of HZ cases [20]. Some investigators have proposed that childhood varicella vaccination will alter the incidence figures considerably when it is more widely adopted. It is thought that the significant reduction in the incidence of varicella resulting from vaccination reduces the chance of exposure of the elderly to the exogenous viral antigen pool needed to boost their cell-mediated immunity. This fact combined with the rapid increase in the number of the elderly and immunocompromised patients is likely to lead to a short-term increase in herpes zoster cases [5]. However, if adult HZ vaccination becomes widely practiced as is expected, the long-term outcome is likely to be a significant reduction in HZ incidence.

Postherpetic neuralgia is the most common complication of herpes zoster. Estimates of its incidence come from both prospective community-based or large retrospective population-based studies. Hall and others evaluated data from the computerized UK general practice records and reported an annual incidence of 40 per 100,000 person-years [2]. This is higher than the incidence calculated from GP records in London of 11 per 100,000 person years [22] but similar to another British population study [23]. In line with incidence of HZ, PHN at 1 month was reported far more frequently by people aged 65–74 (11%) or over 75 (18%) than those 45–54 (4%) [1]. PHN usually resolves spontaneously, leaving a small percentage of patients to suffer from chronic pain.

Before the era of antiviral treatments, reports of the presence of PHN pain sufficient to induce a visit to the physician were 5–7% at 3 months, 3–5% at 6 months and 2–4% at 12 months [18, 24, 25]. Newer data obtained while antivirals were widely available suggest even lower figures. Helgason and co-authors collected data over a 6-year period on 421 patients representing a rural region in Iceland with approximately 100,000 inhabitants [26]. Only 2% of those under 60 years of age reported pain at 3 months which in all cases was mild. Thirty percent of patients over 70 reported pain at 3 months, 11% moderate or severe. At 12 months one patient (1%) in the 60–69 age group and one (2%) patient in the over-70 group reported moderate pain, and none had severe pain. At 12 months 3.3% reported pain, mostly mild. Two patients (0.5%) reported moderate pain. Of note, only 4% received antivirals [26]. Similar results were reported from two opportunistic patient populations. Haanpää *et al.* reported that at 6 months five of their original sample of 113 patients of all ages with HZ had pain of moderate or severe intensity [27]. Similarly, Thyregod and co-workers found at 6 months following the original rash that only two of the original 94 patients had clinically meaningful pain, which they defined at >3/10 [4]. These examples do not reflect the reality seen in many pain clinics who manage patients with intractable PHN. The incidence in the era of antivirals of this extreme form of PHN remains unknown but in all likelihood is very low. Nevertheless, as HZ remains a very common condition (with a 30% lifetime risk in developed countries [28]), there are likely to be a sufficient number of patients with disabling PHN who need specialized help and active pain management.

The prevalence of postherpetic neuralgia in the general population is unknown. One retrospective study based on GP records of patients of all ages in London estimated the lifetime prevalence for PHN (defined as pain at 1 month after the rash) to be 0.7 (95% confidence interval (CI) 0.4–1.0) per 1000 population [22]. Bowsher based his estimate on the personal histories obtained from a community survey of a cohort of 1071 people aged 64–99, and arrived at a figure of 25/1000 in that age group [29]. No estimate of severity of pain was attempted. An example of the difference of pain reported in surveys and those leading patients to seek help from their doctors comes from another study. In a prospective study of 598 patients with acute HZ and aged over 50, 16% had pain of any severity at 6 months, and 10% still reported it at 4 years [30]. However, severe pain was reported by 2% at 6 months and 0.7% (1 out of 139) at 4 years, underlining the vast difference between clinically relevant and other pain.

Prevention of postherpetic neuralgia

A large number of studies show that age is positively correlated with the risk of developing PHN [31]. Most studies also suggest that the severity of inflammation, measured from the extent and intensity of the rash, intensity of early pain and sensory abnormalities, independently adds to the risk of prolongation of PHN pain [31]. No clinical formula exists to predict the minority who after contracting shingles go on to develop the most chronic form of PHN.

Several approaches have been used in an attempt to curb the inflammatory impact of HZ early on. Studies on antivirals conducted in the 1990s have been subjected to four systematic reviews, which have reached somewhat different conclusions [32–35]. One meta-analysis included four trials with 692 patients [33] and another five trials with 792 patients [34]. Wood *et al.* carried out an analysis of the efficacy of aciclovir using Cox's proportional hazards model to test for the significance in group differences in the cessation of herpetic pain, in a pooled population of 691 patients with HZ. The combined overall hazard ratio was 1.79 (95% CI 1.34–2.39) and in the over-50s 2.13 (95% CI 1.42–3.19) (some unpublished data were included). Pain reduction in those receiving acyclovir was greater at 3 and 6 months [34]. Jackson included data from five studies and measured the risk of "any pain" at 6 months. The odds ratio for the incidence was 0.54 (95% CI 0.34–0.81) [33]. In a single multicenter double-blind placebo-controlled trial, famciclovir reduced the duration of postherpetic pain from 119 days (placebo) to 63 days (1500 mg/day) or 61 days (2250 mg/day) [36]. Comparison studies with valaciclovir and brivudin showed no difference [37, 38]. Although the overall evidence is limited [39], recommendations from expert panels favor commencement of antiviral in the first 72 hours after the onset of rash, among other things to maximize the speed of resolution of pain [5]. It is clear from existing data that prompt use of antivirals cannot guarantee freedom from chronic pain in severe cases.

Other treatments proposed and apparently commonly used in clinical practice do not seem to affect the course of HZ or alter the incidence of PHN. Many are based on no evidence or evidence from poor quality studies only. Better-quality studies tend to offer satisfactory evidence against the usefulness of interventions other than antiviral treatment. Early uncontrolled studies published in the 1970s and 1980s suggested some benefit from corticosteroids while small controlled trials did not. These were followed by two large randomized double-blind parallel group trials, with 349 and 241 patients, in which the effect of a week-long tapered prednisolone was evaluated [40, 41]. Both failed to show benefit, for pain at either 21 days or 6 months after rash. Two systematic reviews, one focusing on the two above studies and one evaluating four controlled trials, concurred that corticosteroids given in the early stages do not prevent PHN [35, 42]. A further recommendation was given against their use in the acute setting [39]. An expert panel, however, formulated a statement that their use in HZ can be contemplated for acute pain relief [5]. A single shot epidural steroid injection does not prevent PHN better than epidural saline despite providing temporary pain relief [43].

In a complex study [44] 600 patients over 55 years of age with severe HZ pain (>7/10) were randomized to receive either (a) aciclovir 30 g/kg/day and methylprednisolone 60 mg/day intravenously for 9 days, followed by oral prednisolone in tapering doses for 12 days or (b) epidural 0.25% bupivacaine 2–4 times a day and methylprednisolone 40 mg twice a week, administered over a period of 7 days; the cycle was repeated once or twice if pain persisted. Outcome measures were presence of pain, presence of abnormal sensations and complete recovery. Whether an independent assessor was used is not mentioned. An intention-to-treat analysis showed superiority of the epidural treatment with differences evident from the first month. In the aciclovir group 22% reported pain at 6 months and 22% at 12 months whereas the figures in the methylprednisolone group were significantly lower, 4% and 2% respectively. A similar pattern was seen with regard to sensory abnormalities. The authors based their explanation of the positive effect on reduced axonal transportation of viral inflammation due to bupivacaine; the role of corticosteroids was not discussed [44]. The successful recruitment in 3 years from two centers in Northern Italy of such a high number of patients fulfilling the inclusion criteria and willing to take part in this complicated study is an extraordinary achievement. The poor response to aciclovir and high percentage of patients with clinically meaningful PHN (22% with pain, range on VAS 2.5–7.5 with a mean of 4 after 1 year) in this group is surprising. Even accepting that the patients enrolled in the study had severe symptoms, and hence a higher risk of developing prolonged pain, the percentage of those who did so is higher than all epidemiologic studies to date would suggest. An expert panel took the view that despite the dramatic results, the epidural steroid approach (especially without concomitant antivirals) cannot be recommended without a confirmatory study employing stringent safety measures [5].

In a retrospective review of a nonrandomized case series where the treatment protocol changed over time, patients were divided into three groups: those receiving epidural saline and intermittent 1% mepivacaine and oral aciclovir or vidarabine; those receiving primarily intermittent epidural mepivacaine and only on-demand epidural mepivacaine infusion; and those receiving a priori epidural bupivacaine infusion with epidural bupivacaine top-ups as needed. This arrangement required an in-hospital admission for up to 3 months in severe cases [45]. In the bupivacaine infusion group the pain reduction occurred to a minimal level (20/100) sooner (12.4 (9.1–16.8) days versus

16.6 (10.9–25.2) days and 15.3 (11.6–20.3) days) in the severe pain group. The lack of randomization, sequential recruitment of patients and unusual design make this study difficult to interpret and the actual gain from this very arduous and expensive treatment approach seems to be of modest value.

Sympathetic blockade was suggested to reduce the risk of PHN in large uncontrolled case series [46]. However, only one controlled prospective trial has been published, with methodologic flaws preventing clinical conclusions being drawn from its marginal effect [47]. Two reviews conclude that sympathetic blockade plays no role in prevention of PHN – not surprising considering that all major pathophysiologic studies have hypothesized that the somatic afferents and their central connections are at the core of the pathophysiology of PHN [48, 49].

A small randomized double-blind study evaluated the effect of amitriptyline 25 mg/day compared to placebo in prevention of PHN [50]. The study setting was unusual in that it was co-ordinated by one investigator who recruited patients over 60 years of age through 39 local GP surgeries. GPs were provided with packages of amitriptyline or matching placebo to be distributed to patients with acute HZ of less than 48 hours duration. Patients were to take medication for 90 days. Antiviral treatment was not controlled and the prescribing happened at the participating GP's discretion. The primary outcome measure was the percentage of patients free of pain, based on the patient reporting to the investigator in a telephone discussion 6–8 months later. At 6 months, 32/38 (84%) patients on amitriptyline versus 22/34 (65%) on placebo were free of pain (P < 0.05). A post hoc analysis based on patients who received aciclovir (nine in the amitriptyline group, 17 in the placebo group) also indicated a significant difference [51]. However, several methdodologic flaws associated with the small number of patients recruited render the results unreliable. No attempt was made to ensure the groups were matched, the effect of aciclovir was not controlled, no ITT analysis was carried out, sampling of the information was based on the patient's recollection, and the aberrant outcomes in the placebo group were overlooked. As an example of the latter, 9/17 (53%) of patients randomized to receive placebo and aciclovir reported pain at 3 months, and 8/17 (47%) at 6 months, figures that are many times

higher than those in any recent community-based epidemiologic survey. In this small underpowered study the aberration is so substantial that it would negate the difference obtained between both groups. Similarly, three patients in both groups reported very slight pain. If these six are removed from the analysis, the group-wise difference disappears.

Vaccination

Boosting declining immunity in the elderly could in theory prevent HZ and subsequent PHN. In the first program of its kind, nearly 39,000 immunocompetent subjects over 60 years of age with a history of childhood varicella were randomized to receive live attenuated Oka VZV virus or placebo [3]. The incidence of HZ in the vaccinated group was 51.6% lower than in the placebo group during the mean follow-up of 3 years. There were fewer cases of PHN in the vaccine group than placebo group (0.46 case versus 1.38 cases, respectively, P < 0.001). PHN was defined as pain and discomfort >3/10. Adverse effects were more common in the vaccine group, and were mostly experienced at the injection site. No increase was seen in serious side effects. The cost-effectiveness of this prevention has divided opinion [52–54]. Other vaccination projects are under way in Europe.

Box 18.1 Prevention of postherpetic neuralgia

Interventions supported by evidence
Oral antivirals (within 72 hours of onset of rash)
Vaccine (in healthy people over 60)

Interventions refuted by evidence
Corticosteroids
Single shot epidural steroids
Topical antivirals

Uncertain – inconsistent or insufficient data
Epidural infusion of corticosteroids
Epidural infusion of local anesthetic
Sympathetic blockade
Amitriptyline

Treatment of postherpetic neuralgia

Since the 1970s, a large number of studies of varying quality have been published on pharmacotherapy of PHN. These have been subjected to two major systematic reviews of published clinical trials up to January 2004 and October 2004, respectively [55, 56]. In addition, Cochrane reviews on selected treatments of PHN also exist, including antidepressants, gabapentin, opioids, and topical lidocaine, with review dates ranging from 2005 to 2007 [57–60]. These extensive data are presented here with additional papers and observations regarding conclusions so far as they pertain to PHN. As for guidelines, the reader is advised to turn to a consensus paper commissioned by the European Federation of Neurological Sciences (EFNS) [61] in which treatments for neuropathic pain are recommended, with PHN singled out. General consensus papers based on systematic reviews on neuropathic pain also exist [62, 63].

The two comprehensive systematic reviews on the treatment of PHN differ somewhat in their inclusion and exclusion criteria, although their conclusions are fairly similar [55, 56]. Dubinsky *et al.* [55] followed the Practice Parameter guidelines of the American Academy of Neurology. They included papers based on trials which were of a minimum of 8 weeks duration, provided detailed methodology with a clear outcome measure, and consisted of therapy feasible for an outpatient setting. The quality of papers was based on the AAN criteria. These stipulate that to earn a Class I status, the paper has to be a prospective, randomized, controlled clinical trial with a masked outcome assessment and conducted in a representative population and, in addition, must fulfill other criteria to reduce bias. At the other end of the scale, Class IV studies represent evidence from uncontrolled trials, case series and case reports. Hempenstall *et al.*, by contrast, used the five point "Jadad" scoring system [56, 64]. Studies were included if they achieved a score of three or more on this scale and if they analyzed more than 10 patients [56].

Tricyclic antidepressants

Clinical trials in PHN have been conducted on the efficacy of amitriptyline, nortriptyline, desipramine, and maprolitine. Hempenstall and co-workers included

seven, Saarto & Wiffen eight and Dubinsky and coworkers six studies for their analysis [55–57]. The total number of patients entered into the reviewed studies ranged from 297 to 386. All reviews published show superiority of tricyclics over placebo, with a pooled number needed to treat (NNT) calculated at 2.64 (95% CI 2.1–3.54) or 2.2 (95% CI 1.6–3.1) [56, 57].

In the first randomized, double-blind, cross-over trial, amitriptyline was compared to placebo in 24 patients who all completed the study [65]. The mean dose of amitriptyline was 75 mg/day. Good to excellent pain relief was found in 16/24 patients during the 3-week amitriptyline treatment, significantly better than placebo, although the efficacy of the latter was not detailed [65]. Sleep improved more in the amitriptyline group. Two other studies on amitriptyline that were placebo controlled, albeit also including an active comparator, similarly demonstrated the superiority of amitriptyline [66, 67]. While in one study doses above 100 mg/day did not seem to improve outcome, in the other there was a clear dose-dependent response up to 150 mg/day [66, 67]. Co-morbidity was not adequately addressed. Two other studies, both involving 31 patients, compared amitriptyline with either maprolitine or nortriptyline [68, 69]. The maintenance doses used ranged from 10 to 150 mg/day for amitriptyline, 20–160 mg/day for nortriptyline and 50–150 mg/day for maprolitine. Amitriptyline appeared as effective as nortriptyline but was associated with a higher incidence of intolerable adverse effects (30% versus 15%). In group-wide comparison, maprolitine was less effective than amitriptyline; however, there were seven (20%) patients with pain unresponsive to amitriptyline who reported relief from maprolitine [68]. Sleep and disability improved and concomitant analgesic use decreased to a similar degree with both drugs [68, 69]. Twenty-six patients randomized to desipramine (mean dose 167 mg/day) or placebo, 19 of whom completed both arms of the double-blind cross-over study, reported greater pain relief at the end of the 6-week period compared to placebo [70]. The analysis was both per protocol and ITT with the same conclusion. The weakness of this study is that no washout period was used. Saarto & Wiffen [57] also included in their analysis a study on prevention of PHN [51], although the design of the study and follow-up arrangements were not adequate for the purpose.

The conclusion from all reviews is that tricyclic antidepressants are effective in postherpetic neuralgia. There is no obvious major difference between them in terms of efficacy of pain relief (especially taking into account patients' individual responses). Co-morbidity appears to improve in a similar manner across all drugs tested. Because of better tolerability, guidelines favor nortriptyline over amitriptyline [61]. No studies had been published by 2007 on SNRIs (venlafaxine, duloxetine) in PHN.

Tricyclic antidepressants have a relatively poor side effect profile, especially in the elderly who are at most risk for PHN. Common side effects are central and cholinergic: dry mouth, sweating, disturbed vision, dizziness, sedation, palpitations, orthostatic hypotension and urinary retention. An association between tricyclics in doses higher than 100 mg/day and sudden cardiac death has been described [71]. Guidelines vary in their recommendations on the use of ECG to detect subclinical conduction abnormalities prior to commencement of treatment using a tricyclic antidepressant [61, 62].

Gabapentin

Two double-blind placebo-controlled trials demonstrated superior efficacy of gabapentin over placebo in PHN [72, 73]. In the first, with 229 participants, gabapentin or placebo was titrated up to 3600 mg/day, following which the dose remained stable. The minimum dose accepted for the patient to remain in the trial was 1200 mg/day. Previous stable antidepressant and analgesic medication was allowed. The primary outcome measure was change in the average daily pain scored on a scale of 0–10. Just over 80% of randomized patients completed the study. Of those on gabapentin, 65% received 3600 mg/day and 83% at least 2400 mg/day. Gabapentin reduced pain by 33.3% compared to 7.7% achieved on placebo; 43% receiving gabapentin reported their pain as much or moderately improved versus 12% on placebo. Gabapentin also improved several dimensions of quality of life (measured using the SF-36) and mood (measured using the POMS)[72].

In the second study, 334 patients with PHN were randomized to either 2400 mg/day or 1800 mg/day of gabapentin or placebo, using a forced titration schedule which comprised a stepwise dose escalation to the target dose over 16 days [73]. Those unable to tolerate the regimen were withdrawn from the study. Previous failure to respond to gabapentin at ≤1200 mg/day was an exclusion criterion. Permissible medications during the trial included mild opioids and antidepressants. The primary outcome measure was reduction in daily pain score, while secondary outcome measures comprised a numerical rating scale (0–10) of sleep, Clinician and Patient Impression of Change, SF McGill Pain Questionnaire (SF-MPQ) and SF-30 as the measure of quality of life [73]. Just over 81% of the patients completed the trial. The daily pain score decreased 34.4% in the 1800 mg/day group, 34.5% in the 2400 mg/day group and 15.7% in the placebo group – a treatment difference of 18.8% (95% CI 10.7–26.7; $P < 0.001$). The difference between placebo and gabapentin was observed from the first week onwards. All parameters of SF-MPQ improved more on both doses of gabapentin than placebo. Gabapentin was also superior in improving sleep and some dimensions of quality of life [73].

Both studies reported similar adverse events. Withdrawals due to adverse effects were more common in those receiving any dose of gabapentin (13–18%) or placebo (6–10%). The most common side effects were dizziness, somnolence, ataxia, peripheral edema, asthenia, dry mouth and diarrhea, reported by >5% of participants [72, 73]. The combined NNT from these studies was calculated to be 4.4 (95% CI 3.3–6.10).

A slightly different picture emerges from a study involving 305 patients with neuropathic pain of various etiologies among whom there were 43 with PHN [74]. The inclusion and exclusion criteria were similar to those of Rice et al. [73]. The trial lasted a total of 8 weeks including an uptitration phase of 2–5 weeks during which dose escalation continued until patients reported a reduction in daily pain by at least 50% or the final target dose of 2400 mg/day was reached. Of the 305 entered, 234 (77%) completed the study. The authors report that the study demonstrates the superiority of gabapentin over placebo, with the mean daily pain score for the previous 7 days reduced 1.5 in the active drug group versus 0.5 in the placebo group (rank-based ANCOVA, $P = 0.048$). The treatment difference of 0.5 is amongst the lowest ever reported in studies showing efficacy in neuropathic pain. The authors also state that at weeks 7 and 8 there was no difference between placebo and gabapentin. Self-reports of allodynia, hyperalgesia, burning pain and shooting pain did not show a difference between the study groups. However, the Patient and Clinician Global Impression of Change favored gabapentin. Of the SF-36 measures, emotional role and social functioning improved more in the gabapentin group. A *post hoc* analysis showed similar responses to gabapentin in each pain syndrome included in the study, allowing the results to be extrapolated to PHN.

Gabapentin has a mode of action that seems to be restricted to the voltage-gated calcium channels (and specifically mediated by the $\alpha 2\delta$ subunit) of the receptors which are expressed in dorsal root ganglia and central terminals of neurones in neuropathic pain [75] with little effect on other ion channels or opioid receptors. Combining treatments with medications from different classes is regular clinical practice but controlled trials are few. Gilron and co-authors [76] devised a randomized four-way cross-over study in which gabapentin alone, morphine alone, combination of the two and active placebo (lorazepam) were compared. There were 57 patients with either PHN (n = 22) or painful diabetic neuropathy (n = 35). Each treatment arm lasted 5 weeks during which the drugs were uptitrated to the maximum tolerated dose. The gabapentin-morphine combination (mean daily dose of gabapentin: 1705 ± 38 mg; morphine: 34.4 ± 2.6 mg) was more effective than morphine alone (45.5 ± 3.9 mg/day) or gabapentin alone (2207 ± 89 mg/day), while all three active treatments were superior to placebo. Combined gabapentin and morphine caused more constipation than gabapentin alone and more dry mouth than morphine alone [76].

Pregabalin

As far as the pharmacologic properties of pregabalin are concerned, there are few differences between gabapentin and pregabalin, as both block the $\alpha 2\delta$ subunit of the voltage-gated calcium channel to prevent neurotransmitter release. The significant differences relate to better pharmacokinetics of pregabalin, with a need for no more than two administrations per day. Three multicenter, fixed-dose, parallel-group trials with a similar design consistently showed superiority of pregabalin over placebo [77–79]. The duration of the trials ranged from 8 to 13 weeks. Previous lack of response to gabapentin was an exclusion criterion. Concomitant analgesia was allowed (including opioids, antiepileptic and antidepressant drugs), and the primary efficacy measure was change in pain at

the end of the study. Sleep, mood and quality of life were measured as secondary outcomes. In the first study, the dose was force titrated to 600 mg/day (with one-third remaining on 300 mg/day due to low creatinine clearance). Reduction in mean pain scores was significantly greater in the pregabalin than placebo group (mean treatment difference –1.69 (95% CI –2.33 to –1.05). Of the secondary outcome measures, sleep and mood improved but quality of life did not (apart from general health perception and, inevitably, bodily pain) [77]. In another multicenter trial of 8 weeks' duration, 238 patients were randomized to receive pregabalin 150 mg day, 300 mg/day or placebo. The reduction in daily pain was significantly greater with pregabalin than placebo in both the 150 mg/day (mean difference -1.20 (95% CI 11.81 to -0.58)) and 300 mg/day groups (mean difference -1.57 (95% CI -2.20 to -0.95)). Sleep and mood, but not quality of life, improved significantly as well [78].

In the third study, 370 patients with PHN were randomized to receive either placebo or three doses of pregabalin, 150 mg/day, 300 mg/day and 600 mg/day, in a 13-week trial (including a 1-week titration phase) [79]. Pregabalin showed an increase in effect with increasing dosage. Weekly mean pain scores rated on an 11-point scale improved steadily in all groups and were greatest in the 600 mg/day group. Sleep improved in all active drug groups more than in the placebo group.

Gabapentin and pregabalin are, generally speaking, well tolerated although there are significant individual variations. The side effect profiles are identical, with dizziness, somnolence, dry mouth, weight gain, peripheral edema, blurred vision and constipation. Also cognitive problems and injuries due to falls are reported in some studies [77–79].

Opioids

Oxycodone titrated up to 60 mg/day was reported to reduce pain more than placebo in a double-blind cross-over study in which 50 patients were recruited [80]. Other stable analgesic medication was allowed, and 30% of the patients were on antidepressant medication. Of the total of 50 patients enrolled, 12 (24%) failed to complete the study, with one patient withdrawing because of side effects, the rest due to lack of efficacy. Oxycodone reduced steady pain, short-lived pain and allodynia more than placebo [80]. From the dichotomous data provided, the NNT was calculated to be 2.5 (95% CI 1.7–5.1). Controlled-release morphine was evaluated against nortriptyline (or desipramine) in a three-way double-blind cross-over study. Of the 76 patients initially randomized, 44 completed all three treatment arms [81]. Morphine (or, in case it was not tolerated methadone) reduced pain more than did tricyclic antidepressants (see paper) with an NNT of 2.79 (95% CI 2.0–4.6) versus NNT for tricyclics 3.73 (95% CI 2.43–7.99). In this study patients also expressed preference for opioids over tricyclics despite more frequent side effects.

In a controlled trial lacking placebo, high (0.75 mg/day) and low (0.15 mg/day) doses of levorphanol were compared in a group of patients with various neuropathic pains, of which 18 had PHN [82]. The pain reduction was 42% in the high and 10% in the low levorphanol group. IV morphine (0.3 mg/kg infused over 1 hour) reduced ongoing pain.

One placebo-controlled parallel-group trial was published in 2003, involving 127 patients who received flexible dosing between 100 mg and 400 mg/day of tramadol over 6 weeks [83]. Both per protocol and ITT analyses were reported. The mean daily dose in the tramadol group was 276(90) mg/day. Sixteen (25%) patients in the tramadol group and five (8%) in the placebo group prematurely discontinued the trial. Tramadol was reported to be superior to placebo, with an NNT of 4.7 (95% CI 2.9–19) in the ITT analysis. The wide 95% CI is noteworthy, and caution is recommended in drawing conclusions about its usefulness without corroboration from other studies [56].

Well-known side effects associated with the use of opioids are constipation, sedation, dizziness, nausea and vomiting, pruritus and urinary retention. Prophylactic use of antiemetics and laxatives may be considered. The risk for addiction in the general pain population appears low in long-term follow-up studies [84, 85] but there are no data relating specifically to patients with PHN. International guidelines recommend chronic opioids as second- or third-line treatments, reflecting these concerns.

Topical lidocaine

Three studies have evaluated the efficacy of topical lidocaine in patients with PHN [86–88]. Hempenstall and co-authors included only results published in

original full communications, whereas Khaliq and co-authors also included a randomized study that had only appeared as an abstract (with added data obtained from the US Food and Drug Administration) [56,60]. Both reviews concluded that topical lidocaine is superior to placebo. Further support for its efficacy comes from a double-blind, vehicle-controlled, two-way, cross-over trial conducted in patients with diverse peripheral neuropathic pains [89]. Of the participants, 55% had PHN. Each treatment arm lasted 7 days and was provided as an add-on to existing medication. Lidocaine plaster was superior to the vehicle patch, with a moderate effect size of 0.4 and an NNT (50%) of 4.4 (95% CI 2.1–17.5) for pain and 8.4 (3.5–α) for allodynia [89]. Lidocaine patches are well tolerated, with local irritation of the skin emerging as the only significant side effect. If not used over broken skin, systemic absorption is considered negligible [60]. The European Federation of Neurological Sciences Task Force recommends lidocaine plasters as the first-line treatment in focal painful neuropathies (such as PHN), and it is licensed for this indication in some European countries [61].

Other pharmacotherapies

A single RCT of 8 weeks duration reported valproic acid (1000 mg/day) to be highly efficacious compared to placebo in 42 patients with PHN. The treatment difference was −2.4 at the end of the trial, with 48% reported to be much or moderately improved versus 15% on placebo, leading to an NNT of 2.1 (95% CI 1.4–4.2). Only one patient withdrew due to an adverse event (vertigo) and only mild and transient central nervous system side effects were reported by three other patients. This small study with such promising results needs corroboration; however, guidelines on neuropathic pain recommend valproate as a second-, third- or fourth-line option [61–63].

The two systematic reviews and individual Cochrane reviews reach similar conclusions and recommendations on a number of drugs in the management of PHN, including tricyclic antidepressants, gabapentin, pregabalin, certain opioids, topical lidocaine, and moderate evidence for tramadol (Table 18.1) [55–60]. Other agents that have been subjected to smaller and lower quality trials require considerable discretion on the part of the reviewers, and it is in these circumstances that the reviewing panels

Table 18.1 Efficacy of treatments estimated from systematic reviews*

Agent	NNT**	NNH***
Tricyclic antidepressants	2.6 (2.1–3.5)	5.7 (3.3–18.6)
Gabapentin	4.4 (3.3–6.1)	4.1 (3.2–5.1)
Pregabalin	4.9 (3.7–7.6)	4.3 (2.8–9.2)
Strong opioids	2.7 (2.1–3.8)	3.6 (2.2–10.2)
Tramadol	4.8 (2.6–27.0)	
Topical lidocaine	2.0 (1.4–3.3)	
Topical capsaicin	3.3 (2.3–5.9)	3.9 (2.5–8.6)
IT methylprednisolone	1.1 (1.1–1.2)	
Sodium valproate	2.1 (1.4–20.6)	

*Hempenstall et al. [56] modified; **NNT numbers needed to treat for 50% pain relief compared to placebo; ***NNH, numbers needed to harm (minor harm).

reach different conclusions. Hempenstall and co-workers took the view that capsaicin has the potential to provide pain relief whereas Dubinsky *et al.* considered the magnitude of improvement too small for clinical usefulness [55, 56]. The efficacy of topical aspirin was considered possibly effective in one but not the other review [55, 56]. Both panels, however, agree on the lack of efficacy of NMDA antagonists, lorazepam, topical indomethacin, iontophoresis of vincristine, epidural morphine, and epidural methylprednisolone. There is also some difference in how the reviewers classified treatments as either "proven ineffective" or "inadequately tested," e.g. vitamin E, zimeldine, subcutaneous cronaissal and intravenous lidocaine [55, 56]. Over the years very large numbers of treatments have been advocated but not subjected to any form of critical analysis and these are not discussed further here.

Finally, a controversial paper was published on the efficacy of intrathecal methylprednisolone in chronic intractable PHN [90]. None of the systematic reviews or existing guidelines accept the results to the point of recommending this therapy in spite of the dramatic results reported. In this multicenter study from Japan published in 2000, 277 patients with intractable PHN were randomized to receive four intrathecal injections of methylprednisolone (60 mg) and 3% lidocaine, or 3% lidocaine. Control patients received no injections. Pain and allodynia at the end of the treatment period, 4 weeks, 1 year and 2 years consistently and substantially favored IT methylprednisolone. Concentration

of interleukin-8 in the cerebrospinal fluid halved during the treatment and this change correlated with pain relief. No complications were reported and MRI taken at the end of the intrathecal injections and a year later showed no change in the spinal cord. There has been little enthusiasm in the pain community to take up this practice and a corroborative study with a focus on safety measurement is very much in demand.

Adverse effects

Adverse effects have been presented in several different ways. It is probably not useful to generalize from individual studies considering the methodologic differences of data collection, estimation of severity, dosaging, inclusion and exclusion criteria and policies of patient withdrawal. A crude method adopted by Hempenstall and co-workers was to calculate number needed to harm (NNH) based on withdrawals from studies due to side effects [56]. An abbreviated list is presented in Table 18.1.

Detailed information is readily available for the pharmacokinetics and side effect profiles of individual drugs, their indications and contraindications in different patient populations and different age groups. The reader is strongly advised to use such material to become fluent with the pharmacologic properties of the drugs they choose to prescribe.

Cost-effectiveness

Relatively few studies have been published on relative costs of pharmacologic therapies. Because the costs are not stable, many reports are obsolete by the time they are published. From the reader's viewpoint, a confusing feature is the variability of of criteria for economic costings and economic models used. Depending on the authors, all recommended pharmacologic agents emerge as cost-effective from the analyses [91–95]. Regarding treatments in the UK in late 2007, the following were inexpensive: all tricyclics, gabapentin, tramadol, morphine, methadone, sodium valproate, whereas oxycodone was moderately expensive and pregabalin and lidocaine plasters expensive.

Nonpharmacologic treatments

Two studies appear to have been published on the use of neurostimulation in PHN. In 62 patients weekly acupuncture was compared to mock TENS over eight sessions [96]. No difference in pain relief was found between the two groups: in both, approximately one-fifth reported improvement irrespective of the treatment. Genuine TENS was inferior to combined clomipramine and carbamazepine in a moderate-quality study involving 29 patients (odds ratio 0.15; 95% CI 0.03–0.7) [97]. There is currently insufficient evidence to support the use of either acupuncture or TENS in PHN.

Although controlled studies demonstrate that spinal cord stimulation (SCS) is effective in some neuropathic conditions, none have been published on PHN. In one case series of 28 patients good results were reported from SCS in 82% of patients with PHN [98]. Patients were those responding to a sympathetic block and did not have sensory deficits. The effect of SCS was tested at times by switching off the stimulator. There were 10 patients who recovered, five who developed progressive dementia and one who only reported pain at 2/10 during 60 hours of nonstimulation. Unequivocal long-term benefit was therefore seen in 12/28 (40%) in this carefully chosen patient population. A properly controlled trial seems warranted in view of these results.

For neuroablative surgical interventions, several small case series have been published. These range from neurectomy to dorsal root entry zone ablation, spinal trigeminal nucleotractotomy and stereotactic radiosurgery of the trigeminal root [99]. The reported outcomes suggest satisfactory pain relief lasting 2 or 3 years. These results are highly contentious and almost certainly represent a small number of surgical interventions attempted with a strong publication bias. The data are far too limited and methodologic flaws too significant in the reports to allow any recommendation on the use of neurodestructive procedures.

Author's recommendations

The author is an advocate of use of combination medication in PHN. Although properly controlled studies are few [76], most well-controlled studies have allowed the continuation of stable analgesia throughout trials, in effect assessing efficacy of add-on treatment. The mode of action of topical lidocaine, gabapentinoids, tricyclics and opioids is sufficiently different to justify their combined use. The finding by Raja et al. that patients with PHN would respond differently to tricyclics and opioids is in line with this thinking [80].

The author's practice is based on sequential addition of medication with a firm target set in mixture of several agents to optimize pain relief with acceptable side effects. Choice of pharmacologic agents follows the recommendations of the EFNS [61]. The treatment is commenced with topical lidocaine (except in case of severe deafferentation) in conjunction with a gabapentinoid. A tricyclic antidepressant (occasionally an SNRI) is added if not contraindicated in most cases, as soon as the effect of the gabapentinoid is established. Ineffective treatment is stopped whereas in refractory cases low-dose strong opioids are introduced. It is critical

---

Box 18.2   Treatment of established postherpetic neuralgia

Interventions supported by evidence

Tricyclic antdepressants
Gabapentin
Pregabalin
(Strong) opioids
Topical lidocaine
Tramadol
Capsaicin (0.075%)

Interventions refuted by evidence

Epidural morphine
Epidural methylprednisolone
NSAIDs
NMDA antagonists
Lorazepam
Intravenous lidocaine
Acupuncture
Vincristine by iontophoresis

Uncertain – inconsistent or insufficient data

Intrathecal methylprednisolone
Sympathetic blockade
Spinal cord stimulation
TENS
Topical aspirin
Sodium valproate
Carbamazepine
Paracetamol
Mild opioids (codeine, dihydrocodeine)

Modified from Dubinsky et al. [55]), Hempenstall et al. [56], Saarto & Wiffen [57], Wiffen et al. [58], Eisenberg et al. [59], Khaliq et al. [60], Attal et al. [61].

to engage the patient in understanding the target of achieving the best benefit/adverse effect ratio rather than excellent pain relief. A key aspect of patient education is to provide a decent prognosis for the recovery, discussed in this chapter. Very refractory cases are very rare so an element of optimism and hope can be offered while gently curtailing the patient's expectations with realism.

Many treatments I have seen colleagues endorse, e.g. local injections, TENS, desensitization therapy, continuing search for an effective drug, hypnosis, herbal treatment or other forms of complementary therapy, are not in my armamentarium. I have used spinal cord stimulation with variable success and in relatively young (<70 years) patients who have been refractory (or more commonly entirely intolerant of most medications). Most patients with refractory PHN, however, are elderly and have relative contraindications to spinal cord stimulation, so its use in general is very limited. I remain reluctant to recommend either neuroablation or demanding neuromodulation, such as deep brain stimulation. Although depression and anxiety are common in this condition, psychiatric treatment rarely helps as colleagues are easily overwhelmed by the patient's pain presentation, and I believe that a sympathetic clinician with some understanding of and tolerance toward psychologic distress will be able to help their patient more.

Research priorities

Although successful programs have been initiated to vaccinate children against chickenpox and elderly people against HZ, we are far from globally eradicating the virus and in all likelihood will be treating patients with PHN during the next few decades. Much research will be needed to establish how effectively PHN can be prevented through immunization. Interventions during HZ to prevent PHN are too little researched, partially due to limited understanding of the pathophysiology of prolonged pain. A better understanding of the transition of HZ to PHN may reveal a new target for preventive treatment. Whereas highly invasive interventions possibly have a potential to lessen the development of PHN [44, 45], they are not practical in the clinic, and lesser interventions are not helpful [43]. We need studies to establish whether substantial pain relief *per se* (irrespective of

the method used) in the acute stage is sufficient to prevent PHN or whether a more precise alteration in neural signaling is required. As is the case with other neuropathic pain conditions, better treatment outcomes for chronic PHN will require a leap in pharmacologic development. The goal of mechanically based treatment of neuropathic pain remains realistic but advances toward it have been slow.

References

1. Opstelten W, Mauritz JW, de Wit NJ, *et al.* Herpes zoster and postherpetic neuralgia: incidence and risk indicators using a general practice research database. *Fam Pract* 2002; **19**: 471–475.
2. Hall GC, Carroll D, Parry D, McQuay HJ. Epidemiology and treatment of neuropathic pain: the UK primary care perspective. *Pain* 2006; **122**: 156–162.
3. Oxman MN, Levin MJ, Johson GR, *et al.* A vaccine to prevent herpes zoster and postherpetic neuralgia in older adults. *N Engl J Med* 2005; **352**: 2271–2284.
4. Thyregod HG, Rowbotham MC, Peters M, Possehn J, Berro M, Petersen KL. Natural history of pain following herpes zoster. *Pain* 2007; **128**: 148–156.
5. Dworkin RH, Johnson RW, Breuer J, *et al.* Recommendations for the management of herpes zoster. *Clin Infect Dis* 2007; **44**(suppl 1): S1–26.
6. Zacks W, Lanfitt TW, Elliott FA. Herpetic neuritis: a light electron microscopic study. *Neurology* 1964; **14**: 744–750.
7. Haanpää M, Dastidar P, Weinberg A, *et al.* CSF and MRI findings in patients with acute herpes zoster. *Neurology* 1998; **51**: 1405–1411.
8. Denny-Brown D, Adams RD, Fitzgerald PJ. Pathologic features of herpes zoster. *Arch Neurol Psychiatr* 1944; **57**: 216–231.
9. Watson CPN, Deck JH, Morshead C, van Kooy D, Evans RJ. Postherpetic neuralgia: further post-mortem studies of cases with and without pain. *Pain* 1991; **44**: 105–117.
10. Oaklander AL, Romans K, Horasek S, Stocks A, Hauer P, Meyer RA. Unilateral postherpetic neuralgia is associated with bilateral sensory neuron damage. *Ann Neurol* 1998; **44**: 789–795.
11. Nurmikko T. Clinical features and pathophysiological mechanisms of postherpetic neuralgia. *Neurology* 1995; **45**(suppl 8): S54–S55.
12. Rowbotham MC, Fields HL. The relationship of pain, allodynia and thermal sensation in post-herpetic neuralgia. *Brain* 1996; **119**: 347–354.
13. Pappagallo M, Oaklander AL, Qutrano-Piancentini AL, Clark MR, Raja SR. Heterogeneous patterns of sensory dysfunction in postherpetic neuralgia suggest multiple pathophysiological mechanisms. *Anesthesiology* 2000; **92**: 691–698.
14. Nurmikko T, Bowsher D. Somatosensory findings in postherpetic neuralgia. *J Neurol Neurosurg Psychiatry* 1990; **53**: 135–141.

15. Petersen KL, Fields HL, Brennum J, Sandroni P, Rowbotham MC. Capsaicin evoked pain and allodynia in post-herpetic neuralgia. *Pain* 2000; **88**: 125–133.

16. Baron R, Saguer M. Postherpetic neuralgia. Are C-nociceptors involved in signalling and maintenance of tactile allodynia? *Brain* 1993; **116**: 1477–1496.

17. Field HL, Rowbotham MC. Postherpetic neuralgia: irritable nociceptors and deafferentation. *Neurobiol Dis* 1998; **5**: 209–227.

18. Ragozzino MW, Melton LJ III, Kurland LT, Chu CP, Perry HO. Population-based study of herpes zoster and its sequelae. *Medicine* 1982; **61**: 310–316.

19. Donahue JG, Choo PW, Manson J, Platt R. The incidence of herpes zoster. *Arch Intern Med* 1995; **155**: 1605–1609.

20. Yawn BP, Saddier P, Wollan PC, Sauver JL, Kurland MJ, Sy LS. A population-based study of the incidence of herpes zoster and complication rates before zoster vaccine introduction. *Mayo Clin Proc* 2007; **82**: 1341–1349.

21. Scott F, Leedham-Green ME, Barrett-Muir WY, *et al.* A study of shingles and the development of postherpetic neuralgia in East London. *J Med Virol* 2003; **70**: S24–S30.

22. MacDonald BK, Cockerell OC, Sander JWAS, Shorvon SD. The incidence and lifetime prevalence of neurological disorders in a prospective community-based study in the UK. *Brain* 2000; **123**: 665–676.

23. Cockerell OC, Goodridge DM, Brodie D, Sander JW, Shorvon SD. Neurological disease in a defined population: the results of pilot study in two general practices. *Neuroepidemiology* 1996; **15**: 73–82.

24. Burgoon CF, Burgoon JS, Baldridge GD. The natural history of herpes zoster. *JAMA* 1957; **164**: 265–269.

25. Hope-Simpson RE. The nature of herpes zoster: a long-term study and anew hypothesis. *Proc R Soc Med* 1965; **58**: 9–20.

26. Helgason S, Petursson G, Gudmundsson S, Sigurdsson JA. Prevalence of postherpetic neuralgia after a first episode of herpes zoster: prospective study with long term follow up. *BMJ* 2000; **321**: 794–796.

27. Haanpää M, Laippala P, Nurmikko T. Allodynia and pinprick hypesthesia in acute herpes zoster, and the development of postherpetic neuralgia. *J Pain Symptom Manage* 2000; **20**: 50–58.

28. Scott FT, Johnson RW, Leedham-Green M, Davies E, Edmunds WJ, Breuer J. The burden of herpes zoster: a prospective population based study. *Vaccine* 2006; **24**: 1308–1314.

29. Bowsher D. The lifetime occurrence of herpes zoster and prevalence of post-herpetic neuralgia: a retrospective survey in an elderly population. *Eur J Pain* 1999; **3**: 335–341.

30. van Wijck AJM, Opstelten W, van Essen GA, Verheij TJM, Moons KGM, Kalkman CJ. Long-term follow up of herpes zoster patients. In: van Wijck AJM (ed) *Postherpetic Neuralgia*. Febodruk BV, Enschede, 1996: 61–70 .

31. Jung BF, Johnson RW, Griffin DRJ, Dworkin RH. Risk factors for postherpetic neuralgia in patients with herpes zoster. *Neurology* 2004; **62**: 1545–1551.

32. Lancaster T, Silagy C, Gray S. Primary care management of acute herpes zoster: systematic review of evidence from randomized controlled trials. *Br J Gen Pract* 1995; **45**: 39–45.

33. Jackson JL, Gibbons R, Meyer G, *et al.* The effect of treating herpes zoster with oral acyclovir: a meta-analysis. *Arch Intern Med* 1997; **157**: 909–912.

34. Wood MJ, Kay R, Dworkin RH, *et al.* Oral acyclovir therapy accelerates pain resolution in patients with herpes zoster: a meta-analysis of placebo-controlled trial. *Clin Infect Dis* 1996; **22**: 341–347.

35. Alper BS, Lewis PR. Does treatment of acute herpes zoster prevent or shorten postherpetic neuralgia? *J Fam Pract* 2000; **49**: 255–264.

36. Tyring S, Barbarash RA, Nahlik JE, *et al.* Famciclovir vor the treatment of acute herpes zoster: efects on acute disease and postherpetic neuralgia: a randomized, double-blind, placebo-controlled trial. *Ann Intern Med* 1995; **123**: 89–96.

37. Tyring SK, Beutner KR, Tucker BA, Anderson WC, Crooks RJ. Antiviral therapy for herpes zoster: randomized controlled clinical study of valacyclovir and famciclovir therapy in immunocomptenet patients 50 and older. *Arch Fam Med* 2000; **9**: 863–869.

38. Wassilew SW. Brivudin compared with famciclovir in the treatment of herpes zoster effects in acute disease and chronic pain in immunocompetent patients. *J Eur Acad Dermatol Venereol* 2005; **19**: 47–55.

39. Wareham D. Postherpetic neuralgia. *Clin Evid Online* 2007; Aug 1: 0905.

40. Wood MJ, Johnson RW, McKendrick MW, *et al.* A randomized trial of acyclovir for 7 days or 21 days with and without prednisolone for treatment of acute herpes zoster. *N Engl J Med* 1994; **330**: 896–900.

41. Whitley RJ, Weiss H, Gnann JW, *et al.* Acyclovir with and without prednisolone for the treatment of herpes zoster. *Ann Intern Med* 1996; **125**: 376–383.

42. MacFarlane LL, Simmons MM, Hunter MH. The use of corticosteroids in the management of herpes zoster. *J Am Board Fam Pract* 1998; **11**: 224–228.

43. van Wijck AJM, Opstelten W, Moons KGM, *et al.* The PINE study of epidural steroids and local anaesthetics to prevent postherpetic neuralgia: a randomized controlled trial. *Lancet* 2006; **367**: 219–224.

44. Pasqualucci A, Pasqualucci G, Galla F, *et al.* Prevention of postherpetic neuralgia: acyclovir and prednisolone versus epidural local anesthetic and methylprednisolone. *Acta Scand Anaesthesiol* 2000; **44**: 910–918.

45. Manabe H, Dan K, Hirata K, *et al.* Optimum pain relief with continuous epidural infusion of local anesthetics shortens the duration of zoster-associated pain. *Clin J Pain* 2004; **20**: 302–308.

46. Winnie AP, Hartwell WP. Relationship between time of treatment of acute herpes zoster with sympathetic blockade and prevention of postherpetic neuralgia: clinical support for a new theory of the mechanism by which sympathetic blockade provides therapeutic benefit. *Reg Anesth* 1993; **18**: 277–282.

47. Tenicela R, Lovasik D, Eaglstein W. Treatment of herpes zoster with sympathetic blocks. *Clin J Pain* 1985; **1**: 63–67.

48. Wu CL, Marsh A, Dworkin RH. The role of sympathetic nerve blocks in herpes zoster and postherpetic neuralgia. *Pain* 2000; **87**: 121–129.

49. Opstelten W, van Wijck AJ, Stolker RJ. Interventions to prevent postherpetic neuralgia: cutaneous and percutaneous techniques. *Pain* 2004; **107**: 202–206.

50. Bowsher D. The effects of pre-emptive treatment of postherpetic neuralgia with amitriptyline: a randomized, double-blind, placebo-controlled trial. *J Pain Symptom Manage* 1997; **13**: 327–331.

51. Dworkin RH. Prevention of postherpetic neuralgia. *Lancet* 1999; **353**: 1636–1637.

52. Hornberger J, Roberts K. Cost-effectiveness of a vaccine to prevent herpes zoster and postherpetic neuralgia in older adults. *Ann Intern Med* 2006; **145**: 317–325.

53. Rothberg MB, Virapongse A, Smith KS. Cost effectiveness of a vaccine to prevent herpes zoster and postherpetic neuralgia in older adults. *Clin Infect Dis* 2007; **44**: 1200–1208.

54. Brisson M, Pellissier J, Levin MJ. Cost-effectiveness of herpes zoster vaccine: flawed assumptions regarding efficacy against postherpetic neuralgia. *Clin Infect Dis* 2007; **45**: 1527–1529.

55. Dubinsky RM, Kabbani H, El-Chami Z, Boutwell C, Ali H. Practice Parameter: treatment of postherpetic neuralgia. An evidence-based report of the Quality Standards Committee of the American Academy of Neurology. *Neurology* 2004; **63**: 959–965.

56. Hempenstall K, Nurmikko TJ, Johnson RW, A'Hern RP, Rice AS. Analgesic therapy in postherpetic neuralgia: a quantitative systematic review. *PLoS Med* 2005; **2**: e164.

57. Saarto T, Wiffen PJ. Antidepressants for neuropathic pain. Cochrane Database of Systematic Reviews 2007, Issue 4. Art. No.: CD005454. DOI: 10.1002/1465858.CD005454.pub2.

58. Wiffen PJ, McQuay HJ, Edwards JE, Moore RA. Gabapentin for acute and chronic pain. Cochrane Database of Systematic Reviews 2005, Issue 3. Art. No.: CD005452. DOI: 10.1002/14651858.CD005452.

59. Eisenberg E, McNicol E, Carr DB. Opioids for neuropathic pain. Cochrane Database of Systematic Reviews 2006, Issue 3. Art. No.: CD006146. DOI: 10.1002/14651858.CD006146.

60. Khaliq W, Alam S, Puri N. Topical lidocaine for the treatment of postherpetic neuralgia. Cochrane Database of Systematic Reviews 2007, Issue 2. Art. No.: CD004846. DOI: 10.1002/14651858.CD004846.pub2.

61. Attal N, Cruccu G, Haanpää M, et al. EFNS guidelines on pharmacological treatment of neuropathic pain. *Eur J Neurol* 2006; **13**: 1153–1169.

62. Moulin DE, Clark AJ, Gilron I, et al. Pharmacological management of chronic neuropathic pain – consensus statement and guidelines from the Canadian Pain Society. *Pain Res Manage* 2007; **12**(1): 13–21.

63. Dworkin RH, O'Connor AB, Backonja M, et al. Pharmacologic management of neuropathic pain: evidence based recommendations. *Pain* 2007; **132**: 237–251.

64. Jadad AR, Moore RA, Carroll D, et al. Assessing the quality of reports of randomized clinical trials: is blinding necessary? *Control Clin Trials* 1996; **17**: 1–12.

65. Watson CP, Evans RJ, Reed K, Merskey H, Goldsmith L, Warsh J. Amitriptyline versus placebo in postherpetic neuralgia. *Neurology* 1982; **32**: 671–673.

66. Max MB, Schafer SC, Culnane M, et al. Amitriptyline, but not lorazepam, relieves postherpetic neuralgia. *Neurology* 1998; **38**: 1427–1432.

67. Graff-Radford SB, Shaw LR, Naliboff BN. Amitriptyline and fluphenazine in the treatment of postherpetic neuralgia. *Clin J Pain* 2000; **16**: 188–192.

68. Watson CPN, Chipman M, Reed K, Evans RJ, Birkett N. Amitriptyline versus maprolitine in postherpetic neuralgia: a randomized, double-blind, crossover trial. *Pain* 1992; **48**: 29–36.

69. Watson CPN, Vernich L, Chipman M, Reed K. Nortriptyline versus amitriptyline in postherpetic neuralgia. *Neurology* 1998; **51**: 1166–1171.

70. Kishore-Kumar R, Max MB, Schafer SC, et al. Desipramine relieves postherpetic neuralgia. *Clin Pharm Ther* 1990; **47**: 305–312.

71. Ray WA, Meredith S, Thapa PB, et al. Cyclic antidepressants and the risk of sudden cardiac death. *Clin Pharmacol Ther* 2004; **75**: 234–241.

72. Rowbotham M, Harden N, Stacey B, Bernstein P, Magnus-Miller L. Gabapentin for the treatment of postherpetic neuralgia: a randomized controlled trial. *JAMA* 1998; **280**: 1837–1842.

73. Rice ACR, Maton S, Postherpetic Neuralgia Study Group. Gabapentin in postherpetic neuralgia: a randomized, double-blind, placebo-controlled study. *Pain* 2001; **94**: 215–224.

74. Serpell MG, Neuropathic Pain Study Group. Gabapentin in neuropathic pain syndromes: a randomized, double-blind, placebo-controlled trial. *Pain* 2002; **99**: 557–566.

75. Field MJ, Cox PJ, Stott E. Identification of the α-2-δ subunit of voltage dependent calcium channels as a molecular target for pain mediating the analgesic actions of pregabalin. *PNAS* 2006; **46**: 17537–17542.

76. Gilron I, Bailey JM, Tu D, et al. Morphine, gabapentin or their combination for neuropathic pain. *N Engl J Med* 2005; **13**: 1324–1334.

77. Dworkin RH, Corbin AE, Young JP Jr, et al. Pregabalin for the treatment of postherpetic neuralgia: a randomized, placebo-controlled trial. *Neurology* 2003; **60**: 1274–1283.

78. Sabatowski R, Galvez R, Cherry DA, et al. Pregabalin reduces pain and improves sleep and mood disturbances in patients with post-herpetic neuralgia: results of a randomized, placebo-controlled clinical trial. *Pain* 2004; **109**: 26–35.

79. van Seventer R, Feister HA, Young JP Jr, et al. Efficacy and tolerability of twice-daily pregabalin for treating pain and related sleep interference in postherpetic neuralgia: a 13 week, randomized trial. *Curr Med Res Opin* 2006; **2**: 375–384.

80. Raja SN, Haythornthwaite JA, Pappagallo M, et al. Opioids versus antidepressants in postherpetic neuralgia. A randomized, placebo-controlled trial. *Neurology* 2002; **59**: 1015–1021.

81. Watson CPN, Babul N. Efficacy of oxycodone in neuropathic pain. A randomized trial in postherpetic neuralgia. *Neurology* 1998; **50**: 1837–1841.

82. Boureau F, Legallicier P, Kabir-Ahmadi M. Tramadol in post-herpetic neuralgia: a randomized, double-blind, placebo-controlled trial. *Pain* 2003; **104**: 323–331.

83. Watson CPN, Watt-Watson JH, Chipman ML. Chronic non-cancer pain and the long term utility of opioids. *Pain Res Manage* 2004; **9**: 19–24.

84. Jensen MK, Thomsen AB, Højsted J. 10-year follow-up of chronic non-malignant pain patients: opioid use, health related quality of life and health care utilization. *Eur J Pain* 2006; **10**: 423–433.

85. Rowbotham MC, Davies PS, Verkempinck C, Galer BS. Lidocaine patch: double-blind controlled study of a new treatment method for post-herpetic neuralgia. *Pain* 1996; **65**: 39–44.

86. Rowbotham MC, Davies PM, Fields HL. Topical lidocaine gel relieves postherpetic neuralgia. *Ann Neurol* 1995; **37**: 246–253.

87. Galer BS, Rowbotham MC, Perander J, Friedman E. Topical lidocaine patch relieves postherpetic neuralgia more effectively than a vehicle topical patch: results of an enrichment enrollment study. *Pain* 1999; **80**: 533–538.

88. Rowbotham MC, Twilling L, Davies PM, Reisner L, Taylor K, Mohr D. Oral opioid therapy for chronic peripheral and central neuropathic pain. *N Engl J Med* 2003; **348**: 1223–1232.

89. Kochar DK, Garg P, Bumb RA, *et al.* Divalproex sodium in the management of post-herpetic neuralgia: a randomized double-blind placebo-controlled study: *Q J Med* 2005; **98**: 29–34.

90. Kotani N, Kushikata T, Hashimoto H, *et al.* Intrathecal methylprednisolone for intractable postherpetic neuralgia. *N Engl J Med* 2000; **343**: 1514–1549.

91. Smith KJ, Roberts MS. Sequential medication strategies for postherpetic neuralgia a cost-effectiveness analysis. *J Pain* 2005; **8**: 369–404.

92. Tarride J-E, Gordon A, Vera-Llonch M, Dukes E, Rousseau C. Cost effectiveness of pregabalin in the management of neuropathic pain associated with diabetic neuropathy and postherpetic neuralgia: a Canadian experience. *Clin Ther* 2006; **28**: 1922–1934.

93. Cepeda MS, Farrar JT. Economic evaluation of oral treatments for neuropathic pain. *J Pain* 2006; **7**: 119–128.

94. Dakin H, Nuijten M, Liedgens H, Nautrup BP. Cost-effectiveness of a lidocaine 5% medicated plaster relative to gabapentin for postherpetic neuralgia in the United Kingdom. *Clin Ther* 2007; **29**: 1491–1507.

95. O'Connor AB, Noyes KN, Holloway RG. A cost-effectiveness comparison of desipramine, gabapentin and pregabalin for treating postherpetic neuralgia. *J Am Ger Soc* 2007; **55**: 1176–1184.

96. Lewith GT, Field J, Machin D. Acupuncture compared with placebo in postherpetic pain. *Pain* 1983; **17**: 361–368.

97. Gerson GR, Jones RB, Luscombe DK. Studies on concomitant use of carbamazepine and clomipramine for the relief of postherpetic neuralgia. *Postgrad Med J* 1977; **53**(suppl 4): 104–109.

98. Harke H, Gretenkort P, Ladleif HU, Koester P, Rahman S. Spinal cord stimulation in postherpetic neuralgia and in acute herpes zoster pain. *Anesth Analg* 2002; **94**: 694–700.

99. Nurmikko T, Haanpää M. Treatment of postherpetic neuralgia. *Curr Pain Head Rep* 2005; **9**: 161–167.

CHAPTER 19

Phantom limb pain

Lone Nikolajsen

Department of Anaesthesiology and Danish Pain Research Center, Aarhus University Hospital, Aarhus, Denmark

Introduction

Virtually all amputees experience phantom-phenomena following limb amputation. The patients feel that the missing limb is still present, and some may have vivid sensations of shape, length, posture and movement. Such nonpainful phantom sensations rarely pose any clinical problem, but 60–80% of all amputees also have painful sensations located to the missing limb. Stump pain is another consequence of amputation, but in most patients the pain subsides within a few weeks. However, some patients develop chronic pain located to the stump. Phantom limb sensation, phantom limb pain and stump pain often co-exist in the same patient and the elements may be difficult to separate.

The present chapter will focus on phantom limb pain. The following definitions will be used.

- Phantom limb sensation: any sensation of the missing limb, except pain.
- Phantom limb pain: painful sensations referred to the missing limb.
- Stump pain: pain referred to the amputation stump.

Pathophysiology

The mechanisms underlying phantom limb pain are not fully known despite extensive research in the area. The development of animal models that mimic

Evidence-Based Chronic Pain Management. Edited by C. Stannard, E. Kalso and J. Ballantyne. © 2010 Blackwell Publishing.

neuropathic pain and research in other neuropathic pain conditions have, however, contributed significantly to the understanding of phantom limb pain. It is now clear that nerve injury is followed by a number of morphologic, physiologic and chemical changes in both the peripheral and central nervous systems, and that these changes are likely to play a role in the induction and maintenance of phantom limb pain [1]. An overview of the mechanisms involved is presented in Figure 19.1.

Peripheral factors

Several clinical studies support the notion that mechanisms in the periphery (i.e. in the stump or in central parts of the sectioned afferents) play a role in the phantom limb concept.

- Phantom limb pain is significantly more frequent in amputees with long-term stump pain than in those without persistent pain [2].
- Stump pathology with altered stump sensibility is a common feature.
- Phantom pain and pressure pain thresholds at the stump are inversely correlated early after amputation [3].
- Phantom sensations can be modulated by various stump manipulations [4].
- Tapping of neuromas may increase phantom pain.
- Phantom limb sensations are temporarily abolished after local stump anesthesia.
- Changes in blood flow may alter the phantom limb perception.

These clinical observations are supported by experimental studies. Following a nerve cut, formation of neuromas is seen universally. Such neuromas show spontaneous and abnormal evoked activity following

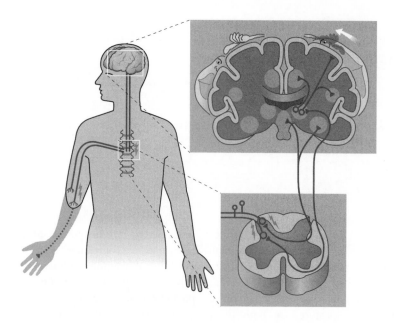

Figure 19.1 A schematic diagram of the areas involved in the generation of phantom limb pain and the main peripheral and central mechanisms.

mechanical or chemical stimulation. The ectopic and increased spontaneous and evoked activity from the periphery is assumed to be the result of an increased expression of sodium channels. In the dorsal root ganglion (DRG) cells, changes also occur following a complete nerve cut. Cell bodies in the DRG show abnormal spontaneous activity and increased sensitivity to mechanical and neurochemical stimulation. The sympathetic nervous system may also play an important role. From animal studies it is known that application of noradrenaline at the stump or activation of the postganglionic sympathetic fibers excites and sensitizes damaged but not normal nerve fibers.

Spinal factors

Clinical observations show that spinal factors must be involved in the generation of phantom limb pain. For example, phantom limb pain may appear or disappear following spinal cord neoplasia. Aydin *et al.* [5] described a woman who suffered from phantom limb pain following lower limb amputation at the age of 5 years. At the age of 65 years, the pain gradually disappeared, paralleling the evolution of cauda equina compression due to an intraspinal tumor. The phantom limb pain gradually reappeared after surgical removal of the tumor. Case reports have suggested that spinal analgesia may provoke phantom limb pain

and that spinal analgesia should be contraindicated in amputees. However, in a prospective study of 17 patients with previous lower limb amputation undergoing 23 spinal anesthetics, only one patient developed phantom limb pain [6].

Experimental and human studies confirm that spinal factors are involved in the generation of phantom limb pain. The increased barrage from neuromas and from DRG cells is thought to induce long-term changes in centrally projecting neurones in the dorsal horn, including spontaneous neuronal activity, induction of immediate early genes, increases in spinal metabolic activity and expansion of receptive fields. Another type of reorganization may also be present and contribute to central sensitization. Substance P is normally expressed in small afferent fibers but following nerve injury, substance P may be expressed in large Aß fibers. This phenotypic switch of large Aß fibers into nociceptive-like nerve fibers may be one of the reasons why non-noxious stimuli can be perceived as painful. The pharmacology of spinal sensitization involves an increased activity in N-methyl-D-aspartate (NMDA) receptor-operated systems, and many aspects of the central sensitization can be reduced by NMDA receptor antagonists. In human amputees, the evoked stump or phantom pain caused by repetitively stimulating the stump can be reduced by the NMDA antagonist ketamine [7].

Supraspinal factors

Amputation produces a cascade of events in the periphery and in the spinal cord. It is reasonable to assume that these changes will eventually sweep more centrally and alter the neuronal activity in cortical and subcortical structures. Also the phantom limb concept, with its complex perceptual qualities and its modification by various internal stimuli (e.g. attention, distraction or stress), shows the phantom image to be a product of the brain.

Animal studies have demonstrated functional plasticity of the primary somatosensory cortex after amputation. After dorsal rhizotomy, a lowered threshold to evoked activity in the thalamus and cortex can be demonstrated, and adult monkeys display cortical reorganization in which the mouth and chin invade cortices corresponding to the representation of the arm and digits that have lost their normal afferent input [8–9].

Studies in humans have also documented cortical reorganization after amputation using different cerebral imaging techniques. In a series of studies Flor et al. [10, 11] showed a correlation between phantom pain and the amount of reorganization in the somatosensory cortex. Birbaumer et al. [12] studied the effect of regional anesthesia on cortical reorganization in upper limb amputees and found that a brachial plexus blockade abolished pain and reorganization in three out of six amputees. Huse et al. [13] showed in a small group of amputees that cortical reorganization and pain were reduced during treatment with morphine.

Changes have also been observed at more subcortical levels. Using neuronal recording and stimulation techniques, thalamic neurones that do not normally respond to stimulation in amputees begin to respond and show enlarged somatotopic maps [14]. In addition to functional plasticity, structural alterations also follow amputation. Draganski et al. [15] recently demonstrated a decrease in the gray matter of the thalamus in 28 amputees. The decrease was correlated with the time span after the amputation and explained as a structural correlate of the loss of afferent input.

Epidemiology

Phantom limb pain

The reported prevalence of phantom pain varies much in the literature. Very early studies claimed that the prevalence was 2–4%, but today most studies agree that 60–80% of all amputees experience phantom pain following amputation. The prevalence of phantom pain seems to be independent of age in adults, gender, side or level of amputation and cause (nontraumatic versus traumatic) of the amputation. Interestingly, phantom limb pain is more frequent when the amputation occurs in adulthood, less frequent in child amputees and virtually nonexistent in congenital amputees.

Prospective studies in patients amputated mainly because of peripheral vascular disease have shown that the onset of phantom pain is usually within the first week after amputation [16, 17]. Amputees who do not experience phantom pain in the first days or weeks after amputation are less likely to develop phantom pain later in the course. Richardson et al. [17] prospectively examined the incidence of phantom pain in 52 amputees. Phantom pain was reported by 92.3% in the first week after amputation and by 78.8% after 6 months. The onset of phantom pain, however, can be delayed for months or even years. In some cases a trauma to the stump can elicit phantom pain in a previously pain-free individual. The exact long-term course of phantom limb pain is unclear because no prospective studies with long-term (many years) follow-up exist. Some prospective studies with a maximum follow-up period of 2 years have reported a slight decline in the proportion of patients affected over time.

Phantom limb pain is episodic in nature, and only few amputees are in constant pain. Diary studies have shown that most amputees report pain attacks to occur daily or at daily or weekly intervals.

The reported intensity of phantom pain varies between studies. In a recent study of 57 amputees, the average phantom pain intensity was 2.05 on a numeric rating scale (0–10) 24 months after the amputation [18]. In another recent study of 914 amputees, pain was classified into three categories: 38.9% experienced severe pain intensity (rating 7–10), 26.4% experienced moderate pain intensity (rating 5–6) and 34.7% experienced mild pain intensity (rating 1–4) [19].

Phantom limb pain can have several different qualities and is often described as shooting, pricking, stabbing, throbbing, burning, pin and needles, tingling, crushing or cramping. The pain seems to be more intense in the distal portions of the missing limb: fingers and palm in upper limb amputees, toes, foot and ankle in lower limb amputees. In a prospective study of 52 amputees, the position of phantom pain within the phantom limb was in the toes or the foot in 66.7% of cases [20]. These distal parts of the limbs are represented by a larger area in the sensory cortex compared to more proximal parts, and this may play a role in the more frequent phantom experience of hands and feet.

Phantom limb sensations

Phantom sensation is experienced by almost everyone who undergoes limb amputation, but it rarely represents a clinical problem. Immediately after the amputation, the phantom limb often resembles the preamputation limb in shape, size and volume. The sensation can be very vivid and often includes feelings of posture and movement. The phantom sensation may fade over time. One hundred and twenty-four upper limb amputees were asked about the frequency of phantom sensations a median time of 19 years after amputation. Forty percent experienced phantom sensations always, another 20% had phantom sensations daily, and the rest had sensations at intervals of weeks, months or even years [2].

In some patients, a phenomenon called telescoping occurs when the distal parts of the phantom are gradually felt to approach the residual limb, and eventually they may even be experienced within the stump. It has been suggested that phantom pain prevents telescoping, but Montoya et al. [20] failed to find such a relation: 12/16 patients with phantom pain and 5/10 patients without pain reported telescoping.

Stump pain

Not surprisingly, stump pain is common in the early postoperative period, but in most patients it subsides with healing. In some patients, however, stump pain persists beyond the stage of surgical healing. The prevalence of chronic stump pain is reported to vary between 5% and 100%. In a survey of 78 traumatic amputees, 14.1% suffered from severe and constant pain in the stump [21]. Similar results have been found by others in patients who have undergone amputation for different reasons, including medical.

Stump pain may be described as pressing, throbbing, burning, squeezing or stabbing. Some patients have spontaneous movements of the stump, ranging from slight, hardly visible jerks to severe contractions.

Careful sensory examination of amputation stumps may reveal areas with sensory abnormalities such as hypoesthesia, hyperalgesia or allodynia. However, it is not clear whether there is any correlation between phantom pain and the extent and degree of sensory abnormalities in the stump. Hunter et al. [22] carefully examined the stump in 12 traumatic upper limb amputees but failed to find any simple relation between psychophysical thresholds and phantom phenomena.

Stump pain and phantom pain are strongly correlated. Carlen et al. [23] noted that phantom pain was decreased by the resolution of stump-end pathology. In a survey of 648 amputees, stump pain was present in 61% of amputees with phantom pain, but in only 39% of those without phantom pain [24]. Similar results have been found in other studies.

Risk factors

Preamputation pain

Both retrospective and prospective studies have pointed to preamputation pain as a risk factor for phantom pain. The hypothesis is that preoperative pain may sensitize the nervous system, thus making the individual very susceptible to the development of phantom pain.

In a study by Houghton et al. [25], there was a significant relationship in vascular amputees between preamputation pain and phantom pain. In traumatic amputees, phantom pain was only related to preamputation pain immediately after the amputation. In a study of mostly vascular amputees, a correlation was found between preoperative pain and phantom pain 1 week and 3 months after the amputation, but not after 6 months. However, some patients with severe preoperative pain never developed phantom pain, while others with traumatic amputations who never experienced pain before the amputation developed phantom pain to the same extent as patients with long-standing preamputation pain amputated for medical reasons [16].

In a recent prospective study, the associations of preamputation pain and acute postoperative pain with chronic amputation-related pain were examined in 57 lower limb amputees. The acute postamputation pain intensity was the only significant independent predictor of chronic phantom pain at 6 and 12 months after amputation, whereas the preamputation pain intensity was the only significant predictor of chronic phantom at 24 months [18].

Another issue concerns the extent to which phantom pain is a revivification of pain experienced before the amputation. Remarkable case reports show that phantom pain may mimic the pain experienced before the amputation in both character and localization. For example, Hill *et al.* [26] described a woman who had her left leg amputated because of recurrent wound infection. The most distressing preoperative pain was invoked by the treatment carried out on the open drainage site on the calf, which required cleaning and repacking twice daily. Immediately after the amputation, the patient experienced phantom pain localized to the open drainage site that was no longer there.

In a retrospective study by Katz & Melzack [27], 68 patients were questioned about preamputation pain and phantom pain from 20 days to 46 years after amputation. A very large proportion (57%) of amputees with preamputation pain claimed that their present phantom pain resembled the pain they had before the amputation. Prospective studies, however, in which pain is described before and at intervals after the amputation suggest that preamputation pain only persists as phantom pain in very few cases. In a study by Nikolajsen *et al.* [16], 56 patients were interviewed before and at specific time intervals after the amputation about the character and localization of the pain. This was done using different word descriptors: the McGill Pain Questionnaire and their own words. About 42% of the patients reported that their phantom pain resembled the pain they had experienced at the time of the amputation. There was, however, no relation between the patients' own opinion about similarity between the preamputation pain and the phantom pain and the actual similarity found when comparing pre- and postoperative recordings of the pain. The patients significantly overestimated the preamputation pain intensity after 6 months. Thus, retrospective memories about pain should be judged carefully because of the type of assessment and potential errors in retrospective reports. It is likely that pain experienced preoperatively may survive as phantom pain in some patients, but this is not the case in the vast majority of patients.

Psychologic factors

Losing a limb is a traumatic experience and amputees often exhibit a range of psychologic symptoms such as depression, anxiety, self-pity and isolation. It has previously been proposed that complaints of persisting pain were related to patients with a rigid, self-reliant personality and to unemployment or retirement. There is, however, no evidence that phantom pain represents a psychologic disturbance. It has been shown that coping strategies are important for the experience of phantom pain and as in other chronic pain conditions, phantom pain may be triggered and exacerbated by psychosocial factors.

Desmond *et al.* [28] recently investigated psychologic distress among 582 amputees with long-term amputations and showed that distress was related to residual limb pain. In another recent study, depressive symptoms were found to be a significant predictor of the level of pain intensity and bothersomeness [19].

Others have looked at pain-related disability and rehabilitation. A study in The Netherlands examining the occupational situation of people with lower limb amputations found that amputees experiencing a long delay between the amputation and their return to work had difficulty in finding suitable jobs and had fewer opportunities for promotion [29].

Other factors

Evidence is growing that the individual's genetic predisposition to develop neuropathic pain may be important. On the other hand, Schott described an interesting case in which five members of a family sustained traumatic amputations of their limbs. The development of phantom pain was unpredictable despite their being first-degree relatives [30]. An inherited component is not always a feature of phantom pain.

Phantom pain may also be related to several internal and external factors, such as attention, emotional stress, anxiety and autonomic reflexes such as coughing and urination. A certain position or movement of the phantom and manipulation of the stump can affect the phantom pain, and pain may also be elicited or exacerbated by a range of physical factors, for example weather changes.

Interventions

Treatment of chronic postamputation pain represents a major challenge to the clinician, in particular the treatment of phantom pain. There is only little evidence from randomized trials to guide clinicians with treatment, and most studies dealing with phantom pain suffer from major methodologic errors: samples are small, randomization and blinding are either absent or inappropriate, controls are often lacking and follow-up periods are short. Halbert *et al.* [31] performed a systematic literature search (Medline 1966–99) to determine the optimal management of phantom pain. The authors identified 186 articles, but after exclusion of letters, reviews, descriptive trials without intervention, case reports and trials with major methodologic errors, only 12 articles were left for review. Since then, some well-designed studies have been published. Until more clinical data become available, guidelines in analogy with treatment regimens used for other neuropathic pain conditions are probably the best approximation, especially for the treatment of stump pain. A combination of medical and nonmedical treatment may be advantageous. In general, treatment should be noninvasive. Surgery on the peripheral or central nervous system always implicates further deafferentation and thereby an increased risk of persistent pain.

Medical treatment

Tricyclic antidepressants

A large number of randomized controlled trials have shown a beneficial effect of tricyclic antidepressants in different neuropathic pain conditions. Only few controlled data are available for phantom pain, but the drugs are generally believed to be effective, at least in some patients.

A recent study examined the effect of tricyclic antidepressants on phantom pain. Thirty-nine patients were randomized to receive either amitriptyline or active placebo during a 6-week trial period. The dosage of amitriptyline was increased until the patient reached the maximum tolerated dose or 125 mg/day. Unfortunately, this study showed no effect of amitriptyline on pain intensity or secondary outcome measures such as satisfaction with life [32]. In contrast, Wilder-Smith *et al.* [33] found excellent pain relief of amitriptyline (mean dose 55 mg) on both stump and phantom pain. Ninety-four post-traumatic amputees were randomized to receive amitriptyline, tramadol or placebo for 1 month. The administration of tramadol and placebo was blinded; amitriptyline was given

nonblinded as open comparison. Nonresponders (less than 10 mm pain relief on a VAS from baseline on day 3) were switched to the alternative active treatment, e.g. tramadol to amitriptyline treatment and vice versa. Placebo nonresponders were switched to tramadol or amitriptyline. Both tramadol and amitriptyline almost abolished stump and phantom pain at the end of the treatment period.

Gabapentin

Bone *et al.* [34] examined the effect of gabapentin in a well-designed cross-over study including 19 patients with phantom pain. The dose of gabapentin was titrated in increments of 300 mg to a maximum dosage of 2400 mg per day. After 6 weeks of treatment, gabapentin was better than placebo in reducing phantom pain. Smith *et al.* [35] administered gabapentin or placebo for 6 weeks to 24 amputees in a double-blind cross-over fashion. The maximum dose given was 3600 mg. Gabapentin did not decrease the intensity of pain significantly, but the participants rated the decrease of pain as more meaningful during the treatment period with gabapentin All the abovementioned studies examined the effect of gabapentin on established phantom pain. In a recent study, 46 lower limb amputees were randomized to receive either gabapentin or placebo for the first 30 days after amputation. The first dose of 300 mg gabapentin/placebo was given on the first postoperative day, and the dosage was gradually increased until a maximum of 2400 mg was reached. The intensity, frequency and duration of phantom pain attacks were recorded daily in the first 30 days and after 3 and 6 months. The intensity of stump pain was also recorded and sensory testing of the stump was performed. The two treatment groups were similar as regards all outcome parameters. Thus, early treatment with gabapentin started before the phantom pain becomes established did not seem to affect outcome [36].

Opioids

Failure to provide efficient pain relief should not be accepted until opioids have been tried. In a randomized, double-blind, cross-over study with active placebo, 31 amputees received a 40-minute infusion of lidocaine (lignocaine), morphine or diphenhydramine. Compared with placebo, morphine reduced both stump and phantom pain, whereas lidocaine decreased only stump pain [37]. In another placebo-controlled, cross-over study including 12 patients, a significant reduction of phantom pain during treatment with oral morphine was found [13]. Case reports have suggested that methadone may reduce phantom pain.

NMDA receptor antagonists

The effect of NMDA receptor antagonists has been examined in different studies. In a double-blind, placebo-controlled study, intravenous ketamine reduced pain, hyperalgesia and wind-up like pain in 11 amputees with stump and phantom pain [7]. Three other trials have examined the effect of memantine, an NMDA receptor antagonist available for oral use. In all studies, memantine was administered in a blinded, placebo-controlled, cross-over fashion to patients with established stump and phantom pain. Memantine at doses of 20 or 30 mg per day failed to have any effect on spontaneous pain, allodynia and hyperalgesia [38–40]. Schley et al. [41] recently randomized 19 patients with traumatic amputations to receive either memantine or placebo in combination with a continuous brachial plexus blockade in the immediate postoperative phase. The dose of memantine was increased from 10 to 30 mg during the 4-week treatment period. Treatment with memantine resulted in a decrease of phantom pain at 4-week and 6-month follow-up, but not at 12-month follow-up. Dextromethorphan, another NMDA receptor antagonist, has also been suggested to be effective in the treatment of phantom limb pain.

Other drugs

Calcitonin significantly reduced phantom pain when used intravenously in the early postoperative phase [42]. A large number of other treatments, for example β-blockers, the oral congener of lidocaine (lignocaine), topical application of capsaicin, intrathecal opioids, various anesthetic blocks, injection of botulinum toxin and topiramate, have been claimed to be effective in phantom pain, but none of them has proved to be effective in well-controlled trials with a sufficient number of patients.

Nonmedical treatment

A recent survey of treatments used for phantom pain revealed that after pharmacologic treatments, physical therapy was the treatment modality most often used. Physical therapy involving massage, manipulation and passive movements may prevent trophic changes and vascular congestion in the stump. Other treatments, such as transcutaneous electrical nerve stimulation, acupuncture, ultrasound and hypnosis, may in some cases have a beneficial effect on stump and phantom pain. At least three studies have examined the effect of transcutaneous electrical nerve stimulation on phantom pain, but the results are not consistent. One study showed an effect of a Farabloc, a metal-threaded sock to be worn over the stump [43]. It has been suggested that visual feedback with a mirror can eliminate painful phantom limb spasms. In a larger clinical trial of 80 amputees, however, Brodie et al. [44] failed to find any significant effect of mirror treatment on phantom limb pain, sensation, and movement. Flor et al. [4] demonstrated that sensory discrimination training obtained by applying stimuli at the stump reduced pain in five upper limb amputees. The advantage of most of the above-mentioned methods is the absence of side effects and complications, and the fact that the treatment can be easily repeated. However, most of these studies are uncontrolled observations.

Surgical and other invasive treatment

Surgery on amputation neuromas and more extensive amputation previously played important roles in the treatment of stump and phantom pain. Today, stump revision is probably performed only in cases of obvious stump pathology, and in properly healed stumps there is almost never any indication for proximal extension of the amputation because of pain. The results of other invasive techniques such as, for example, dorsal root entry zone lesion sympathetectomy and cordotomy have generally been unfavorable, and most of them have been abandoned. Surgery may produce short-term pain relief but the pain often reappears. Spinal cord stimulation and deep brain stimulation are probably effective for the treatment of phantom limb pain. As the methods are invasive and associated with considerable costs, they should only be used for carefully selected patients.

Prevention of phantom pain

The idea of a pre-emptive analgesic effect in postamputation pain was prompted by observations that the phantom pain in some cases seemed to be similar to the pain experienced before the amputation, and that the presence of severe pain before the amputation was associated with a higher risk of postamputation phantom pain. These observations led to the theory that preamputation pain created an imprint in memorizing structures of the central nervous system, and that such an imprint could be responsible for persistent pain after amputation.

Inspired by this, Bach *et al.* [45] carried out the first study on the prevention of phantom pain. Twenty-five patients were randomized by birth year to either epidural pain treatment 72 hours before the amputation or conventional analgesics. All patients had spinal or epidural analgesia for the amputation, and both groups received conventional analgesics to treat postoperative pain. Blinding was not described. After 6 months, the incidence of phantom pain was lower among patients who had received the preoperative epidural blockade.

Jahangiri and co-workers examined the effect of perioperative epidural infusion of diamorphine, bupivacaine and clonidine on postamputation stump and phantom pain. Thirteen patients received epidural treatment 5–48 h preoperatively and for at least 3 days postoperatively. A control group of 11 patients received opioid analgesia on demand. All patients had general anesthesia for the amputation. The incidence of severe phantom pain was lower in the epidural group 7 days, 6 months and 1 year after amputation [46]. The study was not randomized or blinded.

Nikolajsen *et al.* carried out a randomized, double-blind and placebo-controlled study in which 60 patients scheduled for lower limb amputation were randomly assigned to one of two groups: a blockade group that received epidural bupivacaine and morphine before the amputation and during the operation (29 patients) and a control group that received epidural saline and oral or intramuscular morphine (31 patients). Both groups had general anesthesia for the amputation, and all patients received epidural analgesics for postoperative pain management. Patients were interviewed about preamputation pain on the day before the amputation and about stump and phantom pain after 1 week and 3, 6 and 12 months. The median duration of preoperative epidural blockade was 18 hours. After 1 week, the percentage of patients with phantom pain was 51.9% in the blockade group and 55.6% in the control group. Subsequently, the percentages were

(blockade/control): at 3 months, 82.4%/50%; at 6 months, 81.3%/55% and at 12 months, 75%/68.8%. The intensity of stump and phantom pain and the consumption of opioids were similar in the two groups at all four postoperative interviews [47].

Others have examined the effect of peri- or intraneural blockade on phantom limb pain. For example, Pinzur and co-workers prospectively randomized 21 patients to continuous postoperative infusion of either bupivacaine or saline, but failed to find any difference between the two groups with regard to the incidence of phantom pain after 3 and 6 months [48].

Lambert *et al.* [49] compared two techniques of regional analgesia. Thirty patients were randomized to receive either epidural bupivacaine and diamorphine started 24 h before the amputation and continued 3 days postoperatively or an intraoperative perineural catheter for intra- and postoperative administration of bupivacaine. All patients had general anesthesia for the amputation. The pre-, peri- and postoperative epidural pain treatment was not superior to the intra- and postoperative perineural pain treatment in preventing phantom pain, as the incidence of phantom pain was similar in the two groups after 3 days and after 6 and 12 months.

The aim of pre-emptive treatment is to avert spinal sensitization by blocking, in advance, the cascade of intraneuronal responses that takes place after peripheral nerve injury. A true pre-emptive approach is probably not possible in patients scheduled for amputation. Many have suffered from ischemic pain for months or years and are likely to present with pre-existing neuronal hyperexcitability. It cannot be excluded that a preoperative regional blockade for a longer period would prevent phantom pain from developing. However, this would be very inconvenient from a practical point of view as the decision to amputate is often not taken until the day before.

In conclusion, regional blocks are effective in the treatment of preoperative ischemic pain and postoperative stump pain. At present, no studies of sufficient methodologic quality have provided evidence that regional blocks have any beneficial effect in preventing phantom pain. It cannot be excluded that other approaches may be effective. For example, it has been suggested that peri- and postamputation administration of NMDA receptor antagonists such as ketamine [50] and memantine [41] reduces phantom limb pain.

Future research

There is still a need for well-controlled studies examining the effect of different medical and nonmedical interventions. Also, it would be of interest to explore the extent to which cortical reorganization depends on alterations in the periphery, the spinal cord or the genetic constitution.

Author recommendations for the management of phantom pain

Treatment of phantom pain is very difficult. Medical treatment should follow the guidelines for other neuropathic pain conditions. Since medical treatment may not always be successful, combinations of medical and nonmedical treatment should be tried. Alternative treatments should be considered if conventional treatment is inadequate.

Box 19.1 Interventions for the management of phantom limb pain

Supported by evidence (ranked according to evidence level)
Gabapentin
Tricyclic antidepressants
Opioids (morphine, tramadol)
Ketamine (IV)
Calcitonin (IV) (acute phase only)
Use of a Farabloc (a metal threaded sock)
Sensory discrimination training

Refuted by evidence
Memantine (20–30 mg/day)
Epidural treatment (started 18 h before amputation)
Perineural blocks (started postoperatively)

Commonly used interventions currently unproven
Pregabalin
Various anticonvulsants (except gabapentin)
Antidepressants (except tricyclic antidepressants)
Opioids (methadone, oxycodone)
Physical therapy
Acupuncture
Hypnosis
Mirror treatment
Spinal cord stimulation

References

1. Flor H, Nikolajsen L, Jensen TS. Phantom limb pain: a case of maladaptive CNS plasticity? *Nature Rev Neurosci* 2006; **7**: 873–881.
2. Kooijman CM, Dijkstra PU, Geertzen JHB, *et al.* Phantom pain and phantom sensations in upper limb amputees: an epidemiological study. *Pain* 2000; **87**: 33–41.
3. Nikolajsen L, Ilkjær S, Jensen TS. Relationship between mechanical sensitivity and postamputation pain: a prospective study. *Eur J Pain* 2000; **4**: 327–334.
4. Flor H, Denke C, Schaefer M, *et al.* Effect of sensory discrimination training on cortical reorganization and phantom limb pain. *Lancet* 2001; **357**: 1763–1764.
5. Aydin MD, Cesur M, Aydin N, Alici HA. Disappearance of phantom limb pain during cauda euina compression by spinal meningioma and gradual reactivation after decompression. *Anesth Analg* 2005; **101**: 1123–1126.
6. Tessler MJ, Kleiman SJ. Spinal anaesthesia for patients with previous lower limb amputations. *Anaesthesia* 1994; **49**: 439–441.
7. Nikolajsen L, Hansen CL, Nielsen J, *et al.* The effect of ketamine on phantom pain: a central neuropathic disorder maintained by peripheral input. *Pain* 1996; **67**: 69–77.
8. Florence SL, Kaas JH. Large-scale reorganization at multiple levels of the somatosensory pathway follows therapeutic amputation of the hand in monkeys. *J Neurosci* 1995; **15**: 8083–8095.
9. Pons TP, Garraghty PE, Ommaya AK, *et al.* Massive cortical reorganization after sensory deafferentation in adult macaques. *Science* 1991; **252**: 1857–1860.
10. Flor H, Elbert T, Knecht S. Phantom limb pain as a perceptual correlate of cortical reorganization following arm amputation. *Nature* 1995; **375**: 482–484.
11. Flor H, Elbert T, Mühlnickel W. Cortical reorganization and phantom phenomena in congenital and traumatic upper-extremity amputees. *Exper Brain Res* 1998; **119**: 205–212.
12. Birbaumer N, Lutzenberger W, Montoya P, *et al.* Effects of regional anesthesia on phantom limb are mirrored in changes in cortical reorganization in upper limb amputees. *J Neurosci* 1997; **17**: 5503–5508.
13. Huse E, Larbig W, Flor H, *et al.* The effect of opioids on phantom limb pain and cortical reorganization. *Pain* 2001; **90**: 47–55.
14. Davis KD, Kiss ZH, Luo L. Phantom sensations generated by thalamic microstimulation. *Nature* 1998; **391**: 385–387.
15. Draganski B, Moser T, Lummel N, *et al.* Decrease of thalamic gray matter following limb amputation. *NeuroImage* 2006; **31**: 951–957.
16. Nikolajsen L, Ilkjær S, Krøner K, *et al.* The influence of preamputation pain on postamputation stump and phantom pain. *Pain* 1997; **72**: 393–405.
17. Richardson C, Glenn S, Nurmikko T, Horgan M. Incidence of phantom phenomena including phantom limb pain 6 months after major lower limb amputation in patients with peripheral vascular disease. *Clin J Pain* 2006; **22**: 353–358.

18. Hanley MA, Jensen MP, Smith DG, *et al.* Preamputation pain and acute pain predict chronic pain after lower extremity amputation. *J Pain* 2007; **8**(2): 102–109.

19. Ephraim PL, Wegener ST, MacKenzie EJ, *et al.* Phantom pain, residual limb pain, and back pain in amputees: results of a national survey. *Arch Phys Med Rehabil* 2005; **86**: 1910–1919.

20. Montoya P, Larbig W, Grulke N. Relationship of phantom limb pain to other phantom limb phenomena in upper extremity amputees. *Pain* 1997; **72**: 87–93.

21. Pezzin LE, Dillingham TR, Mackenzie EJ. Rehabilitation and the long-term outcomes of persons with trauma-related amputations. *Arch Phys Med Rehabil* 2000; **81**: 292–300.

22. Hunter JP, Katz J, Davis KD. Dissociation of phantom limb phenomena from stump tactile spatial acuity and sensory thresholds. *Brain* 2005; **128**: 308–320.

23. Carlen PL, Wall PD, Nadvorna H, *et al.* Phantom limbs and related phenomena in recent traumatic amputations. *Neurology* 1978; **28**: 211–217.

24. Sherman R, Sherman C. Prevalence and characteristics of chronic phantom limb pain among American veterans: results of a trial survey. *Am J Phys Med* 1983; **62**: 227–238.

25. Houghton AD, Nicholls G, Houghton AL, *et al.* Phantom pain: natural history and association with rehabilitation. *Ann Roy Coll Surg Engl* 1994; **76**: 22–25.

26. Hill A, Niven CA, Knussen C. Pain memories in phantom limbs: a case story. *Pain* 1996; **66**: 381–384.

27. Katz J, Melzack R. Pain 'memories' in phantom limbs: review and clinical observations. *Pain* 1990; **43**: 319–336.

28. Desmond DM, Maclachlan M. Affective distress and amputation–related pain among older men with long-term, traumatic limb amputations. *J Pain Symptom Manage* 2006; **31**: 362–368.

29. Schoppen T, Boonstra A, Groothoff JW, *et al.* Employment status, job characteristics, and work-related health experience of people with a lower limb amputation in The Netherlands. *Arch Phys Med Rehabil* 2002; **82**: 239–245.

30. Schott G D. Pain and its absence in an unfortunate family of amputees. *Pain* 1986; **25**: 229–231.

31. Halbert J, Crotty M, Cameron ID. Evidence for the optimal management of acute and chronic phantom pain: a systematic review. *Clin J Pain* 2002; **18**: 84–92.

32. Robinson LR, Czerniecki JM, Ehde DM, *et al.* Trial of amitriptyline for relief of pain in amputees: results of a randomized controlled study. *Arch Phys Med Rehabil* 2004; **85**: 1–6.

33. Wilder-Smith CH, Hill LT, Laurent S. Postamputation pain and sensory changes in treatment-naive patients: characteristics and responses to treatment with tramadol, amitriptyline, and placebo. *Anesthesiology* 2005; **103**: 619–628.

34. Bone M, Critchley P, Buggy DJ. Gabapentin in postamputation phantom limb pain: a randomized, double-blind, placebo-controlled, cross-over study. *Region Anesth Pain Med* 2002; **27**: 481–486.

35. Smith DG, Ehde DM, Hanley MA, *et al.* Efficacy of gabapentin in treating chronic phantom limb and residual limb pain. *J Rehabil Res Dev* 2005; **42**: 645–654.

36. Nikolajsen L, Finnerup NB, Kramp S, *et al.* A randomized study of the effects of gabapentin on postamputation pain. *Anesthesiology* 2006; **105**: 1008–1015.

37. Wu CL, Tella P, Staats PS, *et al.* Analgesic effects of intravenous lidocaine and morphine on postamputation pain. *Anesthesiology* 2002; **96**: 841–848.

38. Nikolajsen L, Gottrup H, Kristensen AGD, *et al.* Memantine (a N-methyl D-aspartate receptor antagonist) in the treatment of neuropathic pain following amputation or surgery: a randomized, double-blind, cross-over study. *Anesth Analg* 2000; **91**: 960–966.

39. Maier C, Dertwinkel R, Mansourian N, *et al.* Efficacy of the NMDA-receptor antagonist memantine in patients with chronic phantom limb pain – results of a randomized double-blinded, placebo-controlled trial. *Pain* 2003; **103**: 277–283.

40. Wiech K, Kiefer RT, Töpfner S, *et al.* A placebo-controlled randomized crossover trial of the N-methyl-d-aspartic acid receptor antagonist, memantine, in patients with chronic phantom limb pain. *Anesth Analg* 2004; **98**: 408–413.

41. Schley M, Topfner S, Wiech K, *et al.* Continuous brachial plexus blockade in combination with the NMDA receptor antagonist memantine prevents phantom pain in acute traumatic upper limb amputees. *Eur J Pain* 2007; **11**(3): 299–308

42. Jaeger H, Maier C. Calcitonin in phantom limb pain: a double-blind study. *Pain* 1992; **48**: 21–27.

43. Conine TA, Herschler C, Alexander ST, *et al.* The efficacy of Farabloc in the treatment of phantom limb pain. *Can J Rehabil* 1993; **6**: 155–161.

44. Brodie EE, Whyte A, Niven CA. Analgesia through the looking-glass? A randomized controlled trial investigating the effect of viewing a 'virtual' limb upon phantom limb pain, sensation and movement. *Eur J Pain* 2007; **11**(4): 428–436.

45. Bach S, Noreng MF, Tjéllden NU. Phantom limb pain in amputees during the first 12 months following limb amputation after preoperative lumbar epidural blockade. *Pain* 1988; **33**(3): 297–301.

46. Jahangiri M, Jayatunga AP, Bradley JWP, *et al.* Prevention of phantom pain after major lower limb amputation by epidural infusion of diamorphine, clonidine and bupivacaine. *Ann Roy Coll Surg Engl* 1994; **76**: 324–326.

47. Nikolajsen L, Ilkjær S, Krøner K, *et al.* Randomized trial of epidural bupivacaine and morphine in prevention of stump and phantom pain in lower-limb amputation. *Lancet* 1997; **350**: 1353–1357.

48. Pinzur MS, Garla PGN, Pluth T, *et al.* Continuous postoperative infusion of a regional anaesthetic after an amputation of the lower extremity. *J Bone Joint Surg* 1996; **78:** 1501–1505.

49. Lambert AW, Dashfield AK, Cosgrove C, *et al.* Randomized prospective study comparing preoperative epidural and intraoperative perineural analgesia for the prevention of postoperative stump and phantom limb pain following major amputation. *Region Anesth Pain Med* 2001; **26:** 316–321.

50. Dertwinkel R, Heinrichs C, Senne I, *et al.* Prevention of severe phantom limb pain by perioperative administration of ketamine – an observational study. *Acute Pain* 2002; **4:** 9–13.

CHAPTER 20

Complex regional pain syndrome

Andreas Binder and Ralf Baron

Division of Neurological Pain Research and Therapy, Kiel, Germany

Introduction

Complex regional pain syndrome (CRPS), usually occurring in a distal extremity, is clinically characterized by different symptoms and signs comprising pain and sensory abnormalities, abnormal regulation of the blood flow, sweating, trophic changes, edema of skin and subcutaneous tissues and active and passive movement disorders. It is classified into type I (reflex sympathetic dystrophy) and type II (causalgia). In CRPS type I (reflex sympathetic dystrophy), minor injuries or fractures of a limb precede the onset of symptoms without any overt nerve lesion. CRPS type II (causalgia) develops after injury to a major peripheral nerve.

The current understanding of relevant pathophysiology

Sensory abnormalities and pain

In CRPS various forms of hyperalgesia and spontaneous pain develop at the distal extremity that are thought to be generated by processes of peripheral and central sensitization. In addition to positive sensory phenomena, up to 50% of patients with chronic CRPS I develop hypoesthesia and hypoalgesia on an entire half of the body or in the upper quadrant or face ipsilateral to the affected extremity [1–2]. Systematic quantitative sensory testing has shown that patients with these generalized hypoesthesias have

increased thresholds to mechanical, cold, warmth and heat stimuli compared with the responses generated from the corresponding contralateral healthy body side. Patients with these extended sensory deficits tend to have longer disease duration, greater pain intensity, a higher frequency of mechanical allodynia and a higher tendency to develop changes in the somatomotor system than do patients with spatially restricted sensory deficits.

There is increasing evidence that changes in the central representation of somatosensory sensations in the thalamus and cortex are one of the underlying courses of sensory abnormalities. Magnetoencephalographic (MEG) and functional magnetic resonance imaging (fMRI) studies of patients with upper limb CRPS demonstrated a shortened distance between little finger and thumb representations in the primary somatosensory (SI) cortex on the painful side [3–4]. This cortical reorganization was reversible, correlating with pain reduction and improvement of tactile impairment [5–6]. Accordingly, a 6-month behavioral training program led to pain reduction and was paralleled by restoration of two-point discrimination and reorganization of physiologic SI and SII representation [7]. A fMRI study showed reduced contralateral SI and SII activity paralleled with two-point discrimination impairment [7]. Sensory impairment was found to be predicted by mechanical hyperalgesia in CRPS I [8] whereas mechanical hyperalgesia is represented within a network involving the anterior cingulate cortex (ACC), associative somatosenory and frontal affective cortices [9].

Furthermore, there is evidence of central sensitization in CRPS. Positron emission tomography (PET) studies demonstrated adaptive changes in the

Evidence-Based Chronic Pain Management. Edited by C. Stannard, E. Kalso and J. Ballantyne. © 2010 Blackwell Publishing.

thalamus during the course of the disease [10] and using MEG, SI responses were found to be increased on the affected side [11]. Psychophysical and transcranial magnetic stimulation (TMS) studies suggest sensory and motor hyperexcitability within the central nervous system [12]. A PET study revealed an exaggerated metabolism in the somatosensory cortex, ACC, parietal cortex, thalamus and insula [13] while glucose utilization was reduced in prefrontal cortex and primary motor cortex.

Taken together, these studies suggest increasing evidence for dramatic cerebral reorganization and sensitization due to chronic painful input to the brain that in turn leads to sensory and motor deficits (see below). However, the dependency of these phenomena on structural or functional changes in the peripheral nerve system is not known so far. Skin preparations from CRPS I patients showed diminished axonal density [14] and mixed decreased and increased innervation of epidermal and vascular structures as well as sweat glands [15]. The relevance of these findings to distinct pathophysiologic mechanisms remains unclear [16].

Autonomic abnormalities

In general, there is evidence that sympathetic dysfunction can normalize within the course of the disease in mild CRPS [17].

Denervation supersensitivity

A partial nerve lesion is the important preceding event in CRPS II. Therefore, it has generally been assumed that abnormalities in skin blood flow within the territory of the lesioned nerve are due to peripheral impairment of sympathetic function and sympathetic denervation. During the first weeks after transection of vasoconstrictor fibers, vasodilation is present within the denervated area. Later the vasculature may develop increased sensitivity to circulating catecholamines, probably due to upregulation of adrenoceptors.

Central autonomic dysregulation

Sympathetic denervation and denervation hypersensitivity cannot completely account for vasomotor and sudomotor abnormalities in CRPS. First, in CRPS I there is no overt nerve lesion and second, in CRPS II the autonomic symptoms spread beyond the territory of the lesioned nerve. In fact, there is direct evidence for a reorganization of central autonomic

control in these syndromes [18, 19]. Hyperhidrosis, for example, is found in many CRPS patients. Resting sweat output, as well as thermoregulatory and axon reflex sweating, are increased in CRPS I patients [20]. Increased sweat production cannot be explained by a peripheral mechanism since, unlike blood vessels, sweat glands do not develop denervation supersensitivity.

In order to study cutaneous sympathetic vasoconstrictor innervation in CRPS I patients, central sympathetic reflexes were modulated by thermoregulatory (whole-body warming, cooling) and respiratory stimuli [21–23]. Sympathetic effector organ function, i.e. skin temperature and skin blood flow, was measured bilaterally at the extremities by infrared thermometry and laser Doppler flowmetry. Under normal conditions these reflexes do not show interside differences. In CRPS patients three distinct vascular regulation patterns were identified related to the duration of the disorder.

- In the warm regulation type (acute stage, <6 months) the affected limb was warmer and skin perfusion values were higher than contralaterally during the entire spectrum of sympathetic activity. Even massive body cooling failed to activate sympathetic vasoconstrictor neurones [22]. Consistently, direct measurements of norepinephrine levels from the venous effluent above the area of pain show a reduction in the affected extremity [22, 24].
- In the intermediate type temperature and perfusion were either elevated or reduced, depending on the degree of sympathetic activity.
- In the cold type (chronic stage) temperature and perfusion were lower on the affected side during the entire spectrum of sympathetic activity. Norepinephrine levels, however, were still lower on the affected side [23].

These data support the idea that CRPS I is associated with a pathologic unilateral inhibition of cutaneous sympathetic vasoconstrictor neurones leading to a warmer affected limb in the acute stage [21, 25]. The locus of pathophysiologic changes underlying such disturbed reflex activity must be in the central nervous system.

The few microneurographic studies of small sympathetic nerve fascicles that have been performed so far in patients with CRPS have not confirmed the presence of reflex abnormalities; the average skin sympathetic activity, i.e. a combination of vasoconstrictor and sudomotor activity, was not different on the two sides [26]. Assessing autonomic efferent control to the heart, however, tilt table tests demonstrated higher, i.e. impaired, mean heart rates than controls, comparable with patients suffering from postural tachycardia syndrome [27].

Secondary changes in neurovascular transmission may induce severe vasoconstriction and cold skin in chronic CRPS [28, 29]. Accordingly, α-adrenoceptor density has been reported to be increased in skin biopsies of patients with CRPS I [30]. Furthermore, skin lactate was increased in CRPS patients, indicating an enhanced anaerobic glycolysis, probably as a result of vasoconstriction and chronic tissue hypoxia [31, 32]. Moreover, in patients suffering from "cold type" CRPS, iontophoresis of acetylcholine into the skin of the affected and unaffected extremities revealed a decrease of the vasodilatory response in the CRPS extremity [33]. The pathophysiology of the hereby proven endothelial dysfunction in "cold type" CRPS is not known so far. However, it can be assumed that production of free radicals is triggered by tissue hypoxia and tissue acidosis due to peripheral vasoconstriction. Thereby, the production of free radicals is responsible for the observed endothelial function. The vasoconstrictor and nociceptor sensitizing agent endothelin-1 seems not to be involved in CRPS pathophysiology [34].

Neurogenic inflammation and oxidative stress

Some of the clinical features of CRPS, particularly in its early phase, could be explained by an inflammatory process [35]. Consistent with this idea, corticosteroids are often successfully used in acute CRPS [36].

There is increasing evidence that a localized neurogenic inflammation might be involved in the generation of acute edema, vasodilation and increased sweating. Scintigraphic investigations with radiolabeled immunoglobulins show extensive plasma extravasation in patients with acute CRPS I [37]. Analysis of joint fluid and synovial biopsies in CRPS patients have shown an increase in protein concentration and synovial hypervascularity. Furthermore, synovial effusion is enhanced in affected joints as measured with MRI and leukocytes have been demonstrated to accumulate in the affected extremity in acute CRPS I [38].

In acute untreated CRPS I patients, neurogenic inflammation was elicited by strong transcutaneous electrical stimulation via intradermal microdialysis capillaries. Protein extravasation that was simultaneously assessed by the microdialysis system was only provoked on the affected extremity as compared with the normal side. Furthermore, axon reflex vasodilation was increased significantly. The time course of electrically induced protein extravasation in the patients resembled the one observed following application of exogenous substance P (SP) [39] or did not show differences to healthy controls [40]. Additionally, high SP levels may be caused by impaired SP inactivation in acute stages of CRPS [40]. As further support of a neurogenic inflammatory process, systemic calcitonin gene-related peptide (CGRP) levels were found to be increased in acute CRPS but not in chronic stages [41]. In the fluid of artificially produced skin blisters significantly higher levels of endothelin-1, interleukin (IL)-6 and tumor necrosis factor α (TNF-α) were observed in the involved extremity as compared with the uninvolved extremity [42, 43] as well as diminished NO [43]. These findings persisted although pain and signs of CRPS I improved, questioning the direct relation between clinical signs and symptoms and proinflammatory cytokines [44]. However, proinflammatory cytokine levels were also more significantly elevated first, in CRPS patients complaining from mechanical hyperalgesia than in CRPS patients without hyperalgesia [44] and second, in the venous blood of the affected limb compared with the unaffected contralateral extremity [45]. Moreover, analysis of the cerebrospinal fluid in CRPS I and II revealed higher levels of proinflammatory IL-1β and -6, whereas TNF levels did not differ from levels in patients with painful conditions of other origin [46]. Interestingly, as an indirect proof of ongoing oxidative stress in CRPS, preliminary data show efficacy of hyperbaric oxygen therapy on pain, edema and motor dysfunction [47].

Exogenous infections are discussed here as they may partially contribute to the symptoms and signs of CRPS. A significantly higher seroprevalence of erythrovirus (formerly parvovirus) B19 was observed in CRPS I patients [48]. Additionally, studies have discussed whether an exogenous campylobacter infection may trigger autoimmune activation [49, 50]. However, the importance of antecedent infections as well as detected autoantibodies against autonomic nervous system structures [51] in the pathophysiology of CRPS (e.g. in the generation of a facilitated chronic inflammation) is currently not known. Interestingly, erythrovirus B10 IgG were not associated with antiendothelial autoantibodies [50].

In conclusion, evidence indicates that inflammatory processes and oxidative stress are involved in the pathogenesis of early CRPS. However, the exact mechanisms of the initiation and maintenance of these inflammatory reactions are unclear [52]. One central issue is whether the sympathetic nervous system may contribute to the early inflammatory state. *De novo* expression of adrenoreceptors on macrophages after experimental nerve lesion supports this idea, leading to possible interaction of sympathetic fibers, afferent fibers, blood vessels and non-neural cells related to the immune system. However, this concept has yet to be proven in patients with CRPS.

Motor abnormalities

About 50% of patients with CRPS show a decrease of active range of motion, an increased amplitude of physiologic tremor or reduced active motor force of the affected extremity. In about 10% of cases dystonia of the affected hand or foot develops, especially in chronic cases. It is unlikely that these motor changes are related to a peripheral process (e.g. influence of the sympathetic nervous system on neuromuscular transmission and/or contractility of skeletal muscle). These somatomotor changes are more likely generated by changes of activity in the motor neurones, i.e. they have a central origin. Turton *et al.* showed physiological EMG responses to TMS in the CRPS I affected limb when applied with median nerve stimulation, giving evidence for an indirect neural pathway accounting for motor deficits in CRPS [53]. Localized CNS hyperexcitability was shown in another TMS study [12]. Furthermore, kinematic analysis of target reaching and grasping and functional imaging (fMRI) showed reorganization in the central nervous system, predominantly in the parietal cortices, supplementary motor area (SMA) and primary motor cortex [54]. Interestingly, the motor performance is also slightly impaired on the contralateral unaffected side [55]. Furthermore, a sustained disinhibition of the motor cortex was found in CRPS patients on the contralateral as well as the ipsilateral hemisphere [11, 56]. Interestingly, repetitive TMS applied to the motor cortex contralateral to the affected extremity in CRPS I showed potential to modulate, i.e. decrease, pain [4].

According to this view, a neglect-like syndrome was clinically described as being responsible for the disuse of the extremity [57, 58] that is also to a lesser extent detectable in other chronic pain syndromes but may also support the diagnosis of CRPS [59]. Delayed recognition of hand laterality that is related to the duration and pain intensity in CRPS I [60] and impairment of self-perception of the affected extremity that is related to pain intensity, illness duration and extent of sensory deficits [61] may contribute to disuse, impaired motor planning and function. A controlled study also supports an incongruence between central motor output and sensory input as an underlying mechanism in CRPS. Using the method of mirror visual feedback, the visual input from a moving unaffected limb to the brain was able to re-establish the pain-free relationship between sensory feedback and motor execution. After 6 weeks of therapy pain and function were improved as compared with the control group [62, 63]. A study extension comparing the combined therapy regime of hand laterality recognition training, imagination of movements and mirror movements demonstrated the ability to reduce pain and disability [64, 65]. It is thought that limb laterality recognition activates premotor cortex, movement imagination premotor and motor cortex, leading to a training effect. Sensory-motor incongruence might be removed by motor imagery (substraction of command from sensory input of attempted/performed movement leading to error). A 6-month behavioral training program led to pain reduction and restoration of the impaired two-point discrimination at the affected extremity. Additionally, fMRI showed a parallel reorganization of a physiologic representation of the initially shrunk areas SI and SII by regaining normal cortical map size [6].

Additionally, the afferent sensory input to cortical motor centers in CRPS is decreased [66]. Recently Sumitani *et al.* demonstrated a shift of the subjective body midline towards the affected limb that was reversed by deafferentation following peripheral nerve blockade [67]. Moreover, treatment with prism adaptation towards the unaffected extremity combined with target-orientated training tasks of the affected hand relieved CRPS symptoms whereas adaptation towards the affected limb caused an exacerbation [68].

Sympathetically maintained pain

On the basis of experience and recent clinical studies, the term "sympathetically maintained pain" was redefined. Neuropathic pain patients presenting with similar clinical signs and symptoms can clearly be divided into two groups by the negative or positive effect of selective sympathetic blockade or antagonism of α-adrenoceptor mechanisms. The pain component that is relieved by specific sympatholytic procedures is considered to be sympathetically maintained pain (SMP). Thus, SMP is now defined as a symptom or the underlying mechanism in a subset of patients with neuropathic disorders and not a clinical entity. The positive effect of a sympathetic blockade is not essential for the diagnosis. On the other hand, the only way to differentiate between SMP and sympathetically independent pain (SIP) is the efficacy of a correctly applied sympatholytic intervention, indicating high specificity and low sensitivity of this procedure [69]. However, the exact sensitivity and specificity of this test to diagnose or exclude SMP are not known (see below).

Clinical studies in CRPS support the idea that nociceptors develop catecholamine sensitivity [70]. Intraoperative stimulation of the sympathetic chain induces an increase of spontaneous pain in patients with causalgia (CRPS II) but not in patients with hyperhidrosis. In CRPS II, post-traumatic neuralgias, intracutaneous application of norepinephrine, into a symptomatic area rekindles spontaneous pain and dynamic mechanical hyperalgesia that had been relieved by sympathetic blockade, supporting the idea that noradrenergic sensitivity of human nociceptors is present after partial nerve lesion. Also intradermal norepinephrine or phenylepherine, respectively, in physiologically relevant doses, was demonstrated to evoke greater pain in the affected regions of patients with SMP than in the contralateral unaffected limb and in control subjects [71, 72].

Within a study in patients with CRPS I physiologic stimuli of the sympathetic nervous system were used [73]. Cutaneous sympathetic vasoconstrictor outflow to the painful extremity was experimentally activated to the highest possible physiologic degree by whole-body cooling. During the thermal challenge the affected extremity was clamped to 35°C in order to avoid thermal effects at the nociceptor level. The intensity as well as area of spontaneous pain and mechanical hyperalgesia (dynamic and punctate) increased significantly in patients who had been classified as having SMP by positive sympathetic blocks but not in SIP patients. The experimental set-up used in the latter study selectively alters sympathetic cutaneous vasoconstrictor activity without influencing other sympathetic systems innervating the extremities, e.g. sudomotor and muscle vasoconstrictor neurones. Therefore, the interaction of sympathetic and afferent neurones measured here is likely to be located within the skin as predicted by the pain-enhancing effect of intracutaneous norepinephrine injections [71]. Interestingly, the relief of spontaneous pain after sympathetic blockade was more pronounced than changes in spontaneous pain that could be induced experimentally by sympathetic activation. One explanation for this discrepancy might be that a complete sympathetic block affects all sympathetic outflow channels projecting to the affected extremity. It is very likely that in addition to a coupling in the skin, a sympathetic–afferent interaction may also occur in other tissues, in particular in deep somatic domains such as bone, muscle or joints. Supporting this view, these structures in particular are extremely painful in some cases with CRPS. Furthermore, there may be patients who are characterized by a selective or predominant sympathetic–afferent interaction in deep somatic tissues, sparing the skin [22]. Additionally, nonresponsiveness to sympathetic blockades or modulation of sympathetic activity may be explained by the observation that the sympathetic maintained pain component is not a constant phenomenon over time and decreases in the course of the disease [74]. Also sympathetic activity may act independently from the peripheral efferent pathways [75] and therefore account for unresponsiveness.

Pathophysiologic concepts in CRPS following stroke and spinal cord injury

Complex regional pain syndrome may occasionally develop after lesions of the central nervous system [76]. In patients with stroke, visual deficits, neglect, paresis of the shoulder girdle and somatosensory deficits are risk factors for recurrent initiating events (e.g. trauma of the affected extremity) that may self-perpetuate a vicious cycle of CRPS. Accordingly, affected extremities after brain injury are at higher risk of developing CRPS than unaffected.

Complex regional pain syndrome following spinal cord injury is relatively rare, ranging from 5% to 12% in selected cohorts. It develops within a few months, more often unilaterally at the upper extremity in tetraplegic patients. Similar to stroke patients, the association of paresis and limb trauma may initiate a vicious cycle in the pathophysiology. Additionally, CRPS may contribute to contractures in the course of spinal cord injury.

Epidemiology

Incidence and prevalence

A population-based study in the USA on CRPS I calculated an incidence of about 5.5 per 100,000 person-years at risk and a prevalence of about 21 per 100,000 [77]. An incidence of 0.8 per 100,000 person-years at risk and a prevalence of about 4 per 100,000 was reported for CRPS II. In contrast, a European population-based study determined a much higher incidence of 26.2 per 100,000 for CRPS in general when using a different diagnostic approach. However, CRPS I develops more often than CRPS II. The incidence of CRPS II in peripheral nerve injury varies from 2% to 14% in different series, with a mean around 4% [78]. Estimations suggest an incidence of CRPS I of 1–2% after fractures, 12% after brain lesions and 5% after myocardial infarction. However, the latter data for brain lesions and myocardial infarctions are relatively high and have to be interpreted with some care because of the lack of uniform diagnostic criteria in the past. Females are more often affected than males with a female-to-male ratio ranging from 2:1 to 4:1. CRPS shows a distribution over all ages, affecting the upper extremity without side preferences by about 60%, with a mean age peak at diagnosis of 37–50 years and highest incidence rates at 61–70 years. Differences in ethnicity, socio-economics and different diagnostic criteria used may contribute to epidemiologic differences.

Risk factors

No clear risk factors have been identified so far. However, etiology, psychologic state and genetic factors might influence the occurrence, course or recurrence of CRPS.

Course and recurrence

The severity rather than the etiology seems to determine the disease course. Age, sex and affected side are not associated with the outcome [77]. Fractures may be associated with a higher resolution rate (91%) than sprain (78%) or other inciting event (55%) [77]. In 1183 patients [79] the incidence of recurrence was 1.8% per year. The patients with a recurrent CRPS were significantly younger but did not differ in gender or primary localization. The recurrence of CRPS presents more often with few symptoms and signs and spontaneous onset. A low skin temperature at the onset of the disease may predict an unfavorable course and outcome [78, 80]. A retrospective analysis of 1006 CRPS cases, mostly female, and younger patients with CRPS of the lower limb showed an incidence of severe complications in about 7%, such as infection, ulceration, chronic edema, dystonia and/or myoclonus [81].

Psychologic factors

The widely proposed "CRPS personality" as a predisposing factor is clearly unsubstantiated. This assumption was further strengthened since no differences in psychologic patterns were found in patients with radius fracture developing CRPS I in comparison to patients who recovered without developing a CRPS [82]. According to this view, an even distribution of childhood trauma, pain intensity and psychologic distress was confirmed in patients with CRPS in comparison with patients with other neuropathic pain and chronic back pain [83]. Further studies demonstrated a high psychiatric co-morbidity, especially depression, anxiety and personality disorders, in CRPS patients. These findings are also present in other chronic pain patients and are thought to be at least in part more likely a result of the long and severe pain of disease [84]. Compared to patients with low back pain, CRPS patients showed a higher tendency to somatization but did not show any other psychologic differences [85]. In 145 patients, 42% reported stressful life events in close relationship to the onset of CRPS and 41% had a previous history of chronic pain [86]. Thus, stressful life events could be risk factors for the development of CRPS.

Genetics

One of the unsolved features in human pain diseases is the fact that only a minority of patients develop chronic pain after seemingly identical inciting events. Similarly, in certain nerve lesion animal models, differences in pain susceptibility were found to be due to genetic factors. A mendelian law does not seem to impact the incidence and prevalence. However, there is evidence for certain genotypes predisposing to a risk of developing CRPS. Human leukocyte antigen (HLA) associations with different phenotypes have shown an increase in A3, B7 and DR(2) major histocompatibility complex (MHC) antigens in a small group of CRPS patients in whom resistance to treatment was associated with positivity of DR(2). In a cohort of 52 CRPS patients, class I and II MHC antigens were typed. The frequency of HLA-DQ1 was found to be significantly increased compared with control frequencies [87]. In patients with CRPS who progressed towards multifocal

or generalized tonic dystonia, an association with HLA-DR13 was reported [88]. Furthermore, a different locus, centromeric in HLA class I, was found to be associated with spontaneous development of CRPS, suggesting an interaction between trauma severity and genetic factors that describe CRPS susceptibility [89]. However, to date the clinical importance of genetic factors in CRPS is not clear.

Treatment

Only a few evidence-based treatment regimens for CRPS are available so far; these are summarized in Box 20.1. In fact, three literature reviews of outcome studies found discouragingly little consistent information regarding the pharmacologic agents and methods for treatment of CRPS [90–93]. Moreover, the methodology is often poor and patient numbers are low. Although CRPS shows a different phenotype in

---

Box 20.1 Interventions supported by evidence

Modality of pain relief	Analgesics	Administration route	Evidence level
Pharmacologic treatment			
Steroids	Prednisolone	po	B
Calcium-regulating drugs	Calcitonin	IN	B
	Clodronate	IV	B
	Alendronate	IV/po	B
	Pamidronate	IV	B
Free radical scavengers	DMSO	Topical	B
	NAC	po	B
Calcium channel-blocking anticonvulsants	Gabapentin	po	C
Spinal drug application			
GABA agonists	Baclofen	IT (in dystonia)	C
α2-receptor agonist	Clonidine	Epidural	C
Stimulation techniques			
Spinal cord stimulation		Epidural	B
Physical and occupational therapy			B
Physical or occupational therapy, mirror visual feedback treatment, hand laterality recognition training, movement imagination			
Psychologic therapy			B
Cognitive behavioral treatment, graded exposure, disease education			

DMSO, dimethylsulfoxide; GABA, gamma aminobutyric acid; IN, intranasal; IV, intravenous; IT, intrathecal; NAC, N-acetylcysteine; po, oral.

comparison to other neuropathic pain syndromes like postherpetic neuralgia or painful polyneuropathy, clinicians extrapolate the results of clinical trials in these disease entities to guide therapy in CRPS. However, since functional imaging and neuropyhsiologic studies indicate that a reduction of pain does not only reduce the burden of illness but also contributes to the reversibility of cortical reorganization and improvement of function, the standard analgesics to treat neuropathic pain also become part of CRPS therapy.

Pharmacologic therapy

Interventions supported by evidence
Steroids
Orally administered prednisone, 10 mg three times daily, has clearly demonstrated efficacy in the improvement of the entire clinical status (up to 75%) of acute CRPS patients (<13 weeks) [36]. In CRPS I following stroke 40 mg prednisolone for 14 days followed by tapering significantly improved the signs and symptoms compared to piroxicam 20 mg daily [94]. In this randomized controlled trial in 60 patients, baseline scores for sensory, motor and autonomic symptoms improved significantly in the prednisolone group (drop of mean 10.7 to 4.3; score 0–14) whereas piroxicam did not show any significant change when assessed 1 month after therapy initiation.

Calcium-regulating drugs
Calcitonin administered three times daily intranasally demonstrated a significant pain reduction in CRPS patients [95]. In 2001 Perez and co-workers conducted a blinded meta-analysis on randomized trials using calcitonin in CRPS I. The meta-analysis of the five trials available evaluating the efficacy of calcitonin demonstrated a significant analgesic effect [96]. In contrast, the review of Albazaz and co-workers could not show a definite efficacy of calcitonin [97].

Clodronate 300 mg daily IV and daily alendronate 7.5 mg IV or 40 mg orally showed a significant improvement in pain, swelling and movement range in acute CRPS [98, 99]. Alendronate 40 mg daily for 8 weeks and a single infusion of pamidronate showed beneficial effects on pain and physical function [100, 101]. A nonplacebo-controlled trial showed the same efficacy of calcitonin 200 IU/day together with physiotherapy as the combination of paracetamol

1500 mg/day and physiotherapy [102]. The mode of action of these compounds in CRPS is unknown. Bisphosphonates may interact with CRPS-related bone resorption and showed some analgesic effect themselves. However, a recent meta-analysis showed a potential to reduce pain in CRPS associated with bone loss but the authors stated that there are insufficient data to recommend their use in practice [103].

Free radical scavengers
One placebo-controlled trial was performed, using the free radical scavengers dimethylsulfoxide (DMSO) 50% topically or N-acetylcysteine (NAC) orally for the treatment of CRPS I [104]. Both drugs were found to be equally effective; however, DMSO seemed more favorable for "warm" and NAC for "cold" CRPS I. The results were negatively influenced by longer disease duration. A previous trial with DMSO failed to show a positive result in CRPS [105]; however, DMSO applied in patients suffering from CRPS I of the upper extremity has been shown to be more effective than regional blocks with guanethidine in an uncontrolled trial in a small population of CRPS patients [106]. Interestingly, vitamin C has been shown to be effective in the prevention of CRPS after surgery (see below).

Gabapentin
Promising preliminary evidence was revealed by two studies on patients with CRPS that showed an analgesic effect of gabapentin [107–109]. A randomized double-blind placebo-controlled cross-over trial was performed in 58 patients with CRPS I. In half of the patients gabapentin was uptitrated to 600 mg tid and taken for 21 days before washout and placebo intake. The second group received placebo first and gabapentin thereafter. The change of pain intensity, assessed as the primary endpoint, demonstrated a mild but not statistically significant effect of gabapentin on pain compared to placebo. However, gabapentin demonstrated a significant reversal of mechanical hypoesthesia but no superior effect on motor, autonomic and positive sensory signs, such as dynamic mechanical allodynia, compared to placebo [110]. Pregabalin has not been studied in CRPS so far.

Interventions refuted by evidence
Since there is only limited evidence on the pharmacologic treatment of CRPS, there is no clear indication that any specific interventions are ineffective.

Commonly used interventions currently unproven

Nonsteroidal anti-inflammatory drugs (NSAIDs)

Naproxen has not been effective in a very small number of patients [111]. This trial assessed the ratio of bone to soft tissue uptake with scintigraphy in eight patients with CRPS I. After 3 months' intake of 500 mg naproxen bid, the uptake showed no statistically significant improvement. The effect on pain was not assessed properly in this trial. Other NSAIDs have not been investigated in the treatment of CRPS to date. However, clinical experience suggests that they can control mild to moderate pain.

Opioids

Opioids are clearly effective in postoperative, inflammatory and cancer pain. The use of opioids in CRPS has not been studied. In other neuropathic pain syndromes, compounds such as tramadol, morphine, oxycodone and levorphanol are clearly analgesic when compared to placebo. However, there are no long-term studies of oral opioid use regarding efficacy and safety for treatment of neuropathic pain generally or CRPS in particular. Even without solid scientific evidence, derived as an analogy from recent treatment recommendations for neuropathic pain, opioids could be and should be used as part of a comprehensive pain treatment program [112–114]. Opioids enable the clinician to use (potentially) fast-acting potent analgesics that might be necessary in the beginning of therapy, e.g. while uptitrating co-analgesics, but also in the long term. The definite efficacy in CRPS still remains to be determined.

Antidepressants

Tricyclic antidepressants (TCAs) have been intensively studied in different neuropathic pain conditions as published in recent treatment algorithms, but not in CRPS [112–114]. There is solid evidence that reuptake blockers of serotonin and noradrenaline (e.g. amitriptyline) and selective noradrenaline blockers (e.g. desipramine) produce pain relief in neuropathic pain. The effectiveness of selective serotonin reuptake inhibitors in neuropathic pain states is still discussed and the controlled trials conducted so far have shown limited or no efficacy [112–114]. Selective serotonin noradrenaline reuptake inhibitors, however, are effective in painful diabetic polyneuropathy [112–114]. None has been studied in CRPS patients [93].

Sodium channel-blocking agents

Lidocaine administered intravenously is effective in CRPS I and II for spontaneous and evoked pain [115]. Within this randomized double-blind placebo-controlled trial on 16 CRPS patients with predominant mechanical allodynia, lidocaine was infused once intravenously to reach three different plasma levels of 1, 2 and 3 µg/ml in each patient. Compared to baseline, lidocaine achieved a statistically significant reduction of spontaneous pain intensity at the highest plasma level and a decrease of cold and less mechanical hyperalgesia as well as dynamic mechanical allodynia.

The orally administered lidocaine analog mexiletene has not been evaluated in the treatment of CRPS and is not included in the recent therapy algorithms of neuropathic pain due to lack of efficacy or poor tolerability [112–114].

Systemic sodium channel-acting anticonvulsants, such as carbamazepine, oxcarbazepine and lamotrigine, have not been tested in CRPS. However, there is evidence for their effectiveness in various neuropathic pain conditions although recent trials using oxcarbazepine and lamotrigine failed to prove consistent efficacy [112–114].

N-methyl-D-aspartate (NMDA) receptor blockers

Clinically available compounds that are demonstrated to have NMDA receptor-blocking properties and at least in part are effective in neuropathic pain include ketamine, dextromethorphan and memantine [112–114]. An uncontrolled prospective open-label trial using low-dose ketamine infusion (40–80 mg/day) for 10 days reported pain reduction in a heterogeneous group of 40 CRPS I or II patients [116]. A combination of ketamine and midazolam in anesthetic dosages in an ICU setting over 6 days led to a full recovery in the case report of a CRPS I patient [117]. However, the trial results are inconsistent. There are only results of small trials available and accordingly these compounds are only third-line recommendations in neuropathic pain [114]. Further studies that would help clinicians to fully utilize these agents are not yet available.

Immune-modulating drugs

Only one case report showed a favorable effect of a TNF-α antagonist [118]. No solid evidence has been obtained with other immune-modulating therapies except steroids, such as immunoglobulins or immunosuppressive drugs.

Transdermal application of the α2-adrenoceptor agonist clonidine, which is though to prevent the release of catecholamines by a presynaptic action, may be helpful when small areas of hyperalgesia are present [119]. However, this uncontrolled observation was made in a small group of four patients and only three of these reported efficacy.

Invasive interventional therapy

Interventions supported by evidence
Stimulation techniques and spinal drug application
Epidural spinal cord stimulation (SCS) in one randomized study in selected chronic CRPS patients [120] improved pain and health-related quality of life but not functional outcome assessed 2 years later. Interestingly, these patients had previously undergone unsuccessful surgical sympathectomy. The pain-relieving effect was not associated with peripheral vasodilation, suggesting that central disinhibition processes are involved. Sensory detection thresholds were not affected by the stimulation. At a 5-year follow-up pain intensity, global perceived effect, treatment satisfaction and health-related quality of life in the group who received SCS and physiotherapy did not differ from those who received physiotherapy only [121](Figure 20.1). A meta-analysis showed that in selected patients SCS can relieve pain and allodynia and improve quality of life [122] but further studies are warranted since trials on larger groups of patients assessing short- and long-term efficacy on pain and motor functioning are still missing [123]. Moreover, safety data show that about 30% of the patients who received stimulation experienced treatment-related adverse events [121, 123]. Cervical and lumbar devices seem to be equally effective [124]. SCS was also effective in selected CRPS patients with sympathetically maintained pain [125] but further predicting factors beside test stimulations are still under investigation [126]. Other stimulation techniques, e.g. peripheral nerve stimulation with implanted electrodes, repetitive transcranial magnetic stimulation, and deep brain stimulation (sensory thalamus and medial lemniscus, motor cortex), have been reported to be effective in selected cases of CRPS [4, 127, 128]. In summary, there is limited evidence for the use of SCS in selected cases of CRPS but there is no evidence for using other invasive stimulation techniques as part of commonly used therapy algorithms.

Intrathecal baclofen is effective in some patients with CRPS-related dystonia [129]. Within a randomized double-blind placebo-controlled cross-over study in seven female patients with localized or generalized dystonia, baclofen, a potent GABA$_b$ receptor agonist, was applied intrathecally. After receiving 50 and 75 µg baclofen, six patients experienced complete or partial reversal of the dystonic posture of the hands but much less reversal of the dystonic posture of the legs. In these six patients a pump for continuous therapy was implanted. The follow-up showed high variability in long-term efficacy, ranging from nearly complete recovery to fading resolution of dystonia.

In selected patients with severe refractory CRPS, the epidural application of clonidine showed a greater

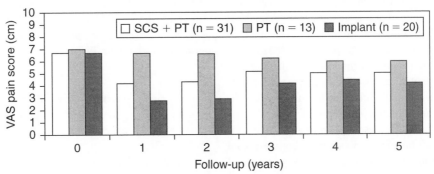

Figure 20.1 Bar graph demonstrating the mean (± SD) VAS pain scores in patients with complex CRPS I. The groups in the main analysis are represented by white and gray bars, whereas the subgroup of patients with an implant at the final follow-up is represented by black bars. Reproduced from Kemler *et al.* [121].

pain reduction in higher dosages (700 µg) than in lower dosages (300 µg) [130]. However, the drug was associated with marked side effects (e.g. sedation and hypotension).

Interventions refuted by evidence

Since proven effectiveness is lacking in large trials of interventional treatment of CRPS, there is no clear evidence for *a priori* omission of specific interventions.

Commonly used interventions currently unproven

Interventional therapy at the sympathetic nervous system level

Currently, two therapeutic techniques for blocking sympathetic activity are used:

- injections of local anesthetic around sympathetic paravertebral ganglia that project to the affected body part (sympathetic ganglion blocks)
- regional intravenous application of guanethidine, bretylium or reserpine (which all deplete noradrenaline in the postganglionic axon) to an isolated extremity blocked with a tourniquet (intravenous regional sympatholysis, IVRS).

Epidural blocks have not been investigated in CRPS within controlled studies so far.

There are many uncontrolled surveys in the literature reviewing the effect of sympathetic interventions in CRPS patients, about 70% of whom report full or partial response [131]. The efficacy of these procedures is, however, still controversial and has been questioned in the past [91, 132]. In fact, the specificity and the long-term results as well as the techniques used have rarely been adequately evaluated.

One controlled study in patients with CRPS I has shown that sympathetic ganglion blocks with local anesthetic have the same immediate effect on pain as a control injection with saline [133]. However, after 24 hours patients in the local anesthetic group were much better, indicating that nonspecific effects are important initially and that evaluating the efficacy of sympatholytic interventions is best done after 24 hours. With these data in mind, the uncontrolled studies mentioned above must be interpreted cautiously. Only 10 out of the 24 studies we reviewed assessed long-term effects.

No improvement compared with baseline was found for reserpine (IVRS) and guanethidine

(IVRS) [134]. No differences were obtained between guanethidine (IVRS) or lidocaine (lignocaine) (IVRS) [135]. Guanethidine and pilocarpine versus placebo showed no difference after application of four blocks [136]. However, stellate blocks with bupivacaine as well as regional blocks with guanethidine (IVRS) demonstrated a significant improvement of pain compared with baseline but no differences between these two therapies [137]. One study demonstrated that IVRS bretylium plus lidocaine (lignocaine) produce significantly longer pain relief than lidocaine (lignocaine) alone [138]. No effect was obtained by droperidol (IVRS) [139]. Hanna & Peat [140] demonstrated a significant improvement in pain due to a single (IVRS) bolus of ketanserin. Bounameaux *et al.* [141] failed to show any significant effect with the same procedure. Bier's block with methylprednisolone and lidocaine in CRPS I did not provide a short- or long-lasting benefit compared to placebo [142].

Although no straightforward conclusion on the efficacy of IVRS in CRPS can be drawn from the above data, the evaluation of this intervention is also limited by small sample sizes ranging from six to 21 only, insufficient trial designs and short observation periods. A meta-analysis of studies assessing the effect of intravenous regional sympathetic blockade for CRPS failed to draw conclusions concerning the effectiveness of this procedure, mainly due to small sample sizes [134].

There is a desperate need for controlled studies that assess the acute as well as the long-term effect of sympathetic blockade and IVRS on pain and other CRPS symptoms, in particular motor function. Although evidence is sparse, interventions at the sympathetic efferent system are part of therapy algorithms in CRPS that are based mainly on clinical experience and on the limited evidence of controlled trials. Well-performed sympathetic ganglion blocks should be performed rather than IVRS [143].

TENS

Transcutaneous electrical nerve stimulation (TENS) may be effective in some cases and has few side effects. No sufficient clinical trials are available.

Surgical sympathectomy

There is only limited evidence regarding the efficacy of thoracoscopic or surgical sympathectomy. Four open studies report partly long-lasting benefits in

CRPS I and II [144–147]. The most important independent factor in determining a positive outcome of sympathectomy is a time interval of less than 12 months between inciting event and sympathectomy [144, 147]. The videoscopic lumbar sympathectomy is as effective as the open surgical intervention [148]. However, one study [149] showed lower efficacy of thoracic sympathectomy in CRPS compared to other diseases. The irreversible sympathectomy may be effective in selected cases. Because of the risk of developing adaptive supersensitivity even on nociceptive neurones and consequent pain increase and prolongation, these procedures should not be recommended on a broad indication basis.

Physical therapy and occupational therapy

Physical therapy and occupational therapy are supported by the results of several trials. It should be stressed that clinical experience clearly indicates that physiotherapy is of the utmost importance in achieving recovery of function and rehabilitation. Standardized physiotherapy has shown long-term relief in pain and physical dysfunction in children [150]. Recent developments of mirror and limb recognition techniques have advanced this field.

Physical and, to a lesser extent, occupational therapy are able to reduce pain and improve active mobility in CRPS I [151]. Lymph drainage provides no benefit when applied together with physiotherapy in comparison with physiotherapy alone [152]. Patients with initially less pain and better motor function are predicted to benefit to a greater degree than others. Physical therapy of CRPS is both more effective and less costly than either occupational therapy or control treatment [153].

Mirror visual feedback treatment in CRPS I has been shown to reduce pain and improve function in a controlled trial in eight patients [62]. After a 6-week treatment phase including no-mirror control phases, pain reduction and gain of function were documented in patients with a disease duration < 1year. Although these results were obtained in a preliminary trial, recent studies have demonstrated that the combination of hand laterality recognition training, imagination of movements and mirror movements, called a motor imagery program, reduces pain and disability in CRPS patients [63–65]. Initially, 13 CRPS I patients were randomly allocated to a motor imagery program or to continuation of their previous treatment. After 12 weeks the control group crossed over to the motor imagery program [65]. As a result, a NNT of 3 for a 6-month period can be achieved. It is important to recognize that the order of training – laterality recognition, movement imagination followed by mirror movements – is important. Thus, adding the motor imagery program might be more effective than physiotherapy sparing these techniques. However, it is important to acknowledge that this conclusion is based on a small sample size only. However, physical and occupational therapy and attentional training have become an important part of successful therapy in CRPS patients.

Psychologic therapy

Although there is evidence of a psychologic impact on CRPS patients, only one study has addressed the efficacy of psychologic treatment. A prospective, randomized, single-blind trial of cognitive behavioral treatment (CBT) was conducted together with physical therapy of different intensities in children and adolescents. Twenty-eight patients were randomly assigned to two groups, both receiving six sessions of CBT, including pain management strategies, relaxation training, biofeedback, guided imagery, and physical therapy once or three times a week within a 6-week treatment period. At the end, long-lasting reduction of all symptoms in both arms in both treatment groups was demonstrated [154]. Fear of injury or reinjury by moving the affected limb is thought to be a possible predictor of chronic disability. Thus, in a small group of patients graded exposure therapy was successful in decreasing pain-related fear, pain intensity and consequent disability [155]. Beside the lack of well-controlled studies, a sequenced protocol for psychologic treatment has been proposed recently by Bruehl & Chung [156]: 1. education regarding the nature of the disease for all patients and their families, 2. if disease duration exceeds 6–8 weeks, patients should be evaluated psychologically and treated with cognitive behavioral techniques, 3. in case of psychiatric co-morbidities or major ongoing life stressors, these issues should be addressed additionally with general CBT [156].

Prevention studies

Only two reliable randomized placebo-controlled prevention studies have been conducted to date. Zollinger

Box 20.2   Commonly used interventions currently unproven

Modality of pain relief	Analgesics	Administration route
Pharmacologic treatment		
NSAIDs	e.g. naproxen, ibuprofen, diclofenac	po
Opioids	e.g. tramadol, morphine, oxycodone	po
Antidepressants	e.g. amitryptiline, desipramine, duloxetine	po
Calcium channel-blocking anticonvulsants	Pregabalin	po
Sodium channel-blocking agents/anticonvulsants	Lidocaine	IV
	Carbamazepine	po
NMDA receptor blockers	Ketamine	po/IV
	Dextrometorphan	po
Immune-modulating drugs	Intravenous immunoglobulin	IV
α2-receptor agonist	Clonidine	Topical
Interventional treatment		
Electrical nerve stimulation	TENS	Local
Intervention at the sympathetic nervous system level	Sympathetic ganglion blocks	Local
	Intravenous regional sympatholysis	IV
	Surgical sympathectomy	

IV, intravenous; NMDA, N-methyl-D-aspartate; NSAIDs, nonsteroidal anti-inflammatory drugs; po, oral; TENS, transcutaneous electrical nerve stimulation.

et al. [157] proved a significantly reduced incidence of CRPS following Colles' fracture with vitamin C (500 mg/day) treatment. In this study, 123 patients who were treated conservatively for wrist fractures were randomized to a double-blind trial receiving 500 mg vitamin C or placebo. Within the observation period of 1 year, only 7% of the treatment group developed a CRPS, compared to 22% in the placebo group. A recent trial confirmed this result and determined 500 mg as a sufficient dosage [158]. Preoperatively administered guanethidine (20 mg, RIS) did not prevent CRPS in patients undergoing fasciotomy for Dupuytren's disease [159].

Cost of treatment and cost-benefit

Treatment costs for patients suffering from neuropathic pain may exceed $100.000. Cost-benefit ratios are not available for most of the pharmacologic treatment options and interventions in CRPS so far. Only one study performed a cost analysis in CRPS I. SCS in combination with physiotherapy produced costs of 9805 Euro, physiotherapy alone was 5741 Euro. After 3 years of treatment, a lifetime cost saving of 58,471 Euro was calculated for SCS and physiotherapy treatment compared to physiotherapy monotherapy [160]. A recent review and therapy recommendations rated venlafaxine, gabapentin, pregabalin opioids and tramadol as more expensive compared to TCA.

How to produce evidence of effectiveness in future

Since the etiology, pathophysiology and clinical picture of CRPS are "complex," putting up a feasible trial protocol is challenging. However, in the light of high rates of chronicity and disability in CRPS, there is a desperate need for controlled studies regarding pharmacologic and interventional therapy in CRPS. To achieve a comprehensive evidence-based treatment algorithm, studies need to be stratified, e.g. by type of CRPS (type I or II), disease duration (acute/chronic CRPS), CRPS with SMP or SIP, and probably by subgroups, e.g. warm, intermediate, cold type. Furthermore, trials that assess the acute as well as the long-term effects, especially of interventional therapy such as sympathetic blocks and IVRS, are warranted. Outcome parameters should not focus on pain but also assess other CRPS symptoms, in particular motor function.

Authors' recommendations

Although trials to determine the best time for treatment initiation are lacking, from the pathophysiologic concerns, it is of the utmost importance that treatment in CRPS should be immediate and most importantly directed toward restoration of full function of the extremity. This view is derived from the evidence in pain research that the duration of pain leads to ongoing changes in the peripheral and central nervous system underlying chronic pain syndromes and possibly predicts less treatment response in the later course of the disease. To achieve a favorable outcome, a comprehensive interdisciplinary setting with particular emphasis on pain management and functional restoration is thought to be best [161, 162].

The severity of the disease determines the therapeutic regime. The reduction of pain is the precondition with which all other interventions have to comply. Interestingly, relative pain reduction of at least 50% and 30 mm on the 100 mm VAS is judged to be the result of a "successful" therapy [90]. All therapeutic approaches must not hurt. At the acute stage of CRPS when the patient still suffers from severe pain at rest and during movement, it is mostly impossible to carry out intensive active therapy. Painful interventions and in particular aggressive physical therapy at this stage often lead to deterioration. Therefore, immobilization, combination of hand laterality recognition training, imagination of movements and mirror movements and careful contralateral physical therapy should be the acute treatments of choice and intense pain treatment should be initiated immediately. Although definite evidence is lacking, first-line analgesics and co-analgesics are opioids, TCA and calcium/sodium channel-acting anticonvulsants. Additionally, corticosteroids should be considered if inflammatory signs and symptoms are predominant. Sympatholytic procedures, preferably sympathetic ganglion blocks, should identify the component of the pain that is maintained by the sympathetic nervous system. For efficacy, a series of blocks should be perpetuated. By block application it might be possible to decrease pain in a step-wise manner and therefore facilitate physiotherapy. Calcium-regulating agents should be used in cases of refractory pain. Despite the limited evidence, the effectiveness of topical agents is still questioned. If resting pain subsides, first passive physical therapy in combination with the motor retuning program (see above) then later active isometric followed by active isotonic training should be performed in combination with sensory desensitization programs until restitution of complete motor function is achieved. Psychologic treatment has to support the regime to strengthen coping strategies and uncover contributing factors. In refractory cases spinal cord stimulation and epidural clonidine could be considered. If refractory dystonia develops, intrathecal baclofen application is worth considering.

Acknowledgments

The authors' work was supported by the German Ministry of Research and Education, German Research Network on Neuropathic Pain (BMBF, 01EM05/04) and an unrestricted research grant (Pfizer, Germany).

References

1. Rommel O, Gehling M, Dertwinkel R, et al. Hemisensory impairment in patients with complex regional pain syndrome. *Pain* 1999; **80**: 95–101.
2. Drummond PD, Finch PM. Sensory changes in the forehead of patients with complex regional pain syndrome. *Pain* 2006; **123**(1-2): 83–89.
3. Maihofner C, Handwerker HO, Neundorfer B, Birklein F. Patterns of cortical reorganization in complex regional pain syndrome. *Neurology* 2003; **61**(12): 1707–1715.
4. Pleger B, Janssen F, Schwenkreis P, Volker B, Maier C, Tegenthoff M. Repetitive transcranial magnetic stimulation of the motor cortex attenuates pain perception in complex regional pain syndrome type I. *Neurosci Lett* 2004; **356**(2): 87–90.
5. Maihofner C, Handwerker HO, Neundorfer B, Birklein F. Cortical reorganization during recovery from complex regional pain syndrome. *Neurology* 2004; **63**(4): 693–701.
6. Pleger B, Tegenthoff M, Ragert P, et al. Sensorimotor retuning in complex regional pain syndrome parallels pain reduction. *Ann Neurol* 2005; **57**(3): 425–429.
7. Pleger B, Ragert P, Schwenkreis P, et al. Patterns of cortical reorganization parallel impaired tactile discrimination and pain intensity in complex regional pain syndrome. *Neuroimage* 2006; **32**(2): 503–510.
8. Maihofner C, Neundorfer B, Birklein F, Handwerker HO. Mislocalization of tactile stimulation in patients with complex regional pain syndrome. *J Neurol* 2006; **253**(6): 772–779.
9. Maihofner C, Handwerker HO, Neundorfer B, Birklein F. Mechanical hyperalgesia in complex regional pain syndrome: a role for TNF-alpha? *Neurology* 2005; **65**(2): 311–313.

10. Fukumoto M, Ushida T, Zinchuk VS, Yamamoto H, Yoshida S. Contralateral thalamic perfusion in patients with reflex sympathetic dystrophy syndrome. *Lancet* 1999; **354**(9192): 1790–1791.

11. Juottonen K, Gockel M, Silen T, Hurri H, Hari R, Forss N. Altered central sensorimotor processing in patients with complex regional pain syndrome. *Pain* 2002; **98**(3): 315–323.

12. Eisenberg E, Chistyakov AV, Yudashkin M, Kaplan B, Hafner H, Feinsod M. Evidence for cortical hyperexcitability of the affected limb representation area in CRPS: a psychophysical and transcranial magnetic stimulation study. *Pain* 2005; **113**(1-2): 99–105.

13. Shiraishi S, Kobayashi H, Nihashi T, *et al.* Cerebral glucose metabolism change in patients with complex regional pain syndrome: a PET study. *Radiat Med* 2006; **24**(5): 335–344.

14. Oaklander AL, Rissmiller JG, Gelman LB, Zheng L, Chang Y, Gott R. Evidence of focal small-fiber axonal degeneration in complex regional pain syndrome-I (reflex sympathetic dystrophy). *Pain* 2006; **120**(3): 235–243.

15. Albrecht PJ, Hines S, Eisenberg E, *et al.* Pathologic alterations of cutaneous innervation and vasculature in affected limbs from patients with complex regional pain syndrome. *Pain* 2006; **120**(3): 244–266.

16. Janig W, Baron R. Is CRPS I a neuropathic pain syndrome? *Pain* 2006; **120**(3): 227–229.

17. Gradl G, Schurmann M. Sympathetic dysfunction as a temporary phenomenon in acute posttraumatic CRPS I. *Clin Auton Res* 2005; **15**(1): 29–34.

18. Janig W, Baron R. Complex regional pain syndrome is a disease of the central nervous system. *Clin Auton Res* 2002; **12**(3): 150–164.

19. Janig W, Baron R. Complex regional pain syndrome: mystery explained? *Lancet Neurol* 2003; **2**(11): 687–697.

20. Birklein F, Sittle R, Spitzer A, Claus D, Neundörfer B, Handwerker HO. Sudomotor function in sympathetic reflex dystrophy. *Pain* 1997; **69**(1-2): 49–54.

21. Baron R, Maier C. Reflex sympathetic dystrophy: skin blood flow, sympathetic vasoconstrictor reflexes and pain before and after surgical sympathectomy. *Pain* 1996; **67**(2–3): 317–326.

22. Wasner G, Heckmann K, Maier C, Baron R. Vascular abnormalities in acute reflex sympathetic dystrophy (CRPS I) – complete inhibition of sympathetic nerve activity with recovery. *Arch Neurol* 1999; **56**: 613–620.

23. Wasner G, Schattschneider J, Heckmann K, Maier C, Baron R. Vascular abnormalities in reflex sympathetic dystrophy (CRPS I): mechanisms and diagnostic value. *Brain* 2001; **124**(Pt 3): 587–599.

24. Harden RN, Duc TA, Williams TR, Coley D, Cate JC, Gracely RH. Norepinephrine and epinephrine levels in affected versus unaffected limbs in sympathetically maintained pain. *Clin J Pain* 1994; **10**(4): 324–330.

25. Birklein F, Riedl B, Neundorfer B, Handwerker HO. Sympathetic vasoconstrictor reflex pattern in patients with complex regional pain syndrome. *Pain* 1998; **75**(1): 93–100.

26. Casale R, Elam M. Normal sympathetic nerve activity in a reflex sympathetic dystrophy with marked skin vasoconstriction. *J Auton Nerv Syst* 1992; **41**(3): 215–219.

27. Meier PM, Alexander ME, Sethna NF, de Jong-de Vos van Steenwijk CC, Zurakowski D, Berde CB. Complex regional pain syndromes in children and adolescents: regional and systemic signs and symptoms and hemodynamic response to tilt table testing. *Clin J Pain* 2006; **22**(4): 399–406.

28. Goldstein DS, Tack C, Li ST. Sympathetic innervation and function in reflex sympathetic dystrophy. *Ann Neurol* 2000; **48**(1): 49–59.

29. Haensch CA, Jorg J, Lerch H. I-123-metaiodobenzylguanidine uptake of the forearm shows dysfunction in peripheral sympathetic mediated neurovascular transmission in complex regional pain syndrome type I (CRPS I). *J Neurol* 2002; **249**(12): 1742–1743.

30. Drummond PD, Finch PM, Gibbins I. Innervation of hyperalgesic skin in patients with complex regional pain syndrome. *Clin J Pain* 1996; **12**(3): 222–231.

31. Birklein F, Weber M, Neundorfer B. Increased skin lactate in complex regional pain syndrome: evidence for tissue hypoxia? *Neurology* 2000; **55**(8): 1213–1215.

32. Koban M, Leis S, Schultze-Mosgau S, Birklein F. Tissue hypoxia in complex regional pain syndrome. *Pain* 2003; **104**(1-2): 149–157.

33. Schattschneider J, Hartung K, Stengel M, *et al.* Endothelial dysfunction in cold type complex regional pain syndrome. *Neurology* 2006; **67**(4): 673–675.

34. Eisenberg E, Erlich T, Zinder O, *et al.* Plasma endothelin 1 levels in patients with complex regional pain syndrome. *Eur J Pain* 2004; **8**(6): 533–538.

35. van der Laan L, Goris RJ. Reflex sympathetic dystrophy. An exaggerated regional inflammatory response? *Hand Clin* 1997; **13**(3): 373–385.

36. Christensen K, Jensen EM, Noer I. The reflex dystrophy syndrome response to treatment with systemic corticosteroids. *Acta Chir Scand* 1982; **148**(8): 653–655.

37. Oyen WJ, Arntz IE, Claessens RM, van der Meer JW, Corstens FH, Goris RJ. Reflex sympathetic dystrophy of the hand: an excessive inflammatory response? *Pain* 1993; **55**(2): 151–157.

38. Tan EC, Oyen WJ, Goris RJ. Leukocytes in complex regional pain syndrome type I. *Inflammation* 2005; **29**(4-6): 182–186.

39. Weber M, Birklein F, Neundorfer B, Schmelz M. Facilitated neurogenic inflammation in complex regional pain syndrome. *Pain* 2001; **91**(3): 251–257.

40. Leis S, Weber M, Isselmann A, Schmelz M, Birklein F. Substance-P-induced protein extravasation is bilaterally increased in complex regional pain syndrome. *Exp Neurol* 2003; **183**(1): 197–204.

41. Birklein F, Schmelz M, Schifter S, Weber M. The important role of neuropeptides in complex regional pain syndrome. *Neurology* 2001; **57**(12): 2179–2184.

42. Huygen FJ, de Bruijn AG, de Bruin MT, Groeneweg JG, Klein J, Zijistra FJ. Evidence for local inflammation in complex regional pain syndrome type 1. *Mediators Inflamm* 2002; **11**(1): 47–51.

43. Groeneweg JG, Huygen FJ, Heijmans-Antonissen C, Niehof S, Zijlstra FJ. Increased endothelin-1 and diminished nitric oxide levels in blister fluids of patients with

intermediate cold type complex regional pain syndrome type 1. *BMC Musculoskelet Disord* 2006; **7**: 91.

44. Munnikes RJ, Muis C, Boersma M, Heijmans-Antonissen C, Zijlstra FJ, Huygen FJ. Intermediate stage complex regional pain syndrome type 1 is unrelated to proinflammatory cytokines. *Mediators Inflamm* 2005; 2005(6): 366–372.

45. Schinkel C, Gaertner A, Zaspel J, Zedler S, Faist E, Schuermann M. Inflammatory mediators are altered in the acute phase of posttraumatic complex regional pain syndrome. *Clin J Pain* 2006; **22**(3): 235–239.

46. Alexander GM, van Rijn MA, van Hilten JJ, Perreault MJ, Schwartzman RJ. Changes in cerebrospinal fluid levels of pro-inflammatory cytokines in CRPS. *Pain* 2005; **116**(3): 213–219.

47. Kiralp MZ, Yildiz S, Vural D, Keskin I, Ay H, Dursun H. Effectiveness of hyperbaric oxygen therapy in the treatment of complex regional pain syndrome. *J Int Med Res* 2004; **32**(3): 258–262.

48. van de Vusse AC, Goossens VJ, Kemler MA, Weber WE. Screening of patients with complex regional pain syndrome for antecedent infections. *Clin J Pain* 2001; **17**(2): 110–114.

49. Goebel A, Vogel H, Caneris O, *et al.* Immune responses to Campylobacter and serum autoantibodies in patients with complex regional pain syndrome. *J Neuroimmunol* 2005; **162**(1-2): 184–189.

50. Gross O, Tschernatsch M, Brau ME, *et al.* Increased seroprevalence of parvovirus B 19 IgG in complex regional pain syndrome is not associated with antiendothelial autoimmunity. *Eur J Pain* 2007; **11**(2): 237–240.

51. Blaes F, Schmitz K, Tschernatsch M, *et al.* Autoimmune etiology of complex regional pain syndrome (M. Sudeck). *Neurology* 2004; **63**(9): 1734–1736.

52. Kingery WS, Davies MF, Clark JD. A substance P receptor (NK(1)) antagonist can reverse vascular and nociceptive abnormalities in a rat model of complex regional pain syndrome type II. *Pain* 2003; **104**(1-2): 75–84.

53. Turton AJ, McCabe CS, Harris N, Filipovic SR. Sensorimotor integration in complex regional pain syndrome: a transcranial magnetic stimulation study. *Pain* 2007; **127**(3): 270–275.

54. Maihofner C, Baron R, DeCol R, *et al.* The motor system shows adaptive changes in complex regional pain syndrome. *Brain* 2007; **130**(Pt 10): 2671–2687.

55. Ribbers GM, Mulder T, Geurts AC, den Otter RA. Reflex sympathetic dystrophy of the left hand and motor impairments of the unaffected right hand: impaired central motor processing? *Arch Phys Med Rehabil* 2002; **83**(1): 81–85.

56. Schwenkreis P, Maier C, Pleger B, *et al.* NMDA-mediated mechanisms in cortical excitability changes after limb amputation. *Acta Neurol Scand* 2003; **108**(3): 179–184.

57. Galer BS, Butler S, Jensen MP. Case reports and hypothesis: a neglect-like syndrome may be responsible for the motor disturbance in reflex sympathetic dystrophy (complex regional pain syndrome-1). *J Pain Symptom Manage* 1995; **10**(5): 385–391.

58. Schattschneider J. Complex regional pain syndrome – are we neglecting neglect? *Nat Clin Pract Neurol* 2007; **3**(1): 16–17.

59. Frettloh J, Huppe M, Maier C. Severity and specificity of neglect-like symptoms in patients with complex regional pain syndrome (CRPS) compared to chronic limb pain of other origins. *Pain* 2006; **124**(1-2): 184–189.

60. Moseley GL. Why do people with complex regional pain syndrome take longer to recognize their affected hand? *Neurology* 2004; **62**(12): 2182–2186.

61. Forderreuther S, Sailer U, Straube A. Impaired self-perception of the hand in complex regional pain syndrome (CRPS). *Pain* 2004; **110**(3): 756–761.

62. McCabe CS, Haigh RC, Ring EF, Halligan PW, Wall PD, Blake DR. A controlled pilot study of the utility of mirror visual feedback in the treatment of complex regional pain syndrome (type 1). *Rheumatology (Oxford)* 2003; **42**(1): 97–101.

63. Moseley GL. Graded motor imagery is effective for long-standing complex regional pain syndrome: a randomised controlled trial. *Pain* 2004; **108**(1-2): 192–198.

64. Moseley GL. Is successful rehabilitation of complex regional pain syndrome due to sustained attention to the affected limb? A randomised clinical trial. *Pain* 2005; **114**(1-2): 54–61.

65. Moseley GL. Graded motor imagery for pathologic pain: a randomized controlled trial. *Neurology* 2006; **67**(12): 2129–2134.

66. Krause P, Foerderreuther S, Straube A. Effects of conditioning peripheral repetitive magnetic stimulation in patients with complex regional pain syndrome. *Neurol Res* 2005; **27**(4): 412–417.

67. Sumitani M, Shibata M, Iwakura T, *et al.* Pathologic pain distorts visuospatial perception. *Neurology* 2007; **68**(2): 152–154.

68. Sumitani M, Rossetti Y, Shibata M, *et al.* Prism adaptation to optical deviation alleviates pathologic pain. *Neurology* 2007; **68**(2): 128–133.

69. Stanton-Hicks M, Janig W, Hassenbusch S, Haddox JD, Boas R, Wilson P. Reflex sympathetic dystrophy: changing concepts and taxonomy. *Pain* 1995; **63**(1): 127–133.

70. Baron R, Levine JD, Fields HL. Causalgia and reflex sympathetic dystrophy: does the sympathetic nervous system contribute to the generation of pain? *Muscle Nerve* 1999; **22**: 678–695.

71. Ali Z, Raja SN, Wesselmann U, Fuchs PN, Meyer RA, Campbell JN. Intradermal injection of norepinephrine evokes pain in patients with sympathetically maintained pain. *Pain* 2000; **88**(2): 161–168.

72. Mailis-Gagnon A, Bennett GJ. Abnormal contralateral pain responses from an intradermal injection of phenylephrine in a subset of patients with complex regional pain syndrome (CRPS). *Pain* 2004; **111**(3): 378–384.

73. Baron R, Schattschneider J, Binder A, Siebrecht D, Wasner G. Relation between sympathetic vasoconstrictor activity and pain and hyperalgesia in complex regional pain syndromes: a case-control study. *Lancet* 2002; **359**(9318): 1655–1660.

74. Schattschneider J, Binder A, Siebrecht D, Wasner G, Baron R. Complex regional pain syndromes: the influence of cutaneous and deep somatic sympathetic innervation on pain. *Clin J Pain* 2006; **22**(3): 240–244.

75. Drummond PD, Finch PM. Persistence of pain induced by startle and forehead cooling after sympathetic blockade in patients with complex regional pain syndrome. *J Neurol Neurosurg Psychiatry* 2004; **75**(1): 98–102.

76. Wasner G, Schattschneider J, Binder A, Baron R. Complex regional pain syndrome – diagnostic, mechanisms, CNS involvement and therapy. *Spinal Cord* 2003; **41**(2): 61–75.

77. Sandroni P, Benrud-Larson LM, McClelland RL, Low PA. Complex regional pain syndrome type I: incidence and prevalence in Olmsted County, a population-based study. *Pain* 2003; **103**(1-2): 199–207.

78. Veldman PH, Reynen HM, Arntz IE, Goris RJ. Signs and symptoms of reflex sympathetic dystrophy: prospective study of 829 patients. *Lancet* 1993; **342**(8878): 1012–1016.

79. Veldman PH, Goris RJ. Multiple reflex sympathetic dystrophy. Which patients are at risk for developing a recurrence of reflex sympathetic dystrophy in the same or another limb [see comments]. *Pain* 1996; **64**(3): 463–466.

80. Vaneker M, Wilder-Smith OH, Schrombges P, de Man-Hermsen I, Oerlemans HM. Patients initially diagnosed as 'warm' or 'cold' CRPS 1 show differences in central sensory processing some eight years after diagnosis: a quantitative sensory testing study. *Pain* 2005; **115**(1-2): 204–211.

81. van der Laan L, Veldman PH, Goris RJ. Severe complications of reflex sympathetic dystrophy: infection, ulcers, chronic edema, dystonia, and myoclonus. *Arch Phys Med Rehabil* 1998; **79**(4): 424–429.

82. Puchalski P, Zyluk A. Complex regional pain syndrome type 1 after fractures of the distal radius: a prospective study of the role of psychological factors. *J Hand Surg [Br]* 2005; **30**(6): 574–580.

83. Ciccone DS, Bandilla EB, Wu W. Psychological dysfunction in patients with reflex sympathetic dystrophy. *Pain* 1997; **71**(3): 323–333.

84. Monti DA, Herring CL, Schwartzman RJ, Marchese M. Personality assessment of patients with complex regional pain syndrome type I. *Clin J Pain* 1998; **14**(4): 295–302.

85. Bruehl S, Husfeldt B, Lubenow TR, Nath H, Ivankovich AD. Psychological differences between reflex sympathetic dystrophy and non- RSD chronic pain patients. *Pain* 1996; **67**(1): 107–114.

86. Birklein F, Riedl B, Sieweke N, Weber M, Neundorfer B. Neurological findings in complex regional pain syndromes – analysis of 145 cases. *Acta Neurol Scand* 2000; **101**(4): 262–269.

87. Kemler MA, van de Vusse AC, van den Berg-Loonen EM, Barendse GA, van Kleef M, Weber WE. HLA-DQ1 associated with reflex sympathetic dystrophy. *Neurology* 1999; **53**(6): 1350–1351.

88. van Hilten JJ, van de Beek WJ, Roep BO. Multifocal or generalized tonic dystonia of complex regional pain syndrome: a distinct clinical entity associated with HLA-DR13. *Ann Neurol* 2000; **48**(1): 113–116.

89. van de Beek WJ, Roep BO, van der Slik AR, Giphart MJ, van Hilten BJ. Susceptibility loci for complex regional pain syndrome. *Pain* 2003; **103**(1-2): 93–97.

90. Forouzanfar T, Koke AJ, van Kleef M, Weber WE. Treatment of complex regional pain syndrome type I. *Eur J Pain* 2002; **6**(2): 105–122.

91. Kingery WS. A critical review of controlled clinical trials for peripheral neuropathic pain and complex regional pain syndromes. *Pain* 1997; **73**(2): 123–139.

92. Perez RS, Kwakkel G, Zuurmond WW, de Lange JJ. Treatment of reflex sympathetic dystrophy (CRPS type 1): a research synthesis of 21 randomized clinical trials. *J Pain Symptom Manage* 2001; **21**(6): 511–526.

93. Rowbotham MC. Pharmacological management of complex regional pain syndrome. *Clin J Pain* 2002; **22**(5): 425–429.

94. Kalita J, Vajpayee A, Misra UK. Comparison of prednisolone with piroxicam in complex regional pain syndrome following stroke: a randomized controlled trial. *QJM* 2006; **99**(2): 89–95.

95. Gobelet C, Waldburger M, Meier JL. The effect of adding calcitonin to physical treatment on reflex sympathetic dystrophy. *Pain* 1992; **48**(2): 171–175.

96. Perez RS, Kwakkel GS, Zuurmond WW, de Lange JJ. Treatment of reflex sympathetic dystrophy (CRPS type 1): a research synthesis of 21 randomized clinical trials. *J Pain Symptom Manage* 2001; **21**(6): 511–526.

97. Albazaz R, Wong YT, Homer-Vanniasinkam S. Complex regional pain syndrome: a review. *Ann Vasc Surg* 2008; **22**(2): 297–306.

98. Adami S, Fossaluzza V, Gatti D, Fracassi E, Braga V. Bisphosphonate therapy of reflex sympathetic dystrophy syndrome. *Ann Rheum Dis* 1997; **56**(3): 201–204.

99. Varenna M, Zucchi F, Ghiringhelli D, *et al.* Intravenous clodronate in the treatment of reflex sympathetic dystrophy syndrome. A randomized, double blind, placebo controlled study. *J Rheumatol* 2000; **27**(6): 1477–1483.

100. Manicourt DH, Brasseur JP, Boutsen J, Depreseaux G, Devogelaer JP. Role of alendronate in therapy for posttraumatic complex regional pain syndrome type I of the lower extremity. *Arthritis Rheum* 2004; **50**(11): 3690–3697.

101. Robinson JN, Sandom J, Chapman PT. Efficacy of pamidronate in complex regional pain syndrome type I. *Pain Med* 2004; **5**(3): 276–280.

102. Sahin F, Yilmaz F, Kotevoglu N, Kuran B. Efficacy of salmon calcitonin in complex regional pain syndrome (type 1) in addition to physical therapy. *Clin Rheumatol* 2006; **25**(2): 143–148.

103. Brunner F, Schmid A, Kissling R, Held U, Bachmann L. Biphosphonates for the therapy of complex regional pain syndrome I – systematic review. *Eur J Pain* 2008; **13**: 17–21.

104. Perez RS, Zuurmond WW, Bezemer PD, *et al.* The treatment of complex regional pain syndrome type I with free radical scavengers: a randomized controlled study. *Pain* 2003; **102**(3): 297–307.

105. Zuurmond WW, Langendijk PN, Bezemer PD, Brink HE, de Lange JJ, van Loenen AC. Treatment of acute reflex sympathetic dystrophy with DMSO 50% in a fatty cream. *Acta Anaesthesiol Scand* 1996; **40**(3): 364–367.

106. Geertzen JH, de Bruijn H, de Bruijn-Kofman AT, Arendzen JH. Reflex sympathetic dystrophy: early treatment and psychological aspects. *Arch Phys Med Rehabil* 1994; **75**(4): 442–446.

107. Mellick LB, Mellick GA. Successful treatment of reflex sympathetic dystrophy with gabapentin. *Am J Emerg Med* 1995; **13**(1): 96.

108. Mellick GA, Mellick LB. Gabapentin in the management of reflex sympathetic dystrophy. *J Pain Symptom Manage* 1995; **10**(4): 265–266.

109. Serpell MG. Gabapentin in neuropathic pain syndromes: a randomised, double-blind, placebo-controlled trial. *Pain* 2002; **99**(3): 557–566.

110. van de Vusse AC, Stomp-van den Berg SG, Kessels AH, Weber WE. Randomised controlled trial of gabapentin in complex regional pain syndrome type 1 [ISRCTN84121379]. *BMC Neurol* 2004; **4**: 13.

111. Rico H, Merono E, Gomez-Castresana F, Torrubiano J, Espinos D, Diaz P. Scintigraphic evaluation of reflex sympathetic dystrophy: comparative study of the course of the disease under two therapeutic regimens. *Clin Rheumatol* 1987; **6**(2): 233–237.

112. Finnerup NB, Otto M, McQuay HJ, Jensen TS, Sindrup SH. Algorithm for neuropathic pain treatment: an evidence based proposal. *Pain* 2005; **118**: 289–305.

113. Attal N, Cruccu G, Haanpää M, *et al.*. EFNS guidelines on pharmacological treatment of neuropathic pain. *Eur J Neurol* 2006; **13**: 1153–1169.

114. Dworkin RH, O'Connor AB, Backonja M, *et al.* Pharmacologic management of neuropathic pain: evidence-based recommendations. *Pain* 2007; **132**: 237–251.

115. Wallace MS, Ridgeway BM, Leung AY, Gerayli A, Yaksh TL. Concentration-effect relationship of intravenous lidocaine on the allodynia of complex regional pain syndrome types I and II. *Anesthesiology* 2000; **92**(1): 75–83.

116. Goldberg ME, Domsky R, Scaringe D, *et al.* Multi-day low dose ketamine infusion for the treatment of complex regional pain syndrome. *Pain Physician* 2005; **8**(2): 175–179.

117. Kiefer RT, Rohr P, Ploppa A, Altemeyer KH, Schwartzman RJ. Complete recovery from intractable complex regional pain syndrome, CRPS-type I, following anesthetic ketamine and midazolam. *Pain Pract* 2007; **7**(2): 147–150.

118. Huygen FJ, Niehof S, Zijlstra FJ, van Hagen PM, van Daele PL. Successful treatment of CRPS 1 with anti-TNF. *J Pain Symptom Manage* 2004; **27**(2): 101–103.

119. Davis KD, Treede RD, Raja SN, Meyer RA, Campbell JN. Topical application of clonidine relieves hyperalgesia in patients with sympathetically maintained pain [see comments]. *Pain* 1991; **47**(3): 309–317.

120. Kemler MA, Barendse GA, van Kleef M, *et al.* Spinal cord stimulation in patients with chronic reflex sympathetic dystrophy. *N Engl J Med* 2000; **343**(9): 618–624.

121. Kemler MA, de Vet HC, Barendse GA, van den Wildenberg FA, van Kleef M. Effect of spinal cord stimulation for chronic complex regional pain syndrome type I: five-year final follow-up

122. Taylor RS. Spinal cord stimulation in complex regional pain syndrome and refractory neuropathic back and leg pain/failed back surgery syndrome: results of a systematic review and meta-analysis. *J Pain Symptom Manage* 2006; **31**(4 suppl): S13–S19.

123. Turner JA, Loeser JD, Deyo RA, Sanders SB. Spinal cord stimulation for patients with failed back surgery syndrome or complex regional pain syndrome: a systematic review of effectiveness and complications. *Pain* 2004; **108**(1-2): 137–147.

124. Forouzanfar T, Kemler MA, Weber WE, Kessels AG, van Kleef M. Spinal cord stimulation in complex regional pain syndrome: cervical and lumbar devices are comparably effective. *Br J Anaesth* 2004; **92**(3): 348–353.

125. Harke H, Gretenkort P, Ladleif HU, Rahman S. Spinal cord stimulation in sympathetically maintained complex regional pain syndrome type I with severe disability. A prospective clinical study. *Eur J Pain* 2005; **9**(4): 363–373.

126. Eisenberg E, Backonja MM, Fillingim RB, *et al.* Quantitative sensory testing for spinal cord stimulation in patients with chronic neuropathic pain. *Pain Pract* 2006; **6**(3): 161–165.

127. Hassenbusch SJ, Stanton-Hicks M, Schoppa D, Walsh JG, Covington EC. Long-term results of peripheral nerve stimulation for reflex sympathetic dystrophy. *J Neurosurg* 1996; **84**(3): 415–423.

128. Son UC, Kim MC, Moon DE, Kang JK. Motor cortex stimulation in a patient with intractable complex regional pain syndrome type II with hemibody involvement. Case report. *J Neurosurg* 2003; **98**(1): 175–179.

129. van Hilten BJ, van de Beek WJ, Hoff JI, Voormolen JH, Delhaas EM. Intrathecal baclofen for the treatment of dystonia in patients with reflex sympathetic dystrophy. *N Engl J Med* 2000; **343**(9): 625–630.

130. Rauck RL, Eisenach JC, Jackson K, Young LD, Southern J. Epidural clonidine treatment for refractory reflex sympathetic dystrophy. *Anesthesiology* 1993; **79**(6): 1163–1169; discussion 27A.

131. Cepeda MS, Lau J, Carr DB. Defining the therapeutic role of local anesthetic sympathetic blockade in complex regional pain syndrome: a narrative and systematic review. *Clin J Pain* 2002; **18**(4): 216–233.

132. Schott GD. Interrupting the sympathetic outflow in causalgia and reflex sympathetic dystrophy. *BMJ* 1998; **316**(7134): 792–793.

133. Price DD, Long S, Wilsey B, Rafii A. Analysis of peak magnitude and duration of analgesia produced by local anesthetics injected into sympathetic ganglia of complex regional pain syndrome patients. *Clin J Pain* 1998; **14**(3): 216–226.

134. Jadad AR, Carroll D, Glynn CJ, McQuay HJ. Intravenous regional sympathetic blockade for pain relief in reflex sympathetic dystrophy: a systematic review and a randomized, double- blind crossover study. *J Pain Symptom Manage* 1995; **10**(1): 13–20.

135. Ramamurthy S, Hoffman J. Intravenous regional guanethidine in the treatment of reflex sympathetic dystrophy/causalgia: a randomized, double-blind study. Guanethidine Study Group. *Anesth Analg* 1995; **81**(4): 718–723.

136. Livingstone JA, Atkins RM. Intravenous regional guanethidine blockade in the treatment of post-traumatic complex regional pain syndrome type 1 (algodystrophy) of the hand. *J Bone Joint Surg Br* 2002; **84**(3): 380–386.

137. Bonelli S, Conoscente F, Movilia PG, Restelli L, Francucci B, Grossi E. Regional intravenous guanethidine vs. stellate ganglion block in reflex sympathetic dystrophies: a randomized trial. *Pain* 1983; **16**(3): 297–307.

138. Hord AH, Rooks MD, Stephens BO, Rogers HG, Fleming LL. Intravenous regional bretylium and lidocaine for treatment of reflex sympathetic dystrophy: a randomized, double-blind study. *Anesth Analg* 1992; **74**(6): 818–821.

139. Kettler RE, Abram SE. Intravenous regional droperidol in the management of reflex sympathetic dystrophy: a double-blind, placebo-controlled, crossover study. *Anesthesiology* 1988; **69**(6): 933–936.

140. Hanna MH, Peat SJ. Ketanserin in reflex sympathetic dystrophy. A double-blind placebo controlled cross-over trial. *Pain* 1989; **38**(2): 145–150.

141. Bounameaux HM, Hellemans H, Verhaeghe R. Ketanserin in chronic sympathetic dystrophy. An acute controlled trial. *Clin Rheumatol* 1984; **3**(4): 556–557.

142. Taskaynatan MA, Ozgul A, Tan AK, Dincer K, Kalyon TA. Bier block with methylprednisolone and lidocaine in CRPS type I: a randomized, double-blinded, placebo-controlled study. *Reg Anesth Pain Med* 2004; **29**(5): 408–412.

143. Hord ED, Oaklander AL. Complex regional pain syndrome: a review of evidence-supported treatment options. *Curr Pain Headache Rep* 2003; **7**(3): 188–196.

144. AbuRahma AF, Robinson PA, Powell M, Bastug D, Boland JP. Sympathectomy for reflex sympathetic dystrophy: factors affecting outcome. *Ann Vasc Surg* 1994; **8**(4): 372–379.

145. Bandyk DF, Johnson BL, Kirkpatrick AF, Novotney ML, Back MR, Schmacht DC. Surgical sympathectomy for reflex sympathetic dystrophy syndromes. *J Vasc Surg* 2002; **35**(2): 269–277.

146. Schwartzman RJ, Liu JE, Smullens SN, Hyslop T, Tahmoush AJ. Long–term outcome following sympathectomy for complex regional pain syndrome type 1 (RSD). *J Neurol Sci* 1997; **150**(2): 149–152.

147. Singh B, Moodley J, Shaik AS, Robbs JV. Sympathectomy for complex regional pain syndrome. *J Vasc Surg* 2003; **37**(3): 508–511.

148. Lacroix H, Vander Velpen G, Penninckx F, Nevelsteen A, Suy R. Technique and early results of videoscopic lumbar sympathectomy. *Acta Chir Belg* 1996; **96**(1): 11–14.

149. Rizzo M, Balderson SS, Harpole DH, Levin LS. Thoracoscopic sympathectomy in the management of vasomotor disturbances and complex regional pain syndrome of the hand. *Orthopedics* 2004; **27**(1): 49–52.

150. Sherry DD, Wallace CA, Kelley C, Kidder M, Sapp L. Short- and long-term outcomes of children with complex regional pain syndrome type I treated with exercise therapy. *Clin J Pain* 1999; **15**(3): 218–223.

151. Oerlemans HM, Oostendorp RA, de Boo T, van der Laan L, Severens JL, Goris JA. Adjuvant physical therapy versus occupational therapy in patients with reflex sympathetic dystrophy/complex regional pain syndrome type I. *Arch Phys Med Rehabil* 2000; **81**(1): 49–56.

152. Uher EM, Vacariu G, Schneider B, Fialka V. [Comparison of manual lymph drainage with physical therapy in complex regional pain syndrome, type I. A comparative randomized controlled therapy study]. *Wien Klin Wochenschr* 2000; **112**(3): 133–137.

153. Severens JL, Oerlemans HM, Weegels AJ, van 't Hof MA, Oostendorp RA, Goris RJ. Cost-effectiveness analysis of adjuvant physical or occupational therapy for patients with reflex sympathetic dystrophy. *Arch Phys Med Rehabil* 1999; **80**(9): 1038–1043.

154. Lee BH, Scharff L, Sethna NF, et al. Physical therapy and cognitive-behavioral treatment for complex regional pain syndromes. *J Pediatr* 2002; **141**(1): 135–140.

155. de Jong JR, Vlaeyen JW, Onghena P, Cuypers C, den Hollander M, Ruijgrok J. Reduction of pain-related fear in complex regional pain syndrome type I: the application of graded exposure in vivo. *Pain* 2005; **116**(3): 264–275.

156. Bruehl S, Chung OY. Psychological and behavioral aspects of complex regional pain syndrome management. *Clin J Pain* 2006; **22**(5): 430–437.

157. Zollinger PE, Tuinebreijer WE, Kreis RW, Breederveld RS. Effect of vitamin C on frequency of reflex sympathetic dystrophy in wrist fractures: a randomised trial. *Lancet* 1999; **354**(9195): 2025–2028.

158. Zollinger PE, Tuinebreijer WE, Breederveld RS, Kreis RW. Can vitamin C prevent complex regional pain syndrome in patients with wrist fractures? A randomized, controlled, multicenter dose-response study. *J Bone Joint Surg Am* 2007; **89**(7): 1424–1431.

159. Gschwind C, Fricker R, Lacher G, Jung M. Does peri-operative guanethidine prevent reflex sympathetic dystrophy? *J Hand Surg Br* 1995; **20**(6): 773–775.

160. Taylor RS, van Buyten JP, Buchser E. Spinal cord stimulation for complex regional pain syndrome: a systematic review of the clinical and cost-effectiveness literature and assessment of prognostic factors. *Eur J Pain* 2006; **10**(2): 91–101.

161. Stanton-Hicks M, Baron R, Boas R, et al. Complex regional pain syndromes: guidelines for therapy. *Clin J Pain* 1998; **14**(2): 155–166.

162. Stanton-Hicks M, Burton AW, Bruehl SP, et al. An updated interdisciplinary clinical pathway for CRPS: report of an expert panel. *Pain Practice* 2002; **2**(1): 1–16.

CHAPTER 21

Central pain syndromes

Kristina B. Svendsen, Nanna B. Finnerup, Henriette Klit and Troels Staehelin Jensen

Danish Pain Research Center and Department of Neurology, Aarhus University Hospital, Aarhus, Denmark

Introduction

Central pain (CP) is defined by the International Association for the Study of Pain as "pain initiated or caused by a primary lesion or dysfunction in the central nervous system (CNS)" [1]. CP may occur in a wide spectrum of quite different neurologic diseases. The most common and well-described CP conditions are central post-stroke pain (CPSP), central pain in multiple sclerosis (MS) and central pain in spinal cord injury (SCI) including syringomyelia, but any lesion or disease affecting the central somatosensory system (cerebrum, brainstem and spinal cord) may lead to this type of pain.

The diagnosis of central pain may sometimes be difficult. Demonstration of a nervous system lesion is often not difficult in central pain conditions but differentiation from nociceptive types of pain (e.g. shoulder pain in stroke patients) or peripheral neuropathic pain (e.g. at-level pain in SCI) may not always be easy. It is important that the pain has a relevant onset after the CNS lesion or disease and that it is located in areas of sensory changes that are neuroanatomically compatible with the lesion. Central pain may be located diffusely below the level of a spinal cord injury, affect the hemibody in stroke or it may affect only a smaller part of the areas with somatosensory disturbances.

Evidence-Based Chronic Pain Management. Edited by C. Stannard, E. Kalso and J. Ballantyne. © 2010 Blackwell Publishing.

Pathophysiology

It is well known that identical lesions in the CNS may lead to CP in one patient but not in another and the underlying mechanisms of CP are still not clear. Different theories have been proposed to explain pain following CNS lesions, and they probably involve several different mechanisms at different levels in the CNS [2]. In animal models of SCI, changes in glutamate receptors, excessive glutamate release, loss of tonic inhibition by γ-aminobutyric acid (GABA) interneurones, changes in descending inhibition and facilitation, microglia activation, and abnormal expression of sodium and calcium channels have been suggested to contribute to initiation and maintenance of central pain [2]. Central sensitization in parts of the nervous system seems to be an important mechanism of CP. This is supported by the higher prevalence of sensory hypersensitivity in patients with CP [3–5]. Various disinhibition hypotheses have been put forward, including deafferentation in the lateral rapidly conducting spinothalamic tract causing disinhibition of medially located slowly conducting polysynaptic pathways [6] or lesion of a normal inhibitory effect exerted by the lateral cool projection system on the medial system of heat-pinch-cold neurones passing from lamina I to the medial part of the thalamus, resulting in the release of cold allodynia and burning and ongoing pain [7].

Central post-stroke pain

Central post-stroke pain is often continuous and described as burning, aching, pricking, lacerating, and squeezing [4] but may have any pain descriptor.

Over two-thirds of central post-stroke pain patients have allodynia [4, 8, 9]. Tactile, movement and cold allodynia are commonly found [4, 8, 9]. Unilateral face pain, especially periorbital pain, is common in lateral medullary infarctions [10], but otherwise the pain may involve the whole hemibody or smaller parts of the area with sensory abnormality (hypo- or hypersensitivity) as a result of the stroke [9].

Prevalence

Few studies have examined the prevalence of central post-stroke pain. In a prospective study of 207 consecutive stroke patients, 8% developed central post-stroke pain within the first year [4], but prevalence figures range from 1% to 11% in various studies [9].

Risk factors

Both ischemic lesions and hemorrhages may cause CP. The frequency seems to depend on the location of the lesion. Patients with lesions in the thalamus have a higher risk of developing CP than patients with other stroke locations, and patients with lateral medullary infarctions are suggested to have a 25% incidence of CP within 6 months after their stroke [10].

Pharmacologic intervention in CPSP
(Box 21.1)

Diagnosing CPSP is the first important step in the treatment. A few randomized controlled trials have evaluated the efficacy of pharmacologic agents in CPSP. The tricyclic antidepressant amitriptyline has been studied in a three-way cross-over study with amitriptyline 75 mg daily in central post-stroke pain. Amitriptyline significantly relieved pain and the efficacy correlated well with total plasma concentration in a high number of responders with plasma concentrations exceeding 300 nmol/l [11]. In the same study, carbamazepine did not reduce central

---

Box 21.1 Interventions (oral drug treatment) supported or refuted by evidence as well as commonly used interventions currently unproven in central post-stroke pain but with evidence in other neuropathic pain conditions

Level	Drug daily dose	Study	Design	No. of patients	Pain type	Outcome	NNT (95% CI)
Interventions supported by evidence							
Grade B recommendation							
Ib	Amitriptyline 75 mg	Leijon & Boivie 1989 [11]	RCT, D, Pl, cross-over	15	Central pain	ami > pl	1.7 (1.2–3.1)
Ib	Pregabalin up to 600 mg	Vranken *et al.* 2007 [13]	RCT, D, Pl, parallel	20 pre 20 pla*	Central pain	pre > pl	3.3 (1.9–14.3)
Ib	Lamotrigine 200 mg	Vestergaard *et al.* 2001 [14]	RCT, D, Pl, cross-over	30	Central pain	lmt > pl	NA
Interventions refuted by evidence							
Ib	Carbamazepine 800 mg	Leijon & Boivie 1989 [11]	RCT, D, Pl, cross-over	15	Central pain	carb = pl	–
Ib	Citalopram 10–40 mg	Vestergaard *et al.* 1996 [12]	RCT, D, Pl, parallel	9 cit 4 pla	Central pain	cit = pl	–

Interventions commonly used but unproven in central post-stroke pain
Gabapentin
Serotonin noradrenaline reuptake inhibitors
Opioids including tramadol

Rating of evidence was evaluated according to European Federation of Neurological Societies standard [61].
* Included 21 patients with central pain following spinal cord injury and 19 with central post-stroke pain.
ami, amitriptyline; carb, carbamazepine; CI, confidence interval; cit, citalopram; D, double-blinded; lmt, lamotrigine; NNT, number needed to treat for 50% pain relief; pl/PL, placebo-controlled; pre, pregabalin; RCT, randomized clinical trial.

post-stroke pain compared to placebo; however, both amitriptyline and carbamazepine treatments gave a 20% lower mean pain intensity score during the last week of treatment and, based on the relatively small number of patients in this study, a pain-relieving effect of carbamazepine in CPSP cannot be excluded. In a small parallel study, the selective serotonin reuptake inhibitor citalopram did not relieve CPSP [12].

Recently, pregabalin was studied in a parallel group design study in patients with central pain following stroke or spinal cord injury [13]. The etiology was stroke in 19 patients (of these, thalamic lesion in four and brainstem infarction in three) and SCI in 21 patients. The study lasted 4 weeks. Pregabalin significantly relieved pain with no difference in efficacy between the groups with spinal and brain injury. The number needed to treat (NNT) for 50% pain relief was low, at 3.3 (1.9–14.3). Lamotrigine 200 mg daily also reduced pain with a mean reduction of 30% as well as cold allodynia assessed by an acetone droplet [14].

The possibility of preventing CPSP was studied using amitriptyline (10 mg the first day after the onset of stroke was diagnosed titrated to 75 mg within 3 weeks) or placebo administered to 39 stroke patients for 1 year [15]. Within this year, CPSP developed in three patients receiving amitriptyline (VAS 5.0) and in four receiving placebo (VAS 5.4) and more studies with larger samples sizes are needed to establish the role of early treatment in this condition unless certain early predictors for developing CPSP can be identified. In a randomized study with high and low strength levorphanol in peripheral and central neuropathic pain, patients with central pain following stroke were least likely to report benefit, which may partly be explained by the large number of withdrawals in this group (7/10)[16]. In another randomized controlled trial in mixed neuropathic pain which included nine patients with CPSP, dextromethorphan in a relatively small dose had no pain-relieving effect [17].

Spinal cord injury pain

Patients with SCI may experience central pain, peripheral neuropathic pain due to root lesions and nociceptive types of pain such as pain secondary to overuse, painful muscle spasms, and visceral pain [18]. In some patients, the mechanism underlying the pain may be difficult to access and often it is a mixture of different types of pain. Neuropathic pain felt below the level of injury (below-level pain) is considered a central pain, while neuropathic pain felt at the level of injury (at-level pain) in many cases may have both peripheral and central mechanisms.

Central pain in SCI is often a spontaneous ongoing pain described as burning, squeezing, pricking/sticking sensations. It may be accompanied by allodynia, in which non-noxious touch, thermal stimuli, and movement can give rise to pain. Allodynia may occasionally be present without ongoing pain. Other sensations such as paresthesia and dysesthesia may be present spontaneously or evoked, e.g. an ongoing tight sensation or tingling sensations evoked by touching the area.

Prevalence

Only a few studies have evaluated the prevalence of central pain in a SCI population. In a prospective study, 100 patients were followed for 5 years after a SCI and pain was classified based on telephone interview [19]. At 5-year follow-up, 73 patients were available and 52% were classified as having neuropathic pain (34% had below-level pain and 41% at-level neuropathic pain). In a retrospective register study of 402 patients at the SCI Unit at the Karolinska Hospital in Stockholm, Sweden, 40% had neuropathic pain (28% had below-level pain and 12% at-level pain) [20]. Thus the prevalence of central pain is suggested to be between 28% and 52%.

Risk factors

Spinal cord injury at older age seems to be a risk factor for the development of SCI neuropathic pain [20], while no consistent findings have emerged with respect to gender, level or extent (incomplete versus complete) of injury [18]. Sensory hypersensitivity is more common in SCI patients with neuropathic pain [5], while there is no difference in thermal sensitivity and thus spinothalamic tract function in SCI patients with or without central pain.

Pharmacologic intervention in SCI pain

Few randomized controlled studies have been performed in SCI pain (Box 21.2). Gabapentin and pregabalin have been shown to relieve SCI pain. In a small

Box 21.2 Interventions (oral drug treatment) supported or refuted by evidence as well as commonly used interventions currently unproven in central pain following spinal cord injury but with evidence in other neuropathic pain conditions

Level	Drug daily dose	Study	Design	No. of patients	Pain type	Outcome	NNT (95% CI)
Interventions supported by evidence							
Grade A recommendation							
Ib	Pregabalin up to 600 mg	Siddall *et al.* 2006 [23]	RCT, D, Pl, parallel	70 pre 76 pl	Central pain	pre > pl	7.1 (3.9–37)
Ib	Pregabalin up to 600 mg	Vranken *et al.* 2007 [13]	RCT, D, Pl, parallel	20 pre 20 pl*	Central pain	pre > pl	3.3 (1.9–14.3)
Grade B recommendation							
Ib	Gabapentin up to 3600 mg	Levendoglu *et al.* 2004 [22]	RCT, D, Pl, cross-over	20	Neuropathic	gab > pl	NA
Interventions refuted by evidence							
Ib	Amitriptyline 10–125 mg	Cardenas *et al.* 2002** [24]	RCT, D, Pl, parallel	44 ami 40 pl	Nociceptive + Neuropathic	ami = pl	–
Ib	Trazodone 150 mg	Davidoff *et al.* 1987 [25]	RCT, D, Pl, cross-over	18	Neuropathic	tra = pl	–
Ib	Lamotrigine 200–400 mg	Finnerup *et al.* 2002 [26]	RCT, D, Pl, cross-over	22	Neuropathic	lmt = pl	–
Ib	Valproate 600–2400 mg	Drewes *et al.* 1994 [27]	RCT, D, Pl, cross-over	20	Central pain	val = pl	–
Ib	Mexiletine 450 mg	Chiou-Tan *et al.* 1996 [28]	RCT, D, Pl, cross-over	11	Neuropathic	mex = pl	–

Interventions commonly used but unproven in spinal cord injury pain
Antidepressants (serotonin and noradrenaline reuptake inhibitors and tricyclic antidepressants)
Opioids including tramadol

Rating of evidence was evaluated according to European Federation of Neurological Societies standard [61].
Neuropathic pain includes at-level and below-level pain and thus both peripheral and central neuropathic pain.
* Included 21 patients with central pain following spinal cord Injury and 19 with central post-stroke pain.
** Study included nociceptive pain and had no separate evaluation of neuropathic pain.
ami, amitriptyline; CI, confidence interval; D, double-blinded; gab, gabapentin; lmt, lamotrigine; mex, mexiletine; NNT, number needed to treat for 50% pain relief; pl/PL, placebo-controlled; pre, pregabalin; RCT, randomized clinical trial; tra, trazodone; val, valproate.

randomized study including seven patients, there was no statistically significant effect of gabapentin [21] but in a subsequent study including 20 paraplegics with complete SCI, gabapentin up to 3600 mg relieved the intensity and frequency of pain and improved quality of life measures [22]. In a large parallel-group 12-week study, 70 SCI patients with central pain were allocated to pregabalin up to 600 mg daily and 76 SCI patients to placebo [23]. Concurrent pain medication was kept constant during the trial and included tricyclic antidepressants and antiepileptic drugs except gabapentin.

Pregabalin significantly improved pain with a mean pain decrease of -1.53 (-0.92 to -2.15), measured on a numeric rating scale (NRS 0–10), similar to values observed in studies in peripheral neuropathic pain. The effect was significant from week 1 and remained so for the duration of the study. Pregabalin also improved pain-related sleep interference and anxiety. The NNT for 50% and 30% pain relief were 7.1 (3.9–37) and 3.9 (2.5–9.1) respectively. As discussed above, pregabalin also relieved pain in 21 patients with SCI in the mixed central pain study [13]. Other trials performed in SCI pain have all been negative (see Table 21.2), but there is a risk of type II error due to limited number of patients in these studies.

In the study on amitriptyline, patients with mixed neuropathic and nociceptive pains were included and despite a mean serum concentration of 92 ng/ml, there was no significant pain-relieving effect [24]. Intensity of specific types of pain was, however, not recorded and thus an effect on neuropathic pain cannot be excluded. No effect of the antidepressant trazodone was found in a RCT including 18 SCI patients with neuropathic pain [25]. Lamotrigine was suggested to relieve pain in a subgroup of patients with incomplete injury and evoked pain, but this has not been confirmed [26]. Valproate as well as mexiletine failed to relieve CP in SCI patients [27, 28]. The combination of morphine and clonidine given intrathecally, but not the single drugs alone, provided significant pain relief in SCI patients with neuropathic pain [29]. The study suggested that the drugs had to reach either the rostral end of the lesion or supraspinal sites to exert their analgesic effects.

Intravenous drug trials are helpful in understanding mechanisms of SCI pain and such trials suggest that agents with sodium channel or NMDA receptor-blocking effects and maybe also GABA agonists may be useful in SCI pain provided the therapeutic window is large enough for oral long-term treatment (reviewed in references 5, 18). The efficacy of opioids given intravenously is less consistent, but oral opioids are suggested to relieve SCI pain [16].

Central pain in multiple sclerosis

The demyelination seen in the central nervous system in MS is the likely cause of acute and chronic central pain conditions. Acute or chronic recurrent central pain conditions associated with MS disease include trigeminal neuralgia (TN), L'Hermitte's sign, painful tonic seizures and paroxysmal extremity pain. Most commonly, the patients report a chronic ongoing central pain mostly located in the lower extremities [3, 30], but pain may be widespread. About half of the patients experience both superficial and deep pain at the same time and pain descriptors often used are pricking/tingling, aching, tiring, taut, burning and dull [3, 30].

In addition to central pain, nociceptive pain conditions (including spasm-related pain and low back pain) and pain associated with optic neuritis are frequently seen in this population of patients. It may be difficult to differentiate between nociceptive pain conditions and central pain.

Prevalence

Central pain is experienced by around 30–40% of the MS population [30]. In a few patients CP may be the first symptom of the disease and may precede other symptoms for months or even years.

Subtypes of central pain conditions in MS

The prevalence of *trigeminal neuralgia* in MS patients is estimated at 2–5% and is thus much more common than in the background population. In addition, bilateral TN is more frequently seen in MS patients [31] and TN associated with MS has a lower age of onset. TN is characterized by recurrent paroxysms of high pain intensity in the distribution of one or two branches of the fifth cranial nerve and may be triggered by nonpainful stimuli. The pathophysiology of TN pain in MS is not fully explained. The pain condition may be explained by focal demyelination of the sensory nerve fibers within the nerve root or the brainstem [32]. Increased excitability in the trigeminal afferent neurones and altered threshold for repetitive firing may be the consequence of focal demyelination leading to spontaneous firing and pain paroxysms. A close apposition of axons and an absence of intervening glial cells favor ectopic firing and ephaptic conduction.

L'Hermitte's sign is described as an electric/tingling sensation radiating down the limbs and body that may be painful. It may be provoked by neck flexion. Pathophysiologically, this pain syndrome may be explained by demyelinating lesions of sensory axons in the cervical posterior column [33]. Around 5–10% of MS patients may experience painful L'Hermitte's sign [34].

Painful tonic seizures (PTS) are reported in 1–19% of the MS population. PTS are described as paroxysms of uncontrollable uni- or bilaterally dystonic posturing, lasting minutes, preceded and accompanied by a cramp-like, radiating pain [35, 36]. Movements or nonpainful tactile stimulation may provoke PTS. Electroencephalography shows no abnormalities and the patient is conscious during attacks. Unilateral PTS is suggested to be caused by lesions involving the contralateral posterior limb of the internal capsule or cerebral peduncle [36], whereas bilateral PTS is more likely caused by lesions involving pyramidal fibers in the medulla oblongata or medulla spinalis. The underlying mechanism may be explained by transversely spreading ephaptic activation within a demyelinated lesion. It may be argued that pain associated with dystonic posturing in PTS is rather classified as a nociceptive pain condition. However, pain precedes other symptoms in PTS and part of the pain reported by patients is probably of central origin.

Acute paroxysmal extremity pain not associated with PTS has been described as lasting seconds to minutes [37], often located to the extremities. It has been suggested that paroxysmal extremity pain in MS occurs on the basis of ectopic activity at sites of demyelination in CNS [38]. Paroxysmal limb pain occurs in about 1–4% of MS patients [37, 39].

Chronic ongoing central pain is seen in around 25% of MS patients [30]. The pathophysiology of this type of pain is unknown. As chronic CP in MS most often affects the lower extremities and often is bilateral, it may be speculated that medullar lesions (plaques) in particular may give rise to CP conditions [30].

The sensory function in MS patients with pain has only been evaluated in a few studies. Two clinical studies [37, 39] found that almost all MS patients with CP had involvement of the posterior column, whereas not all showed clinical involvement of the spinothalamic tract. Österberg [40] studied 62 MS patients with CP and 16 MS patients with sensory abnormalities but without pain. Quantitative sensory testing (QST) revealed that the temperature sense was more affected in pain patients than in controls. Comparison of sensory function at maximal pain site in 50 MS patients with pain and 50 MS patients without pain [3] showed that the spinothalamic and lemniscal pathways were affected in both groups with no differences in detection or pain thresholds (QST). The MS patients with pain (58% with central pain), however, more frequently reported cold allodynia (acetone), abnormal temporal summation, lower threshold for mechanical pressure and pinprick hyperalgesia. This suggests that MS pain is associated with some degree of hyperexcitability in the CNS.

Risk factors of CP in MS

Longer disease duration, higher age, higher degree of disability (higher Expanded Disability Status Scale (EDSS) score) and a progressive disease course are associated with the presence of general pain in MS [34]. However, it has not been evaluated if these factors also influence the risk of developing central pain.

Pharmacologic intervention in MS associated CP (Box 21.3)

The first-line treatment for both idiopathic and MS-related TN is carbamazepine which in RCT has been shown to reduce TN pain and paroxysms. Alternatively, oxcarbazepine may be used, though with a lower strength of evidence (for review see reference 41). The efficacy of antiepileptics in treating MS-related TN has not been documented so far. Uncontrolled studies including small numbers of patients have reported a reduction of TN pain in MS by lamotrigine [42] and gabapentin [43].

Painful tonic seizures in MS are normally treated with anticonvulsants [44] including carbamazepine, phenytoin and gabapentin. Pain-reducing effect of carbamazepine and diphenylhydantoin has only been reported in randomized trials in individual patients (N of 1 trial) [35]. Both IV lidocaine and mexiletine were found to be superior to placebo in treating PTS in a nonrandomized placebo-controlled study [45].

In a recent randomized placebo-controlled study concerning the effect of cannabinoids on CP in MS [46], seven of the included patients had PTS and the authors stated that treatment response for this subgroup was as good as treatment response for patients with dysesthetic limb pain (see next section).

Chronic and recurrent central pain conditions including paroxysmal limb pain are often treated with antiepileptics or tricyclic antidepressants [44]. However, choosing these medications as first-line treatment of CP is not based on large RCT in MS patients. Österberg [40] conducted a randomized placebo-controlled three-phase trial evaluating the effect of amitriptyline and carbamazepine on CP in MS. A weak effect of amitriptyline (75 mg daily), but not carbamazepine, on nonparoxysmal central pain was found. Many dropouts (in the two active treatment periods) due to side

Box 21.3 Interventions (oral drug treatment) supported or refuted by evidence as well as commonly used interventions currently unproven in multiple sclerosis but with evidence in other neuropathic pain conditions

Level	Drug daily dose	Study	Design	No. of patients	Pain type	Outcome	NNT (95% CI)
Interventions supported by evidence							
Grade B recommendation							
Ib	Dronabinol (THC) 5–10 mg	Svendsen *et al.* 2004 49]	RCT, D, Pl, cross-over	24	Chronic CP	THC > pl	3.5 (1.9–24.8)
Ib	THC:CBD (CBM) 25.9 mg:24 mg	Rog *et al.* 2005 [46]	RCT, D, Pl, parallel	34, CBM 32, pl	Chronic CP (59) PTS (7)	CBM > pl	3.7 (2.2–13.0)
Grade C recommendation							
II	Amitriptyline 75 mg	Österberg 2005** [40]	RCT, D, Pl, three-phase, cross-over	23	Nonparox CP	ami > pl	NA
Interventions refuted by evidence							
II	Carbamazepine 600–800 mg	Österberg 2005*** [40]	RCT, D, Pl, three-phase, cross-over	23	Nonparox CP	carb = pl	–
Interventions commonly used but unproven in multiple sclerosis							
Gabapentin/pregabalin							
Tricyclic antidepressants							
Carbamazepine/oxcarbazepine for TN/PTS							
Lamotrigine for TN/PTS							

Rating of evidence was evaluated according to European Federation of Neurological Societies standard [61].

* Level B recommendation due to possible side effects.

** Seven patients dropped out during amitriptyline phase.

*** Twelve patients dropped out during carbamazepine phase.

ami, amitriptyline; carb, carbamazepine; CBM, cannabis-based medicine; CI, confidence interval; CP, central pain; D, double-blinded; European Federation of Neurological Societies; NNT, number needed to treat for 50% pain relief; pl/PL, placebo-controlled; PTS, painful tonic spasms; RCT, randomized clinical trial; THC, δ-9-tetrahydrocannabinol; TN, trigeminal neuralgia.

effects affected the results of this study. The target dose of carbamazepine had to be reduced (from 800 mg to 600 mg daily).

According to open studies and clinical reports, gabapentin and lamotrigine may be effective analgesics in MS. However, no randomized studies have evaluated this. In an open-label study [47] moderate to excellent pain relief was obtained by gabapentin treatment in 15 of 22 MS patients with a variety of pain syndromes. However, 50% of the patients reported side effects and five had to discontinue treatment.

Different studies suggest that opioids may be used as alternative analgesics in neuropathic pain conditions (for review see reference 41). In MS patients the efficacy of opioids in CP has not been documented. In a nonrandomized, placebo-controlled study [48] it was found that IV morphine only had an analgesic effect in a minority (4/14) of the MS patients with central pain.

The efficacy of cannabinoids in the treatment of central pain in MS has recently been evaluated in two RCT. Svendsen *et al.* [49] conducted a randomized cross-over trial including 24 MS patients with CP. Three weeks' treatment with orally administered synthetic δ-9-tetrahydrocannabinol (THC) (dronabinol) in a maximal dose of 10 mg reduced the intensity of ongoing and paroxysmal pain. In a randomized placebo-controlled parallel trial by Rog *et al.* [46] a whole-plant cannabis-based oromucosal spray (CBM) was administered to MS patients with central pain (including seven with PTS). Also in this study, CBM was found to be effective in reducing CP.

In the same line a large randomized placebo-controlled multicenter study from the UK [50] found an improvement in pain after 15 weeks' treatment with cannabinoids (oral THC or cannabis extract). The primary outcome measure of this study, however, was spasticity and no information was given about subtypes of pain. In a heterogeneous group of neurologic patients (including 14 MS patients, four patients with spinal cord injury and two patients with peripheral nerve injury) a double-blind placebo-controlled cross-over trial [51] found that both cannabidiol and THC were superior to placebo in pain relief.

Intrathecally administered baclofen (50 μg) had a pain-relieving effect in a small randomized trial including four MS patients, one patient with SCI and two patients with transverse myelitis [52]. Both dysesthetic and spasm-related pain were reduced.

Side effects of commonly used drugs in central pain

Gabapentin and pregabalin are structurally related compounds and have similar side effect profiles. They are usually well tolerated with no contraindications except for known hypersensitivity to their components and lack drug interactions although additive side effects may be seen. Dose reduction is needed in patients with impaired renal function. The most common adverse reactions are dose-related somnolence, which seems to be higher in the SCI population (41% in the pregabalin group and 9% in the placebo group [23]) than in peripheral pain trials, and dizziness (occurring in 20–40%). These side effects pose a risk for accidental injury in the elderly. Other adverse reactions include dry mouth, asthenia, blurred vision, ataxia, peripheral edema, and weight gain.

Lamotrigine is also well tolerated but is associated with dizziness, ataxia, diplopia, somnolence, and nausea. The most serious side effects are allergic exanthema and Stevens–Johnson syndrome and therefore, very slow dose escalation is recommended.

Tricyclic antidepressants have common side effects attributed to anticholinergic actions, e.g. dry mouth, constipation, sweating, urinary retention, and blurred vision. There is a risk of somnolence and confusion,

especially in elderly patients and patients treated with concomitant centrally acting drugs, and orthostatic hypotension and gait disturbances are also concerns. TCAs are contraindicated in patients with epilepsy. The most serious side effect is cardiotoxicity and TCAs are contraindicated in patients with heart failure and cardiac conduction blocks and ECG is needed before initiating treatment with TCAs.

The most common side effect of serotonin noradrenalin reuptake inhibitors (SNRI) is nausea. Other side effects include somnolence, dizziness, constipation, anorexia, sweating, and sexual dysfunction. SNRI are safer drugs to use than TCA in patients with cardiac disease.

The most frequently reported side effects of cannabis-based medicine in clinical studies in MS were related to the central nervous system (dizziness, headache, somnolence/tiredness), gastrointestinal tract (dry mouth, constipation, diarrhea) and musculoskeletal system (myalgia, weakness). A few patients reported psychiatric side effects including euphoria and dissociation. Tachycardia is a known side effect of dronabinol. Combination treatment with TCA, antihistamine or anticholinergics increases the risk of tachycardia, hypertension and somnolence. Cannabinoids should be used with caution in patients with a history of heart disese or seizure disorder. Although more studies support the thesis that cannabinoids are effective in treating central pain in MS patients, it should be noted that additional studies are needed to fully determine the safety profile of these drugs. Cannabis use has been shown to be an independent risk factor for psychosis and psychotic symptoms, especially in adolescence, in individuals who have previously experienced psychotic symptoms and in those with genetic predisposition to schizophrenia [53] and therefore cannabis-based medicine should be avoided in these groups of patients. Addiction is not a common problem but has been reported after long-term treatment with high doses in healthy volunteers (Marinol, official FDA information).

The most common adverse effects of opioids are sedation, constipation and nausea and often treatment requires administration of laxatives and antiemetics. Other side effects include confusion, especially in elderly patients, urinary retention, dizziness, dysphoria, and nightmares. Cognitive changes, addiction and tolerance issues as well as unsettled long-term hormonal changes are reasons for not considering opioids as first-line drugs in chronic noncancer pain [54].

Conclusion – evidence-based treatment of central pain

Treatment algorithm in CP

It is difficult to suggest a treatment algorithm based on randomized controlled trials within each of the above-mentioned central pain conditions and impossible in more rare central pain conditions. Peripheral and central pain conditions share common clinical characteristics and it is likely that some of the underlying mechanisms may be similar. Most drugs suggested to be effective in neuropathic pain (TCA, SNRI, gabapentin/pregabalin, opioids and tramadol) are nonspecific and act at multiple sites in both the peripheral and central nervous systems. So far, there is no evidence to suggest that these drugs/drug classes are effective in only some neuropathic pain conditions and it is rational to expect some overlap in efficacy in various central pain conditions and probably also to translate efficacy from peripheral to central pain conditions.

Pregabalin and gabapentin, whose analgesic action is thought to occur via binding to the $\alpha_2\delta$ subunit of voltage-gated calcium channels, have been found effective in both central and peripheral pain syndromes and are normally well tolerated [13, 23, 41]. Therefore we recommend pregabalin/gabapentin as first-line treatment of CP. The efficacy of TCA is documented in peripheral neuropathic pain conditions, whereas the results of randomized trials in different CP conditions are somewhat more conflicting. Amitriptyline reduced CPSP [11] but was ineffective in SCI pain [24]. However, in the SCI trial the primary endpoint was overall pain, not neuropathic pain. The results in peripheral neuropathic pain are very consistent [41] and TCA are therefore recommended here as the second choice of treatment in CP. No RCT have evaluated the efficacy of SNRI in central pain, whereas this class of drugs has shown a moderate effect on pain in painful polyneuropathy [41]. The possible side effects of TCA may limit their use and in patients with cardiac disease, SNRI may be a safer choice.

Lamotrigine has been shown to reduce pain in CPSP in one trial [14] but in SCI pain, there was no effect of lamotrigine although there was some suggestion that it reduced pain in the subgroup of patients with incomplete SCI [26]. Lamotrigine has few side effects and slow dose escalation limits the risk of serious allergic reactions and so it may be considered an alternative analgesic in central pain.

Cannabinoids were shown to be effective in reducing MS-related central pain and were well tolerated in low-dose regimens [46, 49]. However, possible long-term effects including psychiatric symptoms have not been ruled out and cannabinoids are therefore not recommended as first-line treatment in CP. The same is true of opioids and tramadol, in which long-term side effects and drug addiction are concerns. Small studies in CP have failed to document an effect of opioids in stroke patients [16] and MS patients [48]. However, opioids as well as tramadol are effective in reducing peripheral neuropathic pain and may also be considered in refractory CP.

There is a good rationale for combining drugs with different modes of action as this may lower the frequency and severity of side effects and have additive and maybe even synergistic effects but there is little clinical evidence for these assumptions.

Thus, based on efficacy in CP and peripheral neuropathic pain [55], as well as considering side effects and long-tem risks, a treatment algorithm for CP may look as suggested in Figure 21.1.

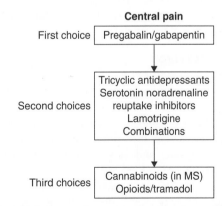

Figure 21.1 Proposed treatment algorithm for central pain conditions (trigeminal neuralgia in MS not included).

Future studies may reveal whether a mechanism-based treatment classification is more useful than the traditional disease-based classification.

Nonpharmacologic treatment of CP

New trials on single and repetitive transcranial magnetic stimulation suggest transient efficacy in central pain (Level B recommendation) and may be predictive of efficacy with implanted motor cortex stimulation [56–58]. Motor cortex stimulation may reduce pain in about 50% of CPSP patients as shown by two class III studies (for review see reference 58). Very few studies have been conducted evaluating the efficacy of deep brain stimulation (DBS) on central pain and the results are conflicting. Therefore the recommendation of the European Federation of Neurological Societies (EFNS) is only to perform DBS in experienced centers with established outcome measures [58].

The difficulties in obtaining optimal pain relief in CP conditions by pharmacologic intervention emphasize the need for a multidisciplinary approach. Nonpharmacologic treatment regimens including physiotherapy, cognitive and behavioral therapy are often used. Norbrink *et al.* [59] performed a non-randomized study, in which a multidisciplinary pain program was evaluated in patients with SCI and neuropathic pain. The 10-week program included educational sessions on pain physiology/pharmacology, behavioral therapy, relaxation techniques and body awareness training and included 27 patients with SCI. A control group consisting of 11 patients with neuropathic pain was included. At 12-month follow-up no effect was seen on pain intensity, but the level of anxiety and depression decreased. Other methods such as hypnosis may also be useful.

Future research

There is a strong need for more randomized clinical studies in optimizing the treatment of CP. Large-scale multicenter studies on both pharmacologic and nonpharmacologic treatments are warranted. Studies evaluating the efficacy of combining different analgesics could give us more information about possible synergistic effects. In the evaluation of treatment efficacy, simple psychometric scales on pain intensity and quality of life measures are recommended [60]. The intensity of different pain qualities (including spontaneous and evoked pain) should be measured separately, enabling us to assess the possibility of a mechanism-based treatment. Functional neuroimaging may in the future give us a better understanding of central pain processing and pathophysiologic differences in spontaneous and provoked pain.

Authors' recommendations

Currently only a few clinical studies are available to guide us in the treatment of the individual patient with CP. However, we recommend that clinicians follow the evidence based treatment algorithm given in Figure 21.1. In our opinion, this is the best treatment option at the time of writing.

It is well known that the outcome of pharmacotherapeutic treatment of neuropathic pain (including CP) is poor. Only 30–40% of patients will achieve a target of at least 50% pain reduction. Therefore, we recommend that a multidisciplinary team (including pain nurses, physiotherapists and psychologists) is established at the pain clinic to help patients to cope with the pain. Invasive procedures such as DBS need further documentation on therapy for CP and are not recommended at this time.

Acknowledgments

Dr Jensen has received research support, consulting fees or honoraria in the past year from Eli Lilly, Lundbeck Research Foundation, Neurosearch, and Pfizer. Dr Finnerup has received research support or honoraria in the past year from Pfizer, Neurosearch, UCB Nordic, Endo Pharmaceuticals, and Mundipharma.

References

1. Merskey H, Bogduk N. *Classification of Chronic Pain: Descriptions of Chronic Pain Syndromes and Definitions of Pain Terms.* IASP Press, Seattle, 1994.
2. Yezierski RP. Pain following spinal cord injury: central mechanisms. In: Cervero F, Jensen TS (eds) *Handbook of Clinical Neurology: Pain.* Elsevier, Amsterdam, 2006: 293–307.
3. Svendsen KB, Jensen TS, Hansen HJ, Bach FW. Sensory function and quality of life in patients with multiple sclerosis and pain. *Pain* 2005; **114**: 473–481.
4. Andersen G, Vestergaard K, Ingeman NM, Jensen TS. Incidence of central post-stroke pain. *Pain* 1995; **61**: 187–193.

5. Finnerup NB, Jensen TS. Spinal cord injury pain – mechanisms and treatment. *Eur J Neurol* 2004; **11**: 73–82.

6. Pagni CA. *Central Pain – A Neurosurgical Challenge*. Edizioni Minerva Medica, Turin, 1998.

7. Craig AD, Chen K, Bandy D, Reiman EM. Thermosensory activation of insular cortex. *Nat Neurosci* 2000; **3**: 184–190.

8. Bowsher D. Central pain: clinical and physiological characteristics. *J Neurol Neurosurg Psychiatry* 1996; **61**: 62–69.

9. Boivie J. Central pain. In: McMahon SB, Koltzenburg M (eds) *Textbook of Pain*. Elsevier Churchill Livingstone, London, 2006: 1057–1074.

10. MacGowan DJ, Janal MN, Clark WC, *et al.* Central post-stroke pain and Wallenberg's lateral medullary infarction: frequency, character, and determinants in 63 patients. *Neurology* 1997; **49**: 120–125.

11. Leijon G, Boivie J. Central post-stroke pain – a controlled trial of amitriptyline and carbamazepine. *Pain* 1989; **36**: 27–36.

12. Vestergaard K, Andersen G, Jensen TS. Treatment of central post-stroke pain with a selective serotonin reuptake inhibitor. *Eur J Neurol* 1996; **3**(suppl. 5): 169.

13. Vranken JH, Dijkgraaf MG, Kruis RM, van der Vegt MH, Hollmann MW, Heesen M. Pregabalin in patients with central neuropathic pain: a randomized, double-blind, placebo-controlled trial of a flexible-dose regimen. *Pain* 2008; **136**(1–2): 150–157.

14. Vestergaard K, Andersen G, Gottrup H, Kristensen BT, Jensen TS. Lamotrigine for central poststroke pain: a randomized controlled trial. *Neurology* 2001; **56**: 184–190.

15. Lampl C, Yazdi K, Roper C. Amitriptyline in the prophylaxis of central poststroke pain. Preliminary results of 39 patients in a placebo-controlled, long-term study. *Stroke* 2002; **33**: 3030–3032.

16. Rowbotham MC, Twilling L, Davies PS, Reisner L, Taylor K, Mohr D. Oral opioid therapy for chronic peripheral and central neuropathic pain. *N Engl J Med* 2003; **348**: 1223–1232.

17. McQuay HJ, Carroll D, Jadad AR, *et al.* Dextromethorphan for the treatment of neuropathic pain: a double-blind randomized controlled crossover trial with integral n-of-1 design. *Pain* 1994; **59**: 127–133.

18. Siddall PJ, Finnerup NB. Pain following spinal cord injury. In: Cervero F, Jensen TS (eds) *Handbook of Clinical Neurology*. Elsevier, Amsterdam, 2006: 689–703.

19. Siddall PJ, McClelland JM, Rutkowski SB, Cousins MJ. A longitudinal study of the prevalence and characteristics of pain in the first 5 years following spinal cord injury. *Pain* 2003; **103**: 249–257.

20. Werhagen L, Budh CN, Hultling C, Molander C. Neuropathic pain after traumatic spinal cord injury – relations to gender, spinal level, completeness, and age at the time of injury. *Spinal Cord* 2004; **42**: 665–673.

21. Tai Q, Kirschblum S, Chen B, Millis S, Johnston M, DeLiza JA. Gabapentin in the treatment of neuropathic pain after spinal cord injury: a prospective, randomized, double-blind, crossover trial. *J Spinal Cord Med* 2002; **25**: 100–105.

22. Levendoglu F, Ogun CO, Ozerbil O, Ogun TC, Ugurlu H. Gabapentin is a first line drug for the treatment of neuropathic pain in spinal cord injury. *Spine* 2004; **29**: 743–751.

23. Siddall PJ, Cousins MJ, Otte A, Griesing T, Chambers R, Murphy TK. Pregabalin in central neuropathic pain associated with spinal cord injury: a placebo-controlled trial. *Neurology* 2006; **67**: 1792–1800.

24. Cardenas DD, Warms CA, Turner JA, Marshall H, Brooke MM, Loeser JD. Efficacy of amitriptyline for relief of pain in spinal cord injury: results of a randomized controlled trial. *Pain* 2002; **96**: 365–373.

25. Davidoff G, Guarracini M, Roth E, Sliwa J, Yarkony G. Trazodone hydrochloride in the treatment of dysesthetic pain in traumatic myelopathy: a randomized, double-blind, placebo-controlled study. *Pain* 1987; **29**:151–161.

26. Finnerup NB, Sindrup SH, Bach FW, Johannesen IL, Jensen TS. Lamotrigine in spinal cord injury pain: a randomized controlled trial. *Pain* 2002; **96**: 375–383.

27. Drewes AM, Andreasen A, Poulsen LH. Valproate for treatment of chronic central pain after spinal cord injury. A double-blind cross-over study. *Paraplegia* 1994; **32**: 565–569.

28. Chiou-Tan FY, Tuel SM, Johnson JC, Priebe MM, Hirsh DD, Strayer JR. Effect of mexiletine on spinal cord injury dysesthetic pain. *Am J Phys Med Rehabil* 1996; **75**: 84–87.

29. Siddall PJ, Molloy AR, Walker S, Rutkowski SB. The efficacy of intrathecal morphine and clonidine in the treatment of pain after spinal cord injury. *Anesth Analg* 2000; **91**: 1–6.

30. Österberg A, Boivie J, Thuomas KA. Central pain in multiple sclerosis – prevalence and clinical characteristics. *Eur J Pain* 2005; **9**: 531–542.

31. Jensen TS, Rasmussen P, Reske-Nielsen E. Association of trigeminal neuralgia with multiple sclerosis: clinical and pathological features. *Acta Neurol Scand* 1982; **65**: 182–189.

32. Love S, Gradidge T, Coakham HB. Trigeminal neuralgia due to multiple sclerosis: ultrastructural findings in trigeminal rhizotomy specimens. *Neuropathol Appl Neurobiol* 2001; **27**: 238–244.

33. Smith KJ, McDonald WI. The pathophysiology of multiple sclerosis: the mechanisms underlying the production of symptoms and the natural history of the disease. *Philos Trans R Soc Lond B Biol Sci* 1999; **354**: 1649–1673.

34. Solaro C, Brichetto G, Amato MP, *et al.* The prevalence of pain in multiple sclerosis: a multicenter cross-sectional study. *Neurology* 2004; **63**: 919–921.

35. Shibasaki H, Kuroiwa Y. Painful tonic seizure in multiple sclerosis. *Arch Neurol* 1974; **30**: 47–51.

36. Spissu A, Cannas A, Ferrigno P, Pelaghi AE, Spissu M. Anatomic correlates of painful tonic spasms in multiple sclerosis. *Mov Disord* 1999; **14**: 331–335.

37. Moulin DE, Foley KM, Ebers GC. Pain syndromes in multiple sclerosis. *Neurology* 1988; **38**: 1830–1834.

38. Raminsky M. Hyperexcitability of pathologically myelinated axons and positive symptoms in multiple sclerosis. In: Waxman SG, Ritchie JM (eds) *Demyelinating Disease: Basic and Clinical Electrophysiology*. Raven Press, New York, 1981: 289–297.

39. Vermote R, Ketelaer P, Carton H. Pain in multiple sclerosis patients. A prospective study using the McGill Pain Questionnaire. *Clin Neurol Neurosurg* 1986; **88**: 87–93.

40. Österberg A. Central pain in multiple sclerosis : clinical characteristics, sensory abnormalities and treatment. Linköping University, thesis, 2005; 903.

41. Attal N, Cruccu G, Haanpää M, *et al.* EFNS Task Force. EFNS guidelines on pharmacological treatment of neuropathic pain. *Eur J Neurol* 2006; **13**: 1153–1169.

42. Lunardi G, Leandri M, Albano C, *et al.* Clinical effectiveness of lamotrigine and plasma levels in essential and symptomatic trigeminal neuralgia. *Neurology* 1997; **48**: 1714–1717.

43. Solaro C, Lunardi GL, Capello E, *et al.* An open-label trial of gabapentin treatment of paroxysmal symptoms in multiple sclerosis patients. *Neurology* 1998; **51**: 609–611.

44. Pollmann W, Feneberg W, Steinbrecher A, Haupts MR, Henze T. [Therapy of pain syndromes in multiple sclerosis – an overview with evidence-based recommendations]. *Fortschr Neurol Psychiatr* 2005; **73**: 268–285.

45. Sakurai M, Kanazawa I. Positive symptoms in multiple sclerosis: their treatment with sodium channel blockers, lidocaine and mexiletine. *J Neurol Sci* 1999; **162**: 162–168.

46. Rog DJ, Nurmikko TJ, Friede T, Young CA. Randomized, controlled trial of cannabis-based medicine in central pain in multiple sclerosis. *Neurology* 2005; **65**: 812–819.

47. Houtchens MK, Richert JR, Sami A, Rose JW. Open label gabapentin treatment for pain in multiple sclerosis. Mult Scler 1997; **3**: 250–253

48. Kalman S, Österberg A, Sorensen J, Boivie J, Bertler A. Morphine responsiveness in a group of well-defined multiple sclerosis patients: a study with i.v. morphine., *Eur J Pain* 2002; **6**: 69–80.

49. Svendsen KB, Jensen TS, Bach FW. Does the cannabinoid dronabinol reduce central pain in multiple sclerosis? Randomized double blind placebo controlled crossover trial, *BMJ* 2004; **329**: 253.

50. Zajicek JP, Fox A, Sanders H, *et al.* Cannabinoids for treatment of spasticity and other symptoms related to multiple sclerosis (CAMS study): multicentre randomized placebo- controlled trial. *Lancet* 2003; **362**: 1517–1526.

51. Wade DT, Robson P, House H, Makela P, Aram J. A preliminary controlled study to determine whether whole-plant cannabis extracts can improve intractable neurogenic symptoms. *Clin Rehabil* 2003; **17**: 21–29.

52. Herman RM, d'Luzansky SC, Ippolito R. Intrathecal baclofen suppresses central pain in patients with spinal lesions. A pilot study. *Clin J Pain* 1992; **8**: 338–345.

53. Semple DM, McIntosh AM, Lawrie SM. Cannabis as a risk factor for psychosis: systematic review. J Psychopharmacol 2005; **19**: 187–194.

54. Kalso E, Allan L, Dellemijn PL, *et al.* Recommendations for using opioids in chronic non-cancer pain. *Eur J Pain* 2003; **7**: 381–386.

55. Finnerup NB, Otto M, McQuay HJ, Jensen TS, Sindrup SH. Algorithm for neuropathic pain treatment: an evidence based proposal. *Pain* 2005; **118**: 289–305.

56. Andre-Obadia N, Peyron R, Mertens P, Mauguiere F, Laurent B, Garcia-Larrea L. Transcranial magnetic stimulation for pain control. Double-blind study of different frequencies against placebo, and correlation with motor cortex stimulation efficacy. *Clin Neurophysiol* 2006; **117**: 1536–1544.

57. Fregni F, Boggio PS, Lima MC, *et al.* A sham-controlled, phase II trial of transcranial direct current stimulation for the treatment of central pain in traumatic spinal cord injury. *Pain* 2006; **122**: 197–209.

58. Gruccu G, Aziz TZ, Garcia-Larrea L, *et al.* EFNS guidelines on neurostimulation therapy for neuropathic pain. *Eur J Neurology* 2007; **14**: 952–970.

59. Norrbrink Budh C, Kowalski J, Lundeberg T. A comprehensive pain management programme comprising educational, cognitive and behavioural interventions for neuropathic pain following spinal cord injury. J Rehabil Med 2006; **38**: 172–180.

60. Gruccu G, Anand P, Attal N, *et al.* EFNS guidelines on neuropathic pain assessment. *Eur J Neurol* 2004; **11**: 153–162.

61. Brainin M, Barnes M, Baron JC, *et al.* Guideline Standards Subcommittee of the EFNS Scientific Committee. Guidance for the preparation of neurological management guidelines by EFNS scientific task forces – revised recommendations 2004. *Eur J Neurol* 2004; **11**: 577–581.

CHAPTER 22

Headache

Peer Tfelt-Hansen

Danish Headache Centre, Department of Neurology, University of Copenhagen, Glostrup Hospital, Glostrup, Denmark

Introduction

Headache disorders are major health problems with great societal and individual impact. Migraine is listed by the World Health Organization (WHO) as the 19th highest cause of disability (12th in women) in the Global Burden of Disease Study from 2000 (www. WHO.int). It is estimated that the total annual cost for migraine is 27 billion euros per year in Europe.

In the last 30 years research, primarily in migraine, has provided new insights into the causes, mechanisms and management of headache disorders. Changes in regional cerebral blood flow linked the migraine aura to spreading depression of Leao in 1981[1], a new specific treatment for migraine, the triptans, was introduced in 1991 [2] and a gene for a subform of migraine was found in 1996 [3].

In this chapter, the epidemiology, clinical features, pathophysiology and drug treatment of the three primary headaches – migraine, tension-type headache, and cluster headache – will be reviewed. Concerning drug treatment, only results based on randomized clinical trials and systematic reviews will be mentioned.

Primary headaches

Epidemiology

Migraine has a uniform worldwide prevalence with a lifetime prevalence of 16% [4,5]. The male/female

ratio varies from 1:2 to 1:3 with a more pronounced female preponderance in migraine without aura than in migraine with aura [6]. In its milder and infrequent forms, tension-type headache is a nuisance rather than a disease, but in its frequent forms, it becomes distressing and socially disturbing like other primary headaches. The prevalence of chronic tension-type headache is quite uniform, 2–3% in most studies [4, 5, 7], and the vast majority of patients with chronic tension-type headache suffer from a daily, almost constant headache.The male:female ratio of tension-type headache is 4:5 indicating that, unlike migraine, females are only slightly more affected [4, 5].

The prevalence of cluster headache is 1% with a male:female ratio of 1:5 [8].

Pain character, severity and location in primary headaches

The typical migraine attack is often dominated by a severe and pulsating, unilateral pain which is aggravated by physical activity [9], although various clinical manifestations are described. The prominent associated symptoms photophobia, phonophobia and nausea, sometimes also vomiting, are often just as incapacitating as the pain itself.

In tension-type headache, patients usually describe their pain as a "dull," "nonpulsating" headache. Terms such as a sensation of "tightness,""pressure" or "soreness" are often employed. Some patients refer to a "band" or a "cap" compressing their heads [10]. The pain of tension-type headache is typically bilateral [11].

In cluster headache there is a severe orbital or periorbital pain lasting 15–180 minutes with accompanying symptoms such as Horner's syndrome, lacrimation, rhinorrhea, and restlessness and agitation.

Evidence-Based Chronic Pain Management. Edited by
C. Stannard, E. Kalso and J. Ballantyne. © 2010 Blackwell Publishing.

The attacks occur in clusters of weeks to months and in a minority of 15% the condition is chronic, going on for years.

Pathophysiology

Migraine

The following pathophysiologic mechanisms behind migraine have been suggested: genetic, neurogenic, vascular, inflammatory or combinations of those. Are the mechanisms peripherally or centrally located or are the interactions between the periphery and the brain altered during the attack? For an update, see Olesen *et al.* [9]).

In the very rare condition familial hemiplegic migraine, mutations in the P/Q calcium channel complex have been described [3]but this gene has so far not been linked to migraine with or without aura [12]. A genetic mechanism is undoubtedly involved as an increased familial risk in first-degree relatives of migraineurs has been described, which varies from 1.9 in migraine without aura to 3.8 in migraine with aura and 14 in cluster headache [13]. Precipitating factors such as stress, mental tension, certain foods, wine and spirits are quite unspecific and are therefore only of limited guidance although the frequent reports of mental and biochemical stressors along with accompanying symptoms as nausea, photo- and phonophobia indicate central mechanisms.

The migraine aura has been linked to a cortical hyperexcitability, and transcranial magnetic stimulation has demonstrated consistently and significantly lowered thresholds and recorded visual symptoms such as phosphenes in all migraine patients, in contrast to only 27.% of controls [14], which suggests an increased excitability. Cortical spreading depression of Leao, which has mainly been demonstrated in animal models and recently in humans after brain injury [15] and during migraine aura [16], is likely to play a fundamental role in the migraine aura [1].

Concerning the peripheral factors, the cranial vessels have been studied extensively. The patients never doubt that their pain is vascular, due to the throbbing, pulsating quality and the transient comfort in a minority (30%) of patients of compressing the temporal artery on the painful site. Dilation of the large intracranial arteries can play a role in the pain process, as dilation of various segments of the middle

cerebral artery can produce referred pain in relevant areas but the pain is transient and not a migraine [9]. Ictally, a strictly unilateral dilation of the temporal artery on the painful site has been demonstrated [17] and there is also indirect evidence of dilation of the middle cerebral artery on the migraine site by means of transcranial Doppler measurements in some [18] but not in all [19] studies. Infusion of the exogenous NO donor glyceryl trinitrate (GTN) causes dilation of the cephalic arteries and a delayed headache indistinguishable from genuine migraine attack is elicited in most migraine patients after 5–6 hours [20, 21]. The NO molecule acts, however, on multiple systems including the cortical and brainstem neurones and the vascular effect may therefore represent an epiphenomenon. Nevertheless, the GTN model is a very useful human model for the study of various aspects of the entire migraine episode [20–22]. The highly prominent vasoconstrictor effect of specific and effective acute migraine drugs such as the triptans, ergotamine, and dihydroergotamine (DHE) also supports a prominent vascular mechanism.

Activation of the trigeminal ganglion and trigeminal nucleus has been intensively studied in animal models [23] and may be involved in the migraine attack, leading to migraine being termed a trigeminovascular disease. Whether the activation of the trigeminal system is primary or secondary to the migraine pain is yet unknown. Calcitonin gene-related peptide (CGRP) in the external jugular measured during migraine attacks was increased in one study [109] but in a recent, controlled study [24] no such increase was found. However, CGRP infusion induces headache in migraine [25] and two CGRP antagonists, BIBN4096BS and MK-0974, were effective in the treatment of migraine attacks [26, 27].

In conclusion, migraine is a transient, complex disorder in otherwise healthy individuals and the most likely mechanism that can unify the numerous existing hypotheses is a neuronal depolarization. This depolarization is probably due to a genetically inherited membrane channel dysfunction in the neurones, either increased excitability or lack of inhibitory transmitters. If a certain number of probably very individual external triggers are present, a migraine attack can be initiated and runs its course when first started. Apart from the attacks, there are no clinical signs of the underlying neuronal dysfunction, as trigger factors are required to start the process. Similarly, the trigger factors alone cannot initiate the migraine attack as a genetic disposition is required. Thus both conditions must be fulfilled. The activation of the trigeminal and the vascular system is most likely to be secondary to the basic migraine process although highly involved in the elicited central–peripheral–central migraine cascade.

At present, acute pharmacologic intervention is quite effective by minimizing and interfering with this cascade reaction but it has no preventive effect on the next attack, indicating that other basic neuronal or transmitter systems are involved. Future studies applying more advanced neurophysiologic and neuroimaging techniques, along with genetic studies, will hopefully shed more light on the basic mechanisms of migraine.

Tension-type headache

The pathophysiology of tension-type headache is also far from being elucidated and has been far less investigated than that of migraine.

The prevalence of tension-type headache is the same in monozygotic and dizygotic twins and it has been concluded that environmental factors are more important than genetic factors in tension-type headache [28].

Tension-type headaches are generally held to occur with emotional conflict and psychosocial stress but the cause–effect relation is not clear. Stress and mental tension are thus the most frequently reported precipitating factors but occur with similar frequency in tension-type headache and migraine [29]. Widely normal personality profiles are found in subjects with episodic tension-type headache, whereas studies of subjects with the chronic form often reveal a higher frequency of depression and anxiety [30, 31].

Increased tenderness in pericranial muscles is the most consistent abnormal physical finding in patients with tension-type headache; it increases with increasing frequency and intensity of the headache [32]. Subjects with the episodic form have increased tenderness compared to migraineurs and healthy controls but are less tender than subjects with chronic tension-type headache [32, 33]. Concerning pain thresholds recorded by pressure algometry, most studies report normal pain thresholds in episodic tension-type headache but decreased values in patients with the chronic form [32, 33]. It is most likely that chronic tension-type headache has a physiologic basis and is caused at least partly by long-term qualitative changes in the central processing of sensory information [33].

The initiating stimulus in tension-type headache may be a condition of mental stress, unphysiologic motor stress, a local irritative process or a combination of these. Secondary to the peripheral stimuli, the supraspinal pain perception structures may become activated, and due to central modulation of the incoming stimuli, a self-limiting process will be the result in most subjects. As most cases of chronic tension-type headache evolve from the episodic form, it is postulated that prolonged peripheral input sensitizes the central nervous system [34] and a disturbance in the complex interaction between peripheral and central mechanisms is therefore likely of major importance for the conversion of episodic into chronic tension-type headache [35].

Cluster headache

Cluster headache is a chronobiologic headache with a tendency for the attacks to occur at a certain time of the day, especially at night. The attacks are most likely generated from the hypothalamus [36]. The pain is most likely a trigeminovascular pain with dilation of large cerebral arteries [36].

Systematic reviews and meta-analyses in migraine

Several systematic reviews with meta-analyses of acute migraine treatment have been published [12, 37–44]. In addition, three systematic reviews of preventive migraine treatment have been published [45–47]. One should distinguish between systematic reviews in which several randomized clinical trials (RCT) of a single drug are evaluated to obtain more precise information about its merits [40, 41, 43–45, 47] and those in which several drugs or administration forms are compared in a meta-analysis [12, 37–40].

In the systematic reviews and meta-analyses of acute migraine treatment [12, 37, 38, 40–44] patients had moderate or severe headache and headache relief was defined as a decrease to none or mild [48]. Headache relief was the primary efficacy measure in most RCTs. Being pain free after 2 hours was also reported in most studies and was evaluated in some meta-analyses [12, 38, 42]. One of the systematic reviews [12, 38] also evaluated sustained pain-free status (pain free after 2 hours, no use of rescue medication and no recurrence within 24 hours). In addition, tolerability versus placebo was evaluated in these systematic reviews.

Systematic reviews of one drug for the treatment of migraine

Naratriptan 2.5 mg was superior to placebo (number needed to treat (NNT) for headache relief 4.6) in a systematic review [43]. For a comment on the magnitude of the effect of naratriptan, see below. Rizatriptan 10 mg was superior to placebo with a NNT of 2.7 (95% confidence interval (CI) 2.4–2.9) [49]. Rizatriptan 10 mg is a first-line drug for the treatment of migraine attacks. Almotriptan 12.5 mg was superior to placebo with a NNT of 3.4 [44]. Both eletriptan 40 mg and 80 mg were superior to placebo [41]. Eletriptan 40 mg is a first-line treatment option in acute migraine attacks with a NNT of 2.9 (95% CI 2.6–3.3 [41] and eletriptan 80 mg (NNT 2.6, 95% CI 2.4–3.0) can be tried in especially severe migraine attacks. In one systematic review the efficacy parameter pain-free response at 2 hours was used [42] and sumatriptan 100 mg was superior to placebo with NNT of 5.1 (95% CI 3.9–7.1). Sumatriptan 50 mg was not superior to placebo for this parameter but only a small number of patients (n = 124) were analyzed [42]. In a large meta-analysis, sumatriptan 50 mg was superior to placebo with a therapeutic gain (TG) (percentage relief with active drug minus percentage relief with placebo) of 18% for pain-free status [12]. In a recent large RCT, sumatriptan 50 mg (49%) taken in the mild phase of a migraine attack was superior to placebo (24%) for pain-free status at 2 hours [50].

Meta-analyses of drugs used for the acute treatment of migraine

One systematic review presented a meta-analysis of the seven oral triptans (sumatriptan, zolmitriptan, naratriptan, rizatriptan, almotriptan, eletriptan, and frovatriptan) and of subcutaneous, intranasal, and rectal sumatriptan [37]. The meta-analysis was based on headache relief, and the mean TG with 95% CI was calculated. Based on this meta-analysis, subcutaneous sumatriptan 6 mg (TG 51%; 95% CI 49–53%) and eletriptan 80 mg (TG 42%; 95% CI 37–47%) were superior to sumatriptan 100 mg (TG 32%; 95% CI

29–34%). In contrast, the mean TG were inferior to sumatriptan 100 mg for naratriptan 2.5 mg (TG 22%; 95% CI 18–26%), and for frovatriptan (TG 16%; 95 CI 8–25%). Similar results were found in two other meta-analyses [39, 49, 51]. For details, see Tfelt-Hansen 2006 [52]. There are minor differences most likely due to differences in the RCT included in the meta-analyses [37, 39, 49].

Based on these three systematic reviews, one can conclude that subcutaneous sumatriptan 6 mg is the most effective triptan. Eletriptan 80 mg (for headache relief and pain-free status), and rizatriptan 10 mg (for pain-free status) are somewhat better than sumatriptan 100 mg, whereas naratriptan 2.5 mg and frovatriptan 2.5 mg are inferior to sumatriptan 100 mg.

A large meta-analysis of 53 RCT with oral triptans was published in *The Lancet* [38] and later in detail in *Cephalalgia* [12]. Unpublished studies were also included in this meta-analysis [38]. Some of the results are shown in Figure 22.1. The authors' interpretation of the meta-analysis combined with evaluated comparative RCT are shown in Table 22.1. Headache relief at 2 hours was the primary per protocol endpoint in nearly all triptan RCT and as illustrated in Figure 22.1A, headache relief after 2 hours, compared with 100 mg sumatriptan, was higher for rizatriptan 10 mg and eletriptan 80 mg, lower for naratriptan 2.5 mg and frovatriptan 2.5 mg. For the placebo-subtracted response, the same as TG, only eletriptan 80 mg was superior to sumatriptan 100 mg. Pain-free status at 2 hours, recommended as the primary efficacy measure by the International Headache Society [53], was a secondary endpoint in most RCT. Compared with sumatriptan 100 mg, naratriptan 2.5 mg showed lower absolute pain-free rates whereas eletriptan 80 mg, almotriptan 12.5 mg, and rizatriptan 10 mg showed higher values. However, only eletriptan 80 mg and rizatriptan 10 mg showed higher values than sumatriptan for TG for pain-free status (placebo-subtracted values) (see Fig. 22.1B). Sustained pain-free status was higher for rizatriptan 10 mg (26%, 95% CI 24–27%), eletriptan 80 mg (25%, 95% CI 23–27%), and almotriptan 12.5 mg (27%, 95% CI 23–30%) compared to sumatriptan 100 mg (20%, 95% CI 18–21%). For adverse events, sumatriptan 100 mg had a mean placebo-subtracted rate of any adverse events of 13% (95% CI 8–18%). Rates for the other triptans overlap, except for lower values for almotriptan 12.5 mg and

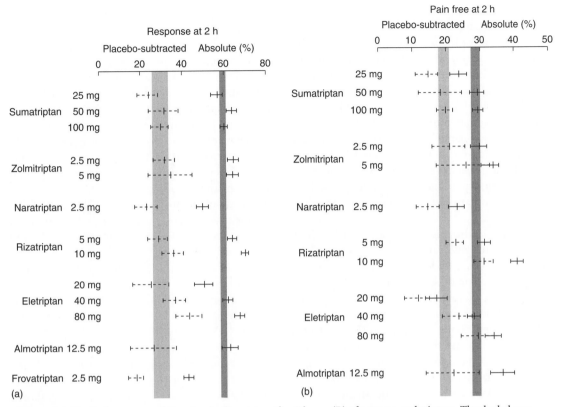

Figure 22.1 Headache response (A) and pain-free status after 2 hours (B) after seven oral triptans. The shaded area indicates the 95% CI for sumatriptan 100 mg for both absolute responses and placebo-subtracted results. From Ferrari *et al.* [38] with permission from the publisher.

Table 22.1 Comparison of the main efficacy and tolerability measures for oral triptans versus sumatriptan 100 mg based on the results of the meta-analysis and direct comparative trials, modified from Ferrari *et al.* 2002 [12]. In bold parentheses is shown my personal judgment of these items for rizatriptan, eletriptan, and almotriptan based on the meta-analysis [12] and some later published comparative RCT [60, 61]

	Initial 2-h relief	Sustained pain-free status	Tolerability
Sumatriptan 50 mg	=	=	=
Sumatriptan 25 mg	−	=/−	+
Zolmitriptan 2.5 mg	=	=	=
Zolmitriptan 5 mg	=	=	=
Naratriptan 2.5 mg	−	−	++
Rizatriptan 5 mg	=	=	=
Rizatriptan 10 mg	+(=/+)	+(−/=)	=(=)
Eletriptan 20 mg	−		=
Eletriptan 40 mg	=/+(+)	=/−(+/=)	=(=)
Eletriptan 80 mg	+(+)(+)	+(+)	−(−)
Almotriptan 12.5 mg	=(=)	+(=)	++(++)

=, no difference when compared with 100 mg sumatriptan; +, better than sumatriptan; −, inferior when compared with sumatriptan.

naratriptan 2.5 mg. The rates for almotriptan and naratriptan did not differ from placebo.

The authors of the meta-analysis concluded that at marketed doses, all oral triptans were effective and well tolerated. Rizatriptan 10 mg, eletriptan 80 mg, and almotriptan 12.5 mg provide the highest likelihood of consistent success [38]. I agree that all triptans are more effective than placebo but the TG for both naratriptan 2.5 mg (22%) [38] and frovatriptan 2.5 mg (18%) [38] are low (see Fig. 22.1A), and lower than the TG for the combination of aspirin plus metoclopramide (31%) [40]. These two triptans are also more costly than this combination.

Rizatriptan 10 mg is rated + for initial 2 hour relief compared with sumatriptan 100 mg (see Table 22.1). The TG for headache relief for rizatriptan 10 mg was similar to sumatriptan (see Fig. 22.1A) and in a large comparative RCT, the two drugs were comparable for this efficacy measure [54]. For pain-free status after 2 hours, however, the TG was higher for rizatriptan 10 mg than for sumatriptan 100 mg. The same was found in a comparative RCT [54]. In addition, rizatriptan 10 mg (n = 1114) was superior (5%: 95% CI 0.6–9%) to sumatriptan 50 mg (n = 1116) for pain-free status after 2 hours in a combined analysis of two trials [55, 56]. Rizatriptan 10 mg was superior to sumatriptan 100 mg for sustained pain-free status [38] but this was not the case in the comparative RCT [12].

After the publication of the meta-analysis [12, 38], a new large placebo-controlled RCT comparing eletriptan 40 mg and sumatriptan 100 mg was published [57]. This study together with two previous RCT [58, 59] constitutes a large head-to-head comparative database [60]. The headache relief rate after 2 hours was higher for eletriptan 40 mg (67%) than for sumatriptan 100 mg (57%) [60] and the 2-hour pain-free response was also higher for eletriptan (35%) than for sumatriptan (25%) [60]. The sustained pain-free response was higher for eletriptan (22%) than for sumatriptan (15%) [60]. The frequency of adverse effects (AE) was similar for the two drugs [60]. In the meta-analysis eletriptan 80 mg, a dose not routinely used, was superior to sumatriptan 100 mg for TG for headache relief, pain-free status after 2 hours (see Fig. 22.1) and sustained pain-free status [12,38]. This was also the case in the comparative studies [12]. Almotriptan 12.5 mg had the same initial 2-hour relief

and TG for pain-free status as sumatriptan 100 mg (see Fig. 22.1).

In one large comparative RCT [61] published after the meta-analysis [38], almotriptan 12.5 mg (18%) was inferior to sumatriptan 50 mg (25%) for pain-free status after 2 hours. Apparently, almotriptan 12.5 mg is better than sumatriptan 100 mg for sustained pain-free status, based on the meta-analysis [12, 38]. This was, however, not the case in a comparative RCT [12] and in a cross-over RCT [61] almotriptan 12.5 mg had a lower sustained pain-free response (12.9%) than sumatriptan 50 mg (17.6%) [62]. The better tolerability of almotriptan 12.5 mg than sumatriptan was confirmed in two trials [61, 63]. In one RCT, treatment-related AE occurred more frequently with sumatriptan 50 mg (15.5%) than with almotriptan 12.5 mg (9.1%) [61] and in another RCT, the incidence of AE was higher with sumatriptan 100 mg (22.2%) than with almotriptan 12.5 mg (8.7%). The incidence of AE was the same for almotriptan as for placebo 12.5 mg (6.1%) [63].

My personal ratings of rizatriptan 10 mg , eletriptan 40 mg and 80 mg, and almotriptan 12.5 mg versus sumatriptan 100 mg are shown in bold parentheses in Table 22.1. Rizatriptan 10 mg should have +/= rating for initial 2-hour relief and for sustained pain-free status whereas the rest of the rating is unchanged. Eletriptan 40 mg should have + for initial relief based on the three comparative RCT [60] and the same is the case for sustained pain-free status. Eletriptan 80 mg is unchanged. Almotriptan 12.5 mg is in my view comparable to sumatriptan 100 mg for initial relief and sustained pain-free status but its better tolerability, comparable to placebo, has been confirmed in two RCTs [61, 63].

Recent results of RCTs with triptans and comparisons with ergotamine

In two recently published RCT [64] with rapid-release/fast-disintegrating tablets, sumatriptan 100 mg (n = 1101) had a TG for headache relief of 30% (95% CI 26–34%) versus placebo (n = 1113), the same as sumatriptan 100 mg in the meta-analysis [12, 38] (see Fig. 22.1A). For pain-free status after 2 hours, the mean TG was 32% (95% CI 28–36%) [64] which is higher than the 20% TG for conventional sumatriptan tablets (see Fig. 22.1B). Unfortunately, there are no

Table 22.2 Clinical efficacy, scientific proof for efficacy, and potential for adverse events, rated on a scale from + to ++++, for some drugs used in acute migraine treatment

Drug	Clinical efficacy[a]	Scientific proof for efficacy	Adverse event potential
Subcutaneous sumatriptan 6 mg	++++	++++*	+++
Sumatriptan 100 mg	+++	++++*	++
Sumatriptan 50 mg	+++	++++*	+
Rizatriptan 10 mg	+++	++++*	++
Zolmitriptan 2.5 mg	+++	++++	++
Naratriptan 2.5 mg	++	++++*	0[b]
Eletriptan 40	+++	++++*	++
Frovatriptan 2.5 mg	++	+++	+
Almotriptan 12.5 mg	+++	++++*	0[b]
Oral ergotamine 2 mg[c]	+	+	++
Rectal ergotamine 2 mg[d]	+++	++	+++
Effervescent aspirin	+++	+++	+
Aspirin plus metoclopramide[e]	+++	+++	+
Naproxen[f]	++	+++	+
Ibuprofen[f]	++	+++	+

* Systematic review available.

[a] Based on a combination of the published literature and personal experience; [b] no more adverse events than placebo; [c] for details, see Tfelt-Hansen *et al.* 2000 [37]; [d] see www.GSK.com; [e] see Tfelt-Hansen *et al.* 1995 [71]; [f] see Tfelt-Hansen & Rolan 2006 [103].

comparative RCT with this new oral formulation of sumatriptan.

Treatment in the mild phase of a migraine attack results in higher TG for 2-hour pain-free status. This measure increased to 48% after rizatriptan 10 mg [65] and 25–44% after sumatriptan 100 mg [50]. It has therefore been suggested that migraine attacks should be treated early.

Finally, in three RCT oral sumatriptan 100 mg, rizatriptan 10 mg, and eletriptan 40 mg and 80 mg were superior to oral ergotamine plus caffeine [66–68]. In contrast, in one RCT rectal ergotamine plus caffeine was superior to rectal sumatriptan 25 mg (Clinical Trial Register, GSK: www.gsk.com).

An overview of acute treatment drugs for migraine is shown in Table 22.2.

Other drugs for migraine

In a consensus paper on ergotamine it was stated that the evidence for its use in migraine is there but is not up to current standards [69]. The oral bio-availability of ergotamine is less than 1% and if used in migraine attacks of long duration, should be administered by the rectal route [69].

The nonsteroidal anti-inflammatories aspirin, tolfenamic acid, naproxen, ketoprofen, ibuprofen, and diclofenac potassium were all superior to placebo in the treatment of migraine attacks [70].

Effervescent aspirin 1000 mg was as effective as sumatriptan 50 mg in one RCT [110].

The combination of lysine acetylsalicylate 1640 mg plus metoclopramide 10 mg was as effective as sumatriptan 100 mg in one placebo-controlled RCT [71]. Diclofenac potassium 100 mg was comparable to sumatriptan 100 mg [111]. Tolfenamic acid 200 mg was inferior to sumatriptan 100 mg [52].

Systematic reviews of drugs for migraine prophylaxis

In one systematic Cochrane review of propranolol [45] it was concluded that propranolol is effective for short-term migraine prophylaxis, evidence on long-term effects is lacking, and propranolol seems to be as effective and safe as a variety of other drugs used for

Table 22.3 Clinical efficacy, scientific proof for efficacy, and potential for adverse events, rated on a scale from + to + + + +, for some drugs used in migraine prophylaxis. Modified from Tfelt-Hansen [104]

Drug	Clinical efficacy[a]	Scientific proof for efficacy	Adverse event potential
β-Blockers (propranolol*, metoprolol, atenolol, nadolol, bisoprolol)	+ + + +	+ + + +	+ +
Antiepileptics			
Sodium valproate /divalproex*	+ + or + + +	+ + +	+ + +
Topiramate*	+ + +	+ + + +	+ + +
Antiserotonin drugs			
Methysergide[b]	+ + + +	+ +	+ + + +
Pizotifen[b]	+ +	+ +	+ + +
Calcium antagonists			
Flunarizine[c]	+ + +	+ + + +	+ + +
Verapamil	+	+	+
NSAIDs			
Naproxen	+ +	+ +	+ +
Tolfenamic acid	+ +	+ +	+ +
Miscellaneous			
Amitriptyline	+ +	+ +	+ + +
Lisinopril	+ +	+ +	+ +
Candesartan	+ +	+ +	+
Clonidine	+	+	+
Dihydroergotamine	+ +	+	+ +

A systematic review is available.

[a] Based on a combination of the published literature and personal experience; [b] for details see Tfelt-Hansen & Saxena 2006 [105–107]; [c] for details, see Toda & Tfelt-Hansen 2006 [108].

migraine prophylaxis. Propranolol is thus a first-line drug for migraine prophylaxis.

In another systematic Cochrane review the efficacy of feverfew in migraine prophylaxis was judged as unproven [46].

Anticonvulsants were evaluated for migraine prophylaxis in one systematic Cochrane review [47]. It was concluded that sodium valproate/divalproex sodium is superior to placebo. Valproate/divalproex sodium are second-line drugs for migraine prophylaxis because of adverse events, sedation and weight gain. There is no RCT comparing valproate with propranolol.

Topiramate has been evaluated in three large RCT and topiramate 100 mg was superior to placebo in all [72–74]. Topiramate 100 mg was comparable to propranolol 160 mg [74]. Topiramate is a second-line drug for migraine prophylaxis. There are, however, adverse events, sedation and cognitive impairment with topiramate and its place in migraine prophylaxis depends on how migraine patients in clinical practice will tolerate the drug.

For a review of preventive therapy in migraine, see Yoon *et al.* 2005 [75]. An overview of the prophylactic drugs for migraine is shown in Table 22.3.

Clinical trials in tension-type headache

Acute treatment of tension-type headache has been investigated in episodic tension-type headache, and in prophylactic treatment of chronic tension-type headache, antidepressant drugs and botulinum toxin have been investigated.

Aspirin and paracetamol are the analgesics used most commonly in the treatment of acute tension-type headache [76]. In the most recent RCT, 452 patients treated episodes of tension-type headache with aspirin (500 mg or 1000 mg), paracetamol (500 mg or 1000 mg) or placebo. Headache relief after 2 hours was 76% after aspirin 1000 mg and 71% after paracetamol 1000 mg. Both were superior to placebo despite a high placebo response of 55%. The following NSAID were superior to placebo in RCT on the treatment of acute tension-type headache: ibuprofen [77], ketoprofen [78, 112] naproxen [79, 80] and diclofenac [81]. Caffeine has long been used as an analgesic adjuvant [76]. In a RCT the combination of aspirin and caffeine was superior to paracetamol and placebo [77]; in another RCT, the combination of caffeine and ibuprofen was superior to ibuprofen and placebo [113]. The combination of caffeine, aspirin and paracetamol was more effective than the single substances in one large RCT.

Antidepressants are the drugs most commonly used in chronic tension-type headache [82]. Amitriptyline was superior to placebo in most RCT [82–86] but in the largest RCT there was no effect of amitriptyline and amitriptylinoxide [87]. Mirtazapine 15–30 mg daily was superior to placebo in one RCT [88] whereas the the selective serotonin reuptake inhibitor (SSRI) citalopram was not more effective than placebo [86].

After positive open studies, botulinum toxin has been studied in chronic tension-type headache but the conclusion of these RCT is that botulinum toxin is not more effective than placebo [89].Thus in the most recent large RCT including 298 randomized patients, botulinum toxin A admistered in doses from 50 U to 150 U was not different from placebo [90].

Clinical trials in cluster headache

In contrast to migraine and tension-type headache, there are very few RCT in cluster headache. This is most likely due to the fact that cluster headache is a rather infrequent disease (see above). There is one RCT demonstrating the superiority of O_2 versus plain air [91]. In one RCT subcutaneous sumatriptan 6 mg was superior to placebo [92]. In another, intranasal sumatriptan 20 mg was superior to placebo [93] and intranasal zolmitriptan 5 mg and 10 mg was superior to placebo in one RCT [94]. Subcutaneous sumatriptan 6 mg is the first-line drug for cluster headache attacks but it is very expensive.

In one prophylactic RCT, verapamil was comparable to lithium [95] and in another, verapamil 360 mg was superior to placebo [96].

Research needed to improve the evidence-based management of migraine

Clinical experience shows that triptans are more effective in migraine than over-the-counter drugs such as aspirin [97]. In RCT, however, triptans and aspirin are comparable [98] and this was also the case in a recent systematic review including 991 migraine attacks [99]. When headache was severe the results were similar [99]. It has been suggested [97] that patients treated with triptans in clinical practice may be relatively more responsive to triptans and relatively less responsive to other agents than those who participate in clinical trials. In patients recruited from general practice, however, the pain-free response [100] was similar to other studies [38]. Thus a selection bias is most likely not the reason for the discrepancy in results in clinical practice and controlled trials. The lack of superiority of triptans in controlled clinical trials has meant that the WHO has not included triptans on the list of essential drugs.

Stricter success criteria [51] have been suggested in order to demonstrate superiority of triptans. It has been recommended to use the criterion of painfree status after 2 hours [53], preferably with administration in the mild phase [65]. This resulted in 70% being pain free after rizatriptan 10 mg [65]. In addition, sustained pain-free status, which occurs in 60% of patients after rizatriptan 10 mg [65], could be used. However, in the systematic review of aspirin versus sumatriptan, these two efficacy measures were quite comparable (pain-free status 27–29% and sustained pain-free status 22–24%) [99]. Based on these results, stepwise care, starting with aspirin, has been recommended [99].

What efficacy can one achieve with a triptan? The highest effect was 87% pain-free status after subcutaneous naratriptan 10 mg [51, 101]. So inherently the triptans as a group are most likely very effective drugs in migraine when the right drug and the optimum form of administration are used. Similarly, subcutaneous sumatriptan (76%) was superior to intravenous acetylsalicylic acid lysinate (44%) for pain-free status after 2 hours [102].

Why the presumed superiority of triptans is not apparent in current RCT remains an enigma. In my opinion, one should probably try the three-way crossover design with a triptan, a NSAID and a placebo. In this design patients can be classified as responding better to one of the active drugs or with equal response. Patients' characteristics in the two groups with active drugs can then be analyzed as possible predictors of response with each drug. If such preferential predictors are identified, they can then be used in clinical practice. In addition, on can ask for preference, a clinically most relevant parameter, with this design.

References

1. Olesen J, Larsen B, Lauritzen M. Focal hyperemia followed by spreading oligemia and impaired activation of rCBF in classic migraine. *Ann Neurol* 1981; **9**: 344–352.

2. Humphrey PP, Feniuk W. Mode of action of the antimigraine drug sumatriptan. *Trends Pharmacol Sci* 1991; **12**: 444–446.

3. Ophoff RA, Terwindt GM, Vergouwe MN, *et al.* Familial hemiplegic migraine and epidodic ataxia type-2 are caused by mutations in the Ca^{2+} channel gene CACNL1A4. *Cell* 1996; **87**: 543–552.

4. Rasmussen BK, Jensen R, Schroll M, Olesen J. Epidemiology of headache in a general population – a prevalence study. *J Clin Epidemiol* 1991; **44**: 1147–1157.

5. Göbel H, Petersen-Braun M, Soyka D. The epidemiology of headache in Germany: a nationwide survey of a representative sample on the basis of the headache classification of the International Headache Society. *Cephalalgia* 1994; **14**: 97–106.

6. Rasmussen BK, Stewart WF. Epidemiology of migraine. In: Olesen J, Tfelt-Hansen P, Welch KMA (eds) *The Headaches*, 2nd edn. Lippincott, Williams and Wilkins, Philadelphia, 2000: 227–233.

7. Schwartz BS, Stewart WF, Simon D, Lipton RB. Epidemiology of tension-type headache. *JAMA* 1998; **279**: 381–383.

8. Goadsby P, Tfelt-Hansen P. Cluster headache: introduction and epidemiology. In: Olesen J, Goadsby PJ, Ramadan NM, Tfelt-Hansen P, Welch KMA (eds) *The Headaches*, 3rd edn. Lippincott, Williams and Wilkins, Philadelphia, 2006: 743–745.

9. Olesen J, Goadsby PJ, Ramadan NM, Tfelt-Hansen P, Welch KMA (eds) *The Headaches*, 3rd edn. Lippincott, Williams and Wilkins, Philadelphia, 2006.

10. Friedman AP. Characteristics of tension headache: a profile of 1420 cases. *Psychosomatics* 1979; **20**: 418–422.

11. Rasmussen BK, Jensen R, Olesen J. A population-based analysis of the diagnostic criteria of the International Headache Society. *Cephalalgia* 1991; **11**: 130–134.

12. Ferrari MD, Goadsby PJ, Roon KI, Lipton RB. Triptans (serotonin, 5-HT$_{1B/1D}$ agonists) in migraine: detailed results and methods of a meta-analysis of 53 trials. *Cephalalgia* 2002; **22**: 633–658.

13. Russell M. Genetic epidemiology of migraine and cluster-headache. *Cephalalgia* 1997; **17**: 683–701.

14. Aurora SK, Welch KMA. Brain hyperexcitability in migraine: evidence from transcranial magnetic stimulation studies. *Curr Opin Neurol* 1998; **11**: 205–209.

15. Fabricius M, Fuhr S, Bhatia R, *et al.* Cortical spreading depression and peri-infarct depolarization in acutely injured human cerebral cortex. *Brain* 2006; **129**: 778–790.

16. Hadjikhani N, Sanchez del Rio M, Wu O, *et al.* Mechanisms of migraine aura revealed by functional MRI in human visual cortex. *Proc Natl Acad Sci USA* 2001; **98**: 4687–4692.

17. Iversen HK, Nielsen TH, Olesen J, Tfelt-Hansen P. Arterial responses during migraine headache. *Lancet* 1990; **336**: 837–839.

18. Friberg L, Olesen J, Iversen HK, Sperling B. Migraine pain associated with middle cerebral artery dilatation: reversal by sumatriptan. *Lancet* 1991; **338**: 13–17.

19. Zwetsloot CP, Caekebeke JF, Ferrari MD. Lack of asymmetry of middle cerebral artery blood velocity in unilateral migraine. *Stroke* 1993; **24**: 1335–1338.

20. Iversen HK, Thomsen LL, Olesen J. Headache induced by a nitric oxide donor (nitroglycerin) responds to sumatriptan. A human model for development of migraine drugs. *Cephalalgia* 1996; **16**: 412–418.

21. Thomsen LL, Kruuse C, Iversen HK, Olesen J. A nitric oxide donor (nitroglycerin) triggers genuine migraine attacks. *Eur J Neurol* 1994; **1**: 73–80.

22. Olesen J, Iversen HK, Thomsen LL. Nitric oxide hypersensitivity. A possible molecular mechanisms of migraine pain. *Neuroreport* 1993; **4**: 1027–1030.

23. Ahn AH, Goadsby PJ. Animal models of headache. In: Olesen J, Goadsby PJ, Ramadan NM, Tfelt-Hansen P, Welch KMA (eds) *The Headaches*, 3rd edn. Lippincott, Williams and Wilkins, Philadelphia, 2006: 221–230.

24. Tvedskov JF, Lipka K, Ashina M, Iversen HK, Schifter S, Olesen J. No increase of calcitonin gene-related peptide in jugular blood during migraine. *Ann Neurol* 2005; **58**: 561–568.

25. Lassen LH, Haderslev PA, Jacobsen VB, Iversen HK, Sperling B, Olesen J. CGRP may play a causative role in migraine. *Cephalalgia* 2002; **22**: 54–61.

26. Olesen J, Diener HC, Husstedt IW, *et al.* Calcitonin gene-related peptide receptor antagonist BIBN 4096 BS for the acute treatment of migraine. *N Engl J Med* 2004; **350**: 1104–1110.

27. Ho T, Mannix L, Rapoport A, *et al.* Efficacy and tolerability of a novel, oral CGRP antagonist, MK-0974, in the acute treatment of migraine. *Cephalalgia* 2007; **27**: 759.

28. Ulrich V, Gervil M, Olesen J. The relative influence of environment and genes in episodic tension-type headache. *Neurology* 2004; **62**: 2065–2069.

29. Rasmussen BK. Migraine and tension-type headache in a general population: precipitating factors, female hormones, sleep pattern and relation to lifestyle. *Pain* 1993; **53**: 65–72.

30. Rasmussen BK. Migraine and TTH in a general population: psychosocial factors. *Int J Epidemiol* 1992; **21**: 1138–1143.

31. Mitsikostas DD, Thomas AM. Comorbidity of headache and depressive disorders. *Cephalalgia* 1999; **19**: 211–217.

32. Jensen R, Rasmussen BK, Olesen J. Cephalic muscle tenderness and pressure pain threshold in headache. A population study. *Pain* 1993; **52**:193–199.

33. Bendtsen L, Jensen R, Olesen J. Decreased pain detection and tolerance thresholds in chronic tension-type headache. *Arch Neurol* 1996; **53**: 373–376.

34. Jensen R, Bendtsen L, Olesen J. Muscular factors are of importance in tension-type headache. *Headache* 1998; **38**:10–17.

35. Jensen R. Pathophysiological mechanisms of tension-type headache. A review of epidemiological and experimental studies. *Cephalalgia* 1999; **19**: 602–621.

36. Goadsby PJ. Pathophysiology of cluster headache: a trigeminal autonomic cephalalgia. *Lancet Neurol* 2002; **1**: 251–257.

37. Tfelt-Hansen P, de Vries P, Saxena PR. Triptans in migraine. A comparative review of pharmacology, pharmacokinetics and efficacy. *Drugs* 2000; **60**: 1259–1287.

38. Ferrari MD, Roon KI, Lipton RB, Goadsby PJ. Oral triptans (serotonin 5-HT$_{1B/1D}$ agonists) in acute migraine: a meta-analysis of 53 trials. *Lancet* 2001; **358**: 1668–1675.

39. Gawel MJ, Worthington I, Maggisano A. A systematic review of the use of triptans in acute migraine. *Can J Neurol Sci* 2001; **28**: 30–41.

40. Oldman AD, Smith LA, McQuay HJ, Moore RA. Pharmacological treatments for acute migraine: quantitative systematic review. *Pain* 2002; **97**: 247–257.

41. Smith LA, Oldman A, McQuay HJ, Moore RA. Eletriptan for acute migraine. Cochrane Database of Systematic Reviews 2007, Issue 1. Art. No.: CD003224. DOI: 10.1002/14651858.CD003224.pub2.

42. McCrory DC, Gray RN. Oral sumatriptan for acute migraine. Cochrane Database of Systematic Reviews 2003, Issue 3. Art. No.: CD002915. DOI: 10.1002/14651858. CD002915.

43. Ashcroft DM, Millson D. Naratriptan for the treatment of acute migraine: meta-analysis of randomised controlled trials. *Pharmacoepidemiol Drug Saf* 2004; **13**: 73–82.

44. Dahlöf CG, Pascual J, Dodick DW, Dowson AJ. Efficacy , speed of action and tolerability of almotriptan in the acute treatment of migraine: pooled individual patient data from four randomized, double-blind, placebo-controlled clinical trials. *Cephalalgia* 2006; **26**: 400–408.

45. Linde K, Rossnagel K. Propranolol for migraine prophylaxis. Cochrane Database of Systematic Reviews 2004, Issue 2. Art. No.: CD003225. DOI: 10.1002/14651858. CD003225.pub2.

46. Pittler MH, Ernst E. Feverfew for preventing migraine. Cochrane Database of Systematic Reviews 2004, Issue 1. Art. No.: CD002286. DOI: 10.1002/14651858.CD002286.pub2.

47. Chronicle EP, Mulleners WM. Anticonvulsant drugs for migraine prophylaxis. Cochrane Database of Systematic Reviews 2004, Issue 3. Art. No.: CD003226. DOI: 10.1002/14651858.CD003226.pub2.

48. Pilgrim AJ. Methodology of clinical trials of sumatriptan in migraine and cluster headache. *Eur Neurol* 1991; **31**: 295–299.

49. Oldman A, Smith LA, McQuay HJ, Moore RA. Rizatriptan for acute migraine. Cochrane Database of Systematic Reviews 2007, Issue 1. Art. No.: CD003221. DOI: 10.1002/14651858.CD003221.pub2.

50. Winner P, Landy S, Richardson M, Ames M. Early intervention in migraine with sumatriptan tables 50 mg versus 100 mg: a pooled analysis of data from six clinical trials. *Clin Ther* 2005; **27**: 1785–1794.

51. Tfelt-Hansen P. Maximum effect of triptans in migraine? A comment. *Cephalalgia* 2008; **28**(7): 767–768.

52. Tfelt-Hansen P. A review of evidence-based medicine and meta-analytic reviews in migraine. *Cephalalgia* 2006; **26**: 1265–1274.

53. International Headache Society Clinical Trial Subcommittee. Guidelines for controlled trials of drugs in migraine. *Cephalalgia* 2000; **20**: 765–786.

54. Tfelt-Hansen P, Teall J, Rodriguez F, *et al*, Rizatriptan 030 Study Group. Oral rizatriptan versus oral sumatriptan: a direct comparative study in the acute treatment of migraine. *Headache* 1998; **38**: 748–755.

55. Goldstein J, Ryan R, Jiang K, *et al*, Rizatriptan Protocol 046 Study Group. Crossover comparison of rizatriptan 5 mg and 10 mg versus sumatriptan 25 mg and 50 mg in migraine. *Headache* 1998; **38**: 737–747.

56. Kolodny A, Polis A, Battisti W, Johnson-Pratt L, Skobieranda F, Rizatriptan Protocol 052 Study Group. Comparison of rizatriptan 5 mg and 10 mg tablets and sumatriptan 25 mg and 50 mg tablets. *Cephalalgia* 2004; **24**: 540–546.

57. Mathew NT, Schoenen L, Winner P, Muirhead N, Sikes CR. Comparative efficacy of eletriptan 40 mg versus sumatriptan 100 mg. *Headache* 2003; **43**: 214–222.

58. Goadsby PJ, Ferrari MD, Olesen J, *et al*, Eletriptan Steering Committee. Eletriptan in acute migraine: a double-blind, placebo-controlled comparison to sumatriptan. *Neurology* 2000; **54**: 156–163.

59. Sandrini G, Färkilä M, Burgess G, Forster E, Haughie S. Eletriptan vs. sumatriptan: a double-blind, placebo-controlled, multiple migraine attack study. *Neurology* 2002; **59**: 1210–1217.

60. Diener HC, Ryan R, Sun W, Hettiarachchi J. The 40-mg dose of eletriptan: comparative efficacy and tolerability versus sumatriptan 100 mg. *Eur J Neurol* 2004; **11**: 125–134.

61. Spierings ELH, Gomez-Mancilla B, Grosz D, Rowland CR, Whaley FS, Jirgens KJ. Oral almotriptan vs oral

sumatriptan in the abortive treatment of migraine. A double-blind, randomized, parallel-group, optimum-dose comparison. *Arch Neurol* 2001; **58**: 944–950.

62. Cabarrocas X. Reply to Tfelt-Hansen. *Cephalalgia* 2004; **24**: 688–689.

63. Dowson AJ, Massiou H, Lainez JM, Cabarrocas X. Almotriptan is an effective and well-tolerated treatment for migraine pain: results of a randomized, double-blind, placebo-controlled clnical trial. *Cephalalgia* 2002; **22**: 453–461.

64. Sheftell FD, Dahlof CG, Brandes JL, Agosti R, Jones MW, Barrett PS. Two replicate randomized, double-blind, placebo-controlled trials of the time to onset of pain relief in the acute treatment of migraine with a fast-disintegrating/rapid-release formulation of sumatriptan tablets. *Clinic Therapeut* 2005; **27**: 407–417.

65. Mathew NT, Kailasam J, Meadors L. Early treatment of migraine with rizatriptan: a placenbo-controlled study. *Headache* 2004; **44**: 669–673.

66. Multinational Oral Sumatriptan and Cafergot Comparative Study Group. A randomized, double-blind comparison of sumatriptan in the acute treatment of migraine. *Eur Neurol* 1991; **31**: 314–322.

67. Christie S, Gobel H, Mateos V, Allen C, Vrijens F, Shivaprakash M. Crossover comparison of efficacy and preference for rizatriptan 10 mg versus ergotamine/caffeine in migraine. *Eur Neurol* 2003; **49**: 20–29.

68. Diener HC, Jansen JP, Reches A, Pascual J, Pieti D, Steiner TJ, Eletriptan and Cafergot Comparative Study Group. Efficacy, tolerability and safety of oral eletriptan and ergotamine plus caffeine (Cafergot) in the acute treatment of migraine: a multicentre, randomized, double-blind, placebo-controlled comparison. *Eur Neurol* 2002; **47**: 99–107.

69. Tfelt-Hansen P, Saxena PR, Dahlof C, *et al.* Ergotamine in the acute treatment of migraine – European consensus. *Brain* 2000; **123**: 9–18.

70. Tfelt-Hansen P, Rolan P. Nonsteroidal antiinflammatory drugs in the acute treatment of migraine. In: Olesen J, Goadsby PJ, Ramadan NM, Tfelt-Hansen P, Welch KMA (eds) *The Headaches*, 3rd edn. Lippincott, Williams and Wilkins, Philadelphia, 2006: 449–457.

71. Tfelt-Hansen P, Henry P, Mulder K, Scheldewaert R G, Schoenen J, Chazot G. The effectiveness of combined oral lysine acetylsalicylate and metoclopramide compared with oral sumatriptan for migraine. *Lancet* 1995; **346**: 923–926.

72. Brandes JL, Saper JR, Diamond M, *et al.* MIGR-002 Study Group. Topiramate for migraine prevention: a randomized controlled trial. *JAMA* 2004; **291**: 965–973.

73. Silberstein SD, Neto W, Schmitt J, Jacobs D, MIGR-001 Study Group. Topiramate in migraine prevention: results of a large controlled trial. *Arch Neurol* 2004; **61**: 490–495.

74. Diener HC, Tfelt-Hansen P, Dahlöf C, *et al.* Topiramate in migraine prophylaxis. Results from a placebo-controlled trial with propranolol as an active control. *Eur Neurol* 2004; **251**: 953–950.

75. Yoon MS, Savidor I, Diener HC, Limmroth V. Evidence-based medicine in migraine prophylaxis. *Exp Rev Neurother* 2005; **5**: 333–341.

76. Mathew NT, Ashina M. Acute pharmacotherapy of tension-type headaches. In: Olesen J, Goadsby PJ, Ramadan NM, Tfelt-Hansen P, Welch KMA (eds) *The Headaches*, 3rd edn. Lippincott, Williams and Wilkins, Philadelphia, 2006: 727–733.

77. Schachtel BP, Furey SA, Thoden WR. Nonprescription ibuprofen and acetaminophen in the treatment of tesion-type headache. *J Clin Pharmacol* 1996; **36**: 1120–1125.

78. van Vergen JMA, Schoemaker RC, Jacobs LD, *et al.* Self-medication of single headache episode with ketoprofen, ibuprofen, or placebo home-monitored with an electronic headache diary. *Br J Clin Pharmacol* 1996; **42**: 475–481.

79. Miller DS, Talbot CA, Simpson W, Korev A. A comparison of naproxen sodium, acetaminophen and placebo in the treatment of muscle contraction headache. *Headache* 1987; **27**: 392–396.

80. Sevelius H, Segre M, Bursick R. Comparative analgesic effects of naproxen sodium, aspirin, placebo. *J Clin Pharmacol* 1980; **20**: 322–329.

81. Kubizek F, Ziegler G, Gold MS, *et al.* Low-dose diclofenac potassium in the treatment of episodic tension-type headache. *Eur J Pain* 2003; **7**: 155–162.

82. Bendtsen L, Mathew NT. Prophylactic pharmacotherapy of tension-type headache, In: Olesen J, Goadsby PJ, Ramadan NM, Tfelt-Hansen P, Welch KMA (eds) *The Headaches*, 3rd edn. Lippincott, Williams and Wilkins, Philadelphia, 2006: 735–741.

83. Lance JW, Curran DA. Treatment of chronic tension headache. *Lancet* 1964; **1**: 1236–1239.

84. Diamond S, Baltes BJ. Chronic tension headache-treated with amitriptyline – a double-blind study. *Headache* 1971; **11**: 110–116

85. Göbel H, Hamouz V, Hansen C, *et al.* Chronic tension-type headache: amitriptyline reduces clinical headache-duration and experimental pain sensitiviity but does not alter pericranial muscle activity readings. *Pain* 1994; **59**: 241–249.

86. Bendtsen R, Jensen R, Olesen J. A non-selective (amitriptyline), but not a selective (citalopram), serotonin reuptake inhibitor is effective in the prophylactic treatment of chronic tension-type headache. *J Neurol Neurosurg Psychiatr* 1996; **61**: 285–290.

87. Pfaffenrath V, Diener HC, Isler H, *et al.* Efficacy and tolerability of amitriptylinoxide in the treatment of chronic tension-type headache: a multi-centre controlled study. *Cephalalgia* 1994; **14**: 149–155.

88. Bendtsen L, Jensen R. Mirtazapine is effective in the prophylactic treatment of chronic tension-type headache. *Neurology* 2004; **62**: 1706–1711.

89. Evers S, Olesen J. Botulinum toxin in headache treatment: the end of the road? *Cephalalgia* 2006; **26**: 789–771.

90. Silberstein SD, Gobel H, Jensen R, *et al.* Botulinum toxin type A in the prophylactic treatment of chronic

tension-type headache: a multicentre, randomized, placebo-controlled, parallel-group study. *Cephalalgia* 2006; **26**: 790–800.

91. Fogan L. Treatment of cluster headache. A double-blind comparison of oxygen v air inhalation. *Arch Neurol* 1985; **42**: 362–363.

92. Ekbom K, Sumatriptan Cluster Headache Study Group. Treatment for acute cluster headache with sumatriptan. *N Engl J Med* 1991; **325**: 322–326.

93. van Vielt JA, Bahra A, Martin V, *et al.* Intranasal sumatriptan in cluster headache: randomized, double-blind placebo-controlled study. *Neurology* 2003; **60**: 630–633.

94. Cittadini E, May A, Straube A, Evers S, Bussone G, Goadsby PJ. Effectiveness of intranasal zolmitriptan in acute cluster headache: a randomized, placebo-controlled, double-blind crossover study. *Arch Neurol* 2006; **63**: 1537–1542.

95. Bussone G, Leone M, Percarisi, *et al.* Double-blind comparison of lithium and verapamil in cluster headache. *Headache* 1990; **30**: 411–317.

96. Leone MJ, d'Amico D, Frediani F, *et al.* Verapamil in the prophylaxis of episodic cluster headache: a double-blind study. *Neurology* 2000; **64**: 1382–1385.

97. Lipton RB, Bigal ME, Goadsby PJ. Double-blind clinical trials of oral triptans vs other classes of acute migraine medication – a review. *Cephalalgia* 2004; **24**: 321–332.

98. Saxena PR, Tfelt-Hansen P. Triptans, 5HT1B/1D agonists in the acute treatment of migraine. In: Olesen J, Goadsby PJ, Ramadan NM, Tfelt-Hansen P, Welch KMA (eds) *The Headaches*, 3rd edn. Lippincott, Williams and Wilkins, Philadelphia, 2006: 469–503.

99. Lampl IC, Voelker M, Diener HC. Efficacy and safety of 1,000 mg effervescent aspirin: individual patient data meta-analysis of three trials in migraine headache and migraine accompanying symptoms. *J Neurol* 2007; **254**: 705–712.

100. Tfelt-Hansen P, Bach F, Daugaard D, Tsiropoulos I, Riddersholm B. Treatment with sumatriptan 50 mg in the mild phase of migraine attacks in patients with infrequent attacks. A randomised, double-blind, placebo-controlled study. *J Headache Pain* 2006; **7**: 389–394.

101. Dahlöf C, Hogenhuis L, Olesen J, Petit H, Ribbat J, Schoenen J *et al.* Early clinical experience with subcutaneous naratriptan in the acute treatment of migraine: a dose-ranging study. *Eur J Neurol* 1998; **5**: 469–477.

102. Diener HC. Efficacy and safety of intravenous acetylsalicylic acid lysinate compared to subcutaneous sumatriptan and parenteral placebo in the acute treatment of migraine. A double-blind, double-dummy, randomized, multicenter, parallel group study. The ASASUMAMIG Study Group. *Cephalalgia* 1999; **19**: 581–588.

103. Tfelt-Hansen P, Rolan P. β-Adrenoceptor blocking drugs in migraine prophylaxis. In: Olesen J, Goadsby PJ, Ramadan NM, Tfelt-Hansen P, Welch KMA (eds) *The Headaches*, 3rd edn. Lippincott, Williams and Wilkins, Philadelphia, 2006: 519–528.

104. Tfelt-Hansen P. Prioritizing prohylactic treatment of migraines. In: Olesen J, Goadsby PJ, Ramadan NM, Tfelt-Hansen P, Welch KMA (eds) *The Headaches*, 3rd edn. Lippincott, Williams and Wilkins, Philadelphia, 2006: 567–568.

105. Tfelt-Hansen P, Saxena PR. Antiserotonin drugs in migraine prophylaxis. In: Olesen J, Goadsby PJ, Ramadan NM, Tfelt-Hansen P, Welch KMA (eds) *The Headaches*, 3rd edn. Lippincott, Williams and Wilkins, Philadelphia, 2006: 529–537.

106. Tfelt-Hansen P, Saxena PR. Antiserotonin drugs in migraine prophylaxis. In: Olesen J, Goadsby PJ, Ramadan NM, Tfelt-Hansen P, Welch KMA (eds) *The Headaches*, 3rd edn. Lippincott, Williams and Wilkins, Philadelphia, 2006: 529–537.

107. Tfelt-Hansen P, Saxena PR. Ergot alkaloids in the acute treatment of migraine. In: Olesen J, Goadsby PJ, Ramadan NM, Tfelt-Hansen P, Welch KMA (eds) *The Headaches*, 3rd edn. Lippincott, Williams and Wilkins, Philadelphia, 2006: 459–467.

108. Toda N, Tfelt-Hansen P. Calcium antagonists in migraine prophylaxis. In: Olesen J, Goadsby PJ, Ramadan NM, Tfelt-Hansen P, Welch KMA (eds) *The Headaches*, 3rd edn. Lippincott, Williams and Wilkins, Philadelphia, 2006: 539–544.

109. Goadsby PJ, Edvinsson L. Human in vivo evidence for trigeminovascular activation in cluster headache. Neuropeptide changes and effects of acute attacks therapies. *Brain* 1994; **117**(3); 427–434.

110. Acute treatment of migraine attacks: efficacy and safety of a nonsteroidal anti-inflammatory drug, diclofenac-potassium, in comparison to oral sumatriptan and placebo. The Diclofenac-K/Sumatriptan Migraine Study Group. *Cephalalgia* 1999; **19**(4): 232–240.

111. Diener HC, Eikermann A, *et al.* Efficacy of 1,000 mg effervescent acetylsalicylic acid and sumatriptan in treating associated migraine symptoms. *Eur Neurol* 2004; **52**(1): 50–56. Epub 2004 Jul 5.

112. Dahlöf CG, Jacobs LD. Ketoprofen, paracetamol and placebo in the treatment of episodic tension-type headache. *Cephalalgia* 1996; **16**(2): 117–123.

113. Diamond S, Balm TK, Freitag FG. Ibuprofen plus caffeine in the treatment of tension-type headache. *Clin Pharmacol Ther* 2000 Sep; 68(3): 312–319.

CHAPTER 23

Chest pain syndromes

Austin Leach and Michael Chester

National Refractory Angina Centre, Royal Liverpool and Broadgreen University Hospital, Liverpool, UK

Introduction

Chest pain is a common presenting symptom. In the UK, two of the most prevalent causes of death are ischemic heart disease and lung cancer. Patients presenting with chest pain often fear a potentially fatal diagnosis; it follows that the pain clinician's skills may be tested to their limits when attempting to help a patient with chest symptoms.

We do not intend to discuss in detail the diagnosis and management of acute chest pain syndromes–these may represent emergency life-threatening situations whose management rightly focuses on interrupting the natural history of the underlying disease rather than symptom control. However, many patients and healthcare professionals may think and behave as if the patient is developing an immediately life-threatening condition such as acute myocardial infarction when, in reality, their symptoms are a manifestation of a chronic pain syndrome. It is important for the patient, and their advisors, to have some basic rules that help to differentiate between fluctuations in stable angina and the development of thrombus-related unstable coronary syndromes (see below).

Managing patients with severe angina can provoke anxiety for the clinician. It is important to note that overall annual all-cause mortality is very low in this population [1]. True unstable angina or myocardial infarction is uncommon in refractory angina and in our experience the majority of patients can distinguish between a fluctuation in stable angina and an infarction.

Persistent (continuous) or episodic (paroxysmal) chest pain is usually a result of pathology of the chest wall. Brief unpredictable episodes of sharp precordial stabbing pains, usually over the anatomic apex of the heart, are common and are rarely associated with underlying pathology. A general sense of chest tightness in the absence of any pathologic process commonly accompanies severe anxiety states. However, a diagnosis of anxiety-related chest tightness should be made with great caution and empathy because anxiety is also a common feature of chest pain of pathologic origin.

Anatomy

The chest, more correctly referred to as the thorax, is an irregularly shaped cylinder with a narrow opening superiorly and a larger opening inferiorly. The superior thoracic opening is in continuity with the neck and the inferior thoracic opening is separated from the abdomen by the diaphragm. The musculoskeletal wall of the thorax is flexible and consists of segmentally arranged vertebrae, ribs, muscles and the sternum. The thoracic cavity enclosed by the thoracic wall is subdivided into three major components: the left and right pleural cavities, each surrounding a lung; the mediastinum, a median, longitudinal soft tissue partition containing the heart, the oesophagus, the trachea, the major systemic blood vessels and a variety of major nerves [2].

The thorax has three main functions.
- Breathing: contraction of the diaphragm and changes in the lateral and anterior dimensions of the thoracic wall caused by movement of the ribs alter the volume of the thoracic cavity – these are key elements in breathing.

Evidence-Based Chronic Pain Management. Edited by C. Stannard, E. Kalso and J. Ballantyne. © 2010 Blackwell Publishing.

- Protection of vital organs.
- The mediastinum acts as a conduit for structures connecting thoracic organs to other body regions, and for structures passing completely through the thorax from one body region to another.

Angina pectoris

The term "angina pectoris" first appeared in print in 1768, in a paper from William Heberden's *Medical Transactions* published by the Royal College of Physicians. The term comes from the Greek word *ankhon* ("strangling") and the Latin *pectus* ("chest"). Commonly omitted from Heberden's original description of the symptoms is the accompanying sensation of *angor animi* (from the Latin for "mental anguish of the animating spirit") which describes the perception of imminent death.

Prevalence

Chronic stable angina is an increasingly common condition affecting approximately 1.3 million UK citizens [3]. Its prevalence closely correlates with the incidence of coronary artery disease (CAD) which is the most common underlying pathologic cause for angina. Although neither condition is "curable," survival with CAD has consistently improved over the past two decades and consequently the prevalence of angina is increasing. Many angina sufferers are successfully managed using a combination of standard medical treatment plus angioplasty and stent (percutaneous coronary intervention (PCI)) or bypass.

The diagnosis of "chronic refractory angina" applies to a subset of stable angina patients for whom PCI or bypass is not suitable. This diagnosis is generally made by interventional cardiologists and surgeons. The prevalence of this painful, disabling and costly problem is hard to quantify because there is a wide range of opinion on the question of when revascularization is not suitable. Many interventionally minded cardiologists consider that revascularization is suitable if it is feasible, whereas there is an emerging body of opinion within cardiology that palliative revascularization should be a last resort and only after the patient has considered the range of alternatives. This latter view is consistent with patient-centered care and necessarily requires the full participation of the informed patient.

In our experience, well-informed patients tend to defer invasive procedures until they have tried low-risk, noninvasive options.

This modern approach to angina management has profound implications for the incidence and prevalence of chronic refractory angina. Using the European Society of Cardiology's disease-centered definition of refractory angina, we conservatively estimate there are at least 50,000+ sufferers in the NHS [4]. The prevalence of refractory angina would be considerably greater if the North American standard of consent were applied since it is reasonable to assume that a prudent patient would wish to know about all available evidence-based alternatives (currently only available to refractory angina patients) before consenting to a potentially lethal palliative revascularization procedure. The proportion of patients who would try relatively noninvasive therapies in preference to invasive therapies can be judged by the very high proportion of patients who "choose" the less effective multivessel PCI option over coronary artery bypass graft (CABG).

Incidence

The estimates of incidence of angina vary in different studies. The Scottish Continuous Morbidity Study estimates that 52,000 men and 43,000 women develop angina across the UK each year [5].

Risk factors

The risk factors for angina are the same as those for CAD and can be divided into reversible and irreversible. The main irreversible risk factors are aging, male gender and a positive family history. There are many reversible risk factors: smoking; raised cholesterol; inadequate physical activity; poor diabetic control; obesity; hypertension; a diet lacking adequate fresh fruit and vegetables, oily fish; inappropriate intake of alcohol.

Pathophysiology of angina

The fact that angina is a symptom rather than a disease in its own right is commonly overlooked. With the rapid rise in the incidence of atheromatous CAD in the latter part of the 20th century, there has been an increasing tendency for many clinicians to mistakenly consider angina to be synonymous with coronary disease. In fact, 100 years ago a patient presenting with typical symptoms of angina would be far likelier to be suffering from aortic valve stenosis or coronary ostial stenosis (with normal coronary arteries) secondary to syphilitic aortitis.

Angina pectoris is a visceral pain. As for other pains of visceral origin, the mechanisms that generate the sensation of angina are poorly understood. In the 17th century, at the dawn of modern medical theory, William Harvey, best known for his description of the circulation, was also considering the nature of sensation and feeling. He was one of the first scientists to consider the blood as a body part, and speculated that the blood itself was capable of feeling: "even if it were devoid of sensation this would not disqualify the blood from forming a part and even a very principal part of a body endowed with sensibility. For neither does the brain nor the spinal marrow nor the crystalline or the vitreous humour of the eye, feel anything, though by common consent these are parts of the body. Nay even the heart itself, the most distinguished part of the body, appears to be insensible." Here Harvey reports the case of the young son of Viscount Montgomery whose heart had been laid bare in consequence of a severe fall in early childhood and tolerated palpation and other forms of stimulation of his heart without discomfort.

There is little evidence for the existence of visceral nociceptors, and the current understanding is that signaling in the "visceral pain pathway" is initiated by sympathetic afferent activity. It is likely that activation of these afferent autonomic nerves results from ischemia in the myocardium and/or the coronary arterial endothelium. Whether the source of sympathetic activation is ischemia or the cellular response to ischemia is uncertain. Furthermore, the gross anatomy of the cardiac autonomic nerve plexuses shows that there is potential for a considerable volume of neurologic "cross-talk" between other visceral inputs to the thoracic sympathetic chain (such as esophagus, stomach and lungs) prior to forming connections within the spinal cord.

Autonomic afferent fibers enter the spinal cord and synapse in laminae 1 and 2. Once again, there is the potential for cross-talk, not only among visceral afferent fibers but also between visceral and somatic afferent fibers. In 1909 Mackenzie postulated that "interconnections" forming between visceral and somatic fibers could explain the phenomenon of

referred pain. This hypothesis remains plausible today. We go further and propose that angina is only possible after such abnormal neurologic pathways develop. Painless or "silent" ischemia is common. Patients who have not experienced prior angina commonly suffer a painless myocardial infarction but subsequently go on to develop exertional angina days, weeks or months later. On detailed questioning, patients often describe an event when they experienced other typical features of a myocardial infarct such as acute dyspnea, nausea and profuse sweating. This observation is consistent with the hypothesis that the sensation of angina requires the development of previously nonexistent or quiescent neurologic connections. However, the neurophysiologic processes that cause new spinal connections to activate between visceral and somatic fibers (i.e. converting "silent" ischemia into "noisy" (painful) ischemia) remain obscure. While elegant animal studies suggest a role for the vagus in afferent cardiac signaling, clinical evidence in humans suggests a far more prominent role for sympathetic tracts [5]. Temporary cardiac sympathectomy has been shown to produce freedom from angina for periods greatly exceeding duration of action of local anesthetic agents. A case of temporary vagus nerve block carried out at the National Refractory Angina Centre, which produced the anticipated tachycardia, did not result in relief from angina [6].

Positron emission tomography studies in patients with angina pectoris show activation of many brain areas that are also active when somatic pain fibers are stimulated: the hypothalamus, the periaqueductal gray matter, thalamus and prefrontal cortex. Silent myocardial ischemia seems to be associated with a failure of transmission of signals from the thalamus to the frontal cortex [7]. Once cortical stimulation has occurred there will be a conscious perception of pain. The pain will seem to originate in the part of the body represented by the area of sensory cortex that has been activated, and the emotional response generated will depend upon the significance of the sensation attached by the limbic system. It is likely, though unproven, that the sensation of *angor animi* arises from activity in the amygdalo-hippocampal apparatus. In part, this seems responsible for the (physiologically entirely inappropriate) increase in catecholamine activity that invariably accompanies an episode of anginal pain.

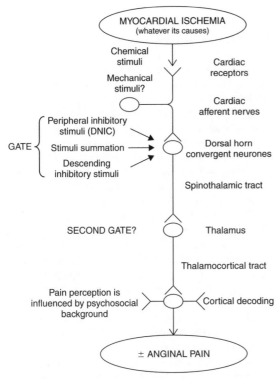

Figure 23.1 Proposed neural pathway for angina perception.

Because of the common assumption that the presence of angina means the existence of coronary atheroma, it is but a short step to assume that severe angina equals severe (i.e. dangerous, life-threatening) coronary disease. The fact that angina is a visceral pain is commonly forgotten by patients and healthcare professionals alike, who apply overly simplistic "rules" regarding somatic pain, i.e. a more or less proportional relationship between injury, signal intensity and perception.

Angiographic studies demonstrate that there is no correlation between the severity, or otherwise, of the pathologic process and the intensity of the sensation of angina that is generated. It is estimated that up to one-third of myocardial infarctions are painless. There is no evidence for the existence of cardiac nociceptors, and it is illogical to presume that the heart alone among the viscera should develop them. The "rules" that appear to govern nociception (i.e. that there is a relationship between stimulus intensity and perception) do not apply in angina.

Normal coronary arteries are end arteries. In the normal condition, myocytes subtended by a coronary artery are entirely dependent on that artery and cannot "borrow" from a neighboring artery. In the abnormal condition of ischemia, myocytes release vascular growth factors (neovascularization) and change cellular activity to minimize the effect of ischemia (ischemic preconditioning) [8]. New vessel growth and the development of collateral blood supply in ischemic muscle, be it skeletal or myocardial, have long been recognized. In cases of ischemic heart disease, coronary angiography may show total proximal occlusion of a main coronary whilst radionuclide studies show normal myocardial perfusion and no evidence of myocardial damage. This can only be possible with full collateralization of the coronary circulation that has been achieved prior to occlusion of the native artery. The processes of full collateralization and ischemic preconditioning take time which may explain why young, apparently fit men drop dead from the first infarct while elderly patients with a long history of angina tend to have small surviveable infarcts.

Cardiac syndrome X

Cardiac syndrome X affects around 2% of postmenopausal women and is rarely seen in younger women and men. The diagnosis of cardiac syndrome X requires a triad of typical angina, objective evidence of ischemia, e.g. positive treadmill test, nuclear scan or stress echo and angiographically "normal" coronary arteries. Ironically, because the orthodox simplistic cardiac view of angina arising from obstructing coronary disease was not applicable, angina arising in the absence of coronary atheroma has attracted disproportionate academic attention. Unfortunately, the general understanding of the condition remains poor and there is no consensus on a clear and effective therapeutic strategy. Consequently sufferers usually feel neglected or even dismissed by their healthcare advisors.

Syndrome X patients typically describe painful, disabling angina that is often triggered by physical or emotional stress. The level of effort required to trigger an episode of pain is often highly variable with clusters of "good" and "bad" periods. Most syndrome X sufferers who experience significant angina have, at one time or another, been left with the impression that their doctors do not believe them. This creates an additional emotional burden that is easily recognized by healthcare professionals who understand pain.

The genesis of ischemia in syndrome X remains obscure. Clinicians may describe microvascular angina, often telling patients that "the small arteries are diseased." While there is evidence of some abnormalities in the endothelium of a large proportion of syndrome X patients, this benign problem may be misunderstood by patients who frequently imagine a continuous blocking up of blood vessels that are too small to operate on. A second problem in syndrome X relates to the way ischemic signals are handled, with an apparent failure to control transmission at the thalamus where gating of ascending pain signals usually takes place [8]. Confusion and a lack of empathy from healthcare professionals experienced by syndrome X sufferers often exaggerate maladaptive responses at a higher cortical level.

Syndrome X-like angina

It is important to appreciate that the diagnostic criteria for true syndrome X were invoked to assist in research and there is a large subset of angina sufferers who just fail to fulfil the diagnostic criteria for true syndrome X. Thus patients with mild coronary disease, ischemia and typical angina are often excluded. Similarly, we see many patients with classic symptoms and angiographically normal arteries but in whom ischemia has not been demonstrated. These patients feel, and often are, neglected. They often respond well to a sympathetic hearing and a working diagnosis of syndrome X- like angina.

As with all forms of pain of presumed cardiac origin, education and demystification form the core of good management.

Prinzmetal angina – vasospastic angina

This rare angina variant is characterized by angina with ECG changes that mimic acute myocardial infarction. As its name suggests, the cause is coronary spasm and is usually self-limiting, though case examples of spasm proceeding to myocardial infarction have been described. Vasospasm is often calcium channel dependent and patients usually respond to a combination of education, demystification, relaxation training and high-dose calcium channel blockade. Some colleagues have reported using temporary sympathectomy despite the theoretical risks of inducing spasm with this technique.

Case scenario

A 53-year-old plumber has recently experienced a return of his symptoms of a sensation of pressure in the central region of his chest. Over the past 4 months it has increased in frequency and now he has daily episodes of pain. As the sensation begins, it is relatively mild but builds progressively over 2–3 minutes until it reaches a plateau. It can remain for between 5 and 20 minutes. It varies in severity and when severe, it is accompanied by an ache in his mandible, pallor, sweating and shortness of breath. It is sometimes provoked by effort, sometimes by emotion, and occasionally develops without any obvious associated activity. When the pain appears without provocation it is accompanied by anxiety that borders on panic.

The sensation is identical to the symptoms he originally experienced 6.5 years earlier when he had mistakenly supposed that he had indigestion. The "indigestion" had persisted for 2 weeks until one night when it had become intolerable and his wife, concerned about his pallor and general appearance, had called for an ambulance. On arrival at the Accident and Emergency department, an acute myocardial infarction had been diagnosed, and after thrombolysis and a period of observation, first on the Coronary Care Unit and subsequently on a general ward, he had been allowed home. He was advised to stop smoking, which he did.

Subsequently, a treadmill test following the modified Bruce protocol showed signs of easily inducible myocardial ischemia in the anterior and lateral chest leads, and an echocardiogram demonstrated a dyskinetic apical segment. Coronary angiography and ventriculography showed mildly impaired left ventricular function with an ejection fraction of 50% and a number of significant (i.e. >70% luminal occlusion) coronary narrowings affecting the left main stem and left anterior descending artery proximal to the first diagonal branch. The right coronary system had minor atheromatous disease. He was referred for urgent coronary artery bypass graft surgery which was carried out a few weeks later. He made an excellent recovery from his surgery and was delighted to find that his symptoms of angina had completely disappeared. Four months after his surgery he was able to return to work.

Six years on, he is distressed by the return of his symptoms. He had been told that the bypass operation "would last 10 years" and he fears that he will be forced into early retirement, which has implications regarding his pension arrangements and his ability to help subsidize his daughter's university course fees. A number of tests are carried out. He has taken aspirin and a statin daily since his original presentation, and he makes sure that he eats the recommended daily five helpings of fruit and vegetables, and some mackerel or salmon once or twice a week. His serum cholesterol is 4.3 mmol/l and echocardiography shows his left ventricular function is normal, with an ejection fraction of 60%. After coronary angiography (which shows that two of the three bypass grafts are still functioning well), he is told that another bypass operation is not feasible and that the only treatment to be offered is drug therapy.

He feels that the cardiac specialist has told him, in code, that there is "nothing more that can be done for him" (besides giving him more pills), which he finds a depressing outlook. Each episode of chest pain he experiences reminds him that he is "living on borrowed time" and he believes that the pain represents ongoing damage to his heart muscle. He recalls that when he was an inpatient 6 years previously a nurse had told him that each episode of anginal pain was "a bit like a mini heart attack." His feelings of hopelessness are increased when his cardiologist suggests a visit to the pain clinic for advice regarding control of his symptoms.

Management of angina pectoris

The presentation of angina is often dramatic and occasionally life threatening. Unheralded myocardial infarction due to coronary occlusion following atheromatous plaque rupture may be the first symptomatic manifestation of coronary disease, but more commonly the initial presentation is with increasing effort-related angina. Few patients correctly self-diagnose angina and their first medical diagnosis is often incorrect. In our 12-year experience of conducting detailed interviews with over 1500 chronic refractory angina patients, only three correctly self-diagnosed the origin of their "anginal" symptoms as cardiac. In many cases medical professionals also misdiagnose chest pain [9]. The initial diagnosis is based on the history and depends heavily on the location of symptoms. The assessment of risk of sudden death from myocardial infarction

following acute coronary occlusion is the priority following the diagnosis of angina. Such assessment, after taking a detailed history and conducting a full clinical examination, generally includes some form of exercise testing with ECG and/or echocardiographic analysis and if there is evidence of significant reversible myocardial ischemia, assessment of the coronary anatomy, generally by performing angiography.

The European Society of Cardiology summarizes the aims of treatment as:
- to improve prognosis by preventing myocardial infarction and death
- to minimize or abolish symptoms *and/or their effects*.

Prognostic interventions

There is overwhelming consensus based on large studies that prognostic improvement may be brought about by appropriate lifestyle behaviors such as: optimizing weight; adoption of a "Mediterranean" diet comprising at least five portions of fresh fruit and vegetables daily and 2–3 portions of oily fish weekly; smoking cessation; programmed exercise (30 minutes of moderate to strenuous exercise five times a week); blood pressure control [10]. In addition, statins and antiplatelet drugs have been shown to improve prognosis in patients with coronary artery disease and are recommended as standard in all CAD patients [11]. In patients with impaired ventricular function or diabetics with well-preserved ventricular function, angiotensin-converting enzyme inhibitors (ACEI) are also strongly recommended [11, 12]. Current guidelines recommend the use of ß-blocking agents for the first year following myocardial infarction (MI) and in patients with heart failure.

It is important to recognise thrombotic plaque events because emergency treatment to restore coronary flow during a thrombotic occlusion event will reduce the size of MI and death. Early referral is important and there are well-established care pathways for suspected MI that are triggered by a 999 call. Increasingly angioplasty is replacing intravenous thrombolytic therapy as the treatment of choice for acute myocardial infarction but there is a limited window of opportunity and reopening an occluded vessel more than 48 hours later increases adverse outcomes [12]. The characteristic clinical presentation of MI (suddenly worsening angina coupled with nausea, sweating, breathlessness and *angor animi*) is often difficult to distinguish from severe prolonged angina episodes. Current guidelines recommend that a prolonged episode of angina that does not show signs of subsiding after 15–20 minutes should be treated as a myocardial infarction.

In patients with atheromatous coronary disease, only CABG surgery has strong supporting evidence for prognostic improvement. Three large multicenter randomized trials, the Veterans Administration Cooperative Study (VA Study) [12], the European Coronary Surgery Study (ECSS) [14], and the Coronary Artery Surgery Study (CASS) [15], have compared the strategy of initial bypass surgery with that of initial medical management in regard to long-term survival and symptoms for patients with mild or moderate symptoms. A meta-analysis of these three major randomized trials as well as other smaller trials has confirmed the survival benefit achieved by surgery at 10 postoperative years for patients with three-, two- or even one-vessel disease that included a stenosis of the proximal left anterior descending (LAD) coronary artery [16]. The survival rate of these patients was improved by surgery whether they had normal or abnormal left ventricle (LV) function. For patients without a proximal LAD stenosis, bypass surgery improved the mortality rate only for those with three-vessel disease or left main stenosis.

Many patients presenting with refractory angina have previously undergone bypass surgery and no randomized studies have been undertaken to determine whether repeat bypass surgery improves prognosis.

There is no evidence that prognosis is improved by angioplasty in chronic stable angina.

Symptomatic interventions

Since the latter half of the 20th century the symptomatic management of angina pectoris has concentrated on drug therapies and revascularization. Only a small number of drugs have been shown to improve prognosis in coronary disease (see above). Several classes of drugs are effective in relieving angina without altering prognosis; the use of these drugs is often limited by unpleasant side effects.

Following the development of cardiopulmonary bypass techniques, CABG using autologous vessels became a useful and effective method of relieving symptoms. As described above, CABG improves prognosis in selected patients.. However, it is an expensive and time-consuming procedure which carries a notable perioperative morbidity and mortality. The introduction of coronary angioplasty and the development of stent placement techniques have failed to live up to initial expectations of improved prognosis and fewer symptoms. The proven reduction in angina associated with angioplasty is short-lived and there is no benefit in terms of reduced cardiovascular risk or need for further revascularization [17,18]. Two large randomized controlled trials (RITA-2 and COURAGE) compared initial angioplasty strategies with conservative management. RITA-2 showed that patients randomized to angioplasty experienced less angina at 3 months following randomization but were no better off at 3 years [18]. However, this temporary improvement was paid for by a substantially increased risk (78%) of experiencing a major adverse cardiac event. The recent COURAGE trial compared PCI plus intensive pharmacologic therapy and lifestyle intervention (optimal medical therapy) with optimal medical therapy alone in 2287 patients [19]. Like RITA-2, the patients randomized to PCI benefited initially but these benefits were not sustained. COURAGE is important because it demonstrates that PCI is no better than optimal medical therapy (OMT) in preventing major adverse cardiac events and that it is safe for stable angina patients who do not require prognostic bypass surgery to defer a decision to undergo PCI until a trial of OMT. In a recent cost-effectiveness analysis, the cost per quality-adjusted life-year (QALY) for angioplasty was £47,000, greatly exceeding the widely used "justification for treatment" threshold of £30,000 per QALY [19]. Importantly, it is now commonly accepted that, for stable angina patients, a decision for angioplasty can be safely deferred until conservative management has been tried.

This has led to a reappraisal of the management of chronic stable angina where no prognostic gain can be made by revascularization. By considering angina as a pain management problem rather than an ischemia problem, and by applying evidence-based pain management interventions, significant improvements in quality of life can be made. The American College of Cardiology (ACC) makes reference to this fact in its *Guidelines for the Management of Stable Angina*:

> Because the presentation of ischemic heart disease is often dramatic and because of impressive recent technological advances, healthcare providers tend to focus on diagnostic and therapeutic interventions, often overlooking critically important aspects of high quality care. Chief among these neglected areas is the education of patients [20].

A recent Health Care Commission audit confirmed that many cardiac patients leave hospital without receiving basic education [21]. Hard data on the effectiveness of education are hard to obtain because it is part of routine medical care, recommended by all clinical guidelines and GMC professional standards guidelines.

Patient-centered management of angina

Modern healthcare systems encourage health professionals to practice "patient-centered medicine." Much confusion exists about what this much-used (and much-abused) phrase actually means. We understand it to mean that patients should be enabled to define the objectives of treatment, and the doctor and other healthcare professionals should form a "therapeutic alliance" with patients to help them achieve those objectives. This should necessarily include education about the condition and the various treatment options so that patients can be active participants in their long-term management. This approach to therapy will be familiar to most practitioners in pain medicine.

If the annual expenditure on coronary disease is considered, surprisingly little evidence exists in support of the many and varied recommended treatments for control of anginal symptoms.

Most patients agree that the fundamental objectives of treatment of angina pectoris are to survive as long as possible, with as high a quality of life as possible. When questioned, the majority stated a preference for a shorter, happier life rather than a longer, more miserable one. This approach is highly relevant to patients who, for example, develop intolerable muscular fatigue and pain caused by statins. The majority of patients taking statins are not significantly affected, although there is a multivariate odds ratio of 1.5 for any muscular

pain for those taking statins when compared to those who do not [22]. Although complex lipid-lowering strategies may be suggested [23], some patients may, after appropriate deliberation, choose to accept a small increase in risk by stopping statin therapy (which may be offset by other lifestyle changes) for a reduction in unpleasant statin-related side effects.

Harmful misconceptions are common amongst angina suffers and their family and friends [2,23]. The majority of patients and carers believe that each episode of pain represents ongoing myocardial damage. In the face of such a widespread and damaging misunderstanding about angina, it is unsurprising that many angina patients and their carers seek to protect themselves by avoiding circumstances that might provoke angina. Mistaken beliefs are often reinforced by concentrating therapy exclusively on the "biologic" component, i.e. the coronary narrowing. Identifying and correcting the patient's misunderstandings is a vital first step.

In that telling quotation from the ACC's guidelines (see above), it is clear that in modern cardiologic practice, much valuable advice regarding lifestyle, weight loss, smoking cessation and fitness improvement is overlooked in favor of a "disease-centered" approach to revascularization. In fact, many palliative revascularization procedures may be avoided once the patient understands the absence of prognostic gain. With an emphasis on optimizing quality of life and using the available evidence, a simple and pragmatic algorithm can be constructed (Fig. 23.2).

Patient education

The rewards achievable with patient education should not be underestimated. Changing harmful misconceptions improves quality of life [24] and it has been known for some time that cognitive rehabilitation programs improve symptoms and produce worthwhile reductions in palliative coronary revascularization. In the 1990s Lewin *et al.* found that the majority of patients listed for bypass surgery improved so much that they changed their minds after attending a cognitive behavioral rehabilitation program [24]. Similarly, Ornish showed that 70% of patients successfully avoided palliative revascularization by enrolling in a comprehensive rehabilitation program. This compared favorably with a control group of patients who had recently undergone "successful" revascularization in whom only 75% avoided further revascularization [25].

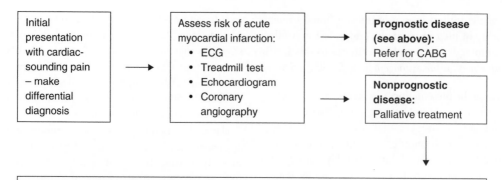

Figure 23.2 National Refractory Angina Centre (NRAC) treatment algorithm.

In our center a brief cognitive intervention delivered to 69 consecutive refractory angina patients resulted in a clinically and statistically significant improvement in symptoms, anxiety and depression and quality of life [26]. In a larger consecutive series of 271 patients enrolled over a 5-year period we compared admissions and myocardial infarct rates before and after enrolment. A rising admission rate of 15.5 days per patient per year fell to 10 days per patient per year within a month of enrolment (P < 0.001). Thirty two MIs were recorded in the year prior to enrolment compared to eight after (P < 0.001) [27].

The key to brief cognitive intervention is mutual respect and a shared understanding of the patients' experiences and objectives [28]. It must not be so brief as to compound patients' and carers' confusion by adding new information to pre-existing misconceptions. It is crucial to identify core beliefs by asking straightforward open-ended questions, taking time to gently explore the patients' and carers' beliefs, and the provenance of those beliefs. Challenging beliefs and offering evidence-based alternatives or opinion should be underpinned by an understanding of the patient's beliefs. Not only does this time-consuming approach represent a worthwhile and effective intervention in terms of quality of life improvement for angina sufferers, it also offers potentially enormous cost savings in terms of reduction in unscheduled admissions, avoidable palliative revascularization, with concomitant reduction in periprocedural complications such as stroke, myocardial infarction and death.

Current all-comer mortality for first-time bypass surgery is 1.7% [29]. Major adverse event rate following planned PCI is difficult to determine with precision because myocardial infarctions that are not associated with the development of a Q wave on the ECG are not routinely recorded. Excluding these important events reduces the PCI complication rates to around 0.5% [30]. In the North West of England, the Cheshire and Merseyside and North Wales Cardiac Network introduced Stable Angina Guidelines in October 2007 that emphasize the importance of incorporating cognitive intervention into routine rehabilitation before medication and palliative revascularization [31].

Lifestyle advice
Relaxation training. Catecholamine release invariably accompanies angina and contributes to worsening of the symptoms (pain, breathlessness, nausea and sweating). Calming techniques that enable patients to reduce endogenous adrenaline release and increase

endogenous endorphin can effectively abort episodes of angina and/or prevent them becoming severe. Research shows that cardiac events (mostly revascularization) were significantly less likely in patients trained in relaxation techniques. Learning a technique of stress management was associated with a relative risk of 0.26 of a cardiac event compared with control patients receiving usual care [32].

Trust and understanding are required before some patients will accept advice on calming techniques, especially if they have formed the suspicion that doctors think their symptoms are "all in the head." Fortunately, most patients will have worked out for themselves that "getting worked up" worsens episodes of angina and many will have already adopted basic relaxation techniques through trial and error.

Exercise. Many patients and their carers mistakenly believe that undertaking exercise is more dangerous than remaining sedentary and it is important to recognize and challenge irrational fears about exercise. Patients and carers will often relate stories of being told to "take things easy" or "avoid overdoing it" following a heart attack and will talk of otherwise fit acquaintances who "dropped dead while jogging" as confirmation of their view that exercise is best avoided. The overwhelming expert consensus view is that regular exercise reduces cardiovascular risk and enhances well-being. The standard advice of 30 minutes of moderate to strenuous exercise five times a week should be given, with additional advice on a slow progressive symptom-avoiding program using pacing and goal-setting techniques [11]. Patients who understand their condition and the wide-ranging beneficial effects of exercise on pain, weight, blood pressure, well-being and cardiovascular risk are more likely to adhere to advice.

Diet. A healthy diet is important. Most patients think that a regimen that avoids saturated fat is adequate. The current recommendations focus on the importance of a cardioprotective diet of at least five portions of fresh fruit and vegetables a day and two portions of oily fish a week. Compared with teetotallers and moderate to heavy drinkers, a daily consumption of modest amounts of alcohol (1–2 units for women and 2–3 units for men) is associated with the lowest cardiovascular risk. Of these, the most controversial is alcohol. There is a clear dose-dependent relationship between alcohol intake and blood pressure [33]. On a population basis, the relationship between alcohol intake and coronary mortality is a U or J shape. A recent long-term study of 45–64 year olds showed that the 6% who took up moderate alcohol were 38% less likely to develop CAD compared to their persistently nondrinking counterparts [34]. The consistent association between moderate alcohol intake (2 units a day for women and 3 units a day for men) and cardiovascular risk reduction is attributed to beneficial effects on HDL-cholesterol, fibrinogen and glucose intolerance [35]. Despite these positive attributes, the European Society of Cardiology guidelines on cardiovascular disease (CVD) prevention do not recommend moderate alcohol intake to prevent the development of CVD. The reason for this appears to relate to concerns about abuse and toxicity.

Smoking. All the evidence points to a direct causal relationship between inhaled cigarette smoke and an increased risk of major cardiovascular events. Unlike some lung diseases and cancers, cardiovascular risk is not linearly related to dose and a single cigarette significantly increases risk of MI. Patients and carers should be urged to consider complete cessation. Passive smoking should be discouraged.

Optimizing medication

Many patients have fundamental misunderstandings about their antianginal medication. In many cases they mistakenly believe that symptomatic treatments carry an additional prognostic benefit. The only groups of drugs for which there is clear evidence that myocardial infarction and cardiac death rates are reduced are antiplatelet drugs (aspirin or clopidogrel) and statins [5]. β-Blockers and ACEI improve prognosis if there is measurable left ventricular dysfunction. β-Blockers are indicated for a year following an uncomplicated MI but there is no evidence of risk reduction beyond a year after infarction. Thus for the majority of stable angina patients with normal ventricular function, most prescribed drugs (i.e. calcium channel blockers; nitrates; potassium channel blockers; the new I_ϕ channel blocker ivabradine) and opioids are for symptom palliation only.

It is important that the prescription of palliative therapy should be subjected to a "cost–benefit" analysis with respect to symptomatic improvement measured against unpleasant side effects. Because most antianginal drugs operate through their vasodilating properties, there is potential for drug interaction causing unpleasant side effects such as postural hypotension, dependant edema and persistent headache. The patient should be encouraged and helped to determine for himself whether his quality of life has been enhanced or reduced by a particular drug. With care, and a logical approach to therapeutic trial, drug intake can be limited to only those medications which control symptoms effectively with an acceptable side-effect profile. *Maximal* medication is often confused with *optimal* medication. It may take some months for patients to optimize their medication successfully.

Transcutaneous electrical nerve stimulation (TENS)
In the 1960s Wall & Melzack proposed the gate control theory of pain transmission based on their observations of neural activity in the dorsal horn of the spinal cord [34]. Since then TENS has become a popular, safe and effective method of controlling various types of pain. Its benefits in treating angina pain are well established, although its use is not widespread in the UK. This may be due to a widely held, although totally fallacious belief that TENS is potentially hazardous to angina sufferers because of potential interference in the heart's conduction pathways.

There is evidence that TENS improves quality of life in patients with angina, and that it has been shown to increase coronary flow. Three groups of patients with heart conditions (34 with syndrome X, 15 with CAD, 16 following heart transplant) had coronary blood flow velocity (CBFV) estimated following TENS. The first two groups showed significant increases in CBFV, but the third group did not, leading the researchers to conclude that TENS-related changes in CBFV were mediated by neural mechanisms [35]. This adds to the earlier observation (in two groups of 13 and 23 patients) that TENS therapy applied in three 1-hour daily sessions increases work capacity, reduces ST segment depression during exercise, reduces frequency of angina episodes and reduces nitrate consumption [36].

Transcutaneous electrical nerve stimulation is less successful in abolishing or reducing pain when the primary area of pain referral extends beyond the chest wall. Episodes of angina that begin in the chest and extend to other areas may be controlled or abolished by TENS with appropriately positioned skin electrodes. A case report describes how TENS may compromise respiratory function in debilitated patients and leads should not be applied to the throat [37]. TENS for angina is most successful when the area of pain referral can be encapsulated by four skin electrodes (personal communication, D Trenbath). Frequency and amplitude need to be adjusted to individual preference.

Temporary sympathetic nerve block
In 1920 Jonnesco published a case report describing the beneficial effect on intractable angina of surgical extirpation of the left stellate ganglion. This treatment was used to treat patients with severe angina and heart failure. Because of high surgical morbidity the procedure was subsequently modified to alcohol ablation, a treatment which remained in use until the 1960s. The reason for the abandonment of this low-risk and effective symptomatic treatment is obscure.

The growing recognition of neural plasticity in the peripheral and central nervous system has led to techniques causing a permanent neurologic lesion becoming less popular among pain clinicians, especially in the knowledge that an anesthesia dolorosa pattern may develop with time. The well-recognized phenomenon of local anesthetic nerve block producing pain relief of a duration far exceeding the longevity of the drug has led to a re-examination of temporary stellate ganglion block and upper thoracic paravertebral block in the management of chronic stable angina. Temporary cardiac sympathectomy may result in many weeks of freedom from pain with low risk of serious complications without requiring fluoroscopy. Following an initial case report confirming prolonged relief from angina following stellate ganglion block, a 2-year unblinded prospective audit examined the effects of a total of 227 stellate ganglion blocks performed on 46 patients with coronary artery disease and refractory angina. Mean duration of freedom from pain was 3.5 weeks (although one patient reported more than 40 pain-free weeks), with a low complication rate (2%). Only one patient required overnight hospitalization following a complication, and no permanent harm was suffered [38, 39]. Although a long-term commitment between pain clinician and patient is required for repeated nerve blocks to be a valid method of symptom control, some patients find it an acceptable strategy.

Opioid drugs

Most health professionals are accustomed to treating chest pain in patients admitted as an emergency with strong opioid analgesics. There is a growing acceptance that it is appropriate to treat patients with severe chronic nonmalignant pain with oral modified-release preparations of opioid drugs. This notion was first presented in the 1980s by Portenoy and was initially regarded as controversial. Concerns among physicians and patients of inducing dependence, addiction and ever-escalating doses have been extensively considered [40]. There remains a reluctance to prescribe opioids among some groups of physicians. An American study showed that geriatricians were more likely than internal medicine specialists to prescribe opioids to elderly patients in pain [41]. The British Pain Society has published evidence-based guidelines about the prescription of strong opioid drugs in chronic nonmalignant pain [42]. The principles described may be applied as effectively in angina management as in any other chronic opioid-sensitive pain condition. Side effects often limit the usefulness of opioids and some authorities have suggested that this may be overcome by delivering opioids intrathecally because lower doses are required.

As more is understood about endogenous opioid cell membrane receptors and their interactions with intracellular processes, it is becoming clearer that the mechanisms of tolerance, dependence and addiction are varied and complex [43]. The use of terms such as "addiction" and "dependence" may become emotive, and the inclusive phrase "problem drug use" has been preferred in some quarters. The growing list of publications on this topic demonstrates that there is a small incidence of problem drug use in chronic pain patients prescribed strong opioids. A recent review of 67 publications on this issue has suggested an incidence of around 0.2% risk of addiction and about 0.6% risk of aberrant drug-related behavior following the prescription of opioids to a chronic pain patient with no previous history of drug or alcohol misuse. In patients who have previous history of alcohol and/or drug misuse, the incidences of addiction and abberrant behavior were higher (3% and 11% respectively) [44].

It is important to include the patient as an equal partner in decision making when considering the use of these drugs in managing long-term pain problems [45].

Intrathecal opioid therapy. Implantable pumps delivering microvolumes of analgesic drugs have been developed since the 1990s. The principle behind their use is the ability to directly target drugs to their site of action rather than relying on intermediary mechanisms of transport. There are a number of drawbacks to the use of these devices.

- Implantation of the drug delivery system requires an invasive procedure.
- The patient and doctor are committed to a long-term relationship which can damage patient autonomy.
- A lengthy titration period may be necessary while previous medication is adjusted to allow the new drug – and route of administration – to "bed in."
- Equipment costs are considerable and pump replacement may be required.
- Intrathecal granuloma formation at the catheter tip, which may cause spinal cord compression, has been reported. The overall incidence is unclear, but in a series describing 41 cases of catheter tip granuloma in chronic pain patients receiving intrathecal drugs, the use of high concentrations of morphine was most strongly linked to granuloma development [46].
- Long-term outcomes are uncertain. A prospective case study followed 38 intrathecal pump recipients for 3 years after implantation and concluded that although intrathecal analgesic administration may improve pain, mood and function, this group of patients continue to experience severe symptoms [47].

Importantly, there is little evidence of overall benefit to chronic angina patients using intrathecal infusion pumps and worldwide experience is limited to a very small number of specialist units [48]. Overall, our own experience (at the National Refractory Angina Centre) of eight implants is discouraging. Intractable nausea, inadequate pain control and testicular suppression are among the problems encountered.

Spinal cord stimulation (SCS)

Following the development of TENS after Melzack & Wall's pioneering work on spinal gating, interest in other neurostimulation techniques quickly gained ground. Analgesia was observed following direct stimulation of the spinal cord by a wire placed in the posterior epidural space. Spinal cord simulation has since become an established treatment for neuropathic pain.

In the opinion of the authers, SCS can be an effective technique in the control of refractory angina, but there is insufficient evidence to support its cost effectiveness in the UK (see NICE puplication: www.nice.org.uk). For a more detailed examination of the role of SCS in pain medicine see Chapter 29.

External enhanced counterpulsation (EECP)

External counterpulsation by the use of sequentially inflated ECG-co-ordinated high-pressure cuffs around calves, thighs and buttocks has been investigated since the 1960s as a noninvasive method of replicating the effects of intra-aortic balloon pumping. Initially it was developed as a treatment for cardiogenic shock. In a randomized controlled trial EECP has been shown to benefit chronic refractory angina patients and has FDA approval [49]. Nevertheless, the evidence for cost-effectiveness of EECP in the routine care of refractory angina patients is lacking and a health technology assessment is under way. In our practice, EECP is reserved for patients who would otherwise be candidates for redo bypass surgery or spinal cord stimulation. EECP's major advantage over the alternatives is that it can be tried without significant risk and withdrawn if it is intolerable. Funding involves a time-consuming process in England and requires approval from the patient's Primary Care Trust specialist commissioning group.

Treatment involves attending for regular sessions to allow a total of 35 hours of therapy. This is a major commitment and limits EECP's usefulness because it is only available in a few centers across the UK. A recent review of data from a long-term follow-up registry suggests that clinically significant benefits are seen in 70% of patients up to 3 years after the initial treatment [50]. There is no doubt that EECP increases coronary perfusion during augmentation but why the effect lasts for so long after completion of the course of treatments is unclear. Whatever the mechanism, EECP is a useful noninvasive treatment option and is often preferred to invasive therapies such as palliative surgery or spinal cord stimulation.

Managing changes in symptoms

It is important to appreciate that coronary atheroma progresses in a nonlinear fashion. Lesions may remain stable for years before an unpredictable plaque disruption event produces sudden progression or, less often, regression of the lesion. Rapid worsening in the severity of a coronary lesion causes ischemia at low workloads, resulting in more frequent and severe angina, and it is important to have a plan to deal with such an event. It is sensible to negotiate with local cardiologists in advance so that a subsequent sudden deterioration in symptoms is handled in the preferred manner. Generally speaking, cardiologists have a low threshold for investigating and treating patients who they suspect may have a fresh clot in a coronary artery.

Even if the deterioration is related to an occlusive event, it need not cause a myocardial infarction. Very severe narrowings are at high risk of occlusion and such events are often associated with an abrupt deterioration in frequency and severity of symptoms. However, severe lesions usually occlude without causing myocardial infarction because of the development of coronary collaterals [51]. In practice, worsening angina is more commonly the result of physical stress, such as chest or urinary infections. Emotional stress plays a major role in otherwise inexplicable deteriorations and is often underplayed by patients who are too embarrassed to mention personal matters. An effective therapeutic alliance will avoid such problems.

Chest wall pain

The chest wall comprises skin, subcutaneous tissues, bony structures linked by symphysis, fibrocartilaginous and synovial joints, muscle, nerves, blood vessels and parietal pleura. Many conditions may present with chest pain, descriptions of which are beyond the scope of this chapter. The most common clinical situations encountered by the pain clinician result from some kind of physical insult to one or more tissue types. This may be accidental trauma, postsurgical or as a consequence of infection.

Chest wall trauma is common. Causes range from road traffic accidents to falls and brawls. The original traumatic event may easily be forgotten if there is a delay between the event and the onset of pain. We have met patients who were unwilling to mention their suspicions that an earlier trauma might be related to their current pain because a doctor had previously dismissed the idea. If rib fracture occurs, the inflammatory process will cause the area to be painful until the bone has healed. Injury to adjacent structures is common following trauma. Fibromyalgia can result from traumatized soft tissues, including muscle and periosteum, and because the neurovascular bundle is so close to the rib its structures may easily be damaged by jagged bone fragments. It has been well established that long-term pain experience can be influenced by the reported level of pain during the acute phase [52].

If lung laceration or contusion has complicated the injury the parietal pleura will be involved in the inflammatory process, and there is an increased risk of local or generalized lung infection. Persistent cough due to pleural or lung injury immediately following trauma is likely to be a determining factor in pain experience during the acute phase.

Chest wall pain after surgery

Pain following surgery to the chest wall is common and frequently under-reported. As with accidental trauma, persistent pain may arise from a variety of sources, and it may be extremely difficult to elucidate the precise cause of pain. Furthermore, there may be a tendency to misdiagnose a new postoperative chronic pain as a recurrence of the original condition. For example, it is well known that chest wall dysesthesia is common following CABG surgery. In a retrospective study of a 2-year cohort of CABG patients, 44% of 380 responders to a questionnaire admitted to persistent dysesthesia of the chest wall [53]. This dysesthesia may be related to the harvesting of the internal mammary artery as part of the revascularization procedure, although incidence of pain is similar at 1 year (approximately 30%) with or without use of the mammary artery and regardless of surgical technique, which were the findings of a prospective study of 349 consecutive patients undergoing CABG. Fourteen (4%) of these patients rated their pain as persistently greater than 50 mm on a visual analog scale [54].

Because there may be a significant delay between time of surgery and onset of pain, and because CABG is often successful in abolishing anginal symptoms for a variable period, a proportion of cases of chest wall pain following CABG will be misdiagnosed as recurrent angina pectoris, and the patient may be subjected to a series of unnecessary and potentially hazardous investigations.

Around 5% of 1000 refractory angina patients referred with a supposed diagnosis of postrevascularization recurrent angina were found to have other causes for their chest pain. A carefully taken history invariably revealed significant differences in the characteristics of their preoperative angina and the presenting pain. When recurrent angina happens, even if it has not been present for many years, it almost always follows the same pattern as it did before surgery. On careful questioning, postbypass patients with noncardiac chest pain will often admit to experiencing their "old" angina under conditions of physical or emotional stress. This will help distinguish true recurrent post-CABG angina from other chest wall pain syndromes.

Other categories of surgery that commonly result in chronic chest wall pain are thoracotomy and breast surgery. Although there are numerous anecdotes and references to the frequency of occurrence, there is a relative lack of accurate published data. A recent retrospective review of a cohort of 255 patients undergoing thoracotomy in a 2-year period received 149 (58%) responses. The overall incidence of chronic chest wall pain was 52% (32% rated "mild," 16% rated "moderate," 3% rated "severe") [55]. These pain syndromes frequently have a significant neuropathic component, and may be helped by the various treatments for neuropathic pain described elsewhere.

Since the mid 1990s an incidence of around 40% of pain after breast surgery has been accepted as accurate. A cohort of 138 women previously reporting pain after breast surgery was reviewed at a mean of 9 years (SD 1.8 years) after initial operation; 113 (82%) women responded, of whom 59 (52%) reported persistent pain [56].

Future directions for research

Despite calls for a comprehensive health strategy going back over a decade, refractory angina remains in the shadows of stable angina. The clinical and financial implications of the condition are poorly understood and a comprehensive epidemiologic review is urgently needed. The lack of interest by independent funding bodies has resulted in the creation of an artificial evidence base funded by the manufacturing and pharmacology industries that appears to support physical and pharmacologic interventions.

No industry-sponsored trial in refractory angina has required patients to have undergone optimal rehabilitation. Similarly, none has used rehabilitation as a comparator. Randomized controlled trials that compare one expensive intervention with another will not provide evidence of cost-effectiveness and are of questionable value.

It is hoped that the current UK NHS practice-based commissioning reforms, enabling primary care practitioners to identify cost-effective services that are best suited to the needs of their patients, will lead to an expansion of noninvasive pain management strategies for the treatment of this complex and disabling chronic pain condition.

Authors' recommendations

After 12 years of developing the UK's first comprehensive refractory angina service, we are convinced that fear and confusion dominate the clinical picture. Parallel lines of research demonstrate the critical importance of setting aside time to take a detailed biopsychosocial history that identifies and deals with misconceptions. However, few are prepared or able to spend the 2–3 hours that we have found necessary to begin the process of changing long-held damaging beliefs. We urge colleagues who plan to treat refractory angina patients to resist management pressure to fall in line with existing outpatient arrangements. Make your clinic patient friendly and insist on at least 2 hours initial assessment for a new patient clinic. In our experience this time is invaluable in preventing patients progressing to time-consuming and costly interventions such as sympathectomy and spinal cord stimulation.

References

1. Drake R, Vogl W, Mitchell A (eds). *Gray's Anatomy for Students* Elsevier, Philadelphia, 2005.

2. http://www.heartstats.org/datapage.asp?id=6799.

3. Mannheimer C, Camici P, Chester MR, *et al.* The problem of chronic refractory angina; report from the ESC Joint Study Group on the Treatment of Refractory Angina. *Eur Heart J* 2002; **23**: 355–370.

4. http://www.heartstats.org/uploads/documents%5C2007. chapter2.pdf.

5. Foreman RD. Mechanisms of cardiac pain. *Annu Rev Physiol* 1999; **61**: 143–167.

6. Rosen SD, Camici PG. The brain–heart axis in the perception of cardiac pain: the elusive link between ischaemia and pain. *Ann Med* 2000; **32**(5): 350–364.

7. Yellon D, Downey J. Preconditioning the myocardium: from cellular physiology to clinical cardiology. *Physiol Rev* 2003; **83**(4): 1113–1151.

8. Sekhri N, Feder GS, Junghans C, Hemingway H, Timmis AD. How effective are rapid access chest pain clinics? Prognosis of incident angina and non-cardiac chest pain in 8762 consecutive patients. *Heart* 2007; **93**: 458–463.

9. European guidelines on cardiovascular disease prevention in clinical practice. *Eur J Cardiovasc Prev* 2007; **14**(suppl 2): S1–S113.

10. European Society of Cardiology. Guidelines on the management of stable angina pectoris: executive summary. *Eur Heart J* 2006; **27**: 1341–1387.

11. Hochman JS, Lamas GA, Buller CE, *et al.*, Occluded Artery Trial Investigators. Coronary intervention for persistent occlusion after myocardial infarction. *N Engl J Med* 2006; **355**(23): 2395–2407.

12. VA Coronary Artery Bypass Surgery Cooperative Study Group. Eighteen-year follow-up in the Veterans Affairs Cooperative Study of Coronary Artery Bypass Surgery for stable angina. *Circulation* 1992; **86**: 121–130.

13. Varnauskas E. Twelve-year follow-up of survival in the randomized European Coronary Surgery Study. *N Engl J Med* 1988; **319**: 332.

14. Passamani E, Davis KB, Gillespie MJ, Killip T. A randomized trial of coronary artery bypass surgery. Survival of patients with a low ejection fraction. *N Engl J Med* 1985; **312**: 1665–1671.

15. Yusuf S, Zucker D, Peduzzi P, *et al.* Effect of coronary artery bypass graft surgery on survival: overview of 10-year results from randomised trials by the Coronary Artery Bypass Graft Surgery Trialists Collaboration [published erratum appears in *Lancet* 1994; **344**: 1446]. *Lancet* 1994; **344**: 563–570.

16. RITA-2 Trial Participants. Coronary angioplasty versus medical therapy for angina: the second Randomised Intervention Treatment of Angina (RITA-2) trial. *Lancet* 1997; **350**: 461–468.

17. Boden WE, O'Rourke RA, Teo KK, *et al.* Optimal medical therapy with or without PCI for stable coronary disease. *N Engl J Med* 2007; **356**: 1503–1516.

18. Griffin SC, Barber JA, Manca A, *et al.* Cost effectiveness of clinically appropriate decisions on alternative treatments for angina pectoris: prospective observational study. *BMJ* 2007; **334**: 624.

19. Gibbons RJ, Chatterjee K, Daley J, *et al.* ACC/AHA/ACP-ASIM guidelines for the management of patients with chronic stable angina: a report of the American College of Cardiology/ American Heart Association Task Force on Practice Guidelines (Committee on Management of Patients With Chronic Stable Angina). *J Am Coll Cardiol* 1999; **33**(7): 2092–2197.

20. Heart patient survey shows too many people are leaving hospital without aftercare and advice, June 2005. www. healthcarecommission.org.uk/newsandevents/pressreleases. cfm/widCall1/customWidgets.content_view_1/cit_id/1998.

21. Buettner C, Davis R, Leveille S, Mittleman M, Mukamal K. Prevalence of musculoskeletal pain and statin use. *J Gen Intern Med* 2008; **23**(8): 1182–1186.

22. Jacobsen T. Towards pain-free statin prescribing: a clinical algorithm for diagnosis and managment of myalgia. *Mayo Clin Proc* 2008; **83**(6): 687–700.

23. Furze G, Lewin R, Murberg TA, Bull P, Thompson D. Does it matter what patients think? The relationship between changes in patients' beliefs about angina and their psychological and functional status. *J Psychosom Res* 2005; **59**: 323–329.

24. Lewin B, Cay E, Todd I, Soryal I, Goodfield N, Bloomfield P, Elton R The angina management programme: a rehabilitation treatment. *Br J Cardiol* 1995; **2**(8): 221–226.

25. Ornish D. Avoiding revascularization with lifestyle changes: the Multicenter Lifestyle Demonstration Project. *Am J Cardiol* 1998; **82**(10B): 72T–76T.

26. Moore RK, Groves D, Bateson S, Barlow P, Hammond C, Leach AA, Chester MR. Health related quality of life of patients with refractory angina before and one year after enrolment onto a refractory angina program. *Eur J Pain* 2005; **9**: 305–310.

27. http: //heartsurgery.healthcarecommission.org.uk/Survival.aspx.

28. http://www.bcis.org.uk/resources/audit/audit_2006.

29. http://www.cmcn.nhs.uk/guidelines/stable_angina.htm.

30. Blumenthal JA, Jiang W, Babyak MA, *et al.* Stress management and exercise training in cardiac patients with myocardial ischemia: effects on prognosis and evaluation of mechanisms. *Arch Intern Med* 1997; **157**: 2213–2223.

31. Xin X, He J, Frontini MG, Ogden LG, Motsami OI, Whelton PK. Effects of alcohol reduction on blood pressure: a meta-analysis of randomised controlled trials. *Hypertension* 2001; **38**: 112–117.

32. King DE, Mainous AG 3rd, Geesey ME. Adopting moderate alcohol consumption in middle age: subsequent cardiovascular events. *Am J Med* 2008; **121**: 201–206.

33. Mukamal KJ, Jensen MK, Grønbaek M, *et al.* Drinking frequency, mediating biomarkers, and risk of myocardial infarction in women and men. *Circulation* 2005; **112**(10): 1406–1413.

34. Melzack R, Wall PD. Pain mechanisms: a new theory. *Science* 1965; **150**(699): 971–979.

35. Chauhan A, Mullins PA, Thuraisingham SI, Taylor G, Petch MC, Schofield PM. Effect of transcutaneous electrical nerve stimulation on coronary blood flow. *Circulation* 1994; **89**: 694–702.

36. Mannheimer C, Carlsson C-A, Emanuelsson H, Vedin A, Waagstein F, Wilhelmsson C. The effects of transcutaneous electrical nerve stimulation in patients with severe angina pectoris. *Circulation* 1985; **71**: 308–316.

37. Mann CJ. Respiratory compromise: a rare complication of transcutaneous electrical nerve stimulation for angina pectoris. *J Accident Emerg Med* 1996; **13**: 68.

38. Chester M, Hammond C, Leach A. Long-term benefits of stellate ganglion block in severe chronic refractory angina. *Pain* 2000; **87**: 103–105.

39. Moore R, Groves D, Hammond C, Leach A, Chester MR. Temporary sympathectomy in the treatment of chronic refractory angina. *J Pain Symptom Manage* 2005; **30**(2): 183–191.

40. Ballantyne JC, LaForge KS. Opioid dependence and addiction during opioid treatment of chronic pain. *Pain* 2007; **129**(3): 235–255.

41. Lin JJ, Alfandre D, Moore C. Physician attitudes toward opioid prescribing for patients with persistent non-cancer pain. *Clin J Pain* 2007; **23**(9): 799–803.

42. Recommendations for the appropriate use of opioids for persistent non-cancer pain, 2005. www.britishpainsociety.org.

43. Christie MJ. Cellular neuroadaptations to chronic opioids: tolerance, withdrawal and addiction. *Br J Pharmacol* 2008; **154**(2): 384–396.

44. Fishbain DA, Cole B, Lewis J, Rosomoff HL, Rosomoff RS. What percentage of chronic non-malignant pain patients exposed to chronic opioid analgesic therapy develop abuse/addiction and/or aberrant drug-related behaviours? A structured evidence-based review. *Pain Med* 2008; **9**(4): 444–459.

45. Blake S, Ruel B, Seamark C, Seamark D. Experiences of patients requiring strong opioid drugs for chronic non-cancer pain: a patient-initiated study. *Br J Gen Pract* 2007; **57**(535): 101–108.

46. Coffey RJ, Burchiel K. Inflammatory mass lesions associated with intrathecal drug infusion catheters: report and observations on 41 patients. *Neurosurgery* 2002; **50**(1): 78–87.

47. Thimineur MA, Kravitz E, Vodapally MS. Intrathecal opioid treatment for chronic non-malignant pain: a 3 year prospective study. *Pain* 2004; **109**(3): 242–249.

48. Cherry DA, Gourlay GK, Eldredge KA. Management of chronic intractable angina – spinal opioids offer an alternative therapy. *Pain* 2003; **102**(1-2): 163–166.

49. Arora RR, Chou TM, Jain D, *et al.* The multicenter study of enhanced external counterpulsation (MUST-EECP): effect of EECP on exercise-induced myocardial ischemia and anginal episodes. *J Am Coll Cardiol* 1999; **33**(7): 1833–1840.

50. Loh PH, Cleland JG, Louis AA, *et al.* Enhanced external counterpulsation in the treatment of chronic refractory angina: a long-term follow-up outcome from the International Enhanced External Counterpulsation Patient Registry. *Clin Cardiol* 2008; **31**(4): 159–164.

51. Davies MJ. The pathophysiology of acute coronary syndromes. *Heart* 2000; **83**: 361–366.

52. Curran N, Brandner B. Chest pain following trauma. *Trauma* 2005; **7**(3): 123–131.

53. Bar-El Y, Gilboa B, Unger N, Pud D, Eisenberg E. Skeletonized versus pedicled internal mammary artery: impact of surgical technique on post CABG surgery pain. *Eur J Cardiothorac Surg* 2005; **27**(6): 1065–1069.

54. Meyerson J, Thelin S, Gordh T, Karlsten R. The incidence of chronic post-sternotomy pain after cardiac surgery – a prospective study. *Acta Anaesthesiol Scand* 2001; **45**(8): 940–944.

55. Pluijms WA, Steegers MA, Verhagen AF, Scheffer GJ, Wilder-Smith OH. Chronic post-thoracotomy pain: a retrospective study. *Acta Anaesthesiol Scand* 2006; **50**(7): 804–808.

56. Macdonald L, Bruce J, Scott NW, Smith WC, Chambers WA. Long-term follow-up of breast cancer survivors with post-mastectomy pain syndrome. *Br J Cancer* 2005; **92**(2): 225–230.

PART 3

Cancer pain

CHAPTER 24

Oncologic therapy in cancer pain

Rita Janes and Tiina Saarto

Department of Oncology, Helsinki University Hospital, Helsinki, Finland

Background

Cancer pain becomes more frequent as the malignancy progresses, with one-third reporting pain at the time of diagnosis and 60–80% of patients with advanced cancer. Tumor growth and metastasis can cause pain in any organ but no single site is predestined to be painful. The skeleton is the most common site of cancer pain because several of the most prevalent malignancies, i.e. breast, prostate and lung cancer, have a propensity for bone secondaries and more than half of those who have skeletal disease experience bone pain. Mechanisms by which cancer causes pain include tissue damage and inflammation, nerve compression and infiltration, increased intracranial pressure, obstruction of hollow organs and distension of capsules surrounding internal organs such as the liver and spleen.

Analgesics are the mainstay for treating cancer pain. Specific cancer therapies including surgery, cancer medicine and radiotherapy rarely relieve pain quickly enough to render the use of analgesics needless. Oncologic treatments alleviate cancer pain mainly by removing or downsizing pain-causing tumors. The anti-inflammatory effect of some treatment modalities such as corticosteroids, radiotherapy and bisphosphonates is also of significance in relieving cancer-related pain. Radiotherapy is the single most effective oncologic treatment of cancer pain. In the treatment of bone metastases, the pain-relieving efficacy of both external radiotherapy and systemic radionuclide

Evidence-Based Chronic Pain Management. Edited by
C. Stannard, E. Kalso and J. Ballantyne. © 2010 Blackwell
Publishing.

therapy is well documented. Radiotherapy is effective also in treating pain caused by soft tissue tumors. The pain-relieving effect of bisphosphonates in the treatment of bone metastases is relatively low, but they are used to slow down progression of bone metastases and prevent skeletal complications including pain, hypercalcemia, fractures and spinal cord compression.

In this chapter we will focus on evidence for the use of radiotherapy, radionuclides and bisphosphonates in treating malignant bone pain and that of radiotherapy in the treatment of pain caused by soft tissue tumors.

Epidemiology

Cancer pain affects the majority of patients with advanced cancer. At the time of diagnosis one in three patients report cancer-related pain whereas 74% (53–100%) of those with advanced malignancy have cancer pain [1]. Pain syndromes were assessed in a prospective study of 2266 cancer patients; 30% presented with one, 39% with two and 31% with three or more distinct pain syndromes. The majority of patients had pain caused by cancer (85%) or antineoplastic treatment (17%) and 9% had pain not related to cancer. Pain could be classified as originating from nociceptors in the bone (35%), soft tissue (45%) or visceral structures (33%) or otherwise of neuropathic origin (34%). In most patients, pain syndromes were located in the lower back (36%), abdominal region (27%), thoracic region (23%), lower limbs (21%), head (17%) and pelvic region (15%) [2].

Bone is the third most common metastatic site after the lung and liver [3]. Several of the most prevalent malignancies, i.e. breast, prostate and lung cancer, have a propensity for bone [3]. More than two-thirds of patients with metastatic breast or prostate cancer and 30–50% of those with lung cancer will develop metastatic bone disease. Skeletal metastases are often present also in thyroid and renal cancer and multiple myeloma. The median survival after the appearance of bone metastases varies between 2 and 4 years for patients with cancer arising from the breast, prostate or thyroid and those with multiple myeloma, while the prognosis for lung and renal cancer is shorter, less than a year. Five to 40% are alive at 5 years depending on the tumor histology and tumor burden [4]. Approximately 65–75% of patients with bone secondaries suffer from bone pain [5].

The incidence of pain arising from nonosseous metastases is also high, though less well documented [6]. Among soft tissue tumors, the prevalence of pain in lung cancer is best recorded. Approximately 60% (25–62%) of patients with locally advanced inoperable primary lung cancer suffer from chest pain; almost one half have moderate to severe pain [7]. Anecdotally, in one series 84% of pancreatic cancer patients with inoperable disease suffered from pain [8].

Current understanding of relevant pathophysiology

Cancer pain is caused by various mechanisms including tissue damage and inflammation, nerve compression and infiltration, increased intracranial pressure, obstruction of hollow organs and distension of capsules surrounding internal organs such as the liver and spleen. Pain caused by tissue damage, i.e. (somatic or visceral) nociceptive pain, is the most common type of cancer pain. Pure neuropathic pain is less common, even though neuropathy as a part of the pain is seen in every third cancer patient suffering from pain. This chapter focuses on the pathophysiology of bone pain.

Skeletal metastases are one of the most common causes of cancer pain [3]. Bone pain is often a dull continuous ache that increases in intensity with time. In addition, many patients suffer from incident pain i.e. pain exacerbated by pressure or movement, which may be difficult to control with analgesics alone due to the quick changes in the level of pain from one moment to another along the course of a day. This leads to impaired mobility.

Bone metastases are either osteolytic, i.e. there is increased osteoclast activity and bone resorption, or osteosclerotic, i.e. osteoblast activity and bone formation are increased. In multiple myeloma, bone lesions are osteolytic whereas osteosclerotic metastases predominate in prostate cancer. Patients with other cancers usually present with mixed bone lesions. Bone secondaries are seldom solitary, with the exception of renal cancer. More than 80% of bone metastases are found in the axial skeleton [6]. The most commonly affected areas are the spine, pelvis, ribs, proximal thigh, upper arm bone and skull [3, 4]. As metastatic bone destruction progresses, the risk of pathologic fracture increases. Eight to 30% of patients with skeletal metastases suffer from pathologic fractures [4, 5]. The underlying malignancy is most often multiple myeloma or breast cancer because of the osteolytic nature of the metastases and the relatively long prognoses [6]. Affected areas include the ribs, pelvis, long bones and vertebrae. Spinal cord compression occurs in 5–10% of patients with skeletal disease and may cause severe neuropathic pain [3–5, 9].

The pathophysiologic mechanism of pain in patients with bone metastases not associated with fracture or spinal cord compression is poorly understood. Not all bone metastases are painful. About two-thirds of demonstrated sites of bone metastases are painless and every sixth to every third of patients with bone metastases do not suffer from pain [5, 9]. The presence of pain does not correlate with the type of tumor, location, number or size of metastases [9]. It is poorly understood why pain patterns vary between patients and even within a patient. Various factors contribute in causing bone pain: mechanical stress of the weakened bone, direct destruction of the bone, microfractures, periosteal distension, nerve entrapment and tumor pressure on adjacent tissues. The mechanisms underlying bone cancer pain also involve changes in osteoclastic activity leading to increased bone resorption, and inflammatory activity provoked by cytokine and prostaglandin production by the cancer cells [10]. Thus bone cancer pain appears to be driven simultaneously by different mechanisms including tumorigenic, inflammatory and neuropathic mechanisms. The healthy bone is constantly undergoing a complex process of remodeling characterized by two opposing actions: the resorption of old bone by osteoclasts and the formation of new bone by osteoblasts. When healthy, there is a steady-state balance or "coupling" of osteoclastic bone resorption and osteoblastic bone formation. This balance is lost when tumor cells enter the bone microenvironment. The tumor induces excessive osteoclast bone resorption. In lytic bone metastases, increased osteoclast activity and bone resorption decrease bone density and disrupt the skeletal architecture, either at focal sites or generally throughout the skeleton.

Actively resorbing bone releases a number of bone-derived growth factors and cytokines, e.g. prostaglandins, bradykinin, substance P, cytokines (e.g. interleukin (IL)-1, IL-6 and tumor necrosis factor (TNF)), which attract circulating cancer cells to the bone surface and facilitate the tumor cells' growth and proliferation [9, 11]. Also sensory neurons are excited and/or sensitized by these growth factors. Malignant cells secrete prostaglandins, cytokines and growth factors, which increase inflammatory activity and may also directly excite primary afferent nociceptors located in bone [9, 11]. This vicious cycle causing multidirectional interactions between tumor cells, bone cells and nociceptors leads to increased tumor growth, osteolysis and pain.

Radiotherapy

Radiotherapy uses high-energy X-rays, γ rays or electrons to deliver ionizing radiotherapy. Ionizing radiation causes DNA damage, leading to cell death. While tumor cell death is responsible for shrinkage of the tumor and thus improvement of pain, the precise mechanism of action by which radiation results in pain relief remains uncertain. Tumor cell kill and shrinking of the tumor bulk in bone promote bone healing by enabling osteoblastic repair and restored integrity of the damaged bone. There is evidence of degeneration and necrosis of cancer cells followed by replacement with proliferative fibrous tissue, which then aggregates and becomes calcified, filling in an osteolytic lesion [12]. This is evident on a plain X-ray where recalcification of osteolytic lesions is seen in 65–85% of treated sites [13]. However, it takes several months for osteolytic bone lesions to heal whereas the pain-relieving effect is usually seen within a few weeks and in some cases within a few days [11]. The rapid onset of pain relief cannot be explained by the tumor cell kill and shrinking of the tumor mass alone [11]. The perceived absence of a dose response relationship also suggests that downsizing of the tumor may not

be the most important mechanism. Significant tumor shrinkage would not be expected when using the relatively low total doses (e.g. 4 Gy) which have been shown to relieve bone pain. Further evidence comes from the absence of a clear relationship between radiosensitivity of the primary tumor and the analgesic effect [9, 11]. Mechanisms which explain the rapid pain response may include the inhibitory effect radiotherapy has on osteoclast activity and other relevant host cells such as macrophages, resulting in down-regulation of the release of chemical mediators of the inflammatory response [6, 9].

External beam radiotherapy using linear accelerators or cobalt machines is the most common way to deliver radiotherapy either, as in most cases, to a local field or, when treating painful disseminated bone metastases, to a wide field. Bone-seeking radioisotopes, samarium-153 and strontium-89, are used to treat disseminated symptomatic bone disease. Several clinical trials have shown that external beam radiotherapy and systemic radionuclide therapy are effective in treating painful bone metastases. There are only a limited number of studies that address the question of how efficient radiotherapy is in relieving pain caused by soft tissue tumors.

Local field radiotherapy in the treatment of bone metastases

Radiation therapy alleviates metastatic bone pain efficiently in the majority of patients. It is particularly useful in treating metastatic bone pain that is not controlled with adequate pain medication and is often of particular help in controlling pain exacerbated by pressure or movement.

In two large controlled studies, complete or partial pain relief was obtained in 30–60% and 70–80% of patients, respectively. The onset of pain relief varied from a few days to 4 weeks and the duration of pain relief between 3 and 6 months [14, 15]. In the Bone Pain Trial Working Party prospective randomized trial, 765 patients with painful skeletal metastases requiring palliative radiotherapy were entered into a study comparing 8 Gy single fraction with a multi-fraction regimen of 20 Gy in five fractions or 30 Gy in 10 fractions. At baseline 29% of patients had mild pain, 44% moderate and 23% severe pain. There were no differences in pain relief: 78% of patients both in the single fraction and multifraction schedules obtained at least 50% pain reduction, and 57% and 58% had a complete response. There were no differences in the time to first improvement in pain, time to complete pain relief or time to first increase in pain at any time up to 12 months from randomization, nor in the class of analgesics used. Retreatment was twice as common after a single fraction compared with multifraction therapy. There were no significant differences in the incidence of nausea, vomiting, spinal cord compression or pathologic fracture between the two groups. Overall survival at 12 months was 44% [15].

A Dutch study randomized 1171 patients to receive either a single 8 Gy fraction (n = 585) or 24 Gy in six fractions (n = 586). The primary tumor was in the breast in 39% of the patients, prostate 23%, lung 25% and other locations 13%. Bone metastases were located in the spine (30%), pelvis (36%), femur (10%), ribs (8%), humerus (6%) and other sites (10%). The main endpoint was pain measured on a pain scale from 0 (no pain at all) to 10 (worst imaginable pain). Median survival was 7 months. Response was defined as a decrease of at least two points compared to the initial pain score. The difference in response between the two treatment groups proved not significant. Overall, 71% experienced a response at some time during the first year. With regard to pain medication, quality of life and side effects, no differences between the two treatment groups were found. The total number of retreatments was 188 (16%), with 147 (25%) in the single fraction and 41 (7%) in the multi-fraction group. It was shown that the level of pain was an important reason for retreatment. There were also indications that doctors were more willing to re-treat patients in the single fraction group because time to retreatment was substantially shorter in this group and the preceding pain score was lower. Unexpectedly, more pathologic fractures were observed in the single fraction group, but the absolute percentage was low. In a cost analysis, the costs of the 24 Gy in six fractions and the 8 Gy single fraction treatment schedules were calculated at 2305 and 1734 euros respectively. Including the costs of retreatment reduced this 25% cost difference to only 8%. The saving of radiotherapy capacity, however, was considered a major economic advantage of the single dose schedule [14].

In a Cochrane analysis, radiotherapy produced complete pain relief at 1 month in 395/1580 (25%) patients, and at least 50% relief in 788/1933 (41%)

patients at some time during the trials. There were no differences in the proportions of patients achieving these outcomes between single or multiple fraction schedules. The number needed to treat (NNT) to achieve complete relief at 1 month was 4.2 (95% confidence interval (CI) 3.7–4.7). No pooled estimates of speed of onset of relief, or of its duration, could be obtained. In the largest trial (759 patients) 52% of those who had complete relief had achieved it within 4 weeks, and the median duration of complete relief was 12 weeks. Adverse effect reporting was poor. There were no obvious differences between the various fractionation schedules in the incidence of nausea and vomiting, diarrhea or pathologic fractures. The authors concluded that radiotherapy is clearly effective at reducing pain from painful bone metastases. There was no evidence of any difference in efficacy between different fractionation schedules, nor indeed of a dose response with total dose of radiation [16].

Another 949 patients with breast or prostate cancer and moderate to severe pain in 1–3 locations were entered into a randomized phase III study that compared 8 Gy single fraction with 30 Gy 10 fraction schedule. Median survival was 9 months. No differences were seen in total or partial pain relief (15% versus 18% and 50% versus 48%, respectively). Acute grade II–IV toxicity was more common among the patients receiving 30 Gy (17% versus 10%); late toxicity was rare in both arms (4%). The incidence of subsequent pathologic fracture was 5% for the 8 Gy arm and 4% for the 30 Gy arm. The retreatment rate was statistically significantly higher in the 8 Gy arm (18%) than in the 30 Gy arm (9%) (P < 0.001) [17].

The efficiency of reirradiation for painful bone metastases

Two groups have reported on reirradiation as part of the treatment of painful bone metastases. Jeremic *et al.* investigated the effectiveness of 4 Gy single fraction given for retreatment after previous single fraction radiotherapy and arrived at the conclusion that the single fraction was effective and well tolerated. Of the 135 patients retreated, 109 patients were treated because of pain relapsing after 4 Gy (group I, n = 34), 6 Gy (group II, n = 39) or 8 Gy (group III, n = 36), while 26 patients were reirradiated after initial nonresponse (group I, n = 12; group II, n = 8; group III, n = 6). Of the 109 patients reirradiated for pain relapse, 74% responded and 31% had complete response. Patients with previous complete response were more likely to achieve complete response. It is worth noting that among the 26 patients who initially did not respond, there were 12 (46%) responses. There were no differences between the three initial treatment groups regarding the efficiency of second radiotherapy. Toxicity was low and only gastrointestinal [18].

The Dutch Bone Metastasis Study mentioned above studied the effect of 8 Gy single fraction versus 24 Gy in six fractions on painful bone metastases [14]. In this study, 24% of patients received retreatment after single fraction versus 6% after multiple fractions (P < 0.001). A new study evaluated factors influencing retreatment and its effect on response. Of the 137 patients who had received a single fraction and were retreated, 33% were given 8 Gy single fraction and 67% 24/4 Gy. The 36 patients having first had multiple fraction therapy received single fraction 8 Gy in 75% of cases and multiple fraction therapy 24/4 Gy in 25%. Among the randomized 1171 patients, the response to initial treatment was 71% after single and 73% after multiple fraction radiotherapy (P = 0.84). Retreatment raised response to 75% for single fraction; multiple fraction remained unaltered (P = 0.54). The response status after initial treatment did not predict occurrence of retreatment: 35% single fraction versus 8% multiple fraction nonresponders and 22% single fraction versus 10% multiple fraction patients with progressive pain were retreated. Logistic regression analyses showed the randomization arm and the pain score before retreatment to significantly predict retreatment (P < 0.001), i.e. intensive pain and single fraction treatment predicted retreatment. Retreatment for nonresponders was successful in 66% after single fraction versus 33% after multiple fractions (P = 0.13); retreatment for progression was successful in 70% after single fraction versus 57% after multiple fractions (P = 0.24). Overall, retreatment was effective in 63%. Irrespective of response to initial treatment, physicians were more willing to retreat after a single fraction [19].

Radiotherapy in the treatment of neuropathic pain due to bone metastases

There are very few data on radiotherapy for bone metastases causing pain with a neuropathic component. The Trans-Tasman Radiation Oncology Group undertook a randomized trial comparing the efficacy of a single 8 Gy fraction with 20 Gy in five fractions for this type of pain. Two hundred and seventy two patients from 15 centers were randomized. Eligible patients had radiologic evidence of bone metastases from a known malignancy, no other metastases along the distribution of the neuropathic pain and no clinical or radiologic evidence of cord/cauda equina compression. Primary endpoints were pain response within 2 months of commencement of radiotherapy and time to treatment failure (TTF).

The most common primary cancers were lung (31%), prostate (29%) and breast (8%); index sites were spine (89%), rib (9%), other (2%). The median overall survival was 4.8 months. The intention-to-treat overall response rates (95% CI) for 8 Gy single fraction versus 20 Gy in five fractions were 53% (45–62%) versus 61% (53–70%) (P = 0.18). Corresponding figures for complete response were 26% (18–34%) versus 27% (19–35%) (P = 0.89). The estimated median TTF (95% CI) were 2.4 mo (2.0–3.3 mo) versus 3.7 mo (3.1–5.9 mo) respectively. The hazard ratio (95% CI) for the comparison of TTF curves was 1.35 (0.99–1.85), log-rank P = 0.056. There were no statistically significant differences in the rates of retreatment, cord compression or pathologic fracture by arm [20].

Wide-field radiotherapy and systemic radionuclide therapy in the treatment of disseminated painful bone metastases

Wide-field radiotherapy and radio-isotopes are used to alleviate pain caused by widespread painful skeletal metastases. They may also be administered with prophylactic intent to reduce the number of new symptomatic sites.

Wide-field radiotherapy

Scattered painful skeletal lesions may be treated with single fraction and fractionated wide-field or half-body irradiation to the upper, lower or mid-body, depending on the extent of metastases and symptoms. A single fraction of 6 Gy is given to the upper half-body field in order to avoid pulmonary toxicity and 8 Gy to the lower half-body field. Half-body irradiation relieves pain as effectively as local external radiotherapy. Response rates up to 73% have been reported with 20% of patients reporting complete pain relief. Because half-body irradiation is usually given to patients with far advanced disease, more than half stay free from pain. Half of those who respond obtain pain relief within 48 hours and 80% within a week [21].

Half-body irradiation has also been administered with prophylactic intent. When compared to local external radiotherapy, there is significantly less need for radiotherapy to new painful sites following half-body irradiation [22, 23].

The side-effects caused by large single fractions include nausea, vomiting, diarrhea, fever, transient increase in bone pain, hematologic toxicity and, rarely, pneumonitis [21]. Patients are usually admitted to hospital for intravenous hydration and premedication consisting of antiemetics and corticosteroids. These side effects may be especially taxing for patients with poor performance status. An interval of at least 4 weeks is recommended before administering the other half-body treatment or continuing chemotherapy to avoid severe hematologic toxicity.

Salazar et al. continued to explore fractionated half-body irradiation to determine whether it was more efficient and less toxic compared to a single dose. They concluded that fractionating half-body irradiation eliminated the need for extensive premedication and patient monitoring required for single fraction [24].

A phase III trial for widespread symptomatic bone cancer from various primaries was carried out in 156 patients to find the fastest and most efficient method of delivery fractionated half-body irradiation. There were three half-body (HBI) arms: (A) 15 Gy/5 fractions/5 days; (B) hyperfractionation 8 Gy/2 fractions/1 day; (C) accelerated hyperfractionation 12 Gy/4 fractions/2 days. Pain relief was seen in 91% of patients (45% complete response and 46% partial response) within 3–8 days. Sixty three percent of patients in arm A obtained complete pain response, compared to 43% and 32% in arms C and B, which was significant between arms A and B (P = 0.016). Pain-free survival was 174 (A), 150 (B), and 122 (C) days. Toxicity was acceptable (41% none, 50% mild/moderate, 12% severe but transitory); more was seen with upper HBI [25]. The authors concluded that, for most primary tumor types (except prostate), delivering two HBI daily doses of 3 Gy on 2 consecutive days is as effective as delivering a daily dose of 3 Gy for 5 consecutive days. Thus, this is a faster and much more convenient HBI schedule for the palliation of pain in widespread cancer.

Systemic radionuclide therapy

Radionuclides, including strontium-89, samarium-153, rhenium-186 and rhenium-188, combined with bone-seeking agents have been used to deliver ionizing radiation to widespread skeletal metastases. Most clinical experience has been gained using strontium-89 and samarium-153, which are administered intravenously, are localized in sites of active bone turnover, emit short-range β particles, are well tolerated and can be administered on an outpatient basis. Indications include multiple painful bone secondaries that are positive on bone scan from prostate, breast and lung cancer, i.e. primaries with sclerotic or mixed bone secondaries. Finlay et al. concluded in their systematic review that radio-isotopes are effective in providing pain relief with response rates between 40% and 95%. Pain relief starts 1–4 weeks after treatment, continues up to 18 months, and is associated with a reduction in analgesic use in many patients. Thrombocytopenia and neutropenia are the most common toxic effects, but they are generally mild and reversible. Repeat doses are effective in providing pain relief in many patients. The effectiveness of systemic radionuclide therapy may be greater when it is combined with chemotherapeutic agents such as cisplatin [26].

Strontium-89

Finlay et al. identified 38 observational studies reporting on the use of strontium-89 for the management of metastatic bone cancer; of these, 16 studies were prospective and had more than 20 patients and were analyzed. Pain was the main outcome measure but the differing criteria used complicated the analysis of the data, although complete response and lack of response were straightforward to define. The proportion classified as complete responders to strontium-89 ranged from 8% to 77% (mean 32%), and the proportion showing no response ranged from 14% to 52% (mean 25%). Within this range, 44% of patients had some degree of response to strontium-89 treatment, giving a mean overall response of 76%. Delay in the start of response was between 4 days and 28 days, with a response duration up to 15 months. Although a reduction in analgesic use was a major criterion for assessing pain response, quantification of this variable was poorly reported in the studies. In those that did report on this variable, a reduction of between 71% and 81% was observed [26].

Buchali *et al.* carried out a double-blind, randomized controlled trial of 49 patients with skeletal metastases from prostatic carcinoma. Patients were assigned to three injections of 75 MBq (2 mCi) strontium-89 with intervals of 1 month (25 patients) or to saline as placebo. There was no significant difference in pain relief between the two groups, which might reflect the suboptimum treatment regimen with a lower than usual dose per injection of strontium-89 used [27]. Another study randomly assigned 26 patients with hormone-refractory prostate cancer to strontium-89 150 MBq (4 mCi) or to stable strontium as a placebo. This study assessed response to treatment by scoring the patients' general condition, mobility, analgesic intake, and pain analysis. Strontium-89 was substantially more effective than placebo, both in patients receiving a single dose (P = 0.01) and in patients allocated to repeated doses (P = 0.03). Complete responses were observed only in patients receiving radio-active strontium. The absolute risk reduction for patients achieving pain relief with strontium-89 was 0.321 (95% CI −0.035 to 0.678) [28].

The combination of external beam radiotherapy and radio-isotopes has been studied. In a double-blind, controlled, randomized trial in Canada, 126 patients with hormone-refractory prostate cancer received local-field radiotherapy and were randomly assigned to strontium-89 or saline placebo. Strontium-89 was given as a single injection of 399.6 MBq (10.8 mCi), 2.5 times that approved by the US Food and Drug Administration. There was a significant reduction in analgesic use at 3 months in patients assigned to strontium-89, and significantly fewer new active sites were recorded. As could be expected, the groups did not differ in pain reduction at the index site [29]. A second placebo-controlled, randomized trial reported contrasting results. This study assessed the effectiveness of concurrent strontium-89 150 MBq (4 mCi) or saline placebo with palliative external radiotherapy in 95 patients with skeletal metastases from various primaries. The endpoint was physician-assessed response at 3 months, which took into consideration the pain score, dose of analgesics, performance status and additional pain treatment. At 3 and 6 months, no differences between treatment arms were observed. The pretreatment use of opiates was independently associated with short progression-free survival, i.e. patients need to be treated before the skeletal disease is too far progressed [30].

A third randomized study, performed by the European Organization for Research and Treatment of Cancer Genitourinary Group, compared strontium-89 150 MBq (4 mCi) with palliative local-field radiotherapy in 203 patients with hormone-refractory prostate cancer and found no difference in subjective response (pain score, dose of analgesics, performance status) [31].

Quilty *et al.* compared the effect of strontium-89 200 MBq (5.4 mCi) local-field or half-body radiotherapy. Two hundred and eighty four patients with prostate cancer and painful bone secondaries were first stratified according to suitability for local or half-body radiotherapy, then randomly allocated that form of treatment or strontium-89. After 4, 8 and 12 weeks pain sites were mapped, toxicity monitored, and all additional palliative treatments recorded. All treatments provided effective pain relief at the index sites; improvement was sustained to 3 months in 63.6% after half-body radiotherapy compared with 66.1% after strontium-89, and in 61% after local radiotherapy compared with 65.9% in the comparable strontium-89 group. Fewer patients reported new pain sites after strontium-89 than after only external radiotherapy local or half-body radiotherapy (P < 0.05). Radiotherapy to a new site was required by 12 patients in the local radiotherapy group compared with two after strontium-89 (P< 0.01); there was no significant difference between half-body radiotherapy (six patients) and strontium-89 (nine patients) in this respect. Platelets and leukocytes fell by an average 30–40% after strontium-89 but sequelae were uncommon, and other symptoms rare [23]. Dearnaley *et al.* compared retrospectively the pain response of 27 prostate cancer patients receiving half-body irradiation with 51 patients receiving strontium-89 and found no difference. Performance status and extent of disease on bone scan were of over-riding importance in determining outcome [32].

The outcome data presented by these studies for strontium-89 are conflicting, although they generally imply similar subjective response rates to external radiotherapy. Variation in the definition of efficacy criteria and the differences in the populations of patients recruited could contribute to the inconsistencies reported.

There have been efforts to improve pain response and possibly survival by adding chemotherapy to strontium-89. Sciuto *et al.* assessed the efficacy of strontium-89 with or without low-dose cisplatin in 70 patients with hormone-refractory prostate cancer in a prospective, randomized controlled trial. The proportion of patients reporting pain relief and the duration of response were significantly higher with combined treatment. Overall pain relief occurred in 91% of patients in the combined arm versus 63% (P < 0.01) with the median duration of 120 days versus 60 [33].

Samarium-153

Resche et al. assessed the therapeutic efficacy of two doses of samarium-153 in alleviating metastatic bone pain from cancers of the prostate (n = 67), breast (n = 36), lung (n = 2), and other primaries (n = 9). Fifty five were randomly assigned to a single dose of 18.5 MBq/kg (0.5 mCi/kg) and 59 patients to 37 MBq/kg (1.0 mCi/kg). Treatment produced improvement from baseline in all patient-rated efficacy assessments, including degree of pain, level of daytime discomfort, quality of sleep and pain relief. During the first 4 weeks after dose administration, when the patients evaluated efficacy daily, there were statistically significant changes from baseline with the 1.0 mCi/kg dose but not with the 0.5 mCi/kg dose. The difference between doses in visual analog pain scores was statistically significant at week 4 (P = 0.0476). Values for platelets and white blood cells reached nadirs at 3 or 4 weeks with both doses and recovered by 8 weeks. Even at their lowest point, the values were generally higher than those associated with infectious or hemorrhagic complications [34].

Serafini et al. assessed the efficacy of two doses of samarium-153 versus placebo; 118 patients with painful metastases secondary to prostate, breast or lung cancers were randomly assigned to 18.5 MBq/kg (0.5 mCi/kg), 37 MBq/kg (1.0 mCi/kg) or placebo. Pain intensity was assessed by patients and clinicians. An improvement in pain relief was reported for both doses compared with the placebo group, but the improvement was significantly greater in the 37 MBq/kg group than in the 18.5 MBq/kg group at 4 weeks (67% versus 42%, absolute risk reduction 0.256; 95% CI 0.043–0.47). Persistence of pain relief was seen through week 16 in 43% of patients receiving the higher dose. Pain relief was observed within 1 week in the majority of patients who responded. Analgesic consumption progressively rose in the placebo group compared with the prestudy rate, whereas there was a reduction in both active treatment groups over 4 weeks after treatment. Mild, transient myelosuppression was the only side effect [35].

Sartor et al. enrolled 152 men with hormone-refractory prostate cancer and painful bone secondaries into a prospective, randomized, double-blind trial comparing radioactive samarium-153 with nonradioactive samarium. Patients were randomized (2:1) to the radioactive agent. Patients' diaries were used to record analgesic use and metastatic bone pain, which was assessed with a visual analog scale and a pain descriptor scale. Nonresponders were informed of the treatment received after 4 weeks of treatment and, if initially treated with placebo, were allowed to receive samarium-153 in an open-label fashion. Pain was measured using validated patient-derived visual analog scales and pain descriptor scales. At 3–4 weeks, analgesic consumption significantly decreased in patients assigned to active samarium compared with those assigned placebo (P = < 0.05). Furthermore, both the visual analog scale and the pain descriptor scale showed significant improvements in the treatment group at 2–4 weeks, which correlated with the reduction in analgesic use (P = 0.0004). The absolute risk reduction for complete responders at 4 weeks was 0.29 (95% CI 0.08–0.36). Because nonresponders were unblinded at week 4, statistical comparisons between the arms beyond week 4 were not possible. Mild and transient myelosuppression was the only clinically important toxic effect associated with active samarium [36].

The different radionuclides have been compared to each other and no significant differences have been found. Liepe et al. investigated samarium-153, strontium-83, rhenium-186 and rhenium-188 to determine their efficacy and toxicity in pain palliation of bone metastases. Seventy nine patients (18 with breast and 61 with prostate cancer) were treated (31 patients with rhenium-188, 15 each with rhenium-186 and samarium-153, and 18 with strontium-83). All patients were interviewed using standardized sets of questions before and after therapy weekly for 12 weeks. Blood counts were taken weekly for 6 weeks and after 12 weeks. In total, 73% of patients reported pain relief (77% after rhenium-188, 67% after rhenium-186, 73% after samarium-153, and 72% after strontium-83). Fifteen percent of patients could discontinue their analgesics and were pain free. Pain showed a decrease from 3.6+/−1.7 to a maximum of 2.2+/−1.8 at visual analog scale in 10 steps (P < 0.01). There were no significant differences in the inducement of flare symptoms or marrow toxicity [37].

Radiotherapy in the treatment of pain caused by soft tissue tumors

Radiotherapy effectively relieves not only pain secondary to bone metastases, but also pain arising from soft tissue tumors. Among soft tissue tumors, palliative radiotherapy for inoperable lung cancer is best documented. Approximately 60% (25–62%) of patients with locally advanced inoperable primary lung cancer suffer from chest pain; almost one half have moderate to severe pain [7]. The other typical local symptoms of inoperable lung cancer are dyspnea in 80–90% (13–90%), cough in 80–90% (24–95%), and hemoptysis in every third patient (13–47%). Radiotherapy alleviates local symptoms in two-thirds (48–94%) of patients. Complete symptom relief is seen in every third patient. Hemoptysis is alleviated in most of the patients (72–97%), chest pain in two-thirds (44–88%), and dyspnea (46–72%) and cough (38–82%) approximately in every second patient. The duration of symptom control lasts approximately 2–3 months [7, 38–44].

Palliative radiotherapy is widely used also in the alleviation of pain from other soft tissue tumors. Whereas the clinical impression is that radiotherapy is effective in reducing pain caused by soft tissue tumors from various primaries, adequate studies are lacking.

Side effects of external beam radiotherapy and radio-isotopes

Palliative radiotherapy for bone pain and pain-causing soft tissue tumors is relatively well tolerated. Side effects are related to total dose, fraction size and the size of the irradiated field. Side effects arise both from adjacent healthy tissues and the tumor. In the latter case, a flare of previous symptoms may occur and dying tumor cells may affect the patient's fluid and electrolyte balance and kidney function. Pelvic irradiation may cause transient nausea and diarrhea resulting from bowel irritation and large pelvic fields may cause myelosuppression; treatment to the cervical or thoracic spine is associated with irritation of the throat and esophagus. Side effects associated with treating nerve compression or brain metastases are increase of pain and associated neurologic symptoms caused by radiotherapy-induced edema; prophylactic corticosteroids are used.

The side effects caused by large single fractions to wide fields such as upper, mid or lower body include nausea, vomiting, diarrhea, fever, transient increase in bone pain, hematologic toxicity and, rarely, pneumonitis [21]. Patients are usually admitted to hospital for intravenous hydration and premedication consisting of antiemetics and corticosteroids. These side effects may be especially taxing for patients with poor performance status. An interval of at least 4 weeks is recommended before administering the other half-body treatment or continuing chemotherapy to avoid severe hematologic toxicity. Toxicity caused by half-body irradiation may be more acceptable with fractionated schedules [25].

Patients close to death should be given adequate medication and good care; they are not candidates for radiotherapy.

Serious late side effects are rarely seen. This is due both to the short prognosis of patients and the low doses used in palliative care. Spinal cord injury is a dreaded late side effect. The risk of myelopathy is low with conventional fractionation schedules 1.8–2 Gy given to a total dose of 45 Gy [45]. It is less clear how safe higher single fractions are. According to Macbeth et al., the cumulative risk of myelopathy was 0.6% at 1 year and 2.2% at 2 years following two 8.5 Gy fractions administered 1 week apart. A single 8 Gy fraction appears to be safe with regard to myelopathy [46].

Systemic radionuclide therapy is usually well tolerated. Thrombocytopenia and neutropenia are the most common toxic effects, but they are generally mild and reversible. For example, in a cohort of men with prostate cancer treated with samarium-153, white cell counts fell by about 45% and platelet counts fell by 40%, with corresponding nadirs at 3–4 weeks of $3.8 \times 10^9/l$ for the white cell count and $127 \times 10^9/l$ for the platelet count. Normal counts of white cells and platelets were observed by week 8 [36]. Hematologic toxicity should be taken into consideration when treating extensively pre-treated patients, and in patients requiring chemotherapy, because bone marrow capacity may be limited.

Pain flares and complications of metastatic bone disease such as spinal cord compression have not been over-represented. In the work by Sartor mentioned above where active samarium-153 was compared with inactive samarium, pain flares were seen in 6% of patients in both groups. Spinal cord compression occurred at the same frequency in both groups (5.9%) [36].

Bisphosphonates

Mechanism of action

Bisphosphonates are potent inhibitors of osteolysis and bone resorption. They are synthetic analogs of natural pyrophosphates. In contrast to the natural pyrophosphates, bisphosphonates are resistant to breakdown by enzymatic hydrolysis. Bisphosphonates act specifically on bone because of their strong affinity for calcium phosphate. According to their structure, bisphosphonates can be divided into those resembling the natural pyrophosphates, or nonaminobisphosphonates (clodronate and etidronate), and those with a nitrogen-containing side chain, aminobisphosphonates (pamidronate, alendronate, zoledronic acid, risedronate, ibandronate). Bisphosphonates inhibit bone resorption by a variety of mechanisms. When osteoclasts ingest bisphosphonate-containing bone, their cytoskeleton becomes disrupted and the apoptosis of the osteoclasts is activated. The nonaminobisphosphonates act as analogs of adenosine triphosphate (ATP) and inhibit ATP-dependent intracellular enzymes, leading to apoptosis and death of the osteoclasts. The aminobisphosphonates, on the other hand, inhibit enzymes of the mevalonate pathway by disrupting the signaling functions of key regulatory proteins and lead to osteoclast apoptosis. Bisphosphonates also inhibit the development of osteoclasts from monocyte precursors by diminishing the recruitment and activity of osteoclasts. These effects on the osteoclasts lead to a decrease in bone turnover that is secondary to the inhibition of bone resorption [47].

The mechanism by which bisphosphonates alleviate pain is not known. According to preclinical data, they inhibit bone resorption and reduce tumor burden at skeletal sites. Bisphosphonates may have some anti-inflammatory and antinociceptive effects [48, 49]. All these mechanisms might contribute to pain relief.

Bisphosphonates in treatment of metastatic cancer

Bisphosphonates have successfully been used in the treatment of malignant hypercalcemia and skeletal metastases [50–53]. The use of bisphosphonates in addition to systemic treatment of malignant disease (chemotherapy or hormone therapy) reduces the risk of developing skeletal events, i.e. new skeletal lesions, progression of existing bone lesions, hypercalcemia, pain, pathologic fractures, need for palliative radiotherapy or surgery, but no survival benefit has been demonstrated. The strongest evidence for the effectiveness of bisphosphonates is found in breast cancer and multiple myeloma. There is some evidence of their efficacy, especially zoledronic acid, in treatment of advanced prostate cancer and other solid tumors.

Bisphosphonates in treatment of pain secondary to bone metastases

The Cochrane review of bisphosphonates (clodronate, pamidronate and etidronate) for the relief of pain secondary to bone metastases includes 30 randomized controlled trials reported before January 2000 [50]. Of those, five studies were designed with pain relief as a primary endpoint and six studies were placebo controlled. Twenty-five studies were available to address the primary objective of the review, but only eight studies (771 patients from six placebo-controlled and two open-controlled studies) were included in the analyses of "the best pain response within 12 weeks." Number needed to treat (NNT) was 11 (95% CI 6–36) at week 4 and 7 (95% CI 5–12) at week 12. Odds ratio of 2.37 (95% CI 1.61–3.5) for "the best pain response within 12 weeks" was in favor of the bisphosphonate group. In double-blinded studies the NNT was somewhat higher (NNT 8). Four other placebo- or open-controlled studies including 619 patients reported no pain-relieving effect with bisphosphonates, but the data were not in usable form for the review. The other 14 placebo- or open-controlled studies had no data on the proportion of patients with pain relief during the time frame of interest. Average drug reactions were generally mild. The number needed to harm (NNH) was 16 (95% CI 12–27) for adverse drug reactions requiring discontinuation of therapy.

Despite the large number of randomized controlled studies, these conclusions are based on a limited number of studies and patients due to methodologic problems in measuring and reporting pain. The reviewers concluded that the evidence suggests that bisphosphonates provide modest pain relief for patients with painful bony metastases [50].

Rosen *et al.* compared zoledronic acid to pamidronate in patients with multiple myeloma and breast cancer [54]. No difference was found between these two bisphosphonates in pain-relieving effect.

Another Cochrane review by Pavlakis *et al.* summarizes the studies of bisphosphonates in breast cancer [51]. The review was updated in 2005. It included 11 studies (seven placebo-controlled and three open studies) that tested the effects of bisphosphonates (compared with placebo or no bisphosphonate) on pain in women with advanced breast cancer and existing bone metastases, using a reference pain scale. In six studies (two placebo-controlled studies of IV pamidronate 90 mg, one placebo-controlled study of IV ibandronate 6 mg, one pooled study of oral ibandronate 50 mg, one oral clodronate 1600 mg, and one open study of oral pamidronate 300 mg), a significant difference was seen in pain in favor of the bisphosphonate group. One study compared zoledronic acid to pamidronate and found no differences between these two bisphosphonates in pain-relieving effect [54]. There were, however, methodologic weaknesses in measuring and reporting the pain-relieving effects.

The Cochrane review of multiple myeloma included 11 trials published before June 2001 [52]. Bisphosphonates statistically significantly ameliorated pain in multiple myeloma. From eight eligible studies (four clodronate, four pamidronate, two etidronate and one ibandronate studies) with a total of 1281 patients, there were 276 out of 657 patients who reported pain on bisphosphonates versus 318 out of 624 controls, 0.59 (95% CI 0.46–0.76, P = 0.00005). The absolute risk reduction was 9% and the NNT to prevent one patient experiencing pain was 11 (95% CI 7–28). However, analysis of the effect of bisphosphonates on pain was based on clinically heterogeneous data and must be interpreted with caution. The benefit was most apparent with clodronate and pamidronate. The review included only one ibandronate study, where ibandronate was given at a dose of 2 mg intravenously, monthly, without any significant pain-relieving effect. However, the dose of ibandronate was suboptimal when compared to the dose used in breast cancer (6 mg intravenously) [55]. No studies of zoledronic acid were available.

In the Rosen study zoledronic acid was compared to pamidronate in patients with multiple myeloma and breast cancer, but myeloma patients have not been reported separately [54].

In the Cochrane review of bisphosphonates in the treatment of skeletal metastatic prostate cancer, no significant pain-relieving effect was seen, even though there was a trend towards it. The review included 1955 patients with skeletal metastatic prostate cancer from 10 controlled trials published up to June 2005. In seven trials pain was the primary endpoint. Clodronate was used in seven trials, pamidronate, etidronate and zoledronic acid in one study each. Pain relief was demonstrated in 27.9% of the patients in the bisphosphonate group and in 21.1% of the controls in 416 patients from three clodronate and one etidronate studies. The odds ratio for pain response was 1.54 (95% CI 0.97–2.44, P = 0.07), showing a trend of improved pain relief in the bisphosphonate group, although this was not statistically significant. Mean pain change was reported in one zoledronic acid study (643 patients) and one pamidronate study (350 patients). The baseline brief pain inventory score was 2.0 (standard deviation (SD) 2.0) in the 4 mg zoledronic acid group, 2.5 (SD 2.1) in the 8/4 mg group and 2.1 (SD 2.0) in the placebo group. The mean changes within 15 months were +0.58 (−0.29 to 0.87), +0.43 (−0.16 to 0.70) and +0.88 (−0.61 to 1.15), respectively. The difference between zoledronic acid 4 mg and placebo was not statistically significant (P = 0.134), while zoledronic acid 8/4 mg was statistically significantly better than placebo (P = 0.026). After combining the two zoledronic acid groups, the mean pain change did not alter during the zoledronic acid therapy −0.04 (SD 0.21), while it increased in the placebo group +0.42 (SD 0.22). No change was seen with pamidronate: the mean pain change decreased by −0.61 (SD 0.17) with pamidronate and −0.44 (SD 0.16) with placebo [53].

In a study of zoledronic acid in the treatment of skeletal metastatic lung cancer and other solid tumors in 773 patients, no significant pain-relieving effect was demonstrated, even though the proportion of skeletal-related events (radiation, surgery, pathologic fracture, spinal cord compression, hypercalcemia of malignancy) was significantly reduced by zoledronic acid [56].

In two open-label pilot studies the analgesic effect of ibandronate loading doses has been studied [57, 58]. Twenty-five hormone-refractory prostate cancer patients participated in an open prospective nonrandomized clinical study. Ibandronate was given 6 mg intravenously on 3 consecutive days at the study entry and 6 mg IV every 4 weeks thereafter [57]. Significant reduction in pain score measured by visual analog scale from 6.5 (5–10) to 2.0 (0–4) was achieved in 23 (92%) patients; nine patients (39%) become completely pain free. Only two patients did not respond. On average, the first analgesic effect was observed at day 3 (1–5). In another study 18 patients were treated with IV ibandronate 4 mg on 4 consecutive days (total dose 16 mg) [58]. Within 7 days there was a significant reduction in bone pain that remained below baseline at 42 days. However, these are preliminary results from open studies and no phase III controlled randomized studies are available.

Dosing and treatment schedules

In clinical phase III studies the onset of the analgesic effect of bisphosphonates has started within 4 weeks and the maximal analgesic effect has been achieved within 8–12 weeks [59–62]. The analgesic effect has been demonstrated with IV pamidronate, oral and IV clodronate, oral and IV ibandronate, and IV zoledronic acid. The best evidence of the pain-relieving effect of pamidronate has been reported with the dose of 90 mg intravenously every 4 weeks. In dose-finding studies of pamidronate, lower doses from 45 to 60 mg have also had some pain-relieving effect, but 90 mg was the most effective dose [50, 51]. The maximum bone-resorbing effect is obtained using oral clodronate at the dose level 1600–3200 mg. The optimal analgesic dose is not known [63]. The corresponding IV doses are either a single dose of 1500 mg or 300 mg on 5 consecutive days [50]. Ibandronate 2 mg intravenously was not effective in the treatment of multiple myeloma whereas 6 mg IV infusion and 50 mg oral ibandronate significantly alleviated pain in breast cancer [59]. Four milligrams of zoledronic acid intravenously is used in clinical practice instead of 8 mg because of renal safety issues. There are only a few direct comparisons between different bisphosphonates. Zoledronic acid has been demonstrated to be as effective as pamidronate [54]. In a small study of 51 patients IV pamidronate 90 mg seemed to alleviate pain more effectively than oral (1600 mg) or intravenous (1500 mg) clodronate [64].

Safety of bisphosphonate treatment

Bisphosphonate therapy is generally well tolerated. According to the Cochrane review on pain relief, the NNH was 16 for adverse drug reactions requiring discontinuation of therapy [50]. Intravenous administration of the aminobisphosphonates can induce transient flu-like symptoms with fever, myalgia and arthralgia. Oral administration of bisphosphonates in turn may be accompanied by gastrointestinal discomfort, nausea, dyspepsia, vomiting, diarrhea and even esophageal ulceration [65]. Some deterioration of renal function is reported in patients treated with bisphosphonates [54, 65, 66]. Forty two patients from a group of 446 who were treated with a total of 3115 zoledronic acid doses experienced renal deterioration [66]. Eight out of 446 patients required discontinuation of zoledronic acid therapy. Predictive factors for the development of renal deterioration were age, diagnosis of myeloma or renal cell carcinoma, cumulative number of doses, concomitant therapy with NSAID and current or prior therapy with cisplatin. Though the renal complications during bisphosphonate therapy are often mild and apparent only as transient increases in serum creatinine, serum electrolyte and creatinine levels should be monitored during bisphosphonate therapy. The probability of acute toxicity due to hypocalcemia is greater with the use of IV aminobisphosphonates and supplementation with calcium and vitamin D is recommended [65].

Osteonecrosis of the jaw is a recently described rare yet severe adverse side effect of bisphosphonates [67, 68]. Patients treated with IV nitrogen-containing bisphosphonates (pamidronate or zoledronic acid) represent 94% of published cases. Of interest, clodronate, a nonaminobisphosphonate, has not been implicated in the development of osteonecrosis. Most patients (85%) have myeloma or breast cancer. The cumulative incidence of osteonecrosis appears to be 1% within the first year, increasing with the prolongation of treatment (3-year cumulative incidence ranging between 4% and 21%), being higher with zoledronic acid than pamidronate treatment. The typical presentation of osteonecrosis is a "nonhealing" extraction socket or exposed jawbone with localized swelling and purulent discharge. The mandible is affected twice as often as the maxilla and 60% of cases are preceded by a dental surgical procedure. The remaining cases occurred spontaneously. Oversuppression of bone turnover is probably the primary mechanism with additional contributing co-morbid factors like dental surgery or poor oral hygiene. The management of this side effect is based on awareness of the problem and its prevention. Dental procedures such as extractions should be kept to a minimum during bisphosphonate treatment and when necessary should prompt temporary interruption of treatment until the lesion is healing satisfactorily.

Conclusion

Analgesics are the cornerstone of cancer pain treatment. Effective systemic oncologic treatment, when available, alleviates cancer pain. Radiotherapy is the single most effective oncologic treatment for cancer pain. Approximately 70% of patients with painful bone secondaries obtain significant pain relief and a complete response is seen in every third patient. Oncologic treatments should be implemented early in the disease before irreversible tissue damage has taken place. Local-field external radiotherapy is the recommended treatment of one to a few painful bony metastases, while systemic radionuclide therapy and wide-field radiotherapy are recommended for patients with multiple painful skeletal metastases.

The latter two may also be administered with prophylactic intent. Single fraction radiotherapy is as effective as multiple fraction therapy in relieving metastatic bone pain. Retreatment following single fraction treatment is needed somewhat more often; retreatment is equally effective. Toxicity caused by wide-field radiation may be more acceptable with fractionated schedules. The onset of pain relief following external radiotherapy varies from a few days to 4 weeks and the duration of pain relief is between 3 and 6 months. The response rate seen following systemic radionuclide therapy is similar to that seen after external beam radiotherapy. Treatment is well tolerated, with the exception of mild myelotoxicity. Systemic radionuclide therapy seem to be more effective in treating osteosclerotic and mixed skeletal metastases. The onset of pain relief takes 2–4 weeks. Radiotherapy is a useful tool in treating pain caused by soft tissue tumors, even though this is less well documented.

Pain relief provided by bisphosphonates is modest at most. The evidence is best documented for myeloma and breast cancer, i.e. in osteolytic or mixed metastases. The pain-relieving evidence for prostate and other solid tumors is insufficient (Table 24.1).

Table 24.1 Bisphosphonates in treatment of pain caused by bony metastases

Tumor type	Reference	Studies	Results	Evidence level
All tumor types	Wong & Wiffen [50]	Cochrane review	NNT 7 (95% CI 5–12)	B
	Rosen et al. [54]	RCT	OR 2.37 (95% CI 1.61–3.5) No significant difference between pamidronate and zoledronic acid	
Multiple myeloma	Djulbegovic et al. [52]	Cochrane review	NNT 11 (95% CI 7–28) OR 0.59 (95% CI 0.46–0.76)	B
Breast cancer	Pavlakis et al. [51]	Cochrane review	Six out of 10 studies demonstrated pain relieving effect of bisphosphonates. No significant difference between pamidronate and zoledronic acid	B
Prostate cancer	Yuen et al. [53]	Cochrane review	OR 1.54 (95% CI 0.97–2.44)	B
	Small et al. [69]	RCT	No significant difference between	
	Saad et.al. [70]	RCT	pamidronate and placebo, or zoledronic acid 4 mg and placebo	
Other solid tumors	Rosen et al. [56]	RCT	No significant difference between zoledronic acid and placebo	C

OR, odds ratio; CI, confidence interval.

Authors' recommendations

- Analgesics are the mainstay in treating cancer pain.
- Determine if effective systemic oncologic treatment is available.
- Radiotherapy is effective for metastatic bone pain (A). External beam radiotherapy is very effective in relieving metastatic bone pain. The overall response rate is approximately 70–80% and the complete response rate is 30–60% (A). Single fraction radiotherapy is as effective as multiple fraction radiotherapy in relieving metastatic bone pain (A). Retreatment is effective (B). Radiotherapy is effective in treating pain caused by soft tissue tumors (C/D).
- Radio-isotopes are effective for metastatic bone pain (A).
- Bisphosphonates provide at best modest pain relief for patients with painful bony metastases (B); this effect is best documented for multiple myeloma and breast cancer (B).
- There is insufficient evidence to support the pain-relieving effect of bisphosphonates in prostate cancer (B)

References

1. Hearn J, Higginsson IJ. Cancer pain epidemiology: a systematic review. In: Bruera ED, Portenoy RK (eds) *Cancer Pain, Assessment and Management*. Cambridge University Press, Cambridge, 2003: 19–37.
2. Grond S, Zech D, Diefenbach C, Radbruch L, Lehmann KA. Assessment of cancer pain: a prospective evaluation in 2266 cancer patients referred to a pain service. *Pain* 1996; **64**(1): 107–114.
3. Tubiana-Hulin M. Incidence, prevalence and distribution of bone metastases. *Bone* 1991; **12**(suppl1): S9–S10.
4. Coleman RE. Skeletal complications of malignancy. *Cancer* 1997; **80** (suppl): 1588–1594.
5. Elte JWF, Bijvoet OLM, Cleton FJ, van Oosterom AT, Sleeboom HP. Osteolytic bone metastases in breast carcinoma pathogenesis, morbidity and bisphosphonate treatment. *Eur J Clin Oncol* 1996; **22**: 493–500.
6. Nielsen OS, Munro AJ, Tannock IF. Bone metastases: pathophysiology and management policy. *J Clin Oncol* 1991; **9**(3): 509–524.
7. Hoopwood P, Stephans RJ. Symptoms at presentation for treatment in patients with lung cancer: implications for the evaluation of palliative treatment. *Br J Cancer* 1995; **71**: 633–636.
8. Singh SM, Longmire WP Jr, Reber HA. Surgical palliation for pancreatic cancer. The UCLA experience. *Ann Surg* 1990; **212**: 132–139.
9. Mercadante S. Malignant bone pain: pathophysiology and treatment. *Pain* 1997; **69**: 1–18.
10. Fulfaro F, Casuccio A, Ticozzi C, Ripamonti C. The role of bisphosphonates in the treatment of painful metastatic bone disease: a review of phase III trials. *Pain* 1998; **78**(3):157–169.
11. Poulsen HS, Nielsen OS, Klee M, Rorth M. Palliative irradiation of bone metastases. *Cancer Treatment Rev* 1989; **16**(1): 41–48.
12. Harrington KD. Impending pathologic fractures from metastatic malignancy: evaluation and management. *Instructional Course Lectures* 1986; **35**: 357–381.
13. Garmatis CJ, Chu FCH. The effectiveness of radiation therapy in the treatment of bone metastases from breast cancer. *Radiology* 1978; **126**: 235–237.
14. Steenland E, Leer JW, van Houwelingen H, *et al*. The effect of a single fraction compared to multiple fractions on painful bone metastases: a global analysis of the Dutch Bone Metastasis Study. *Radiother Oncol* 1999; **52**(2): 101–109.
15. Yarnold JR on behalf of the Bone Pain Trial Working Party. 8 Gy single fraction radiotherapy for the treatment of metastatic skeletal pain: randomised comparison with a multifraction schedule over 12 months of patient follow-up. *Radiother Oncol* 1999; **52**: 111–121.
16. McQuay HJ, Collins S, Carroll D, Moore RA. Radiotherapy for the palliation of painful bone metastases. Cochrane Database of Systematic Reviews 1999, Issue 3. Art. No.: CD001793. DOI: 10.1002/14651858.CD001793.
17. Hartsell WF, Scott CB, Bruner DW, *et al*. Randomized trial of short- versus long-course radiotherapy for palliation of painful bone metastases. *J Natl Cancer Inst* 2005; **97**: 798–804.
18. Jeremic B, Shibamoto Y, Igrutinovic I. Single 4 Gy re-irradiation for painful bone metastasis following single fraction radiotherapy. *Radiother Oncol* 1999; **52**: 123–127.
19. van der Linden YM, Lok JJ, Steenland E, *et al*. Dutch Bone Metastasis Study Group. Single fraction radiotherapy is efficacious: a further analysis of the Dutch Bone Metastasis Study controlling for the influence of re-treatment. *Int J Radiat Oncol Biol Phys* 2004; **59**(2): 528–537.
20. Roos DE, Turner SL, O'Brien PC, *et al*. Randomized trial of 8 Gy in 1 versus 20 Gy in 5 fractions of radiotherapy for neuropathic pain due to bone metastases (Trans-Tasman Radiation Oncology Group, TROG 96.05). *Radiother Oncol* 2005; **75**: 54–63.
21. Salazar OM, Rubin P, Hendrickson FR, *et al*. Single-dose half-body irradiation for palliation of multiple bone metastases from solid tumours. *Cancer* 1986; **58**: 29–36.
22. Poulter CA, Cosmatos DH, Rubin P, *et al*. A report of RTOG 8206: a phase III study of whether the addition of single dose half-body irradiation to standard fractionated local field irradiation is more effective than local field irradiation alone in the treatment of symptomatic osseous metastases. *Int J Radiat Oncol Biol Phys* 1992; **23**: 207–214.
23. Quilty PM, Kirk D, Bolger JJ, *et al*. A comparison of the palliative effects of strontium-89 and external beam radiotherapy in metastatic prostate cancer. *Radiother Oncol* 1994; **31**(1): 33–40.

24. Salazar OM, DaMotta NW, Bridgman SM, Cardiges NM, Slawson RG. Fractionated half-body irradiation for pain palliation in widely metastatic cancers: comparison with single dose. *Int J Radiat Oncol Biol Phys* 1996; **36**(1): 49–60.

25. Salazar OM, Sandhu T, da Motta NW, *et al.* Fractionated half-body irradiation (HBI) for the rapid palliation of widespread, symptomatic, metastatic bone disease: a randomized Phase III trial of the International Atomic Energy Agency (IAEA). *Int J Radiat Oncol Biol Phys* 2001; **50**(3): 765–775.

26. Finlay IG, Mason MD, Shelley M. Radio-isotopes for the palliation of metastatic bone cancer: a systematic review. *Lancet Oncol* 2005; **6**: 392–400.

27. Buchali K, Correns HJ, Schuerer M, Schnorr D, Lips H, Sydow K Results of a double blind study of 89-strontium therapy of skeletal metastases of prostatic carcinoma. *Eur J Nucl Med* 1988; **14**: 349–351.

28. Lewington VJ, McEwan AJ, Ackery DM, *et al.* A prospective, randomised double-blind crossover study to examine the efficacy of strontium-89 in pain palliation in patients with advanced prostate cancer metastatic to bone. *Eur J Cancer* 1991; **27**: 954–958.

29. Porter AT, McEwan JB, Powe JE, *et al.* Results of a randomized phase-III trial to evaluate the efficacy of strontium-89 adjuvant to local field external beam irradiation in the management of endocrine resistant metastatic prostate cancer. *Int J Radiat Oncol Biol Phys* 1993; **25**: 805–813.

30. Smeland S, Erikstein B, Aas M, Skovlund E, Hess SL, Fosså SD. Role of strontium-89 as adjuvant to palliative external beam radiotherapy is questionable: results of a double-blind randomized study. *Int J Radiat Oncol Biol Phys* 2003; **56**(5): 1397–1404.

31. Oosterhof GO, Roberts JT, de Reijke TM, *et al.* Strontium(89) chloride versus palliative local field radiotherapy in patients with hormonal escaped prostate cancer: a phase III study of the European Organisation for Research and Treatment of Cancer, Genitourinary Group. *Eur Urol* 2003; **44**: 519–526.

32. Dearnaley DP, Bayly RJ, A'Hern RP, Gadd J, Zivanovic MM, Lewington VJ. Palliation of bone metastases in prostate cancer. Half-body irradiation or strontium-89? *Clin Oncol* 1992; **4**(2): 101–107.

33. Sciuto R, Festa A, Rea S, *et al.* Effects of low-dose cisplatin on 89Sr therapy for painful bone metastases from prostate cancer: a randomized clinical trial. *J Nucl Med* 2002; **43**: 79–86.

34. Resche I, Chatal JF, Pecking A, *et al.* A dose-controlled study of 153Sm-ethylenediaminetetramethylenephosphonate (EDTMP) in the treatment of patients with painful bone metastases. *Eur J Cancer* 1997; **33**: 1583–1591.

35. Serafini AN, Houston SJ, Resche I, *et al.* Palliation of pain associated with metastatic bone cancer using samarium-153 lexidronam: a double-blind placebo-controlled clinical trial. *J Clin Oncol* 1998; **16**(4): 1574–1581.

36. Sartor O, Reid RH, Hoskin PJ, *et al.* Samarium-153-Lexidronam complex for treatment of painful bone metastases in hormone-refractory prostate cancer. *Urology* 2004; **63**: 940–945.

37. Liepe K, Kotzerke J. A comparative study of 188Re-HEDP, 186Re-HEDP, 153Sm-EDTMP and 89Sr in the treatment of painful skeletal metastases. *Nucl Med Commun* 2007 ;**28**(8): 623–630.

38. Simpson JR, Francis ME, Perez-Tamayo R, Marks RD, Rao DV. Palliative radiotherapy for inoperable carcinoma of the lung: final report of a RTOG multi-institutional trial. *Int J Radiat Oncol Biol Phys* 1985; **11**(4): 751–758.

39. Teo P, Tai TH, Choy D, Tsui KH. A randomized study on palliative radiation therapy for inoperable non small cell carcinoma of the lung. *Int J Radiat Oncol Biol Phys* 1988; **14**(5): 867–871.

40. Anonymous. Inoperable non-small-cell lung cancer (NSCLC): a Medical Research Council randomised trial of palliative radiotherapy with two fractions or ten fractions. Report to the Medical Research Council by its Lung Cancer Working Party. *Br J Cancer* 1991; **63**(2): 265–270.

41. Anonymous. A Medical Research Council (MRC) randomised trial of palliative radiotherapy with two fractions or a single fraction in patients with inoperable non-small-cell lung cancer (NSCLC) and poor performance status. Medical Research Council Lung Cancer Working Party. *Br J Cancer* 1992; **65**(6): 934–941.

42. Macbeth FR, Bolger JJ, Hopwood P, *et al.* Randomized trial of palliative two-fraction versus more intensive 13-fraction radiotherapy for patients with inoperable non-small cell lung cancer and good performance status. Medical Research Council Lung Cancer Working Party. *Clin Oncol* 1996; **8**(3): 167–175.

43. Abratt RP, Shepherd LJ, Salton DG. Palliative radiation for stage 3 non-small cell lung cancer – a prospective study of two moderately high dose regimens. *Lung Cancer* 1995; **13**(2): 137–143.

44. Rees GJ, Devrell CE, Barley VL, Newman HF. Palliative radiotherapy for lung cancer: two versus five fractions. *Clin Oncol* 1997; **9**(2): 90–95.

45. Schultheiss TE, Stephens LC. Permanent radiation myelopathy. *Br J Radiol* 1992; **65**: 737–753.

46. Macbeth FR, Wheldon TE, Girling DJ, *et al.* Estimates of risk in 1048 patients in three randomized trails of palliative radiotherapy for non-small-cell lung cancer. *Clin Oncol* 1996; **8**:176–181.

47. Russell RG, Rogers MJ. Bisphosphonates: from the laboratory to the clinic and back again. *Bone* 1999; **25**(1): 97–106.

48. Bonabello A, Galmozzi MR, Bruzzese T, Zara GP. Analgesic effect of bisphosphonates in mice. *Pain* 2001; **91**(3): 269–275.

49. Walker K, Medhurst SJ, Kidd BL, *et al.* Disease modifying and anti-nociceptive effects of the bisphosphonate, zoledronic acid in a model of bone cancer pain. *Pain* 2002; **100**(3): 219–229.

50. Wong RKS, Wiffen PJ. Bisphosphonates for the relief of pain secondary to bone metastases. Cochrane Database of Systematic Reviews 2002, Issue 2. Art. No.: CD002068. DOI: 10.1002/14651858.CD002068.

51. Pavlakis N, Schmidt RL, Stockler MR. Bisphosphonates for breast cancer. Cochrane Database of Systematic Reviews 2005, Issue 3. Art. No.: CD003474. DOI: 10.1002/14651858. CD003474.pub2.

52. Djulbegovic B, Wheatley K, Ross H, *et al.* Bisphosphonates in multiple myeloma. Cochrane Database of Systematic Reviews 2002, Issue 4. Art. No.: CD003188. DOI: 10.1002/14651858.CD003188.

53. Yuen KY, Shelley M, Sze WM, Wilt T, Mason M. Bisphosphonates for advanced prostate cancer. Cochrane Database of Systematic Reviews 2006, Issue 4. Art. No.: CD006250. DOI: 10.1002/14651858.CD006250.

54. Rosen LS, Gordon D, Kaminski M. Zoledronic acid versus pamidronate in the treatment of skeletal metastases in patients with breast cancer or osteolytic lesions of multiple myeloma: a phase III, double-blind, comparative trial. *Cancer J* 2001; **7**(5): 377–387.

55. Body JJ, Diel I, Lichinitser MR. Intravenous ibandronate reduces the incidence of skeletal complications in patients with breast cancer an bone metastases. *Ann Oncol* 2003; **14**(9): 1399–1405.

56. Rosen LS, Gordon D, Tchekmedyian S, *et al.* Zoledronic acid versus placebo in the treatment of skeletal metastases in patients with lung cancer and other solid tumours: a phase III, double-blind, randomized trial – the Zoledronic Acid Lung Cancer and Other Solid Tumours Study Group. *J Clin Oncol* 2003; **21**(16): 3150–3157.

57. Heidenreich A, Elert A, Hofmann R. Ibandronate in the treatment of prostate cancer associated painful osseous metastases. *Prostate Cancer Prostatic Dis* 2002; **5**(3): 231–235.

58. Mancini I, Dumon JC, Body JJ. Efficacy and safety of ibandronate in the treatment of opioid-resistant bone pain associated with metastatic bone disease: a pilot study. *J Clin Oncol* 2004; **22**(17): 3587–3592.

59. Cameron D, Fallon M, Diel I. Ibandronate: its role in metastatic breast cancer. *Oncologist* 2006; **11**(suppl 1): 27–33.

60. Kohno N, Aogi K, Minami H, *et al.* Zoledronic acid significantly reduces skeletal complications compared with placebo in Japanese women with bone metastases from breast cancer: a randomized, placebo-controlled trial. *J Clin Oncol* 2005; **23**(15): 3314–3321.

61. Hortobagyi GN, Theriault RL, Lipton A. Long-term prevention of skeletal complications of metastatic breast cancer with pamidronate. *J Clin Oncol* 1998; **16**: 2038–2044.

62. McCloskey EV, MacLennan IC, Drayson MT, Chapman C, Dunn J, Kanis JA. A randomized trial of the effect of clodronate on skeletal morbidity in multiple myeloma. MRC Working Party on Leukaemia in Adults. *Br J Haematol* 1998; **100**(2): 317–325.

63. O'Rourke N, McCloskey E, Houghton F, Huss H, Kanis JA. Double-blind, placebo-controlled, dose-response trial of oral clodronate in patients with bone metastases. *J Clin Oncol* 1995; **13**(4): 929–934.

64. Jagdev SP, Purohit P, Heatley S, Herling C, Coleman RE. Comparison of the effects of intravenous pamidronate and oral clodronate on symptoms and bone resorption in patients with metastatic bone disease. *Ann Oncol* 2001; **12**(10): 1433–1438.

65. Conte P, Guarneri V. Safety of intravenous and oral bisphosphonates and compliance with dosing regimens. *Oncologist* 2004; **9**(suppl 4):28–37.

66. McDermott RS, Kloth DD, Wang H, Hudes GR, Langer CJ. Impact of zoledronic acid on renal function in patients with cancer: clinical significance and development of a predictive model. *J Support Oncol* 2006; **4**(10): 524–529.

67. Woo SB, Hellstein JW, Kalmar JR. Narrative [corrected] review: bisphosphonates and osteonecrosis of the jaws. *Ann Intern Med* 2006; **144**(10): 753–761.

68. Migliorati CA, Siegel MA, Elting LS. Bisphosphonate-associated osteonecrosis: a long-term complication of bisphosphonate treatment. *Lancet Oncol* 2006; **7**: 508–514.

69. Small EJ, Smith MR, Seaman JJ, Petrone S, Kowalski MO. Combined analysis of two multicenter, randomized, placebo-controlled studies of pamidronate disodium for the palliation of bone pain in men with metastatic prostate cancer. *J Clin Oncol* 2003 Dec 1; **21**(23): 4277–84. Epub 2003 Oct 27.

70. Saad F, Gleason DM, Murray R, Tchekmedyian S, Venner P, Lacombe L, Chin JL, Vinholes JJ, Goas JA, Chen B; Zoledronic Acid Prostate Cancer Study Group. A randomized, placebo-controlled trial of zoledronic acid in patients with hormone-refractory metastatic prostate carcinoma. *J Natl Cancer Inst* 2002 Oct 2; **94**(19): 1458–68.

CHAPTER 25

Cancer pain: analgesics and co-analgesics

Rae Frances Bell

Pain Clinic/Regional Centre of Excellence in Palliative Care, Haukeland University Hospital, Bergen, Norway

Background

Pathophysiology

Pain due to malignancy may be both acute and chronic. Cancer patients commonly experience several types of pain concurrently. In the majority of cases, one or more types of pain are caused by the cancer [1]. Tumor expansion can cause pressure on surrounding organs, while tumor infiltration into nerve plexi and bone, and damage of nerve tissue can cause neuropathic pain. Metastatic spread of cancer to bone is reported to be one of the most common causes of cancer pain [2]and may cause pain both at rest and on movement. Cancer patients may experience muscular pain due to rapid weight loss and other factors. They are potentially subject to painful adverse effects of treatment, such as joint pain following chemotherapy, painful mucositis, and acute and/or persistent neuropathic pain following radio- or chemotherapy. Cancer patients are often exposed to surgical interventions and experience acute and in some cases chronic postoperative pain [3]. In an international survey addressing cancer pain characteristics, 71.6% of cancer patients with pain were judged to have nociceptive pain, 34.7% nociceptive visceral pain and 39.7% had neuropathic pain [1].

Neuropathic pain

Neuropathic pain is difficult to treat with opioids alone and usually requires adjuvant drugs such

as tricyclic antidepressants (e.g. amitriptyline) or anticonvulsants (e.g. gabapentin or pregabalin). Refractory neuropathic pain requires other measures, such as adjuvant treatment with an NMDA receptor antagonist or anesthesiologic techniques such as spinally administered local anesthetic as an adjuvant to opioid.

Intermittent or breakthrough pain

Breakthrough pain is common in cancer patients, with bone pain, local tumor invasion in soft tissue, and brachial plexopathy most frequently reported [6]. Breakthrough pain usually occurs at the site of the background pain and the duration may vary from minutes to hours [7]. Intense, short-lasting pain episodes and movement-related pain are particularly difficult to treat effectively with analgesics. Normal-release oral opioid or oral transmucosal fentanyl citrate have until recently been the most common pharmacologic treatment options for breakthrough pain. Different formulations/routes of administration of opioids such as the fentanyl buccal tablet [8] or adjuvants such as intranasal ketamine [9] are currently under investigation.

The potential complexity of the cancer patient's pain syndrome (see Table 25.1) underscores the importance of repeated clinical assessment and pain diagnosis, together with an individual treatment plan.

Prevalence, epidemiology and risk factors

Pain is common in patients with cancer. A literature review in patients with lung cancer found that pain affected 27% of outpatients (range 8–85%) and 76%

Evidence-Based Chronic Pain Management. Edited by C. Stannard, E. Kalso and J. Ballantyne. © 2010 Blackwell Publishing.

Table 25.1 Cancer pain. Modified from Bell *et al.* [27]

Examples of pain subtypes	Possible pain mechanisms
Tumor related	Sensitization of peripheral nociceptive primary afferents (tumor factors, e.g. enthothelin and prostaglandins, tumor-induced acidosis, inflammation-associated factors); entrapment and nerve injury; invasion of mechanically sensitive tissues (e.g. visceral pain); central sensitization
Metastatic soft tissue pain	Peripheral sensitization due to inflammation. Hyperalgesia due to central sensitization
Metastatic bone pain	Tumor-induced acidosis; injury or infiltration of sensory neurones that innervate the bone marrow; peripheral sensitization of nociceptors [4]; central sensitization [5] osteolysis, pathologic fracture, microfractures
Inflammatory (e.g. mucositis)	Peripheral sensitization due to inflammation. Hyperalgesia due to central sensitization
Neuropathy	Nervous tissue compression or lesion leading to central sensitization. Degeneration of sensory neurones and sensitization of primary nociceptive afferents due to chemotherapeutic agents and release of cytokines [4]
Muscle pain	Tumor factors; central sensitization; bone metastases causing muscle spasm; muscle hypercatabolism; immobilization leading to muscle atrophy; increased muscular tension
Acute postoperative pain	Acute nociception; peripheral sensitization; nerve damage; (central sensitization)
Chronic postoperative pain	Central sensitization; nerve damage (peripheral sensitization)

of patients cared for by palliative care services (range 63–88%) [10]. Pain was caused by cancer in 73% (range 44–87%) and by treatment in 11% (range 5–17%). The most common type of pain was nociceptive, while neuropathic pain accounted for 30%. A study using data from 1021 patients with advanced lung cancer who were enrolled in three randomized trials of chemotherapy found that 74% of patients reported some pain, with 50% of these stating that pain was affecting daily activities [11].

Interventions supported by evidence (ranked according to evidence level)

Very few interventions in cancer pain are well documented. Even the guidelines for cancer pain treatment lack an evidence base. The current evidence for treatment guidelines and commonly used interventions are discussed below.

World Health Organization pain ladder

The World Health Organization (WHO) three-step ladder for cancer pain relief [12] advises that mild cancer pain should be treated with nonopioid analgesics (paracetamol and/or nonsteroidal anti-inflammatory drugs (NSAIDs)), moderate pain with

the addition of weaker opioids, and strong pain with the substitution of stronger for weaker opioids. The utility of the second step on the ladder has been challenged, with suggestions to replace step two opioids with stronger opioids. Morphine is the "gold standard" opioid for cancer pain.

Although these guidelines are recommended and commonly followed, there is restricted evidence for this practice. A systematic review of studies evaluating the effectiveness of the ladder for cancer pain management included eight uncontrolled case series studies [13]. The conclusion was that the evidence did not permit estimation of the effectiveness of the ladder, and the need for randomized controlled efficacy trials was emphasized. One prospective open-label 10-year study has assessed the course of treatment of 2118 cancer pain patients being treated according to WHO guidelines [14].

NSAIDs and paracetamol

A Cochrane qualitative systematic review published in 2003, with the latest Medline search, concluded that NSAIDs are more effective than placebo for the *short-term* treatment of cancer pain [15]. Forty-two trials with 3084 patients were included. Seven of eight trials that compared NSAIDs with placebo demonstrated that NSAIDs had superior efficacy with no difference in adverse effects. Clear evidence to support superior safety or efficacy of one NSAID was lacking. Only one trial has compared paracetamol to placebo [16]. In this 6-hour cross-over study in 29 evaluable patients, there was no significant difference in effect between paracetamol and placebo. A randomized, placebo-controlled, cross-over trial in patients with advanced cancer already receiving a strong opioid regimen found that pain and overall well-being were better for patients receiving paracetamol than for those receiving placebo [17].

It is important to note that the majority of studies on NSAIDs and paracetamol were of less than 7 days' duration, so that the conclusions cannot be generalized to long-term treatment of cancer pain. There do not appear to be any long-term studies of NSAIDs/paracetamol for cancer pain. It is important to remember that cancer patients are often at high risk of NSAID-related adverse effects. In general, for safety reasons, for daily treatment lasting more than 1–2 weeks, paracetamol is to be preferred. If NSAIDs are used for long-term treatment then the lowest effective dose should be used, and co-treatment with a gastroprotective agent (for example, omeprazole) is recommended.

Opioids

Morphine has been shown to be superior to placebo in patients with noncancer-related neuropathic pain (postherpetic neuralgia (PHN), painful diabetic neuropathy (PDN) and phantom limb pain), while oxycodone has been investigated in relation to PHN and PDN and found to have a similar number needed to treat (NNT) to morphine: 2.5 (95% confidence interval (CI) 1.9–4.1) [18].

However, although oral morphine is the "gold standard" opioid for the treatment of cancer pain, it is surprising how few placebo-controlled trials have been performed. In a methodologic review of trials investigating oral opioids for cancer pain, only one trial had a placebo control, while another trial had a placebo control in the pilot phase of the study [19]. In the first of these trials which investigated the effect of a loading dose of morphine elixir added to the first dose of slow-release morphine tablets, a total of 9 patients were treated with a single dose of placebo, the study duration being 12 hours [20]. In the pilot phase of the second trial, where three different formulations of slow-release morphine were compared

to placebo for 7±1 days, a total of 4 patients received placebo treatment [21]. In the majority of the trials included in this review morphine was used as an active comparator. The assumption for using morphine in this way is that it has previously been found effective in cancer pain compared to placebo. But is this the case?

A Cochrane review concluded that oral morphine is effective for cancer pain [22]. This review attempted to bring all the literature together and included data from randomized trials, including open-label trials. The authors remarked that the majority of trials are equivalence studies designed to show that different formulations of morphine have the same effect, and that this makes it difficult to extract information on the effectiveness of morphine *per se*. Furthermore, they underlined that it is unclear whether the trials are sufficiently powered to detect a clinically meaningful difference between treatments. Although the Oxford Quality Scale scores were generally high, with a median of 4, it was noted that the quality of reporting was disappointing, especially in regard to assessment of pain and pain relief. The trials in this Cochrane review were not scored for validity, and the relevance of a placebo control for the demonstration of efficacy is not specifically addressed.

In a second Cochrane review [23], 11 trials investigating hydromorphone in cancer pain were included, all of which used an active comparator. A recent quantitative systematic review on oxycodone for cancer pain [24] found no placebo-controlled trials. A Cochrane review on methadone for cancer pain identified five randomized, double-blind trials all of which used an active comparator [25]. An Agency for Healthcare Research and Quality (AHRQ) Evidence Report [26] looking at the relative efficacy of analgesics in cancer pain described the need for placebo controls in order to avoid overestimation of treatment effects, at the same time noting that placebo controls in cancer pain trials are "rare." Table 25.2 is a summary of placebo-controlled trials investigating stronger opioids for cancer pain.

Unless there is an as yet unaccessed body of data, these findings raise interesting questions regarding the current efficacy data for oral opioids in cancer pain. Even though opioids appear clinically effective for cancer pain, the question of how effective is not resolved by the literature. Morphine is accepted as the

Table 25.2 Randomized, double-blind trials in cancer pain patients comparing stronger opioid with placebo. Modified from Bell *et al.* [27]

Study	n =	Drug	Route	Duration	Comments
Houde *et al.* [28]	67 (placebo: 28)	Morphine	IM	6 hours	Double-blind
Stambaugh *et al.* [16]	20	Butorphanol (acetaminophen) (B + A)	po	Up to 6 hours	Single dose
Stambaugh *et al.* [29]	30	Meperidine Hydroxyzine M + H	IM	4 days, 1 treatment per day	Single dose
Stambaugh *et al.* [30]	60 (3 groups)	Dezocine Butorphanol	IM	7 days	Double-blind Single and multiple dose study
Stambaugh *et al.* [31]	43 (40 evaluable)	Ciramadol Codeine	po	6 hours	Double-blind Single dose Cross-over
Hoskin *et al.* [20]	20 (19 evaluable) 9 treated with placebo	Morphine	po	12 hours	Double-blind
Broomhead *et al.* [21]	172 (152 final day efficacy data) 4 treated with placebo	Morphine	po	First phase (placebo control): 7 ± 1 days)	Double-blind Placebo control only in first phase of study
Farrar *et al.* [32]	92 (89 assessable, treated with at least one unit of OTFC and one unit of placebo)	Fentanyl citrate (OTFC)	OTM	Titration period ± 10 randomly ordered treatment units (Pain evaluated for 60 minute period)	Double-blind Breakthrough pain

IM, intramuscular; po, oral; OTM, oral transmucosal.
Sources: AHRQ [26], Wiffen *et al.* [22], Quigley [23], Reid [24] and Bell [19]. In addition, searches were performed on PubMed with limits "randomized controlled trial" and search terms "fentanyl AND placebo and cancer" / "methadone AND placebo AND cancer."

gold standard for cancer pain treatment but placebo-controlled efficacy data in cancer pain are lacking.

Opioids for breakthrough pain

A Cochrane review published in 2006 concluded that there is evidence that oral transmucosal fentanyl citrate (OTFC) is an effective treatment in the management of breakthrough pain [33]. Four studies with 393 participants were included. Only one trial compared OTFC to placebo. The literature was small and no trials for other opioids were found. One randomized double-blind, placebo-controlled trial published the same year investigated fentanyl buccal tablet (FBT) (100–800 μg) for breakthrough pain in cancer patients [34]. FBT is an effervescent formulation which has enhanced rate and extent of uptake of fentanyl compared to OTFC. This trial of short duration found the fentanyl buccal tablet to be safe and efficacious.

Antidepressants for neuropathic pain, with special reference to cancer pain

A Cochrane review on antidepressants for neuropathic pain with final search in December 2004 found that antidepressants are effective for the treatment of neuropathic pain, with the best evidence being for tricyclic antidepressants, with amitriptyline having a NNT of 2 (CI 1.7–2.5) [35]. Two small placebo-controlled studies on postoperative neuropathic pain after breast cancer treatment were included in this review. In the first study, a randomized cross-over trial which enrolled 20 patients, amitriptyline 100 mg provided significant pain relief; however, adverse effects such as tiredness compromised treatment and caused four patients to discontinue the trial [36]. In the second study which was also a cross-over study and included 15 patients, venlafaxine 75 mg gave some pain relief and no significance in adverse effects compared to placebo [37].

A second systematic review on drug treatment of neuropathic pain included 105 studies [18]. Cancer pain studies are not specifically described in this review. In peripheral neuropathic pain, the lowest NNT was for tricyclic antidepressants, while there were limited data for central neuropathic pain.

Two recent randomized placebo-controlled trials have reported duloxetine to be effective and well tolerated as a treatment for PDN [38,39]. In the first of these trials, 344 of 457 randomized patients completed the 12-week study period. Duloxetine 60 and 120 mg/d were found to improve pain measures, with a NNT of 4.1 (CI 2.9–7.2), and to improve daily functioning as measured by the Brief Pain Inventory and quality of life measures. Patients with psychiatric disorders, including generalized anxiety disorder and/or major depressive disorder, and patients with mixed pain disorders were excluded from this trial. In the second trial which had similar conclusions, 248 of 334 randomized patients completed the 12-week study period. Since tricyclics are generally poorly tolerated by elderly patients, mainly due to anticholinergic adverse effects, duloxetine may be a more suitable drug for the treatment of neuropathic pain in this patient group. As yet, trials on duloxetine for neuropathic pain in the elderly and in cancer pain are lacking.

Anticonvulsants for neuropathic pain, with special reference to cancer pain

A Cochrane review from 2005 found that gabapentin is effective for PHN and PDN, but does not appear to be superior to carbamazepine, which is a cheaper option [40]. A Cochrane review on gabapentin for acute and chronic pain concludes that there is evidence that gabapentin is effective in neuropathic pain and that approximately two-thirds of patients who take either carbamazepine or gabapentin can expect to achieve good pain relief [41]. Fifteen trials (14 published reports, one reporting on two trials) with 1468 participants were included. Only one study concerned cancer-related neuropathic pain [42]. This was a 10-day randomized, double-blind, placebo-controlled trial in 121 patients where gabapentin was added to existing analgesic treatment. The trial concluded that gabapentin is effective in improving analgesia in patients with neuropathic pain already treated with opioids, However, the trial was of short duration and the magnitude of effect limited compared to placebo [43]. Although pregabalin is currently used for the

treatment of neuropathic cancer pain, there are as yet no published trials on this treatment.

Finnerup et al. performed a systematic review on randomized double-blind placebo-controlled trials of treatment for neuropathic pain [18]. This review found that gabapentin has documented moderate effect on pain and quality of life measures including mood and sleep disturbance in mixed neuropathic pain states, PHN, PDN and spinal cord injury. Pregabalin in PHN and PDN was found to have a combined NNT of 4.2 (CI 3.4–5.4) for doses from 150 mg to 600 mg, comparable to the effect of gabapentin. A subsequent large, randomized study found pregabalin to be effective in PHN and PDN with a NNT of 3.8 (CI 2.6–7.3) [44].

NMDA receptor antagonists for neuropathic pain

The oral NMDA receptor antagonists memantine, dextromethorphan and riluzole have been studied mainly in small trials in neuropathic pain with little or no effect [18]. Randomized placebo-controlled trials in cancer pain are lacking.

Ketamine as an adjuvant to opioids for cancer pain

It is apparent from the literature that this is a common treatment for refractory cancer pain. However, trials are lacking. A Cochrane review published in 2003 found insufficient evidence to support the use of ketamine as an adjuvant to opioids for cancer pain [45]. Only two small placebo-controlled trials with a total of 30 patients could be included. One study with a duration of 3 hours examined the effect of an intravenous bolus of ketamine [46]. The second trial was of longer but unspecified duration, and investigated the co-administration of intrathecal ketamine with intrathecal morphine [47]. This review was updated in 2007 and did not identify additional randomized, controlled trials.

Systemic local anesthetics for neuropathic pain, with special reference to cancer pain

Two systematic reviews have addressed the effect of systemic local anesthetics in chronic pain. The first review, published in 1998, included 17 trials, of which three concerned cancer pain [48]. Two small cross-over trials with 10 patients in each trial investigated the effect of lidocaine 5 mg/kg IV infusion on neuropathic cancer pain [49, 50]. One small trial investigated pain due to bony metastases [51]. Lidocaine 5 mg/kg IV infusion was found to have no significant effect compared to placebo in all three trials. The review concluded that systemic local anesthetics may have an effect in certain types of neuropathic pain, but that cancer-related pain does not seem to respond to this treatment if given in conditions when other strong analgesics are already used. It was suggested that this could also be due to the fact that most difficult cancer-related pains are not purely neuropathic.

A qualitative and quantitative Cochrane review on systemic local anesthetics for neuropathic pain published in 2005 found that intravenous lidocaine and oral mexiletine are more effective than placebo in relieving chronic neuropathic pain in selected patients [52]. This review did not identify additional trials in cancer pain.

Spinal (epidural and intrathecal) treatment of cancer pain

Local anesthetics
Prospective, randomized double-blinded placebo-controlled trials of intrathecal or epidural local anesthetics for cancer pain are lacking.

Opioids
Prospective, randomized double-blinded placebo-controlled trials of intrathecal or epidural opioids for cancer pain are lacking. The few prospective studies compare different routes of administration and are without placebo control. A Cochrane review published in 2005 which investigated the efficacy of epidural, subarachnoid and intracerebroventricular opioids in patients with pain due to cancer did not retrieve any controlled trials [53].

Clonidine
One randomized double-blinded placebo-controlled trial on epidural clonidine included 85 patients with severe cancer pain despite large doses of opioids [54]. This trial concluded that epidural clonidine 30 μg/h may provide effective relief for intractable cancer pain, particularly neuropathic pain.

Ketamine
One small randomized double-blind placebo-controlled trial has investigated the effect of intrathecal ketamine as an adjuvant to opioid in refractory cancer pain [55]. This study found that ketamine had a morphine-sparing effect. The use of spinal ketamine is generally not advised due to unclear toxicity issues [56].

Ziconotide
Ziconotide is a synthetic analog of a conotoxin peptide which is a selective, potent and reversible blocker of neuronal N-type voltage-sensitive calcium channels and which has been introduced as a novel non-opioid treatment of chronic pain. One multicenter randomized, double-blind placebo-controlled trial of intrathecal ziconotide in patients with cancer or AIDS included 111 patients with refractory pain [57]. This trial concluded that intrathecal ziconotide provided clinically and statistically significant analgesia in this patient population. The trial was subsequently criticized due to short (2-week) follow-up, concerns about blinding, and duplicate publication [58, 59].

Capsaicin in neuropathic pain, with special reference to cancer pain
Topical capsaicin cream has been found to relieve pain in PHN, nerve injury pain and mixed neuropathic pain conditions [18]. One randomized placebo-controlled trial in 99 cancer patients found that topical capsaicin cream decreased postsurgical neuropathic pain [60].

The future: how to produce evidence of effectiveness

There is a general lack of efficacy data for the long-term treatment of cancer pain with analgesics and co-analgesics. This is not surprising, given the difficulty of doing good scientific research in seriously ill patients who commonly have multiple unpleasant symptoms and a short life expectancy.

Treatments which are commonly used but which are not scientifically documented include the following.

Corticosteroids
Treatment with corticosteroids is used for the relief of pain due to nerve compression, headache due to raised intracranial pressure and liver capsule distension pain.

There is very little documentation concerning this treatment. A 14-day randomized, placebo-controlled trial compared oral methylprednisolone with placebo for the relief of pain and other symptoms in 40 terminally ill cancer patients and found that 32 mg methylprednisolone daily increased the comfort of terminally ill cancer patients [61].

Neuroleptics

Chlorpromazine and levomepromazine (methotrimeprazine) are often used as adjuvant analgesics. This is principally due to therapy traditions rather than scientific documentation. The use of neuroleptics in pain relief is controversial due to their prominent adverse effects. Olanzapine is reported to have fewer adverse effects than traditional neuroleptics. A limited number of case studies in cancer pain report that adjuvant treatment with olanzapine decreased pain and opioid requirements [62]. Randomized, controlled trials are lacking.

There is a need for well-conducted trials of analgesics and co-analgesics in cancer pain. Since patients in pain respond to placebo, we need placebo-controlled trials to reliably determine analgesic and co-analgesic efficacy. Many researchers consider that it is unethical to use a placebo control in trials of cancer pain. However, it is common to use placebo controls in both acute pain and chronic pain trials. While it is not feasible to use a placebo control in all cancer pain studies, it is possible in certain types of trial. Patients treated with stronger opioids cannot be randomized to a placebo group. However, patients using weaker opioids may well be randomized to a placebo group. Almost half of the studies included in the methodologic review on oral opioids recruited patients being treated with WHO step 2 (weaker) opioids [19]. In these studies, it would have been possible to include a placebo arm, providing the patients had free access to normal-release opioids as rescue medication, and using consumption of rescue medication as the primary outcome measure. This type of study should have a limited duration, for example 14 days, and should not present ethical problems since the treatment is similar to the clinical treatment of

Table 25.3 Commonly used analgesics/co-analgesics

Analgesic/co-analgesic	Evidence level	Comments
Supported by evidence		
NSAIDs	I	Long-term treatment not documented.
Tricyclic antidepressants*	I	Documented for neuropathic pain in general, not cancer pain specifically
Opioids*	I	Documented for chronic noncancer pain, but not for cancer pain. Currently problematic literature. Only one trial where oral morphine is compared to placebo. Small trials, short duration, methodologic weaknesses
Anticonvulsants* (gabapentin, pregabalin, carbamazepine)	I	Documented for neuropathic pain in general, not cancer pain specifically
Currently unproven		
Paracetamol		One 6-hour placebo-controlled cross-over trial in cancer pain (n = 29) found no difference between paracetamol and placebo [16]. One placebo-controlled RCT found paracetamol an effective adjuvant to opioid in cancer pain [17]
Ketamine		Two placebo-controlled RCT [46, 47]. Both trials demonstrated improved analgesia with ketamine. Small number of patients, differing routes of administration
Corticosteroids		RCT lacking
Neuroleptics		RCT lacking

* Randomized placebo-controlled trials in cancer pain lacking.
RCT, randomized controlled trials.

breakthrough pain, and would be expected to give satisfactory pain relief. The ethics of using a placebo control in this kind of design should be compared to the potential ethical dilemma of exposing seriously ill patients to trials which do not produce reliable results due to lack of power or sensitivity, or other methodologic problems.

A number of other methodologic problems were identified in the oral opioid trials, including low trial sensitivity, too small trial size and lack of standardized measures of efficacy. It is important to know which type of pain is being treated. There should be a common definition of analgesic efficacy. Psychologic factors can influence the experience of pain and should be assessed and reported. A number of other factors have the potential for influencing analgesic response, and future research should involve identifying and controlling for such factors.

Conclusion

In conclusion, there is a clear need for standardization and uniformity of design and reporting of trials of analgesics for cancer pain. Trials must be designed to produce reliable results. This cannot be accomplished by a single researcher, but requires the collaboration of experts in several fields. For example, a consensus meeting to establish a standard opioid trial design has been suggested [19]. Standardization of trial design would help researchers to plan trials, improve study quality and validity and enable the combination of data from separate trials.

Given the fact that the documentation of proven efficacy is poor even for opioids in the management of cancer pain, the question of whether conclusions from analgesic studies in chronic noncancer pain may be extrapolated to cancer pain is highly relevant.

Author's recommendations

The proven effectiveness of analgesics and co-analgesics for cancer pain is poorly documented. Efforts should be made to establish efficacy of current treatments. In the absence of such evidence, data from trials in other patient populations, for example non-malignant neuropathic pain, may be helpful.

References

1. Caraceni A, Portenoy R. An international survey of cancer pain characteristics and syndromes. IASP Task Force on Cancer Pain. International Association for the Study of Pain. *Pain* 1999; **82**(3): 263–274.
2. Banning A, Sjøgren P, Henriksen H. Treatment outcome in a multidisciplinary cancer pain clinic. *Pain* 1991; **47**(2): 129–134.
3. Poleshuck E, Katz J, Andrus C, *et al*. Risk factors for chronic pain following breast cancer surgery: a prospective study. *J Pain* 2006; **7**(9): 626–634.
4. Mantyh PW, Clohisy DR, Koltzenburg M, Hunt SP. Molecular mechanisms of cancer pain. *Nat Rev Cancer* 2002; **2**(3): 201–209.
5. Goblirsch M, Zwolak P, Clohisy D. Biology of bone cancer pain. *Clin Cancer Res* 2006; **12**(20 suppl): 6231s–6235s.
6. Hwang SS, Chang VT, Kasimis B. Cancer breakthrough pain characteristics and responses to treatment at a VA medical centre. *Pain* 2003; **101**: 55–64.
7. Svendsen KB, Andersen S, Arnason S, *et al*. Breakthrough pain in malignant and non-malignant diseases: a review of prevalence, characteristics and mechanisms. *Eur J Pain* 2005; **9**: 195–206.
8. Portenoy R, Taylor D, Messina J, Tremmel L. A randomized, placebo-controlled study of fentanyl buccal tablets for breakthrough pain in opioid-treated patients with cancer. *Clin J Pain* 2006; **22**(9): 805–811.
9. Carr DB, Goudas LC, Denman WT, *et al*. Safety and efficacy of intranasal ketamine for the treatment of breakthrough pain in patients with chronic pain: a randomized, double-blind, placebo-controlled, crossover study. *Pain* 2004; **108**(1–2): 17–27.
10. Potter J, Higginson I. Pain experienced by lung cancer patients: a review of prevalence, causes and pathophysiology. *Lung Cancer* 2004; **43**(3): 247–257.
11. Di Maio M, Gridelli C, Gallo C, *et al*. Prevalence and management of pain in Italian patients with advanced non-small-cell lung cancer. *Br J Cancer* 2004; **90**(12): 2288–2296.
12. World Health Organization. Cancer, pain relief and palliative care. WHO Technical Report Series No 408. World Health Organization, Geneva, 1990.
13. Jadad A, Browman G. The WHO analgesic ladder for cancer pain management. Stepping up the quality of its evaluation. *JAMA* 1995; **274**(23): 1870–1873.
14. Zech D, Grond S, Lynch J, Hertel D, Lehmann K. Validation of World Health Organization guidelines for cancer pain relief: a 10 year prospective study. *Pain* 1995; **63**: 65–76.
15. McNicol ED, Strassels S, Goudas L, Lau J, Carr DB. NSAIDS or paracetamol, alone or combined with opioids, for cancer pain. Cochrane Database of Systematic Reviews 2005, Issue 2. Art. No.: CD005180. DOI: 10.1002/14651858.CD005180.
16. Stambaugh JE. Additive analgesia of oral butorphanol/acetaminophen in patients with pain due to metastatic carcinoma. *Curr Therapeut Res* 1982; **31**: 386–392.
17. Stockler M, Vardy J, Pilla A, Warr D. Acetaminophen (paracetamol) improves pain and well being in people with

advanced cancer already receiving a strong opioid regimen: a randomized, double-blind, placebo-controlled crossover trial. *J Clin Oncol* 2004; **22**(16): 3389–3394.

18. Finnerup N, Otto M, McQuay H, Jensen T, Sindrup S. Algorithm for neuropathic pain treatment: an evidence-based proposal. *Pain* 2005; **118**(3): 289–305.

19. Bell RF, Wisløff T, Eccleston C, Kalso E. Controlled clinical trials in cancer pain. How controlled should they be? A qualitative systematic review. *Br J Cancer* 2006; **94**(11): 1559–1567.

20. Hoskin PJ, Poulain P, Hanks GW. Controlled-release morphine in cancer pain. Is a loading dose required when the formulation is changed? *Anaesthesia* 1989; **44**(11): 897–901.

21. Broomhead A, Kerr R, Tester W, *et al.* Comparison of a once-a-day sustained-release morphine formulation with standard oral morphine treatment for cancer pain. *J Pain Symptom Manage* 1997; **14**(2): 63–73.

22. Wiffen PJ, McQuay HJ. Oral morphine for cancer pain. Cochrane Database of Systematic Reviews 2007, Issue 4. Art. No.: CD003868. DOI: 10.1002/14651858.CD003868.pub2.

23. Quigley C. Hydromorphone for acute and chronic pain. Cochrane Database of Systematic Reviews 2002, Issue 1. Art. No.: CD003447. DOI: 10.1002/14651858.CD003447.

24. Reid C, Martin R, Sterne J, Davies A. Oxycodone for cancer-related pain: meta-analysis of randomized controlled trials. *Arch Intern Med* 2006; **166**: 837–843.

25. Nicholson AB. Methadone for cancer pain. Cochrane Database of Systematic Reviews 2007, Issue 4. Art. No.: CD003971. DOI: 10.1002/14651858.CD003971.pub3.

26. Goudas L, Carr DB, Bloch R, *et al.* Management of cancer pain. Evidence Report/Technology Assessment No. 35: AHRQ Publication No. 02–E002. Agency for Healthcare Research and Quality, Rockville, MD: 2001.

27. Bell RF, Wisløff T, Eccleston C, Kalso E. Trial design in cancer pain: oral opioids and the missing placebo. In: McQuay HJ, Kalso E, Moore RA (eds). *Systematic reviews in pain research: methodology refined.* IASP Press, Seattle, 2008: 287–301.

28. Houde RW, Wallenstein SL, Rogers A. Clinical pharmacology of analgesics: a method of assaying analgesic effect. *Clin Pharmacol Therapeut* 1960; **1**(2): 163–174.

29. Stambaugh JE, Lane C. Analgesic efficacy and pharmacokinetic evaluation of meperidine and hydroxyzine, alone and in combination. *Cancer Invest* 1983; **1**: 111–117.

30. Stambaugh JE, McAdams J. Comparison of intramuscular dezocine with butorphanol and placebo in chronic cancer pain: a method to evaluate analgesia after both single and repeated doses. *Clin Pharmacol Therapeut* 1987; **42**: 210–219.

31. Stambaugh JE, McAdams J. Comparison of the analgesic efficacy and safety of oral ciramadol, codeine and placebo in patients with chronic cancer pain. *J Clin Pharmacol* 1987; **27**(2): 162–166.

32. Farrar JT, Cleary J, Rauck R, Busch MA, Nordbrock E. Oral transmucosal fentanyl citrate: randomized, double-blinded placebo-controlled trial for treatment of breakthrough pain in cancer patients. *J Natl Cancer Inst* 1998; **90**: 611–616.

33. Zeppetella G, Ribeiro MDC. Opioids for the management of breakthrough (episodic) pain in cancer patients. Cochrane Database of Systematic Reviews 2006, Issue 1. Art. No.: CD004311. DOI: 10.1002/14651858.CD004311.pub2.

34. Portenoy R, Taylor D, Messina J, Tremmel L. A randomized, placebo-controlled study of fentanyl buccal tablet for breakthrough pain in opioid-treated patients with cancer. *Clin J Pain* 2006; **22**(9): 805–811.

35. Saarto T, Wiffen PJ. Antidepressants for neuropathic pain. Cochrane Database of Systematic Reviews 2007, Issue 4. Art. No.: CD005454. DOI: 10.1002/14651858.CD005454.pub2.

36. Kalso E, Tasmuth T, Neuvonen P. Amitriptyline effectively relieves neuropathic pain following treatment of breast cancer. *Pain* 1996; **64**(2): 293–302.

37. Tasmuth T, Hartel B, Kalso E. Venlafaxine in neuropathic pain following treatment of breast cancer. *Eur J Pain* 2002; **6**(1): 17–24.

38. Goldstein D, Lu Y, Detke M, Lee T, Iyengar S. Duloxetine vs. placebo in patients with painful polyneuropathy. *Pain* 2005; **116**(1–2): 109–118.

39. Wernicke J, Pritchett Y, D'Souza D, *et al.* A randomised controlled trial of duloxetine in diabetic peripheral neuropathic pain. *Neurology* 2006; **67**(8): 1411–1420.

40. Wiffen PJ, Collins S, McQuay HJ, Carroll D, Jadad A, Moore RA. Anticonvulsant drugs for acute and chronic pain. Cochrane Database of Systematic Reviews 2005, Issue 3. Art. No.: CD001133. DOI: 10.1002/14651858.CD001133.pub2.

41. Wiffen PJ, McQuay HJ, Rees J, Moore RA. Gabapentin for acute and chronic pain. Cochrane Database of Systematic Reviews 2005, Issue 3. Art. No.: CD005452. DOI: 10.1002/14651858.CD005452.

42. Caraceni A, Zecca E, Bonnezzi C, *et al.* Gabapentin for neuropathic cancer pain: a randomized controlled trial from the Gabapentin Cancer Pain Study Group. *J Clin Oncol* 2004; **22**(14): 2909–2917.

43. Bennett M. Gabapentin significantly improves analgesia in people receiving opioids for neuropathic cancer pain. *Cancer Treat Rev* 2005; **31**(1): 58–62.

44. Freynhagen R, Strojek K, Griesing T, Whalen E, Balkenohl M. Efficacy of pregabalin in neuropathic pain evaluated in a 12- week, randomised, double-blind, multicentre, placebo-controlled trial of flexible-and fixed-dose regimens. *Pain* 2005; **115**(3): 254–263.

45. Bell RF, Eccleston C, Kalso EA. Ketamine as an adjuvant to opioids for cancer pain. Cochrane Database of Systematic Reviews 2003, Issue 1. Art. No.: CD003351. DOI: 10.1002/14651858.CD003351.

46. Mercadante S, Arcuri E, Tirelli W, Casuccio A. Analgesic effect of intravenous ketamine in cancer patients on morphine therapy: a randomized, controlled, double-blind, crossover, double-dose study. *J Pain Symptom Manage* 2000; **20**(4): 246–252.

47. Yang CY, Wong CS, Chang JY, Ho ST. Intrathecal ketamine reduces morphine requirements in patients with terminal cancer pain. *Can J Anaesth* 1996; **43**(4): 379–383.

48. Kalso E, Tramer M, McQuay H, Moore R. Systemic local-anaesthetic-type drugs in chronic pain: a systematic review. *Eur J Pain* 1998; **2**(1): 3–14.

49. Bruera E, Ripamonti C, Brenneis C, MacMillan K, Hanson J. A randomized double-blind crossover trial of intravenous lidocaine in the treatment of neuropathic cancer pain. *J Pain Symptom Manage* 1992; **7**(3): 138–140.

50. Ellemann K, Sjogren P, Banning A, Jensen T, Smith T, Geertsen P. Trial of intravenous lidocaine on painful neuropathy in cancer patients. *Clin J Pain* 1989; **5**(4): 291–294.

51. Sjøgren P, Banning A-M, Hebsgaard K, Petersen P, Gefke K. Intravenøs lidokain i behandling avf kroniske smerter forrsaget af knoglemetastaser. *Ugeskr Læger* 1989; **151**: 2144–2146.

52. Challapalli V, Tremont-Lukats IW, McNicol ED, Lau J, Carr DB. Systemic administration of local anesthetic agents to relieve neuropathic pain. Cochrane Database of Systematic Reviews 2005, Issue 4. Art. No.: CD003345. DOI: 10.1002/14651858.CD003345.pub2.

53. Ballantyne JC, Carwood C. Comparative efficacy of epidural, subarachnoid, and intracerebroventricular opioids in patients with pain due to cancer. Cochrane Database of Systematic Reviews 2005, Issue 2. Art. No.: CD005178. DOI: 10.1002/14651858.CD005178.

54. Eisenach J, DuPen S, Dubois M, Miquel R, Allin D. Epidural clonidine analgesia for intractable cancer pain. The Epidural Clonidine Study Group. *Pain* 1995; **61**(3): 391–399.

55. Yang C, Wong C, Chang J, Ho S. Intrathecal ketamine reduces morphine requirements in patients with terminal cancer pain. *Can J Anaesth* 1996; **43**(4): 379–383.

56. Eisenach J, Yaksh T. Epidural ketamine in healthy children – what's the point? *Anesth Analg* 2003; **96**: 626–633.

57. Staats P, Yearwood T, Charapata S, *et al.* Intrathecal ziconotide in the treatment of refractory pain in patients with cancer or AIDS: a randomized controlled trial. *JAMA* 2004; **291**(1): 63–70.

58. Bonicalzi V, Canavero S. Intrathecal ziconotide for chronic pain. *JAMA* 2004; **292**(14): 1681–1682.

59. DeAngelis C. Duplicate publication,multiple problems. *JAMA* 2004; **292**(14): 1745–1746.

60. Ellison N, Loprinzi C, Kugler J, *et al.* Phase III placebo-controlled trial of capsaicin cream in the management of surgical neuropathic pain in cancer patients. *J Clin Oncol* 1997; **15**(8): 2974–2980.

61. Bruera E, Roca E, Cedaro L, Carraro S, Chacon R. Action of methylprednisolone in terminal cancer patients: a prospective randomized double-blind study. *Cancer Treat Rep* 1985; **69**(7–8): 751–754.

62. Khojainova N, Santiago-Palma J, Kornick C, Breitbart W, Gonzales G. Olanzapine in the management of cancer pain. *J Pain Symptom Manage* 2002; **23**(4): 346–350.

CHAPTER 26

Psychologic interventions for cancer pain

Francis J. Keefe, Tamara J. Somers and Amy Abernethy
Duke University Medical Center, Durham, NC, USA

Introduction

Recently, there has been growing interest in the role of psychosocial variables in understanding how individuals cope with disease-related pain conditions such as cancer pain [1, 2]. Much of the interest in this area has been generated by the possibility that psychosocial treatment protocols designed to enhance coping efforts may be useful in managing disease-related pain [1]. Over the past two decades, a growing number of randomized clinical trials have tested the efficacy of psychosocial protocols for managing cancer pain.

The goal of this chapter is to analyze the evidence base for psychosocial approaches to cancer pain. The chapter is divided into three sections. In the first section, we describe the conceptual background for psychosocial approaches to cancer pain. In the second section, we summarize empirical evidence on the efficacy of three psychosocial protocols that have been used in the management of cancer pain: imagery and hypnosis-based cognitive behavioral therapy (CBT), comprehensive CBT, and education-focused interventions with brief CBT. In the final section we highlight important clinical and research issues related to the psychosocial management of cancer pain.

Conceptual background

Cancer pain is typically understood and treated using a strictly biomedical model. The primary focus of the biomedical model is on pain and methods of pain relief. The efficacy of the biomedical model is thus based on its ability to produce improvements in pain. The biomedical model maintains that pain is a symptom of underlying tissue damage or injury. There are a number of possible sources of tissue damage or injury in cancer patients. Tissue damage might be due to cancer itself, for example caused by a malignant tumor pressing on a nerve root. Alternatively, medical or surgical interventions designed to treat cancer may produce pain. Persistent neuropathic pain, for example, is common following administration of certain cancer chemotherapy treatment protocols. Radiation therapy can dry or thicken tissues and cause persistent pain. Surgical removal of a tumor may cause nerve damage or swelling that produces persistent pain.

The biomedical model ideally seeks to treat cancer pain by identifying and eliminating its underlying cause. In some patients, surgical treatment of a cancerous tumor effectively alleviates pain. In many cancer patients, however, the underlying biologic factors contributing to pain are multiple and difficult, if not impossible, to eliminate. In such cases, the central goal of treatment is managing pain symptoms by modifying biologic mechanisms (e.g. inflammation, nerve damage) that contribute to pain. Opioid medications are the mainstay of cancer pain management and are used in most patients whose pain persists [1]. Opioids are often supplemented by other medications such as anticonvulsants, psychotropic agents, and corticosteroids. Pain that is refractory to medical management may be treated with specialized surgical, radiation or chemotherapy protocols.

Although the biomedical model is useful in understanding and treating cancer pain, it does have problems [1]. First, cancer pain can be persistent

Evidence-Based Chronic Pain Management. Edited by
C. Stannard, E. Kalso and J. Ballantyne. © 2010 Blackwell
Publishing.

and disabling even when optimal biomedical pain management is provided. Second, commonly used biomedical treatments such as opioids have side effects (constipation, drowsiness) that are sometimes difficult to manage and poorly tolerated by patients. Third, the biomedical approach tends to minimize the important role that psychologic factors (e.g. helplessness) and social factors (e.g. social support) can play in the experience of pain.

Psychosocial approaches to cancer pain are based on a biopsychosocial model of pain. The primary focus of the biopsychosocial approach is on enhancing adjustment to pain. Treatments based on this model seek to produce not only improvements in pain, but also improvements in other important indices of adjustment to pain such as psychologic distress and physical function.

The biopsychosocial model of cancer pain maintains that adjustment to cancer pain is complex and is influenced not only by the biologic factors highlighted in the biomedical model, but also by psychologic factors and social factors. Converging lines of evidence suggest that several psychologic and social factors are especially important in understanding adjustment to cancer pain [1]. First, self-efficacy or the confidence that one has the ability to control pain has emerged as one of the most important psychologic factors in understanding pain [3]. Research has shown that cancer patients who report high levels of self-efficacy for pain control report much lower levels of pain, physical disability, and psychologic distress [4–6]. Second, there is evidence that patients who engage in pain catastrophizing show much poorer adjustment to pain [7]. Pain catastrophizing refers to the tendency to ruminate upon and magnify the threat value of pain sensations. Cancer patients who engage in pain catastrophizing not only report higher levels of pain, but also experience much higher levels of anxiety and interference with daily activities due to pain [8, 9]. Third, recent evidence suggests that cancer patients who hold back on sharing their concerns about pain or who are unwilling to express emotions related to the cancer experience are more likely to experience high levels of pain and lower quality of life [10]. Finally, there is evidence that social factors can influence adjustment to pain [1]. Cancer patients whose spouse is supportive are more likely to experience better adjustment to pain, whereas those whose spouses

are critical or punishing are more likely to experience increased pain and emotional distress [11].

The biopsychosocial model is useful not only in understanding cancer pain but also in developing treatment protocols to enhance adjustment to pain.

Efficacy of psychosocial interventions

The vast majority of randomized clinical trials of psychosocial interventions have tested cognitive behavioral treatment (CBT) protocols. These protocols systematically teach patients cognitive and behavioral strategies for altering psychologic and social factors related to cancer pain and adjustment. To determine the efficacy of cognitive behavioral protocols for cancer pain, we recently conducted a meta-analysis [12]. A total of 21 trials of CBT protocols involving 2296 participants were included in the meta-analysis. CBT protocols were effective in reducing pain in 65% of the studies with an overall average effect size of 0.232 (95% confidence interval (CI) 0.072–0.392; $P = 0.004$). In our meta-analysis we examined the efficacy of CBT across three different types of CBT interventions: imagery and hypnosis-based CBT, comprehensive CBT, and education-focused interventions with brief CBT. For each of these different types of CBT interventions, we provide a brief description, summarize several illustrative studies, and briefly comment on efficacy and ways in which the protocol could be improved.

Imagery- and hypnosis-based CBT

Description
Hypnosis, which induces a state of focused concentration and suspended peripheral awareness, allows the patient to experience relaxation, nonjudgmental attitude, suggestibility, dissociation, and altered time and space perception. In leading the patient through hypnosis, a trained therapist verbally guides the individual to a calm and peaceful state of awareness, refocusing energy away from the source of distress and facilitating a healing process. Imagery, a less passive form of hypnosis, encourages the patient to refocus his/her attention away from the pain itself onto, for example, a safe and pleasant place or an image associated with health, strength, safety, and capability. Unlike with

hypnosis, the therapist utilizing imagery guides the experience but the patient creates the specific visual or perceptual images. Both modalities usually start with relaxation training, and both can be learned by patients for self-use. Because of their similarity, it is often difficult to distinguish between hypnosis and imagery in the pain management research construct and literature.

Illustrative studies

Research studies have demonstrated that hypnosis and imagery are effective in the management of cancer pain, and particularly so for acute procedural pain [13]. In a compelling randomized trial of 80 children undergoing lumbar punctures for hematologic malignancies, the groups who underwent hypnosis or guided imagery peri-procedure (n = 40) experienced less pain, anxiety, and behavioral distress than did those who were randomized to distraction (n = 20) or control (n = 20) [14]. Several years earlier, the same investigators had demonstrated that children undergoing bone marrow biopsy experienced less pain when hypnotized or exposed to cognitive behavioral coping skills than when receiving usual treatment (n = 30; 1:1:1 randomization) [15]. A trend was noted in this study for hypnosis to be superior to CBT (P = 0.20). These results reinforced those of prior studies in the same area [16, 17].

Experiences for adults using hypnosis and/or imagery to manage acute cancer-related pain are similar to those of children. Women randomized to receive hypnosis prior to breast biopsy had less postsurgical pain and distress than did those randomized to the standard care arm (n = 20: 1:1 randomization) [18]. According to a randomized study by Syrjala *et al.* [19], acute mucositis pain associated with bone marrow transplant could be mitigated with hypnosis, whereas CBT was not effective in alleviating this symptom. The hypnosis protocol used in this study was characterized by relaxation and patient-directed imagery prior to the transplant; the authors later changed the name of their intervention to "imagery with relaxation" in order to avoid patients' negative connotations with the word "hypnosis." A 1995 follow-up study by the same team involved 94 participants and found that relaxation and imagery training with or without cognitive behavioral skills training led to reduced pain relative to controls, despite higher

mucositis severity for the intervention groups [20]. The investigators concluded that cognitive behavioral skills training did not provide benefit over relaxation and imagery training alone.

The role of hypnosis and imagery in chronic malignant cancer pain, while less clear, is still promising. Spiegal & Bloom [21] randomized 58 women with metastatic breast cancer to weekly group therapy with or without hypnosis. The hypnosis component lasted 5–10 minutes and taught patients not to fight the pain and to imagine, in the place of their pain, competing positive sensations in the affected area. Hypnosis plus group therapy lead to less pain sensation (P < 0.02) and pain suffering (P < 0.03); the groups did not differ in terms of pain frequency or duration. An obvious limitation of this and other studies of hypnosis and imagery is the fact that they are not recent. Such studies bear repeating in contemporary clinical settings and populations, in order to ensure that the evidence basis is up to date and relevant to patients today.

Comment

In our meta-analysis of CBT interventions we identified seven randomized clinical trials testing the efficacy of imagery and hypnosis-based CBT interventions for cancer pain. Statistically significant effects of imagery- and hypnosis-based CBT on pain were found in 86% of studies. The mean effect size of these interventions was statistically significant (mean 0.419; CI −0.059 to 0.770; P = 0.023). Overall, imagery and hypnosis-based CBT are effective for reducing acute pain in pediatric and adult cancer patients, especially children undergoing short-lived procedures and adults receiving bone marrow transplants. Chronic malignant pain is also likely responsive to hypnosis and imagery, but repeat studies are warranted to firmly establish the impact, effect size, and role of these modalities in the management of chronic cancer pain.

While cancer pain management appears to be an important area of potential impact for the hypnosis practitioner, the value of hypnosis- and imagery-based techniques has yet to be realized by the cancer pain community and their role has yet to be established and integrated into routine clinical care for cancer pain patients. Necessary next steps in advancing these interventions into practice include:

(1) investigation of barriers to uptake, such as the patient and provider associations with terms identified by Syrjala and colleagues; (2) strengthening of the evidence basis through additional studies, particularly investigating the use of hypnosis and imagery for chronic cancer pain management; and (3) dissemination of research findings in well-respected and broadly circulated journals that reach practicing clinicians.

Comprehensive CBT

Description

Comprehensive CBT protocols train cancer patients in a variety of skills for coping with pain. In addition to relaxation training, these protocols often provide training in imagery, activity pacing, goal setting, cognitive restructuring, and problem solving. In comprehensive CBT, imagery typically centers on having the patient imagine a pleasant scene. Activity pacing teaches the patient to avoid overactivity that can lead to extreme pain by breaking down the day into periods of moderate activity and limited rest. In goal setting, patients are taught how to set and then monitor the attainment of realistic and meaningful short- and long-term goals. Cognitive restructuring teaches the patient how to identify and challenge overall negative thoughts (e.g. "I'll never be able to cope with pain," "I am a burden on my family") that work against their abilities to manage pain. Problem solving helps the patient to identify challenging problems (e.g. coping with a pain flare), generate strategies to manage the problem, and evaluate the effectiveness of implemented strategies. Comprehensive CBT protocols are based on a skills model that emphasizes the importance of practicing these skills and incorporating them into everyday life.

Illustrative studies

Syrjala conducted one of the first studies examining the impact of a comprehensive CBT protocol on pain related to bone marrow transplants [20]. The comprehensive CBT protocol included training in relaxation, imagery, cognitive restructuring, distraction, and goal setting. In this study, patients receiving comprehensive CBT reported significantly less pain than those in a usual care control condition. Berglund et al. [22] delivered a comprehensive CBT protocol that included an exercise component to a mixed sample of cancer

patients. Patients receiving the comprehensive CBT intervention reported better pain control for up to 6 months following the intervention. They also reported increases in strength.

Little is known about how tailoring treatment to an individual or including a significant other in treatment might produce additional treatment benefits. Dalton et al. [23] compared standard comprehensive CBT to a comprehensive CBT protocol that was tailored to individual needs. Tailored CBT provided better outcomes immediately after treatment, standard CBT provided more favorable outcomes 6 months following treatment, and both groups were superior compared to usual care.

Keefe and colleagues [24] addressed whether a partner-guided comprehensive CBT protocol could benefit cancer patients who were at the end of life (n = 78). The intervention combined educational pain information with training of patients and partners in cognitive and behavioral pain-coping skills. Following treatment, partners receiving the CBT intervention reported significantly higher ratings of self-efficacy for helping their partner control pain and manage other physical symptoms than patients in the control condition. Partners receiving CBT also reported significant decreases in caregiver strain. The CBT protocol had no significant effects on pain ratings in this very sick, terminally ill population.

Comment

In our meta-analysis of CBT interventions we identified seven randomized clinical trials testing the efficacy of comprehensive CBT interventions for cancer pain. Statistically significant effects of comprehensive CBT on pain were found in 43% of studies. The mean effect size of these interventions did not reach statistical significance (mean 0.148; CI −0.151 to 0.446; P = 0.33).

Although our meta-analysis suggest that studies of comprehensive CBT for cancer pain, as a group, fail to have significant effects on pain, the illustrative studies cited above suggest that this approach to CBT has several advantages. First, since comprehensive CBT encompasses a variety of skills, this approach can be tailored to address the patient's specific pain-related problems. Second, many of the coping skills taught in comprehensive CBT can help patients not only manage their pain, but also cope with other problems they might be experiencing (e.g. other cancer symptoms, emotional distress or problems with engaging in daily activities). Finally, involving a partner or family member in comprehensive CBT may provide benefits to both the patient and the partner or family member.

In addition, as we have noted [12], there are several methodologic issues that arise when comparing studies of comprehensive CBT. These include questions about the appropriate "dosage" of intervention, training of provider delivering treatment (psychologist versus nonpsychologist), small sample sizes, and the type of cancer pain that is treated (acute versus chronic). Perhaps the greatest difficulty in comparing trials of comprehensive CBT for cancer pain is that the combination of behavioral and cognitive pain skills taught varies across studies, making it difficult to evaluate which combinations are most effective.

Education-focused interventions with brief CBT

Description

Over the past 10 years, patient educators working with cancer patients have begun to incorporate some CBT methods into their educational protocols. In most cases, the focus of these protocols remains on providing patients with information on cancer pain, e.g. educational information causes of pain, keeping records of pain, pharmacologic treatments (types, doses, side effects), and communicating about pain with health professionals. The major assumption of these protocols is that when a cancer patient gains a better understanding of educational information, they can become a more active participant in their own pain management [12]. In these protocols, exposure to CBT methods is usually brief and consists of information on the value of nonpharmacologic treatments such as CBT in self-management and brief training in one or more CBT methods (e.g. relaxation training).

Illustrative studies

Dalton [25] conducted one of the first studies to test an educational-focused intervention with brief CBT. She randomized cancer patients having pain to an experimental education condition or a control condition. The education condition consisted of a 1-hour session that provided extensive information about the nature and medical management of pain along with brief training in breathing-based relaxation and the

use of music as a distraction. A 10-minute phone call was made 7–10 days after the educational session to reinforce what was taught. Results indicated significant improvements in knowledge about cancer pain, but no changes in pain medication.

In another study, de Wit et al. [26] examined the efficacy of a pain education program that provided brief exposure to relaxation training. In this study patients were randomly assigned to a patient education intervention or to a control condition. Patients in the education intervention received a 30–60-minute hospital-based session that provided education information about cancer pain and two 15-minute phone-based follow-up sessions. Information and instruction were primarily provided in the hospital-based session and in part of that session patients were told about relaxation and other nonpharmacologic pain management methods (e.g. cold, heat, massage). Results showed that the brief intervention produced a significant increase in knowledge of pain management and a decrease in pain intensity. These results are impressive given the brevity of the treatment. However, the limited time frame for providing training in relaxation makes it unclear how much this CBT technique might have added to the effects obtained.

More recently, Lai et al. [27] investigated the effects of a somewhat more intensive educational protocol that included some exposure to CBT methods. In this study, 30 patients having cancer-related pain were randomly assigned to an experimental group that received 10–15 minutes of pain education per day or to a standard care control condition. The educational information centered on a booklet that covered 11 different topics in the area of pain and pain management, one of which was nonpharmacologic interventions such as relaxation, imagery, and distraction. After completing treatment, patients in the education condition reported significant reductions in pain, negative beliefs about pain medication, and pain catastrophizing and a significant increase in their perceptions of control over pain.

Comment

In our meta-analysis of CBT interventions we identified nine randomized clinical trials testing the efficacy of education-focused interventions with brief CBT. Statistically significant effects of education-focused interventions with brief CBT on pain were found in

56% of studies. The mean effect size of these interventions just missed reaching conventional levels of statistical significance (mean 0.207; CI −0.017 to 0.431; $P = 0.07$).

Education-focused interventions that involve brief CBT have several major strengths. First, these interventions are very brief and designed to be delivered in the context of clinical practice. Second, because they combine information on medical management with CBT they may do a better job of teaching patients how to integrate pharmacologic and CBT methods into pain management than protocols that focus on CBT alone. Third, these interventions are much more likely to reach patients who need them because they are almost always delivered by nurses who have much more access to cancer patients experiencing pain than more traditional CBT providers (e.g. psychologists or mental health professionals).

A number of changes could be used to enhance the efficacy of these interventions. One of the most obvious changes would be to provide more intensive training in CBT methods, particularly imagery-based techniques. To accomplish this, the frequency and duration of sessions of these educational protocols would need to be increased. In addition, the format of individual treatment sessions would need to be more balanced in terms of providing time for educational information versus skills training. Second, greater emphasis could be placed on standardizing the content of the CBT portion of the protocols. Many of these protocols relied on tailoring procedures in which the amount of time educating and training patients in a given CBT method was at the discretion of the therapist. As a result, some patients may have received very abbreviated rationales and training in a CBT method, whereas others might have received more extensive treatment.

Future directions

Randomized clinical trials of psychosocial interventions for pain are a relatively recent development and most of these studies have been conducted in the past 10–15 years. At this point, it seems fair to conclude that these interventions may have some promise in helping cancer patients cope with pain. However, before this promise is fully realized, much more work needs to be done. In this section, we highlight a number of important future directions for clinical and research efforts in this area.

Clinical issues

One of the most important clinical questions is how many sessions of psychosocial treatment is optimal. In published clinical trials, the number of sessions of CBT delivered to cancer patients having pain has ranged from one [28] to 12 sessions [20]. From a clinical perspective, CBT protocols that are delivered in one session are problematic in that they provide little time for instruction, rehearsal, and mastery of pain-coping skills. CBT protocols delivered over months likely place excessive demands on patients who may be quite sick. It probably makes most sense clinically to tailor the number of sessions to the patient's needs. The therapist should evaluate the patient's needs, their ability to comprehend skills instruction, and tolerance for sessions. Our own clinical observations suggest that, for many cancer patients, a 4–6-session protocol is enough to teach and reinforce a set of key coping skills, yet not so lengthy as to overburden the patient.

A second important clinical issue is the timing of intervention. Pain clinicians are increasingly emphasizing the importance of early intervention. Early psychologic intervention is appealing since it provides an opportunity to teach pain-coping skills before maladaptive ways of responding to pain develop. However, early-stage cancer patients may experience relatively low levels of pain or only episodic pain, making them less motivated to pursue treatment. Offering psychologic interventions to patients having pain in the context of advanced cancer makes sense in that these patients tend to experience more severe and frequent pain episodes. CBT interventions delivered with advanced cancer patients, for example, can teach patients and partners coping skills that can be used to enhance their abilities to cope with pain. Although very few studies have examined the efficacy of CBT at end of life, the available evidence suggests these protocols yield significant benefits for partners (e.g. reduced caregiver strain, enhanced self-efficacy) but are less likely to produce reductions in the patient's pain. Clinicians interested in applying CBT or other psychosocial interventions need to be alert to the possibility that, in any given cancer patient, there are likely to be several windows of opportunity in which the patient is experiencing pain-related problems, is open to learning, and has the physical and emotional resources to be actively involved in learning and mastering coping skills.

A third clinical issue relates to involving a patient's partner or caregiver in pain management efforts. There is growing recognition that when cancer pain persists, it can be challenging not only for the patient but also for the partner, and the patient–partner relationship [4]. Clinical observations suggest that many partners and caregivers are actively involved in helping cancer patients manage their pain. In clinical practice, however, very few partners/caregivers report having received any formal training or education in pain management strategies. In clinical settings, instruction in pain management tends to vary a lot and typically centers mainly around the use of pain medications. Over the past 10 years, we have developed and tested protocols that systematically instruct patients and partners in cognitive and behavioral pain-coping skills. We have found these protocols to be beneficial in the management of arthritis pain [29–31] and for cancer pain that occurs at end of life [24]. In the context of cancer pain, these protocols can have a number of benefits. First, there are benefits for patients in terms of enhancing social support for coping efforts and having a partner to coach and guide them in applying coping skills during challenging and difficult time points. Second, there are benefits for partners in terms of increasing their understanding of pain coping, providing them with practical suggestions on managing pain, and giving them skills that can apply in managing their own psychologic distress. Finally, there are benefits for the patient–partner dyad in terms of enhancing their communication and the quality of relationship.

A fourth clinical issue is the background and training needed to deliver psychosocial interventions for cancer pain. To date, most CBT interventions for cancer pain have been delivered by nurses. Nurse-delivered interventions are appealing since they can be easily disseminated into clinical practice. Yet, most nurses have relatively little prior training or background in CBT or other psychosocial interventions. Psychologists, on the other hand, are very familiar with CBT and, because of this, can play an important role in enhancing the ability of other providers of CBT protocols in cancer settings. In the clinical setting, for example, a psychologist could be used to provide initial training and ongoing supervision of nurses who are delivering CBT protocols for pain management.

Another key clinical issue is the need to emphasize the ways in which psychosocial interventions such as CBT can complement and enhance medical approaches to managing cancer pain. Many effective analgesics exist that can help alleviate cancer-related pain. In real-world clinical contexts, for example, CBT is almost always used as an adjunct to analgesics, not as a replacement for them. Patients need to be encouraged by healthcare providers to view pain-coping skills and pain medications as part of a menu of strategies for managing pain. By encouraging patients to combine different pain management strategies (e.g. an opioid medication regimen with regular practice of imagery exercises), providers often can optimize pain management and minimize side effects. Interestingly, in some cases, adequate cancer pain relief is not achieved merely because the patient has difficulty adhering to his/her pain medication regimen. For these patients, CBT that focuses on improving medication adherence either as its central focus or as a corollary issue may be an effective strategy for reducing pain.

Finally, an overarching issue facing the application of psychosocial interventions for cancer pain is that most approaches to cancer pain management are based on a traditional biomedical model that emphasizes pharmacologic or surgical interventions. Patients who might benefit from psychologic interventions for cancer pain are rarely offered treatment [1]. The incorporation of CBT into clinical practice will entail more than simply broadcasting evidence that these interventions are effective in alleviating cancer-related pain. Unless and until these approaches are planted in receptive clinical soil, they are unlikely to take root and flourish. Environmental factors that will support CBT programs' development and integration into clinical practices include: training for nurses and other clinic staff, education of physicians, adequacy of facilities for providing CBT programs, organizational culture that encourages patients and providers to participate in CBT programs, consonance of CBT philosophy and goals with the general dominant care philosophy in the clinic, and funding strategies that allow CBT to flourish.

Research issues

To enhance our understanding of psychosocial interventions, there are several important directions for future research. First, future studies need to test treatment protocols that consistently meet high standards in terms of standardization and quality control. At present, for example, studies of CBT for cancer pain vary considerably in terms of treatment rationales, specific skills being taught, and number and length of treatment sessions. As a result, it is difficult to compare results across studies and to be sure that the treatment delivered was state of the art. Researchers working in this area need to develop consensus-based guidelines for standardizing CBT approaches to cancer pain. Such guidelines could, for example, identify the basic components of CBT for cancer pain management (e.g. rationale, relaxation, activity pacing, cognitive restructuring, and problem solving). They could also specify quality control procedures that should be incorporated into studies to enhance the consistency and competency of interventionists delivering CBT protocols. These quality control procedures could include, for example, audiotaping of sessions, rating of session tapes for therapist adherence and competence, and frequent review/supervision sessions with an individual who is highly experienced in CBT.

Future studies also need to test the efficacy of psychosocial interventions other than CBT in managing cancer pain. There are several novel psychosocial treatments (e.g. emotional disclosure interventions, comprehensive yoga-based therapies, and acceptance and commitment-based treatments) that may benefit cancer patients suffering from pain. Emotional disclosure interventions, first developed by Pennebaker & Beall [32], involve structured sessions (usually four or more) in which individuals are instructed to talk about or write about their deepest feelings and thoughts related to traumatic or very difficult events (e.g. cancer diagnosis or treatment). The results of studies conducted by Stanton and her colleagues suggest that emotional disclosure can enhance pain control in cancer patents. In a study of early-stage patients, Stanton et al. [33] found that women who received an emotional disclosure intervention showed a significant reduction in medical appointments for cancer-related morbidities (e.g. pain) than women who received a control writing intervention.

In a second study, Low et al. [34] reported that an emotional disclosure protocol produced significant reductions in pain in early-stage prostate cancer patients. Although the findings reported by Stanton's research team suggest that emotional disclosure may be beneficial, they need to be replicated in other research labs. Future studies also need to determine whether emotional disclosure protocols can benefit patients who experience pain in the context of advanced cancer.

Recently yoga has become popular and increasingly is being utilized with cancer patients [35]. Currently, however, the term "yoga" is synonomous with a set of physical exercises that represent but one aspect of the yoga tradition. One might expect that more comprehensive yoga protocols that incorporate the broader array of yoga techniques (i.e. physical stretching postures, breathing exercises, meditation techniques, education on pertinent topics, e.g. value of remaining mindful during daily activities, and discussion/sharing of experiences) might be particularly beneficial for cancer pain control. Although we are not aware of randomized clinical trials of comprehensive yoga, we recently conducted an uncontrolled, preliminary study in metastatic breast cancer examining the effects of a comprehensive Yoga of Awareness protocol [35]. Analysis of daily diary data revealed a dose–response relationship showing that on the day after a day during which women practiced more, they experienced significantly less pain and fatigue and significantly higher levels of acceptance, invigoration, and relaxation. These findings are interesting and suggest that further controlled research on comprehensive yoga protocols is warranted.

Acceptance and commitment therapy (ACT) is a relatively new psychologic treatment whose main goals are to help people remain more fully in the present moment and develop psychologic flexibility [36]. ACT helps people commit to actions that better enable them to be in the present, accept moment-to-moment experiences, to understand how verbal constructions of situations influence their behavior, and to focus on long-term values (e.g. family, career, spirituality). ACT has shown benefits in several areas of behavioral medicine including the treatment of diabetes [37] and drug-refractory epilepsy [38]. Research on people having persistent pain has shown that those who report higher levels of acceptance, a key process in ACT, show much lower levels of physical disability and psychologic distress [39]. ACT could help patients suffering from cancer to develop more flexible coping repertoires that enable them to better accept and deal with the challenges of severe or persistent pain. To date, however, the effects of this interesting psychologic intervention on cancer pain and pain-related outcomes have not been tested in controlled studies.

Future trials of psychologic interventions for cancer pain need to include methodologic refinements that enhance study quality. First, more attention needs to be given to control groups. To date, most studies of CBT protocols have compared these protocols to no treatment or routine care. Such control conditions, however, fail to control for therapist contact and attention. Second, to enhance cross-study comparisons, researchers need to consider standardizing the outcome measures used in studies of psychologic interventions for cancer apin. Current large-scale initiatives, of which PROMIS (Patient Reported Outcomes Measurement Information System, a National Institutes of Health Roadmap Initiative) is the largest in scope and vision, seek to develop national metrics that capture the patient's experience of symptoms, psychologic distress, function, and quality of life. PROMIS will result in an outcomes databank and an outcome measures resource bank, both of which will directly support further research on the impact of CBT on cancer pain, and will facilitate cross-study comparisons.

Finally, trials of psychologic interventions for cancer pain often use relatively small sample sizes. Small sample sizes severely limit the statistical power to detect treatment changes and the ability to generalize findings. When designing studies, it is imperative that investigators consider the availability of patients for protocols, the resources they have to conduct thorough research trials, and do appropriate *a priori* power analyses to determine the necessary number of trial participants.

More research is also needed to examine the efficacy of psychosocial intervention in different populations of cancer patients. For example, CBT interventions for cancer pain have varied in terms of types of pain being treated, from procedural pain [20] to pain that occurs at the end of life [24]. Research needs to determine which types of cancer pain are most responsive to intervention. Because not all patients will be equally likely to benefit from specific CBT interventions, future studies will need to stratify results by patient characteristics, thereby defining subpopulations of cancer pain patients who are the most appropriate recipients of specific CBT interventions. Clinical trials should strive for balance between strict eligibility criteria that focus the intervention towards patients most likely to benefit, versus less stringent criteria that may be more generalizable to usual clinical scenarios, at the risk of diluted evidence of effect.

Converging lines of evidence indicate that underserved populations and ethnic minorities may experience specific vulnerabilities in quality of life outcomes (e.g. pain) after a cancer diagnosis [40]. Despite this, few studies of psychologic interventions have addressed cancer pain management issues in ethnic minorities or underserved populations [41]. There are several barriers to the application of psychosocial interventions for underserved and minority populations including accessibility, acceptability, cultural sensitivity, language barriers, costs, and reimbursement. There is evidence that some underserved and minority groups are more amenable to psychosocial interventions while others may not be amenable [41]. Research suggests that Hispanics and African Americans may prefer psychosocial interventions to medication interventions for pain management [42]. On the other hand, Japanese cancer patients tend to repress any emotions associated with their cancer [43] and may be more reluctant to pursue psychosocial interventions for cancer pain [44]. It should be noted, however, that psychosocial interventions trials for cancer-related concerns can be effective in underserved and minority groups [45], although minimal attention has been paid to examining how to decrease the barriers to psychosocial interventions for cancer pain in these groups.

Future studies also need to examine the effects of individual components of psychologic interventions to determine which are most beneficial. It may be that methods that have been shown to be beneficial in managing procedural pain [20] are less appropriate and effective when addressing persistent pain that occurs in patients with advanced cancer.

Traditionally, psychosocial interventions have been delivered in a face-to-face format in a medical setting. There are several barriers to face-to-face treatment for cancer patients including availability of providers and physical limitations such as fatigue, time limitations, work schedules, travel distance, cost, and availability of childcare. A growing number of studies have compared the use of alternative delivery methods for cancer patients, including telephone, audiotape, internet, printed materials, and combinations of these methods, with face-to-face interventions [46, 47]. These methods show some promise for wide application of psychosocial interventions for cancer pain, but more rigorous trials are needed to understand the benefits of nontraditional methods of delivery

To date, psychosocial interventions for cancer pain generally have not been well disseminated. Psychosocial protocols for cancer pain are most often offered within a research context at a major academic medical center. Many patients who might benefit from psychosocial interventions do not have access to them [1]. Cancer Control PLANET is a new online program designed to enhance the quality of life for cancer survivors, sponsored by the National Cancer Institute, the Center for Disease Control, the American Cancer Society, and three other nationally recognized sponsors. The program acknowledges the problem of access to resources that facilitate the transfer of evidence-based research findings into practice. The website provides centralized access to intervention programs that have been rated efficacious. It also offers programs and information about how to tailor evidence-based protocols to meet the needs of specific programs. This program can serve as a centralized location for cancer pain researchers and clinicians to disseminate evidence-based psychosocial cancer pain protocols. The program can be accessed online at http://cancercontrolplanet.cancer.gov/.

Acknowledgments

Preparation of this chapter was supported by the following NIH grants: CA91947-01, CA100734-01, CA107477-01, CA092622-01A2, AG026469-01A1, U01AR052186-01.

References

1. Keefe F, Abernethy A, Campbell L. Psychological approaches to understanding and treating disease-related pain. *Annu Rev Psychol* 2005; **56**: 601–630.

2. Zaza C, Baine N. Cancer pain and psychosocial factors: a critical review of the literature. *J Pain Symptom Manage* 2002; **24**(5): 526–542.

3. Keefe F, Rumble M, Scipio C, Giardano L, Perri L. Psychological aspects of persistent pain: current state of the science. *J Pain* 2004; **5**: 195–211.

4. Keefe F, Ahles T, Porter L, *et al.* The self-efficacy of family caregivers for helping cancer patients manage pain at end-of-life. *Pain* 2003; **103**: 157–162.

5. Manne S, Ostroff J, Norton T, Fox K, Grana G, Goldstein L. Cancer-specific self-efficacy and psychosocial and functional adaptation to early stage breast cancer. *Ann Behav Med* 2006; **31**(2): 145–154.

6. Porter L, Keefe F, McBride C, Pollak K, Fish L, Garst J. Perceptions of patients' self-efficacy for managing pain and lung cancer symptoms: correspondence between patients and family caregivers. *Pain* 2002; **98**: 169–178.

7. Sullivan M, Thorn B, Haythornthwaite J, *et al.* Theoretical perspectives on the relation between catastrophizing and pain. *J Clin Pain* 2002; **17**: 52–64.

8. Keefe F, Lipkus I, Lefebvre H, Clipp E, Smith J, Porter L. The social context of gastrointestinal cancer pain: a preliminary study examining the relation of patient pain catastrophizing to patient perceptions of social support and caregiver stress and negative responses. *Pain* 2003; **103**: 151–156.

9. Lai Y, Chang J, Keefe F, *et al.* Symptom distress, catastrophic thinking, and hope in nasopharyngeal carcinoma patients. *Cancer Nurs* 2003; **26**: 485–493.

10. Porter L, Keefe F, Lipkus I, Hurwitz H. Ambivalence over emotional expression in patients with gastrointestinal cancer and their caregivers: associations with patient pain and quality of life. *Pain* 2005; **177**: 340–348.

11. Manne S, Ostroff J, Winkel G, Grana G, Fox K. Partner unsupportive responses, avoidant coping, and distress among women with early stage breast cancer: patient and partner perspectives. *Health Psychol* 2005; **24**(6): 635–641.

12. Abernethy A, Keefe F, McCrory D, Scipio C, Matchar D. Behavioral therapies for the management of cancer pain: a systematic review. Proceedings of the 11th World Congress on Pain. IASP, Seattle, 2006; 789–798.

13. Syrjala K, Roth-Roemer S. Nonpharmacologic management of pain. In: Berger AM, Portenoy RK, Weissman DE (eds) *Principles and Practice of Palliative Care and Supportive Oncology*, 2nd edn. Lippincott Williams and Wilkins, Philadelphia, 2002:1176.

14. Liossi C, Hatira P. Clinical hypnosis in the alleviation of procedure-related pain in pediatric oncology patients. *Int J Clin Exper Hypnosis* 2003; **51**(1): 4–28.

15. Liossi C, Hatira P. Clinical hypnosis versus cognitive behavioral training for pain management with pediatric cancer patients undergoing bone marrow aspirations. *Int J Clin Exper Hypnosis* 1999; **47**(2): 104–116.

16. Zeltzer L, LeBaron S. Hypnosis and nonhypnotic techniques for reduction of pain and anxiety during painful procedures in children and adolescents with cancer. *J Pediatr* 1982; **101**(6): 1032–1035.

17. Wall V, Womack W. Hypnotic versus active cognitive strategies for alleviation of procedural distress in pediatric oncology patients. *Am J Clin Hypnosis* 1989; **31**(3): 181–191.

18. Montgomery G, Weltz C, Seltz M, Bovbjerg D. Brief presurgery hypnosis reduces distress and pain in excisional breast biopsy patients. *Int J Clin Exper Hypnosis* 2002; **50**(1): 17–32.

19. Syrjala K, Cummings C, Donaldson G. Hypnosis or cognitive behavioral training for the reduction of pain and nausea during cancer treatment: a controlled clinical trial. *Pain* 1992; **48**(2): 137–146.

20. Syrjala K, Donaldson G, Davis M, Kippes M, Carr J. Relaxation and imagery and cognitive-behavioral training reduce pain during cancer treatment: a controlled clinical trial. *Pain* 1995; **63**(2): 189–198.

21. Spiegel D, Bloom J. Group therapy and hypnosis reduce metastatic breast carcinoma pain. *Psychosom Med* 1983; **45**(4): 333–339.

22. Berglund G, Bolund C, Gustafsson U, Sjoden P. One-year follow-up of the 'Starting Again' Group Rehabilitation Programme for Cancer Patients. *Eur J Cancer* 1994; **30A**(12): 1744–1751.

23. Dalton J, Keefe F, Carlson J, Youngblood R. Tailoring cognitive-behavioral treatment for cancer pain. *Pain Manage Nurs* 2004; **4**(1): 3–18.

24. Keefe F, Ahles T, Sutton L, *et al.* Partner-guided cancer pain management at end-of-life: a preliminary study. *J Pain Symptom Manage* 2005; **29**: 263–272.

25. Dalton J. Education for pain management: a pilot study. *Patient Educ Couns* 1987; **9**(2): 155–165.

26. de Wit R, van Dam F, Zandbelt L, *et al.* A pain education program for chronic cancer pain patients: follow-up results from a randomized controlled trial. *Pain* 1997; **73**(1): 55–69.

27. Lai Y, Guo S, Keefe F, *et al.* Effects of brief pain education on hospitalized cancer patients with moderate to severe pain. *Support Care Cancer* 2004; **12**(9): 645–652.

28. Gaston-Johansson F, Fall-Dickson J, Nanda J, *et al.* The effectiveness of the comprehensive coping strategy program on clinical outcomes in breast cancer autologous bone marrow transplantation. *Cancer Nurs* 2000; **23**(4): 277–285.

29. Keefe F, Caldwell D, Baucom D, *et al.* Spouse-assisted coping skills training in the management of osteoarthritis knee pain. *Arthritis Care Res* 1996; **9**: 279–291.

30. Keefe F, Caldwell D, Baucom D, *et al.* Spouse-assisted coping skills training in the management of knee pain in osteoarthritis: Long-term followup results. *Arthritis Care Res* 1999; **12**: 101–111.

31. Keefe F, Blumenthal J, Baucom D, *et al.* Effects of spouse-assisted coping skills training and exercise training in patients with osteoarthritic knee pain: a randomized controlled study. *Pain* 2004; **110**: 539–549.

32. Pennebaker J, Beall S. Confronting a traumatic event: toward an understanding of inhibition and disease. *J Abnormal Psychol* 1986; **95**: 274–281.

33. Stanton A, Danoff-Burg S, Sworowski L, *et al.* Randomized, controlled trial of written emotional expression and benefit finding in breast cancer patients. *J Clin Oncol* 2002; **20**: 4160–4168.

34. Low C, Stanton A, Danoff-Burg S. Expressive disclosure and benefit finding among breast cancer patients: mechanisms for positive health effects. *Health Psychol* 2006; **25**: 181–189.

35. Carson J, Carson K, Porter L, Keefe F, Shaw H, Miller J. Yoga for women with metastatic breast cancer: results from a pilot study. *J Pain Symptom Manage* 2007; **33**: 331–341.

36. Hayes S, Luoma J, Bond F, Masuda A, Lillis J. Acceptance and commitment therapy: model, processes, and outcomes. *Behav Res Ther* 2006; **44**: 1–25.

37. Gregg J, Callaghan G, Hayes S, Glenn-Lawson J. Improving diabetes self-management through acceptance, mindfulness, and values: a randomized controlled trial. *J Consult Clin Psychol* 2007; **75**(2): 336–343.

38. Lundgren T, Dahl J, Melin L, Kies B. Evaluation of acceptance and commitment therapy for drug refractory epilepsy: a randomized controlled trial in South Africa – a pilot study. *Epilepsia* 2006; **47**(12): 2173–2179.

39. McCracken L, Carson J, Eccleston C, Keefe F. Acceptance and change in the context of chronic pain. *Pain* 2004; **109**: 4–7.

40. Aziz N, Rowland J. Cancer survivorship research among ethnic minority and medically underserved groups. *Oncol Nurs Forum* 2002; **29**: 789–801.

41. Moadel A, Morgan C, Dutcher J. Psychosocial needs assessment among an underserved, ethnically diverse cancer patient population. *Cancer* 2007; **109**(2 suppl): 446–454.

42. Dwight-Johnson M, Sherbourne C, Liao D, Wells K. Treatment preferences among depressed primary care patients. *Gen Intern Med* 2000; **15**(8): 527–534.

43. Uchitomi Y, Sugihara J, Fukue M, *et al.* Psychiatric liaison issues in cancer care in Japan. *J Pain Symptom Manage* 1994; **9**: 319–324.

44. Fukui S, Kugaya A, Kamiya M, *et al.* Participation in psychosocial group intervention among Japanese women with primary breast cancer and its associated factors. *Psycho-oncology* 2001; **10**: 419–427.

45. Taylor K, Lamden R, Siegel J, Shelby R, Moran-Klimi K, Hrywna M. Psychological adjustment among African-American breast cancer patients: one-year follow-up results of a randomized psychoeducational group intervention. *Health Psychol* 2003; **22**(3): 316–323.

46. Donnelly J, Kornblith A, Fleishman S, *et al.* A pilot study of interpersonal psychotherapy by telephone with cancer patients and their partners. *Psycho-Oncology* 2000; **9**: 44–56.

47. Sandgren A, McCaul K. Long-term telephone therapy outcomes for breast cancer patients. *Psycho-Oncology* 2007; **16**: 38–47.

CHAPTER 27

Transcutaneous electrical nerve stimulation and acupuncture

Mark I. Johnson

Faculty of Health, Leeds Metropolitan University; and Leeds Pallium Research Group, UK

Introduction

Multimodal management of cancer pain includes multidisciplinary team assessment and holistic care using nonpharmacologic interventions. Peripheral nerve stimulation techniques such as transcutaneous electrical nerve stimulation (TENS) and acupuncture are standard therapy in pain clinics and are becoming more widely used in oncology and palliative care settings [1–4]. In general, TENS and acupuncture are indicated for symptomatic management of pain related to cancer and its treatment and can be used in combination with conventional treatments [5]. Acupuncture also has a role in the management of cancer-related nausea and vomiting, breathlessness, fatigue, xerostomia and vasomotor symptoms [6]. The techniques are safe although they may mask symptoms so tumor progression and disease should be regularly assessed [7]. The effectiveness of TENS and acupuncture has been a matter of much debate.

Transcutaneous electrical nerve stimulation

Context

Transcutaneous electrical nerve stimulation (TENS) is a noninvasive peripheral stimulation technique that is used for symptomatic relief of mild to moderate pain [8]. During TENS, pulsed electrical currents are passed across the intact surface of the skin to activate the underlying nerves. Healthcare professionals use the term TENS to describe currents delivered by a standard TENS device consisting of a hand-held battery-powered current generator and connected by lead wires to self-adhering hydrogel electrode pads. These electrodes are attached to healthy innervated skin where sensation is intact. Users can alter the pulse amplitude, pulse frequency (rate), pulse pattern and pulse duration (width) of currents (Fig. 27.1). In general, TENS is effective when a strong nonpainful electrical paresthesia is generated in dermatomes close to the site of pain [9].

TENS is safe, inexpensive and easy to use. Pain relief is rapid in onset and offset so treatment is administered by patients themselves throughout the day. TENS can be purchased without prescription in the UK although practitioners experienced in TENS should assess and supervise all new patients and provide a point of contact to troubleshoot any problems [10, 11].

Clinical technique

The intention of TENS is to activate different populations of peripheral nerves to produce segmental and extrasegmental pain modulation. Different TENS techniques are used to stimulate different types of peripheral nerve fibers.

Conventional TENS

Conventional TENS is the first treatment option in most situations. The International Association

Evidence-Based Chronic Pain Management. Edited by C. Stannard, E. Kalso and J. Ballantyne. © 2010 Blackwell Publishing.

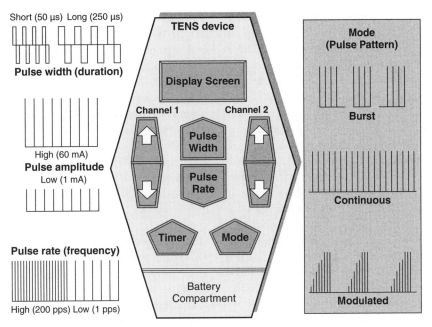

Figure 27.1 A standard TENS device.

for the Study of Pain (IASP) describe conventional TENS as "high frequency (50–100 Hz), low intensity (paresthesia, not painful), small pulse width (50–200 μs)" [12]. The intention of conventional TENS is to stimulate large-diameter non-noxious afferents (i.e. Aβ fibers) in segments related to the painful site as this inhibits second-order nociceptive cell transmission and reduces central sensitization [13–16]. In practice, intensity is titrated until a strong, comfortable, nonpainful TENS paresthesia is experienced around the painful site. Patients are encouraged to experiment with other TENS settings based on patient comfort and symptoms for relief [11, 17, 18]. Electrodes are positioned along nerves proximal to pain if mechanical allodynia exists. Painful TENS paresthesia, indicative of small-diameter noxious afferent activity, is not appropriate.

Acupuncture-like TENS

Acupuncture-like TENS (AL-TENS) is a form of hyperstimulation and was developed to harness the actions of TENS and acupuncture [19]. The IASP describe AL-TENS as currents that are "low frequency (2–4 Hz), higher intensity (to tolerance threshold), [and] longer pulse width (100–400 μs)" [12].

The intention of AL-TENS is to stimulate small-diameter afferents because this produces longer lasting segmental and extrasegmental analgesic effects [20]. In practice, AL-TENS is delivered over painful sites, muscles, trigger points and acupuncture points to generate strong but nonpainful muscle twitching [21]. The resultant small-diameter muscle afferent activity triggers descending pain inhibitory pathways and central release of endogenous opioid peptides [22]. Low-frequency bursts of high-frequency pulses (~2–5 bursts per second of 100 pps) are often used because they are more comfortable for patients than low-frequency single pulses. AL-TENS may benefit patients who do not respond to conventional TENS and some neuropathic pain conditions when it is not possible to position electrodes at the site of pain due to altered skin sensations [23, 24].

Clinical indications

Factors predicting patient success are unknown. Any patient with pain directly or indirectly related to cancer and its treatment may respond [2, 3]. This includes pain from metastatic carcinomas, metastatic bone disease, direct infiltration of nerves, and nerve compression by a neoplasm, vertebral collapse or enlarged organs. TENS may also benefit chemotherapy-related pain, postsurgical pain and postamputation pain. Clinical experience suggests that TENS is useful as a stand-alone treatment for mild to moderate pain and in combination with pharmacotherapy for moderate to severe pain.

Contraindications are cardiac pacemakers and bleeding disorders [25]. TENS can be used in pregnancy and in epilepsy providing electrodes are placed well away from the abdomen, sacrum and neck respectively. It is generally accepted that electrodes should not be positioned over an active tumor in acute oncology settings for a patient whose tumor is treatable [25]. In the palliative setting electrodes can be positioned on areas where there is known disease. No studies have directly assessed the impact of TENS on tumor growth and no detrimental effects on tumor growth have been reported in case series. TENS should not be used on irradiated skin in the immediate weeks after radiotherapy.

Anecdotes of widespread use of TENS in oncology and palliative settings are not supported by the limited amount of published evidence. An assessment of cancer pain treatments used over a 10-year period in an anesthesiology-based palliative care program in Germany revealed that TENS was only used for 3% of 2118 patients sampled [26]. A follow-up survey of 593 cancer patients found that TENS was given to support systemic analgesia in only 1% of patients with nociceptive pain, 6% of patients with neuropathic pain and 6% of patients with mixed nociceptive and neuropathic pain [27]. Audits in the UK also suggest that TENS is used only on selected cancer pain patients [28].

Research evidence

Mechanism of action
TENS causes segmental inhibition of nociceptive information by pre- and postsynaptic mechanisms [13, 14, 29–32]. TENS also reduces inflammation-induced sensitization of dorsal horn neurones in anesthetized rats [16]. TENS antidromically activates peripheral nerves leading to peripheral blockade of afferent impulses arising from noxious stimuli [33–35]. At higher intensities TENS produces longer lasting segmental effects [15, 20] and also extrasegmental effects by activating structures in the descending pain inhibitory pathways such as the periaqueductal gray and ventromedial medulla [36]. It activates diffuse noxious inhibitory controls when delivered at painful intensities as a counterirritant [38, 39]. Deep somatic afferents produce larger effects than skin afferents [39, 40].

The neuropharmacology of TENS is complex. γ-Amino butyric acid (GABA) mediates conventional TENS analgesia [41, 42] and opioids mediate AL-TENS effects [22, 43] although cholinergic [44], adrenergic [45, 46] and serotinergic systems [47] are also involved [14]. μ Opioid receptors are implicated in low-frequency TENS and δ opioid receptors in high-frequency TENS [14, 36].

Clinical effectiveness
TENS for nonmalignant pain
There are numerous clinical trials of TENS but many use an inadequate TENS technique and/or inappropriate outcome measures and this has affected the outcomes of systematic reviews. At present, opinion is divided on the use of TENS for acute pain. Initial systematic reviews on postoperative pain and labor pain concluded that there was evidence of no clinically meaningful effect from TENS [48, 49]. A subsequent meta-analysis of 21 randomized controlled trials (RCT) found that TENS reduced postoperative analgesic consumption providing adequate technique was used [50]. Recent Cochrane reviews on TENS for pain relief in labour [51] and acute pain [52] have been inconclusive. A Cochrane review found that high- but not low-frequency TENS reduced symptoms of primary dysmenorrhea [53].

Systematic reviews of TENS for chronic pain are more positive, although a recent Cochrane review was inconclusive [54]. A review of 38 RCT, of which 29 studies (1227 patients) were suitable for meta-analysis, found that TENS and percutaneous electrical nerve stimulation were effective for chronic musculoskeletal pain [55]. A systematic review of physical interventions in osteo-arthritic knee pain which included a meta-analysis on 11 RCT (414 patients) found that TENS reduced pain by 18.8 mm (95% confidence interval (CI) 9.6–28.1) on a 100 mm visual analog scale (VAS) when compared with placebo [56]. An earlier Cochrane review of seven RCT concluded that TENS was effective for pain and stiffness associated with knee osteo-arthritis [57]. Cochrane reviews on TENS for chronic low back pain [58], rheumatoid arthritis of the hand [59], whiplash and mechanical neck disorders [60], post-stroke shoulder pain [61] and chronic recurrent headache [62] have been inconclusive.

TENS for cancer-related pain

A systematic review of complementary therapies for symptoms in patients near the end of life [63] included one "pilot" RCT [64], one non-RCT [65] and two case series [66, 67] (Table 27.1). The reviewers concluded that TENS may relieve intractable pain in dying patients with cancer.

A Cochrane review on TENS for cancer-related pain identified two RCT which did not meet the criteria for meta-analysis [68, 69]. Robb *et al.* [70] conducted a randomized sham-controlled crossover trial of TENS and transcutaneous spinal electroanalgesia (TSE), which is a TENS-like device which delivers currents that do not produce any appreciable electrical paresthesia. TSE is claimed to reduce central sensitization, although evidence has not been forthcoming [71]. Forty five women with chronic pain associated with breast cancer treatment administered each intervention at home for a 3-week period followed by a 1-week washout. Forty

Table 27.1 Clinical research evidence for TENS

Reference	Condition (n)	Type of research	TENS technique	Results
Robb *et al.* [70]	Chronic pain secondary to treatment for breast cancer (41 completed)	RCT (cross-over) TENS TSE Sham TSE	Conventional TENS	No differences between groups. On completion of study 15 patients requested to continue to use TENS compared to 5 for TSE and 6 for sham
Gadsby *et al.* [64]	Pain from various malignancies in palliative care setting (15)	RCT (parallel group) AL-TENS Sham AL-TENS No treatment control	AL-TENS	Odds ratio AL-TENS 0.5 times greater than placebo and 0.16 times better than no treatment control
Avellanosa & West [65]	Pain from a variety of metastatic carcinomas (60)	Pre/post assessment without control group	Conventional TENS	39/60 patients reported pain relief at 2 weeks and 20/60 at 3 months
Hasun & Marberger [77]	Pain related to advanced cancer of prostate, renal cells or urothelial bladder (45)	Pre/post assessment without control group	Uncertain – galvanic current?	Every other patient responded to TENS
Ostrowski [66]	Pain related to various carcinomas who responded to TENS (9)	Pre/post assessment without control group	Conventional TENS	8/9 patients reported immediate pain relief and 3/9 continued to use TENS at 6 months
Loeser *et al.* [80]	198 chronic pain patients (7 malignancies)	Pre/post assessment without control group	Conventional TENS	3/7 cancer patients reported pain relief
Long [79]	197 chronic pain patients (5 malignancies)	Pre/post assessment without control group	Conventional TENS	3/5 cancer patients reported pain relief
Hardy [81]	53 chronic pain patients (4 malignancies)	Pre/post assessment without control group	Conventional TENS	2/4 cancer patients reported pain relief
Ventafridda *et al.* [73]	Various pains in which cancer was the primary cause (37)	Pre/post assessment without control group	Conventional TENS	36/37 patients reported pain relief in first 10 days but only 4/37 reported pain relief at 30 days

Continued on p. 352

Table 27.1 *Continued*

Reference	Condition (n)	Type of research	TENS technique	Results
Bates & Nathan [82]	161 chronic pain patients (5 malignancies)	Pre/post assessment without control group	Conventional TENS	4/5 cancer patients reported pain relief
Rafter [74] cited in Librach & Rapson [75]	Pain from malignancies predominantly of musculoskeletal origin (49)	Pre/post assessment without control group	Conventional TENS	37/49 patients reported pain relief
Dil'din *et al.* [78]	Pain from malignancies and postoperative procedures (84)	Pre/post assessment without control group	Conventional TENS using a Soviet device	84/84 patients reported pain relief
Reuss & Meyer [72]	Pain predominantly from bony metastasis (60)	Pre/post assessment without control group	Conventional TENS	50/60 patients reported pain relief
Hidderley & Weinel [76]	Pain from head and neck cancers in patients undergoing radiotherapy (4)	Pre/post assessment without control group	TENS on acupuncture points away from the site of pain (TENS intensity very low)	4/4 patients reported pain relief
Wen [67]	Pain from a variety of malignancies (29)	Pre/post assessment without control group	Conventional TENS	Reductions in opioid consumption

one women completed the trial. TENS and TSE reduced pain when compared to baseline but the effect was no greater than that observed with sham TSE. At the end of the study 15 patients selected to continue treatment with TENS compared with five for TSE and six for sham. Gadsby *et al.* [64] conducted a randomized sham-controlled parallel group trial of AL-TENS, sham AL-TENS and no treatment in 15 patients with cancers of the breast, colon, pancreas, kidney, stomach and cervix. Treatment interventions were administered for 30 minutes per day for 5 days and odds ratios suggested that AL-TENS was superior to sham and no treatment (see Table 27.1). However, the study was underpowered so a conclusion about effectiveness is not possible.

Low-quality evidence from uncontrolled trials and case series tends to be positive and may be likely to overestimate TENS effects. Avellanosa & West [65] conducted a nonrandomized controlled trial using 60 patients with pain related to metastatic carcinomas, surgery, irradiation and amputation. TENS reduced pain in 39 patients at 2 weeks but this dropped to 20 patients at 3 months. Reuss & Meyer [72] reported that TENS was beneficial for 50 out of 60 patients, many with painful bony metastasis. Ventafridda *et al.* [73] reported that initially TENS reduced pain in 35 out of 37 patients with a variety of pains arising from compression by large masses over the cervical nerve trunks or neoplastic involvement on maxillofacial tissues. However, only four patients reported benefit at 1 month. Rafter p.72] (cited in Librach & Rapson [76]) reported that TENS provided benefit in 36 out of 49 patients with a variety of malignancies and Ostrowski [66] reported that TENS outcome was good in seven out of nine patients with various carcinomas and metastases in the spine, lung and jaw. Hidderley & Weinel [76] reported that TENS of acupuncture points away from the pain site reduced pain in four out of four patients with head and neck cancers undergoing radiotherapy, and Wen [67] found that TENS and acupuncture reduced severe pain in 18 out of 29 frail cancer patients. Similar findings are available in case series of mixed populations of patients with chronic pain, some of whom have cancer-related pain [77–82]. Recently, a case series reported benefit whilst using TENS for cancer bone pain [83, 84], and a following feasibility trial suggested that TENS has the potential to decrease pain on movement more than pain on rest [85].

There is for the moment insufficient high-quality clinical research evidence to demonstrate the effectiveness of TENS for cancer pain. Indeed, there is no consensus on the optimal use of TENS for many conditions. Yet widespread clinical experience, as reported in noncontrolled clinical trials and case series, suggests that TENS may be useful in both the short and long term. No serious complications from TENS were reported in any of these published trials.

TENS for cancer-related nonpain symptoms
Transcutaneous electrical nerve stimulation over the Pericardium 6 (P6, Neiguan) acupuncture point has been used for chemotherapy-induced and postoperative nausea and vomiting [86, 87]. RCTs provide evidence that transcutaneous electrical acupoint stimulation using a TENS-like device reduces postoperative nausea and vomiting in non-cancer patients [88–90] and a Cochrane review of 24 RCT concluded that nonpharmacologic techniques such as TENS, acupuncture, and electroacupuncture were better than placebo [91]. In contrast, another Cochrane review concluded that noninvasive electrostimulation (TENS) was unlikely to have a clinically meaningful outcome for chemotherapy-induced nausea and vomiting [92]. TENS has been reported to be beneficial for the management of lymphedema when electrodes are placed proximal to the lymphedematous limb [93].

Acupuncture

Context

Acupuncture is the process of inserting needles in the skin at specific points (Latin *acus* "needle", *punctura*, "puncture"). Additional stimulation is achieved by needle manipulation (twirling) or by passing mild electrical currents through pairs of needles (electroacupuncture). Points can also be stimulated using pressure (acupressure), laser, and heat (moxibustion). According to traditional Chinese medicine, acupuncture can alter the flow of "vital energies of life," called Yin and Yang, along "energy channels" called meridians. However, most medical practitioners adopt a neurophysiologic approach to acupuncture using the principles of orthodox medicine for diagnosis.

Clinical technique

Treatment with acupuncture requires a trained specialist (www.medical-acupuncture.co.uk). Acupuncture is administered using fine disposable steel needles (0.2–0.3 mm) at points with properly functioning nerves to stimulate subcutaneous, intramuscular and periosteal tissue [2]. A segmental approach is used by locating needles at dermatomes, myotomes and sclerotomes related to the affected structure. Traditional strong extrasegmental points (e.g. L14) and trigger points are also chosen in certain circumstances. Acupuncture effects are usually slow in onset but usually persist for several days or weeks and may be cumulative over time. Needles are inserted for up to 30 minutes at a time and may be "twirled" to facilitate stimulation. A typical course of acupuncture may last up to 6 weeks and consist of one or two treatments each week. Sensations of heaviness, aching, paresthesia and numbness may be experienced around the needle, called needle sensation or De Qi, and some practitioners believe De Qi is important for outcome.

Practice guidelines [94, 95] and clinical considerations for the use of acupuncture for cancer patients have been published [5, 6, 89, 96–98]. Contraindications include patients with clotting dysfunction, needle phobia and intracardiac defibrillators (electroacupuncture) [7, 99]. Semi-permanent needles are contraindicated for patients with valvular heart disease, neutropenia or after splenectomy. Acupuncture should not be given to limbs with lymphedema, arms following axillary dissection or sampling, tumor nodules, areas of ulceration or on an unstable spine [94]. Cancer patients may be sensitive to acupuncture and may be "strong reactors." Gentle stimulation and close supervision are essential, especially during the first acupuncture treatment. Experts recommend a mix of segmental, extrasegmental and trigger points depending on presenting symptoms.

Clinical indications

Acupuncture is used to manage pain, xerostomia, nausea and vomiting, dyspnea, radiation rectitis, ulcers which fail to heal, intractable fatigue, insomnia and vasomotor symptoms such as hot flushes [94]. It is especially useful for patients whose pain is not satisfactorily managed by conventional analgesia, who are resistant to high-dosage pain medication and/or experiencing unacceptable side effects and who are sensitive to medication.

Up to three-quarters of cancer patients may use complementary therapies although estimates vary widely [100–106]. However, a recent survey of complementary medicine use by 189 women with nonsmall cell lung cancer found that only 2.6% used acupuncture [107]. Once it is integrated into the cancer clinics, patients consider acupuncture as "very important" [108].

Research evidence

The contribution of needling to acupuncture effects has been investigated using sham interventions although some of these are inappropriate, e.g. dummy TENS, dummy laser, "superficial" needling [109]. Sham acupuncture needles which telescope instead of penetrating the skin (e.g. Park sham device) are more appropriate although initial reports that they were indistinguishable from real needles [110] have been challenged [111, 112] because they do cause some degree of acupressure, i.e. are not completely inert.

The contribution of needles positioned on specific points on the body to acupuncture effects has been addressed through comparisons of stimulation at acupuncture points versus nonacupuncture points or acupuncture points not indicated for the condition. Critics of this approach have argued that stimulation of any point on the skin will produce neurophysiologic effects, although the premise still remains that during acupuncture it is important to demonstrate that certain points are superior to others. A critique of controls used in acupuncture trials concluded that it was scientifically unacceptable to summarize the variety of approaches as "placebo control" as is sometimes the case in systematic reviews [113].

Mechanism of action

Acupuncture is a high-intensity stimulus that activates polymodal receptors and high-threshold, small-diameter Aβ, Aδ and C-fibers leading to inhibition of second-order nociceptive transmission cells by segmental and extrasegmental mechanisms [1, 114, 117]. Acupuncture activates structures on the descending pain inhibitory pathways, including the ventromedial medulla and periaqueductal gray (PAG) which have collaterals that project to many levels of the spinal cord [118–120]. Acupuncture

also produces effects similar to those observed during diffuse noxious inhibitory controls [37, 38, 121].

Acupuncture and electroacupuncture upregulate opioid gene production and this may explain why "top-ups" are required to maintain gene expression in a "switched-on" mode [122–124]. Low-frequency electroacupuncture causes preproenkephalin mRNA expression in the rat brain and high-frequency electroacupuncture causes preprodynorphin mRNA expression [125]. The neuropharmacology of acupuncture is complex and involves opioids, serotonin, noradrenaline, adrenocorticotrophic hormone, cholecystokinin, nerve growth factor and oxytocin, to name but a few [1, 116, 126–128].

Recently, brain-imaging studies have demonstrated that acupuncture influences a matrix of structures extending from the cerebrum to the cerebellum [129–131]. Limbic system structures involved in emotion and reward have a critical role and include the anterior cingulate, hippocampus, insula, amygdala and nucleus accumbens [129, 132–135]. They may be responsible for pleasurable feelings sometimes associated with acupuncture and for reports that pain remains but is less unpleasant [136]. Different activation patterns between patients and healthy controls have been reported [137], in line with evidence from animal studies that acupuncture differs in its actions in normal versus inflammatory states [138]. A recent study on heroin addicts suggests that the hypothalamus may be involved in De Qi [139].

Investigators have reported a somatotopic representation of acupuncture points in the primary somatosensory cortex [140, 141] and that deep central areas of the brain appear to respond differently with genuine acupuncture compared with sham [133]. Specific patterns of brain activity are produced when acupuncture is given at different points [142, 143] and durations [144]. The long-lasting analgesic effects of acupuncture have been attributed to a mesolimbic positive feedback loop which perpetuates continuous outflow from descending pain inhibitory pathways [145]. Electroacupuncture produces different brain activation patterns to manual acupuncture [132, 146, 147] and may be dependent on the frequency of the electrical currents [127, 132, 148]. A criticism of brain-imaging studies is that they often use a single measurement and there may be large variability across different sessions within the same subject [149–151].

Evidence for meridians is not convincing although physiologic correlates have been reported, including electrical conductive properties [152, 153] and intermuscular or intramuscular connective tissue planes [154]. Associations between acupuncture points and trigger points [155] and tendinomuscular and tendinofascial structures are tantalizing [156, 157].

Clinical effectiveness

Acupuncture for nonmalignant pain

There are hundreds of RCTs and many systematic reviews on acupuncture and making sense of the research evidence has become a discipline in itself. A systematic review of systematic reviews concluded that there was no robust evidence that acupuncture works for any indication [158]. The Centre for Reviews and Dissemination in the UK concluded that acupuncture was superior to no treatment or waiting list controls in most studies but studies were evenly balanced between acupuncture and sham techniques [159]. A recent critique concluded that acupuncture improves symptoms associated with nausea and vomiting (postoperative and chemotherapy-related), insomnia, fibromyalgia, osteo-arthritis of the knee, nonspecific back pain, dental pain, epicondylitis and idiopathic headache [160].

Two meta-analyses on acupuncture for osteoarthritis of the knee published within 6 months of each other highlight the disparity in interpretation of existing evidence. White *et al.* concluded that "Acupuncture that meets criteria for adequate treatment is significantly superior to sham acupuncture and to no additional intervention in improving pain and function in patients with chronic knee pain" p384) [161]. Manheimer *et al.* concluded that "Sham-controlled trials show clinically irrelevant short-term benefits of acupuncture for treating knee osteoarthritis. Waiting list-controlled trials suggest clinically relevant benefits, some of which may be due to placebo or expectation effects" (p868) [162]. There are indisputable methodologic challenges which hinder RCT design, including inappropriate controls with active therapeutic effects [109, 113] and insufficient doses of acupuncture [160, 163–166].

Acupuncture for cancer-related pain

There is one systematic review of acupuncture for cancer-related pain which concluded there was insufficient evidence to determine effectiveness [167]. Seven trials met the eligibility criteria but only three of these were RCTs [168–170] and four were studies without controls [98, 171–173].

The RCT with the strongest methodologic quality found that auricular acupuncture reduced neuropathic pain arising after cancer treatment by 36% at the 2-month follow-up when compared with sham controls [170] (Table 27.2). The study used 90 patients randomized into one of three possible interventions: auricular acupuncture; auricular acupuncture at nonacupuncture points; and nonpenetrating auricular acupuncture at nonacupuncture points. The other two RCTs were scored low on methodologic quality. Dang & Yang [169] included 48 patients with stomach carcinomas and found no statistical differences between acupuncture using filiform needle, acupuncture point injection with "transfer factor" or conventional analgesics. However, acupuncture had superior long-term effects than conventional analgesics for plasma-leucine-enkephalin concentrations. Xia *et al.* [168] included 72 patients with chest pain related to upper body malignancies and found that acupuncture reduced pain when compared to radiotherapy and chemotherapy alone. The studies without a control group reported benefits from acupuncture on cancer-related neuropathic pain [171], abdominal pain [172], nerve compression pain [173] and breathlessness [98]. It is possible that false-positive findings arose in these studies, with authors possibly overstating the benefit of acupuncture and the role of expectation in the patients being unclear. Some early case series did not meet the eligibility criteria for systematic reviews [67, 97].

Studies published since the reviews are inconclusive. Mehling *et al.* [174] reported that a combination of massage and acupuncture reduced pain and depressive mood when added to usual care in 138 postoperative cancer patients, although differences in outcome were small. Wong & Sager [175] reported that acupuncture reduced chemotherapy-induced peripheral neuropathic pain in five patients. Minton & Higginson [176] attempted to undertake a single-blind RCT of electroacupuncture on cancer-related neuropathic pain but only three patients completed the study.

Reviews of complementary therapies by Bardia *et al.* [177] and Pan *et al.* [63] include the same

Table 27.2 Clinical research evidence for acupuncture

Reference	Condition (n)	Type of research	Acupuncture technique	Results
Lee et al. [167]	Cancer related pain excluding postoperative pain	Systematic review 3 RCT (Jadad scores) Alimi et al. [170] (5/5) Dang & Yang [169] (1/5) Xia et al. [168] (1/5) 4 uncontrolled trials (all 0/5) Alimi et al. [171] Filshie et al. [98] Xu et al. [172] Rico & Trudnowski [173]	Manual acupuncture Auricular acupuncture Electroacupuncture	Insufficient evidence to make conclusion
Alimi et al. [170]	Peripheral/central neuropathic pain after cancer-related treatment (90)	RCT (parallel group) Auricular acupuncture at "true" points Auricular acupuncture at "nonacupuncture" points Sham auricular acupuncture using nonpenetrating needles at "nonacupuncture" points	Auricular acupuncture Point selection: on an individual basis according to electrodermal response. Implanted auricular needles left in situ until fell out Treatment course: needles replaced at 1 month follow-up. Conventional medication continued	Significant reductions in pain for acupuncture compared to nonacupoint and sham at 1 and 2 months
Dang & Yang [169]	Chest, abdomen and back pain related to gastric carcinomas (48)	RCT (parallel group) Acupuncture using filiform needle (16) Acupuncture point injection with "transfer factor aqueous solution" (16) Western medicine (WHO analgesic ladder, 16) [no treatment control (16)]	Manual acupuncture Point selection: individual basis 1 = ST36, Sp6, ST34, P6, LI11, LI4 2 = P2, St19, Sp12, Sp10 Treatment course: 2 months 1 and 2 = 1 × 20 min session per day for 2 weeks; 3 day interval between courses	Effective rate of analgesia All interventions relieved pain with no significant differences between groups
Xia et al. [168]	Chest pain associated with lung, esophageal and stomach cancer (72)	RCT (parallel group) Manual acupuncture (38) Radiotherapy or chemotherapy (38)	Manual acupuncture Point selection: individual basis P6, St36 + others Treatment course: 1 course for 30 days. Conventional medication continued	Reduction in chest pain – no statistical analysis

Minton & Higginson [176]	Neuropathic pain associated with cancer (only 3 completed)	RCT (cross-over) Electroacupuncture Sham acupuncture (Park sham device)	Electroacupuncture (2 Hz and 80 Hz) Point selection: individual basis on recognized acupuncture meridians Treatment course: 1 × 30 min session for 6 weeks followed by 4 week washout and cross-over	No conclusion as only 3 patients completed study
Mehling et al. [174]	Postoperative pain associated with cancer-related surgeries of the breast, abdomen, pelvis, head and neck (138)	RCT (parallel group) Acupuncture, massage and usual care (93) Usual care alone (45)	Manual acupuncture Point selection: core set of points (LI4, Sp6, auricular points) with additional points added Treatment course: 1 × 30 min treatment of acupuncture and 1 × 30 min treatment of "Swedish" massage given each day – sequence and timing variable	Greater pain reduction when acupuncture and massage added to usual care. Cannot separate effects of acupuncture from massage
Wong & Sagar [175]	Pain associated with chemotherapy-induced peripheral neuropathy (5)	Pre/post assessment without control group	Manual acupuncture Point selection: CV6, ST36, LI11, Ba Feng, Ba Xie Treatment course: 1 × 30–45 min session of 6 weeks followed by 4 weeks rest and then repeat 6 week course again	All patients reported pain reduction
Alimi et al. [171]	Peripheral/central neuropathic pain associated with cancer inadequately managed with analgesics (20)	Pre/post assessment without control group	Auricular acupuncture Point selection: on an individual basis according to electrodermal response. Implanted auricular needles left in situ until fell out Treatment course: conventional medication continued	Mean pain decrease over 2 months = 33 mm on 100 mm VAS

Continued on p. 358

Table 27.2 *Continued*

Reference	Condition (n)	Type of research	Acupuncture technique	Results
Filshie et al. [98]	Breathlessness and other symptoms, including anxiety and pain, associated with malignancy (20)	Pre/post assessment without control group	Manual acupuncture Point selection: LI4, ST36, 2 studs on sternum Needles left *in situ* for maximum of 10 minutes Treatment course: 1 treatment Conventional medication continued	No changes in pain were reported but there was a reduction in breathlessness in 14/20 patients which was the primary outcome measure
Xu et al. [172]	Abdominal pain associated with stomach cancer (92)	Pre/post assessment without control group	Manual acupuncture Point selection: ST36 bilateral Treatment course: 14 sessions in 2 weeks. No concurrent medication used	81/90 patients reported complete or much relief at 1 month
Filshie & Redman [97]	Patients with pain from a range of malignancies including breast, bronchus, cervix (146) and also cancer patients with pain unrelated to cancer (37)	Pre/post assessment without control group	Manual acupuncture Point selection: on an individual basis Needles inserted for a maximum of 15 minutes Treatment course: open, on an as-needed basis, after 3 or more weekly intervals Conventional medication continued	52% significant pain relief; 30% some pain relief; 18% no pain relief
Rico & Trudnowski [173]	Poorly managed radiating back pain associated with various malignancies (22)	Pre/post assessment without control group	Electroacupuncture (6–8 Hz) Point selection: unknown Treatment course: 1 × session of unknown duration for 7 days Conventional medication continued	18/22 patients reported benefit
Wen [67]	Various pains associated with cancer and its treatment (29)	Pre/post assessment without control group	Electroacupuncture Point selection: unknown Treatment course: several per day and then on an as-needed basis	Reductions in opioid consumption

acupuncture trials as Lee *et al.* [167] and conclude that acupuncture may be useful in the short term, but recommendations were not possible because of a paucity of rigorous trials.

Acupuncture for cancer-related nonpain symptoms
A meta-analysis of 11 trials (n = 1247) found that acupuncture point stimulation by any method (needles, electrical stimulation, magnets or acupressure) did not reduce chemotherapy-induced nausea severity in cancer patients but did reduce the incidence of acute vomiting [178]. Needle stimulation was better than noninvasive electrical stimulation for acute vomiting but not for nausea severity.

Electroacupuncture was better than manual acupuncture for reducing acute vomiting. Self-administered acupressure reduced acute nausea severity but not acute vomiting.

It is claimed that stimulation of acupuncture points can relieve dyspnea, and RCTs for nonmalignant breathlessness due to chronic obstructive cardiopulmonary disease have been positive [179–181] although one pilot RCT was inconclusive [182]. A pilot RCT using 47 patients with lung or breast cancer with dyspnea found no significant differences between true and sham acupuncture delivered as a single session followed by twice-daily self-administration using studs [183]. A case series of 20 patients found that sternal and LI4 acupuncture reduced cancer-related breathlessness at rest in 14 of the patients [98].

A critical review of complementary therapies for cancer-related fatigue concluded that there were insufficient data to recommend acupuncture [184]. The reviewers found only one trial, a phase II RCT, using 37 patients with fatigue following cytotoxic chemotherapy [185]. Patients received acupuncture either twice per week for 4 weeks or once per week for 6 weeks. Fatigue improved by 31.1% (95% CI 20.6–41.5%).

A systematic review on the efficacy of acupuncture for xerostomia found three articles that met the criteria for inclusion [186]. The reviewers judged that one trial was of high methodologic quality and reported inconclusive findings in patients with radiation-induced xerostomia [187]. The trials of low methodologic quality reported positive outcomes in patients with xerostomia of various causes [188] and negative outcomes in patients with Sjögren's syndrome [189].

The reviewers concluded that evidence was lacking and that a high-quality RCT was needed [186]. The fact that acupuncture helped patients with xerostomia refractory to treatment with pilocarpine is clinically relevant and may merit further testing.

Patients with breast and prostate cancer undergoing anticancer therapy may experience treatment-related vasomotor symptoms. Several RCTs have found that acupuncture reduces menopausal symptoms although evidence from cancer patients is mostly limited to case series [190]. Nedstrand *et al.* evaluated relaxation and electroacupuncture in 38 breast cancer-treated postmenopausal women with vasomotor symptoms and found that hot flushes were reduced by more than 50% in both groups [191]. A retrospective audit of 194 patients with breast and prostate cancer found that 114 (79%) patients achieved 50% or greater reduction in hot flushes [96]. Patients were treated with six weekly acupuncture treatments given at LI4, TE5, LR3 and SP6 and upper sternal points, and instructed to perform weekly self-acupuncture using semi-permanent or conventional needling for up to 6 years. A treatment algorithm for management of vasomotor symptoms has been developed to guide clinical practice.

Conclusion

Transcutaneous electrical nerve stimulation and acupuncture have an increasing clinical role alongside pharmacologic management for cancer-related pain and particularly for patients who have failed to respond to conventional treatment. Much valuable observational work has been performed, yet at present, there is a lack of high-quality evidence to determine more precisely the effectiveness of both modalities. This may be partly due to lack of research funding for nondrug treatments. There is an obvious need for more clinical trials although 46 trials of acupuncture for cancer were listed on the US National Institutes of Health clinical trials register on 1 September 2009 (http: //clinicaltrials.gov).

Acknowledgment
I am most grateful to Jacky Filshie and John Thompson for their assistance in preparing this chapter.

References

1. Barlas P, Lundeberg T. Transcutaneous electrical nerve stimulation and acupuncture. In: McMahon S, Koltzenburg M (eds) *Melzack and Wall's Textbook of Pain*, 5th edn. Elsevier Churchill Livingstone, Philadelphia, 2006: 583–590.

2. Filshie J, Thompson J. Acupuncture and TENS. In: Simpson KH, Budd K (eds) *Cancer Pain Management. A Comprehensive Approach*. Oxford University Press, Oxford, 2000: 188–223.

3. Berkovitch M, Waller A. Treating pain with transcutaneous electrical nerve stimulation (TENS). In: Doyle D, Hanks G, Cherny NI, Calman K (eds) *Oxford Textbook of Palliative Medicine*. Oxford University Press, Oxford, 2005: 405–410.

4. Stannard C. Simulation-induced analgesia in cancer pain management. In: Sykes N, Fallon M, Patt R (eds) *Textbook of Clinical Pain Management*. Hodder Arnold, London, 2002: 245–252.

5. Filshie J. The non-drug treatment of neuralgic and neuropathic pain of malignancy. *Cancer Surv* 1988; **7**(1): 161–193.

6. Cohen AJ, Menter A, Hale L. Acupuncture: role in comprehensive cancer care – a primer for the oncologist and review of the literature. *Integrat Cancer Ther* 2005; **4**(2): 131–143.

7. Filshie J. Safety aspects of acupuncture in palliative care. *Acupunct Med* 2001; **19**(2): 117–122.

8. Walsh D. *TENS. Clinical Applications and Related Theory*. Churchill Livingstone, New York, 1997.

9. Johnson MI. Transcutaneous electrical nerve stimulation. In: Kitchen S (ed) *Electrotherapy: Evidence-Based Practice*. Churchill Livingstone, Edinburgh, 2002: 259–286.

10. Chabal C, Fishbain DA, Weaver M, Heine LW. Long-term transcutaneous electrical nerve stimulation (TENS) use: impact on medication utilization and physical therapy costs. *Clin J Pain* 1998; **14**(1): 66–73.

11. Johnson MI. Transcutaneous electrical nerve stimulation (TENS) – outcomes. In: Schmidt RF, Willis WD (eds) *Encyclopedia of Pain*. Springer-Verlag, Berlin, 2007: 2511–2514.

12. Charlton JE. Task Force on Professional Education (eds). Stimulation-produced analgesia. In: *Core Curriculum for Professional Education in Pain*. IASP Press, Seattle, 2005: 93–96.

13. Garrison DW, Foreman RD. Decreased activity of spontaneous and noxiously evoked dorsal horn cells during transcutaneous electrical nerve stimulation (TENS). *Pain* 1994; **58**(3): 309–315.

14. Sluka KA, Walsh D. Transcutaneous electrical nerve stimulation: basic science mechanisms and clinical effectiveness. *J Pain* 2003; **4**(3): 109–121.

15. Sandkühler J, Chen JG, Cheng G, Randic M. Low-frequency stimulation of afferent Adelta-fibers induces long-term depression at primary afferent synapses with substantia gelatinosa neurons in the rat. *J Neurosci* 1997; **17**(16): 6483–6491.

16. Ma YT, Sluka KA. Reduction in inflammation-induced sensitization of dorsal horn neurons by transcutaneous electrical nerve stimulation in anesthetized rats. *Exper Brain Res* 2001; **137**(1): 94–102.

17. Johnson MI, Ashton CH, Thompson JW. An in-depth study of long-term users of transcutaneous electrical nerve stimulation (TENS). Implications for clinical use of TENS. *Pain* 1991; **44**(3): 221–229.

18. King EW, Sluka KA. The effect of varying frequency and intensity of transcutaneous electrical nerve stimulation on secondary mechanical hyperalgesia in an animal model of inflammation. *J Pain* 2001; **2**(2): 128–133.

19. Eriksson M, Sjölund B. Acupuncture-like electroanalgesia in TNS resistant chronic pain. In: Zotterman Y (ed) *Sensory Functions of the Skin*. Pergamon Press, New York, 1976: 575–581.

20. Sandkühler J. Long-lasting analgesia following TENS and acupuncture: Spinal mechanisms beyond gate control. In: Devor M, Rowbotham MC, Wiesenfeld-Hallin Z (eds) *Progress In Pain Research And Management*, vol 16. IASP Press, Seattle 2000: 359–369.

21. Johnson MI. The analgesic effects and clinical use of acupuncture-like TENS (AL-TENS). *Phys Ther Rev*. 1998; **3**: 73–93.

22. Sjölund B, Terenius L, Eriksson M. Increased cerebrospinal fluid levels of endorphins after electro-acupuncture. *Acta Physiol Scand* 1977; **100**(3): 382–384.

23. Eriksson MB, Sjölund BH, Nielzen S. Long term results of peripheral conditioning stimulation as an analgesic measure in chronic pain. *Pain* 1979; **6**(3): 335–347.

24. Eriksson MB, Sjölund BH, Sundbarg G. Pain relief from peripheral conditioning stimulation in patients with chronic facial pain. *J Neurosurg* 1984; **61**(1): 149–155.

25. Chartered Society of Physiotherapy. *Guidance for the Clinical Use of Electrophysical Agents*. Chartered Society of Physiotherapy, London, 2006.

26. Zech DF, Grond S, Lynch J, Hertel D, Lehmann KA. Validation of World Health Organization Guidelines for cancer pain relief: a 10-year prospective study. *Pain* 1995; **63**(1): 65–76.

27. Grond S, Radbruch L, Meuser T, Sabatowski R, Loick G, Lehmann KA. Assessment and treatment of neuropathic cancer pain following WHO guidelines. *Pain* 1999; **79**(1): 15–20.

28. Hoskin PJ, Hanks GW. The management of symptoms in advanced cancer: experience in a hospital-based continuing care unit. *J Roy Soc Med* 1988; **81**(6): 341–344.

29. Garrison DW, Foreman RD. Effects of transcutaneous electrical nerve stimulation (TENS) on spontaneous and noxiously evoked dorsal horn cell activity in cats with transected spinal cords. *Neurosci Lett* 1996; **216**(2): 125–128.

30. Leem J, Park E, Paik K. Electrophysiological evidence for the antinociceptive effect of transcutaneous electrical stimulation on mechanically evoked responsiveness of dorsal horn neurons in neuropathic rats. *Neurosci Lett* 1995; **192**(3): 197–200.

31. Lee K, Chung J, Willis WD J. Inhibition of primate spinothalamic tract cells by TENS. *J Neurosurg* 1985; **62**(2): 276–287.

32. Urasaki E, Wada S, Yasukouchi H, Yokota A. Effect of transcutaneous electrical nerve stimulation (TENS) on central nervous system amplification of somatosensory input. *J Neurol* 1998; **245**(3): 143–148.

33. Ignelzi RJ, Nyquist JK. Excitability changes in peripheral nerve fibers after repetitive electrical stimulation. Implications in pain modulation. *J Neurosurg* 1979; **51**(6): 824–833.

34. Walsh DM, Lowe AS, McCormack K, Willer JC, Baxter GD, Allen JM. Transcutaneous electrical nerve stimulation: effect on peripheral nerve conduction, mechanical pain threshold, and tactile threshold in humans. *Arch Phys Med Rehabil* 1998; **79**(9): 1051–1058.

35. Nardone A, Schieppati M. Influences of transcutaneous electrical stimulation of cutaneous and mixed nerves on subcortical and cortical somatosensory evoked potentials. *Electroencephalogr Clin Neurophysiol* 1989; **74**(1): 24–35.

36. Kalra A, Urban MO, Sluka KA. Blockade of opioid receptors in rostral ventral medulla prevents antihyperalgesia produced by transcutaneous electrical nerve stimulation (TENS). *J Pharmacol Exper Therapeut* 2001; **298**(1): 257–263.

37. Le Bars D, Dickenson AH, Besson JM. Diffuse noxious inhibitory controls (DNIC). I. Effects on dorsal horn convergent neurones in the rat. *Pain* 1979; **6**(3): 283–304.

38. Morton CR, Du HJ, Xiao HM, Maisch B, Zimmermann M. Inhibition of nociceptive responses of lumbar dorsal horn neurones by remote noxious afferent stimulation in the cat. *Pain* 1988; **34**(1): 75–83.

39. Duranti R, Pantaleo T, Bellini F. Increase in muscular pain threshold following low frequency-high intensity peripheral conditioning stimulation in humans. *Brain Res* 1988; **452**(1–2): 66–72.

40. Radhakrishnan R, Sluka KA. Deep tissue afferents, but not cutaneous afferents, mediate transcutaneous electrical nerve stimulation-Induced antihyperalgesia. *J Pain* 2005; **6**(10): 673–680.

41. Duggan AW, Foong FW. Bicuculline and spinal inhibition produced by dorsal column stimulation in the cat. *Pain* 1985; **22**(3): 249–259.

42. Maeda Y, Lisi TL, Vance CG, Sluka KA. Release of GABA and activation of GABA(A) in the spinal cord mediates the effects of TENS in rats. *Brain Res* 2007; **1136**(1): 43–50.

43. Sjölund BH, Eriksson MB. The influence of naloxone on analgesia produced by peripheral conditioning stimulation. *Brain Res* 1979; **173**(2): 295–301.

44. Radhakrishnan R, Sluka KA. Spinal muscarinic receptors are activated during low or high frequency TENS-induced antihyperalgesia in rats. *Neuropharmacology* 2003; **45**(8): 1111–1119.

45. King EW, Audette K, Athman GA, Nguyen HO, Sluka KA, Fairbanks CA. Transcutaneous electrical nerve stimulation activates peripherally located alpha−2A adrenergic receptors. *Pain* 2005; **115**(3): 364–373.

46. Sluka KA, Chandran P. Enhanced reduction in hyperalgesia by combined administration of clonidine and TENS. *Pain* 2002; **100**(1–2): 183–190.

47. Radhakrishnan R, King EW, Dickman JK, *et al.* Spinal 5–HT(2) and 5–HT(3) receptors mediate low, but not high, frequency TENS-induced antihyperalgesia in rats. *Pain* 2003; **105**(1–2): 205–213.

48. Carroll D, Tramer M, McQuay H, Nye B, Moore A. Randomization is important in studies with pain outcomes: systematic review of transcutaneous electrical nerve stimulation in acute postoperative pain. *Br J Anaesthes* 1996; **77**(6): 798–803.

49. Carroll D, Tramer M, McQuay H, Nye B, Moore A. Transcutaneous electrical nerve stimulation in labour pain: a systematic review. *Br J Obstet Gynaecol* 1997; **104**(2): 169–175.

50. Bjordal JM, Johnson MI, Ljunggreen AE. Transcutaneous electrical nerve stimulation (TENS) can reduce postoperative analgesic consumption. A meta-analysis with assessment of optimal treatment parameters for postoperative pain. *Eur J Pain* 2003; **7**(2): 181–188.

51. Dowswell T, Bedwell C, Lavender T, Neilson JP. Transcutaneous electrical nerve stimulation (TENS) for pain relief in labour. Cochrane Database of Systematic Reviews 2009, Apr 15; (2): CD007214.

52. Walsh DM, Howe TE, Johnson MI, Sluka KA. Transcutaneous electrical nerve stimulation for acute pain. Cochrane Database of Systematic Reviews 2009, Apr 15; (2): CD006142.

53. Proctor M, Smith CA, Farquhar CM, Stones W. Transcutaneous electrical nerve stimulation and acupuncture for primary dysmenorrhoea. Cochrane Database of Systematic Reviews 2002, Issue 1. Art. No.: CD002123. DOI: 10.1002/14651858.CD002123.

54. Nnoaham KE, Kumbang J. Transcutaneous electrical nerve stimulation (TENS) for chronic pain. Cochrane Database of Systematic Reviews 2008, Jul 16; (3): CD003222.

55. Johnson M, Martinson M. Efficacy of electrical nerve stimulation for chronic musculoskeletal pain: a meta-analysis of randomized controlled trials. *Pain* 2007; **130**(1–2): 157–165.

56. Bjordal JM, Johnson MI, Lopes-Martins RA, Bogen B, Chow R, Ljunggren AE. Short-term efficacy of physical interventions in osteoarthritic knee pain. A systematic review and meta-analysis of randomized placebo-controlled trials. *BMC Musculoskelet Disord* 2007; **8**(1): 51.

57. Osiri M, Welch V, Brosseau L, *et al.* Transcutaneous electrical nerve stimulation for knee osteoarthritis. Cochrane Database of Systematic Reviews 2000, Issue 4. Art. No.: CD002823. DOI: 10.1002/14651858.CD002823.

58. Khadilkar A, Milne S, Brosseau L, *et al.* Transcutaneous electrical nerve stimulation for the treatment of chronic low back pain: a systematic review. *Spine* 2005; **30**(23): 2657–2666.

59. Brosseau L, Yonge KA, Welch V, *et al.* Transcutaneous electrical nerve stimulation (TENS) for the treatment of rheumatoid arthritis in the hand. Cochrane Database of Systematic Reviews 2003, Issue 2. Art. No.: CD004377. DOI: 10.1002/14651858.CD004377.

60. Kroeling P, Gross AR, Goldsmith CH. A Cochrane review of electrotherapy for mechanical neck disorders. *Spine* 2005; **30**(21): 641–648.

61. Price CI, Pandyan AD. Electrical stimulation for preventing and treating post-stroke shoulder pain: a systematic Cochrane review. *Clin Rehabil* 2001; **15**(1): 5–19.

62. Brønfort G, Nilsson N, Haas M, *et al*. Non-invasive physical treatments for chronic/recurrent headache. Cochrane Database of Systematic Reviews 2004, Issue 3. Art. No.: CD001878. DOI: 10.1002/14651858.CD001878.pub2.

63. Pan CX, Morrison RS, Ness J, Fugh-Berman A, Leipzig RM. Complementary and alternative medicine in the management of pain, dyspnoea, and nausea and vomiting near the end of life. A systematic review. *J Pain Symptom Manage* 2000; **20**(5): 374–387.

64. Gadsby J, Franks A, Jarvis P, Dewhurst F. Acupuncture-like transcutaneous electrical nerve stimulation within palliative care: a pilot study. *Complement Ther Med* 1997; **5**(1): 13–18.

65. Avellanosa AM, West CR. Experience with transcutaneous electrical nerve stimulation for relief of intractable pain in cancer patients. *J Med* 1982; **13**(3): 203–213.

66. Ostrowski MJ. Pain control in advanced malignant disease using transcutaneous nerve stimulation. *Br J Clin Pract* 1979; **33**(6): 157–162.

67. Wen HL. Cancer pain treated with acupuncture and electrical stimulation. *Mod Med Asia* 1977; **13**: 12–16.

68. Robb KA, Bennett MI, Johnson MI, Simpson KJ, Oxberry SG. Transcutaneous electric nerve stimulation (TENS) for cancer pain in adults. Cochrane Database of Systematic Reviews 2008, Issue 3. Art. No.: CD006276. DOI: 10.1002/14651858.CD006276.pub2.

69. Robb K, Oxberry SG, Bennett MI, Johnson MI, Simpson KH, Searle RD. *J Pain Sympt Manage* 2009; **37**(4): 746–753.

70. Robb KA, Newham DJ, Williams JE. Transcutaneous electrical nerve stimulation vs. transcutaneous spinal electroanalgesia for chronic pain associated with breast cancer treatments. *J Pain Symptom Manage* 2007; **33**(4): 410–419.

71. Macdonald ARJ, Coates TW. The discovery of trancutaneous spinal electroanalgesia and its relief of chronic pain. *Physiotherapy* 1995; **81**: 653–660.

72. Reuss R, Meyer SC. The use of TENS in the management of cancer pain. *Clin Manage* 1985; **5**(5): 26–28.

73. Ventafridda V, Saganzerla EP, Fochi C, Pozzi G, Cordini G. Transcutaneous nerve stimulation in cancer pain. In: Bonica J, Ventafridda V (eds) *Advances in Pain Research and Therapy*. Raven Press, New York, 1979: 509–515.

74. Rafter J. *TENS and Cancer Pain*. Acupuncture Foundation of Canada Congress on Acupuncture Techniques, Toronto, Canada, 1986.

75. Librach S, Rapson LM. The use of transcutaneous electrical nerve stimulation (TENS) for the relief of pain in palliative care. *Palliat Med* 1988; **2**: 15–20.

76. Hidderley M, Weinel E. Clinical practice. Effects of TENS applied to acupuncture points distal to a pain site. *Int J Palliat Nurs* 1997; **3**(4): 185–191.

77. Hasun R, Marberger M. Transdermal electric pain control in urologic cancer patients. *Schmerz Pain Douleur* 1988; **9**(3): 234–238.

78. Dil'din AS, Tikhonova GP, Kozlov SV. [Transcutaneous electrostimulation – method leading to a permeation system of electroanalgesia in oncological practice]. *Vopr Onkologia* 1985; **31**(8): 33–36.

79. Long DM. External electrical stimulation as a treatment of chronic pain. *Minnesota Med* 1974; **57**(3): 195–198.

80. Loeser J, Black R, Christman A. Relief of pain by transcutaneous electrical nerve stimulation. *J Neurosurg* 1975; **42**: 308–314.

81. Hardy RW. Current techniques in the management of pain. *Cleveland Clin Q* 1974; **41**(4): 177–183.

82. Bates JA, Nathan PW. Transcutaneous electrical nerve stimulation for chronic pain. *Anaesthesia* 1980; **35**(8): 817–822.

83. Searle RD, Bennett MI, Johnson MI, Callin S, Radford H. Transcutaneous electrical nerve stimulation (TENS) for cancer bone pain. *Palliat Med* 2008; **22**(7): 878–9.

84. Searle RD, Bennett MI, Johnson MI, Callin S, Radford H. Transcutaneous electrical nerve stimulation (TENS) for cancer bone pain. *J Pain Symptom Manage* 2009; **37**(3): 424–8.

85. Bennett MI, Johnson MI, Brown SR, Searle RD, Radford H, Brown JM. Feasibility study of Transcutaneous Electrical Nerve Stimulation (TENS) for cancer bone pain. *Journal of Pain*, in press.

86. Dundee J, Yang J, McMillan C. Non-invasive stimulation of the P6 (Neiguan) antiemetic acupuncture point in cancer chemotherapy. *J Roy Soc Med* 1991; **84**(4): 210–212.

87. Pearl ML, Fischer M, McCauley DL, Valea FA, Chalas E. Transcutaneous electrical nerve stimulation as an adjunct for controlling chemotherapy-induced nausea and vomiting in gynecologic oncology patients. *Cancer Nurs* 1999; **22**(4): 307–311.

88. Coloma M, White PF, Ogunnaike BO, *et al*. Comparison of acustimulation and ondansetron for the treatment of established postoperative nausea and vomiting. *Anesthesiology* 2002; **97**(6): 1387–1392.

89. Gan TJ, Jiao KR, Zenn M, Georgiade G. A randomized controlled comparison of electro-acupoint stimulation or ondansetron versus placebo for the prevention of postoperative nausea and vomiting. *Anesthes Analges* 2004; **99**(4): 1070–1075.

90. Zarate E, Mingus M, White PF, *et al*. The use of transcutaneous acupoint electrical stimulation for preventing nausea and vomiting after laparoscopic surgery. *Anesthes Analges* 2001; **92**(3): 629–635.

91. Lee A, Done ML. Stimulation of the wrist acupuncture point P6 for preventing postoperative nausea and vomiting. Cochrane Database of Systematic Reviews 2004, Issue 3. Art. No.: CD003281. DOI: 10.1002/14651858.CD003281.pub2.

92. Ezzo J, Streitberger K, Schneider A. Cochrane systematic reviews examine P6 acupuncture-point stimulation for nausea and vomiting. *J Altern Complement Med* 2006; **12**(5): 489–495.

93. Waller A, Bercovitch M. Treatment of lymphoedema with TENS. In: *Lymphoedema*. Radcliffe Medical Press, Oxford, 2000: 27–184.

94. Filshie J, Hester J. Guidelines for providing acupuncture treatment for cancer patients – a peer-reviewed sample policy document. *Acupunct Med* 2006; **24**(4): 172–182.

95. Baum M, Ernst E, Lejeune S, Horneber M. Role of complementary and alternative medicine in the care of patients with breast cancer: report of the European Society of Mastology (EUSOMA) Workshop, Florence, Italy, December 2004. *Eur J Cancer* 2006; **42**(12): 1702–1710.

96. Filshie J, Bolton T, Browne D, Ashley S. Acupuncture and self acupuncture for long-term treatment of vasomotor symptoms in cancer patients – audit and treatment algorithm. *Acupunct Med* 2005; **23**(4): 171–180.

97. Filshie J, Redman D. Acupuncture and malignant pain problems. *Eur J Surg Oncol* 1985; **11**(4): 389–394.

98. Filshie J, Penn K, Ashley S, Davis CL. Acupuncture for the relief of cancer-related breathlessness. *Palliat Med* 1996; **10**(2): 145–150.

99. Cummings M, Reid F. BMAS policy statements in some controversial areas of acupuncture practice. *Acupunct Med* 2004; **22**(3): 134–136.

100. Mansky PJ, Wallerstedt DB. Complementary medicine in palliative care and cancer symptom management. Cancer J 2006; 12(5): 425–431.

101. McEachrane-Gross FP, Liebschutz JM, Berlowitz D. Use of selected complementary and alternative medicine (CAM) treatments in veterans with cancer or chronic pain: a cross-sectional survey. BMC Complement Altern Med 2006; 6: 34.

102. Lengacher CA, Bennett MP, Kip KE, et al. Frequency of use of complementary and alternative medicine in women with breast cancer. *Oncol Nurs Forum* 2002; **29**(10): 1445–1452.

103. Henderson JW, Donatelle RJ. Complementary and alternative medicine use by women after completion of allopathic treatment for breast cancer. *Altern Ther Health Med* 2004; **10**(1): 52–57.

104. Nahleh Z, Tabbara IA. Complementary and alternative medicine in breast cancer patients. *Palliat Support Care* 2003; **1**(3): 267–273.

105. Theron EJ, Vermeulen AM. The utilization of transcutaneous electric nerve stimulation in postoperative ileus. *South Afr Med J* 1983; **63**(25): 971–972.

106. Ernst E, White A. The BBC survey of complementary medicine use in the UK. *Complement Ther Med* 2000; **8**(1): 32–36.

107. Wells M, Sarna L, Cooley ME, *et al.* Use of complementary and alternative medicine therapies to control symptoms in women living with lung cancer. *Cancer Nurs* 2007; **30**(1): 45–55; quiz 56–57.

108. Johnstone PA, Polston GR, Niemtzow RC, Martin PJ. Integration of acupuncture into the oncology clinic. *Palliat Med* 2002; **16**(3): 235–239.

109. Lund I, Lundeberg T. Are minimal, superficial or sham acupuncture procedures acceptable as inert placebo controls? *Acupunct Med* 2006; **24**(1): 13–15.

110. Park J, White A, Stevinson C, Ernst E, James M. Validating a new non-penetrating sham acupuncture device: two randomized controlled trials. *Acupunct Med* 2002; **20**(4): 168–174.

111. White P, Lewith G, Hopwood V, Prescott P. The placebo needle, is it a valid and convincing placebo for use in acupuncture trials? A randomized, single-blind, cross-over pilot trial. *Pain* 2003; **106**(3): 401–409.

112. Tsukayama H, Yamashita H, Kimura T, Otsuki K. Factors that influence the applicability of sham needle in acupuncture trials: two randomized, single-blind, crossover trials with acupuncture-experienced subjects. *Clin J Pain* 2006; **22**(4): 346–349.

113. Dincer F, Linde K. Sham interventions in randomized clinical trials of acupuncture – a review. *Complement Ther Med* 2003; **11**(4): 235–242.

114. Kagitani F, Uchida S, Hotta H, Aikawa Y. Manual acupuncture needle stimulation of the rat hindlimb activates groups I, II, III and IV single afferent nerve fibers in the dorsal spinal roots. *Japan J Physiol* 2005; **55**(3): 149–155.

115. Wang JQ, Mao L, Han JS. Comparison of the antinociceptive effects induced by electroacupuncture and transcutaneous electrical nerve stimulation in the rat. *Int J Neurosci* 1992; **65**(1–4): 117–129.

116. Andersson S, Lundeberg T. Acupuncture – from empiricism to science: functional background to acupuncture effects in pain and disease. *Med Hypotheses* 1995; **45**(3): 271–281.

117. Kawakita K, Okada K. Mechanisms of action of acupuncture for chronic pain relief – polymodal receptors are the key candidates. *Acupunct Med* 2006; **24**(suppl): S58–66.

118. Li G, Liu HL, Cheung RT, *et al.* An fMRI study comparing brain activation between word generation and electrical stimulation of language-implicated acupoints. *Human Brain Map* 2003; **18**(3): 233–238.

119. Guo ZL, Moazzami AR, Longhurst JC. Electroacupuncture induces c-Fos expression in the rostral ventrolateral medulla and periaqueductal gray in cats: relation to opioid containing neurons. *Brain Res* 2004; **1030**(1): 103–115.

120. de Medeiros MA, Canteras NS, Suchecki D, Mello LE. Analgesia and c-Fos expression in the periaqueductal gray induced by electroacupuncture at the Zusanli point in rats. *Brain Res* 2003; **973**(2): 196–204.

121. Bing Z, Villanueva L, Le Bars D. Acupuncture and diffuse noxious inhibitory controls: naloxone-reversible depression of activities of trigeminal convergent neurons. *Neuroscience* 1990; **37**(3): 809–818.

122. Lee JH, Beitz AJ. The distribution of brain-stem and spinal cord nuclei associated with different frequencies of electroacupuncture analgesia. *Pain* 1993; **52**(1): 11–28.

123. Guo HF, Cui X, Hou Y, Tian J, Wang X, Han J. C-Fos proteins are not involved in the activation of preproenkephalin gene expression in rat brain by peripheral electric stimulation (electroacupuncture). *Neurosci Lett* 1996; **207**(3): 163–166.

124. Guo HF, Tian J, Wang X, Fang Y, Hou Y, Han J. Brain substrates activated by electroacupuncture (EA) of different frequencies (II): Role of Fos/Jun proteins in EA-induced transcription of preproenkephalin and preprodynorphin genes. *Brain Res Molec Brain Res* 1996; **43**(1–2): 167–173.

125. Guo HF, Tian J, Wang X, Fang Y, Hou Y, Han J. Brain substrates activated by electroacupuncture of different frequencies (I): Comparative study on the expression of oncogene c-fos and genes coding for three opioid peptides. *Brain Res Molec Brain Res* 1996; **43**(1–2): 157–166.

126. Ulett GA, Han S, Han JS. Electroacupuncture: mechanisms and clinical application. *Biol Psychiat* 1998; **44**(2): 129–138.

127. Han JS. Acupuncture: neuropeptide release produced by electrical stimulation of different frequencies. *Trends Neurosci* 2003; **26**(1): 17–22.

128. Han JS. Acupuncture and endorphins. *Neurosci Lett* 2004; **361**(1–3): 258–261.

129. Hui KK, Liu J, Marina O, *et al.* The integrated response of the human cerebro-cerebellar and limbic systems to acupuncture stimulation at ST 36 as evidenced by fMRI. *Neuroimage* 2005; **27**(3): 479–496.

130. Yoo SS, Teh EK, Blinder RA, Jolesz FA. Modulation of cerebellar activities by acupuncture stimulation: evidence from fMRI study. *Neuroimage* 2004; **22**(2): 932–940.

131. Wang W, Liu L, Zhi X, *et al.* Study on the regulatory effect of electro-acupuncture on hegu point (LI4) in cerebral response with functional magnetic resonance imaging. *Chin J Integr Med* 2007; **13**(1): 10–16.

132. Napadow V, Makris N, Liu J, Kettner NW, Kwong KK, Hui KK. Effects of electroacupuncture versus manual acupuncture on the human brain as measured by fMRI. *Human Brain Map* 2005; **24**(3): 193–205.

133. Yang C, Li B, Liu TS, Zhao DM, Hu FA. [Effect of electroacupuncture on proliferation of astrocytes after spinal cord injury]. *Zhongguo Zhen Jiu (Chinese Acupuncture and Moxibustion)* 2005; **25**(8): 569–572.

134. Hui KK, Liu J, Makris N, *et al.* Acupuncture modulates the limbic system and subcortical gray structures of the human brain: evidence from fMRI studies in normal subjects. *Human Brain Map* 2000; **9**(1): 13–25.

135. Chen AC, Liu FJ, Wang L, Arendt-Nielsen L. Mode and site of acupuncture modulation in the human brain: 3D (124–ch) EEG power spectrum mapping and source imaging. *Neuroimage* 2006; **29**(4): 1080–1091.

136. Lundeberg T. Some of the effects of acupuncture in the knee may be due to activation of the reward system. *Acupunct Med* 2006; **24**(suppl): 67–70.

137. Napadow V, Kettner N, Liu J, *et al.* Hypothalamus and amygdala response to acupuncture stimuli in carpal tunnel syndrome. *Pain* 2007; **130**(3): 254–266.

138. Sekido R, Ishimaru K, Sakita M. Differences of electroacupuncture-induced analgesic effect in normal and inflammatory conditions in rats. *Am J Chin Med* 2003; **31**(6): 955–965.

139. Liu S, Zhou W, Ruan X, *et al.* Activation of the hypothalamus characterizes the response to acupuncture stimulation in heroin addicts. *Neurosci Lett* 2007; **421**(3): 203–208.

140. Nakagoshi A, Fukunaga M, Umeda M, Mori Y, Higuchi T, Tanaka C. Somatotopic representation of acupoints in human primary somatosensory cortex: an FMRI study. *Magnet Reson Med Sci* 2005; **4**(4): 187–189.

141. Li G, Huang L, Cheung RT, Liu SR, Ma QY, Yang ES. Cortical activations upon stimulation of the sensorimotor-implicated acupoints. *Magnet Reson Imag* 2004; **22**(5): 639–644.

142. Zhang WT, Jin Z, Luo F, Zhang L, Zeng YW, Han JS. Evidence from brain imaging with fMRI supporting functional specificity of acupoints in humans. *Neurosci Lett* 2004; **354**(1): 50–53.

143. Yan B, Li K, Xu J, *et al.* Acupoint-specific fMRI patterns in human brain. *Neurosci Lett* 2005; **383**(3): 236–240.

144. Li K, Shan B, Xu J, *et al.* Changes in FMRI in the human brain related to different durations of manual acupuncture needling. *J Altern Complement Med* 2006; **12**(7): 615–623.

145. Han JS, Xuan YT. A mesolimbic neuronal loop of analgesia: I. Activation by morphine of a serotonergic pathway from periaqueductal gray to nucleus accumbens. *Int J Neurosci* 1986; **29**(1–2): 109–117.

146. Kong J, Ma L, Gollub RL, *et al.* A pilot study of functional magnetic resonance imaging of the brain during manual and electroacupuncture stimulation of acupuncture point (LI-4 Hegu) in normal subjects reveals differential brain activation between methods. *J Altern Complement Med* 2002; **8**(4): 411–419.

147. Wu MT, Sheen JM, Chuang KH, *et al.* Neuronal specificity of acupuncture response: a fMRI study with electroacupuncture. *Neuroimage* 2002; **16**(4): 1028–1037.

148. Zhang WT, Jin Z, Cui GH, *et al.* Relations between brain network activation and analgesic effect induced by low vs. high frequency electrical acupoint stimulation in different subjects: a functional magnetic resonance imaging study. *Brain Res* 2003; **982**(2): 168–178.

149. Kong J, Gollub RL, Webb JM, Kong JT, Vangel MG, Kwong K. Test-retest study of fMRI signal change evoked by electroacupuncture stimulation. *Neuroimage* 2007; **34**(3): 1171–1181.

150. Lewith GT, White PJ, Pariente J. Investigating acupuncture using brain imaging techniques: the current state of play. *Evidence-based Complement Altern Med* 2005; **2**(3): 315–319.

151. Campbell A. Point specificity of acupuncture in the light of recent clinical and imaging studies. *Acupunct Med* 2006; **24**(3): 118–122.

152. Ahn AC, Wu J, Badger GJ, Hammerschlag R, Langevin HM. Electrical impedance along connective tissue planes associated with acupuncture meridians. *BMC Complement Altern Med* 2005; **5**: 10.

153. Lee MS, Jeong SY, Lee YH, Jeong DM, Eo YG, Ko SB. Differences in electrical conduction properties between meridians and non-meridians. *Am J Chin Med* 2005; **33**(5): 723–728.

154. Langevin HM, Churchill DL, Wu J, *et al.* Evidence of connective tissue involvement in acupuncture. *Fed Am Soc Exper Biol J* 2002; **16**(8): 872–874.

155. Melzack R, Stillwell DM, Fox EJ. Trigger points and acupuncture points for pain: correlations and implications. *Pain* 1977; **3**(1): 3–23.

156. Moncayo R, Rudisch A, Kremser C, Moncayo H. 3D-MRI rendering of the anatomical structures related to acupuncture points of the Dai mai, Yin qiao mai and Yang qiao mai meridians within the context of the WOMED concept of lateral tension: implications for musculoskeletal disease. *BMC Musculoskelet Disord* 2007; **8**: 33.

157. Moncayo R, Rudisch A, Diemling M, Kremser C. In-vivo visualisation of the anatomical structures related to the acupuncture points Dai mai and Shen mai by MRI: a single-case pilot study. *BMC Med Imag* 2007; **7**: 4.

158. Derry CJ, Derry S, McQuay HJ, Moore RA. Systematic review of systematic reviews of acupuncture published 1996–2005. *Clin Med* 2006; **6**(4): 381–386.

159. National Health Service Centre for Reviews and Dissemination Acupuncture. *Effect Health Care Bull* 2001; **7**(2): 1–12.

160. Ernst E. Acupuncture – a critical analysis. *J Intern Med* 2006; **259**(2): 125–137.

161. White A, Foster NE, Cummings M, Barlas P. Acupuncture treatment for chronic knee pain: a systematic review. *Rheumatology* 2007; **46**(3): 384–390.

162. Manheimer E, Linde K, Lao L, Bouter LM, Berman BM. Meta-analysis: acupuncture for osteoarthritis of the knee. *Ann Intern Med* 2007; **146**(12): 868–877.

163. Ezzo J, Berman B, Hadhazy VA, Jadad AR, Lao L, Singh BB. Is acupuncture effective for the treatment of chronic pain? A systematic review. *Pain* 2000; **86**(3): 217–225.

164. White P, Lewith G, Berman B, Birch S. Reviews of acupuncture for chronic neck pain: pitfalls in conducting systematic reviews. *Rheumatology* 2002; **41**(11): 1224–1231.

165. Linde C, Isacsson G, Jonsson B. Outcome of 6-week treatment with transcutaneous electric nerve stimulation compared with splint on symptomatic temporomandibular joint disk displacement without reduction. *Acta Odontol Scand* 1995; **53**(2): 92–98.

166. Johnson MI. The clinical effectiveness of acupuncture for pain relief – you can be certain of uncertainty. *Acupunct Med* 2006; **24**(2): 71–79.

167. Lee H, Schmidt K, Ernst E. Acupuncture for the relief of cancer-related pain – a systematic review. *Eur J Pain* 2005; **9**(4): 437–444.

168. Xia YQ, Zhang D, Yang CX, Xu HL, Li Y, Ma LT. An approach to the effect on tumors of acupuncture in combination with radiotherapy or chemotherapy. *J Trad Chin Med* 1986; **6**(1): 23–26.

169. Dang W, Yang J. Clinical study on acupuncture treatment of stomach carcinoma pain. *J Trad Chin Med* 1998; **18**(1): 31–38.

170. Alimi D, Rubino C, Pichard-Leandri E, Fermand-Brule S, Dubreuil-Lemaire ML, Hill C. Analgesic effect of auricular acupuncture for cancer pain: a randomized, blinded, controlled trial. *J Clin Oncol* 2003; **21**(22): 4120–4126.

171. Alimi D, Rubino C, Leandri EP, Brule SF. Analgesic effects of auricular acupuncture for cancer pain. *J Pain Symptom Manage* 2000; **19**(2): 81–82.

172. Xu S, Liu Z, Xu M. Treatment of cancerous abdominal pain by acupuncture on zusanli (ST 36) – a report of 92 cases. *J Trad Chin Med* 1995; **15**(3): 189–191.

173. Rico RC, Trudnowski RJ. Studies with electro-acupuncture. *J Med* 1982; **13**(3): 247–251.

174. Mehling WE, Jacobs B, Acree M, *et al.* Symptom management with massage and acupuncture in postoperative cancer patients: a randomized controlled trial. *J Pain Symptom Manage* 2007; **33**(3): 258–266.

175. Wong R, Sagar S. Acupuncture treatment for chemotherapy-induced peripheral neuropathy – a case series. *Acupunct Med* 2006; **24**(2): 87–91.

176. Minton O, Higginson IJ. Electroacupuncture as an adjunctive treatment to control neuropathic pain in patients with cancer. *J Pain Symptom Manage* 2007; **33**(2): 115–117.

177. Bardia A, Barton DL, Prokop LJ, Bauer BA, Moynihan TJ. Efficacy of complementary and alternative medicine therapies in relieving cancer pain: a systematic review. *J Clin Oncol* 2006; **24**(34): 5457–5464.

178. Ezzo J, Vickers A, Richardson MA, *et al.* Acupuncture-point stimulation for chemotherapy-induced nausea and vomiting. *J Clin Oncol* 2005; **23**(28): 7188–7198.

179. Jobst K, Chen JH, McPherson K, *et al.* Controlled trial of acupuncture for disabling breathlessness. *Lancet* 1986; **2**(8521–22): 1416–1419.

180. Wu HS, Wu SC, Lin JG, Lin LC. Effectiveness of acupressure in improving dyspnoea in chronic obstructive pulmonary disease. *J Adv Nurs* 2004; **45**(3): 252–259.

181. Maa SH, Gauthier D, Turner M. Acupressure as an adjunct to a pulmonary rehabilitation program. *J Cardiopulmon Rehabil* 1997; **17**(4): 268–276.

182. Lewith GT, Prescott P, Davis CL. Can a standardized acupuncture technique palliate disabling breathlessness: a single-blind, placebo-controlled crossover study. *Chest* 2004; **125**(5): 1783–1790.

183. Vickers AJ, Feinstein MB, Deng GE, Cassileth BR. Acupuncture for dyspnoea in advanced cancer: a randomized, placebo-controlled pilot trial [ISRCTN89462491]. *BMC Palliat Care* 2005; **4**: 5.

184. Sood A, Barton DL, Bauer BA, Loprinzi CL. A critical review of complementary therapies for cancer-related fatigue. *Integrat Cancer Ther* 2007; **6**(1): 8–13.

185. Vickers AJ, Straus DJ, Fearon B, Cassileth BR. Acupuncture for postchemotherapy fatigue: a phase II study. *J Clin Oncol* 2004; **22**(9): 1731–1735.

186. Jedel E. Acupuncture in xerostomia – a systematic review. *J Oral Rehabil* 2005; **32**(6): 392–396.

187. Blom M, Dawidson I, Fernberg JO, Johnson G, Angmar-Mansson B. Acupuncture treatment of patients with radiation-induced xerostomia. *Eur J Cancer B Oral Oncol* 1996; **32B**(3): 182–190.

188. Blom M, Dawidson I, Angmar-Mansson B. The effect of acupuncture on salivary flow rates in patients with xerostomia. *Oral Surg Oral Med Oral Pathol* 1992; **73**(3): 293–298.

189. List T, Lundeberg T, Lundstrom I, Lindstrom F, Ravald N. The effect of acupuncture in the treatment of patients with primary Sjogren's syndrome. A controlled study. *Acta Odontol Scand* 1998; **56**(2): 95–99.

190. Wymenga AN, Sleijfer DT. Management of hot flushes in breast cancer patients. *Acta Oncol* 2002; **41**(3): 269–275.

191. Nedstrand E, Wyon Y, Hammar M, Wijma K. Psychological well-being improves in women with breast cancer after treatment with applied relaxation or electro-acupuncture for vasomotor symptoms. *J Psychosom Obstet Gynaecol* 2006; **27**(4): 193–199.

PART 4

Treatment modalities: the evidence

CHAPTER 28

Interventional therapies

Anthony Dragovich[1] and Steven P. Cohen[2]

[1]Womack Army Medical Center, Fort Bragg, NC, USA
[2]Johns Hopkins Medical Institutions, Baltimore, USA; and Walter Reed Army Medical Center, Washington, DC, USA

Introduction

Therapeutic interventional techniques used in the management of chronic and malignant pain include various types of neural blockades and minimally invasive surgical procedures. These therapies are employed for a wide range of painful conditions, despite ongoing controversy about their effectiveness. Most of these procedures are performed on patients with chronic pain, which remains a poorly understood, complex clinical state associated with psychiatric, behavioral and neurobiologic implications. Clear, uniform metrics evaluating not only pain relief but other parameters as well, including functional capacity, psychologic well-being and return-to-work status, are evolving but are still in their infancy. However, significant progress has been made in the last 20 years, which forms the foundation for evidence-based pain treatment. The purpose of this chapter is to evaluate systematically the efficacy of interventional therapies with a focus on spinal conditions, discuss the limitations of research methodology, and comment on future directions in interventional pain medicine research.

Epidural injections

Physicians have been injecting medications into the epidural space to relieve pain since the early 1900s. The first reported case of administration of medication

Evidence-Based Chronic Pain Management. Edited by
C. Stannard, E. Kalso and J. Ballantyne. © 2010 Blackwell
Publishing.

into the epidural space was in 1901 by Sicard [1], who injected a dilute cocaine solution through the sacral hiatus to treat lumbago. Numerous studies have since been performed evaluating the efficacy of various solutions and routes of administration.

The rationale behind epidural steroid injections (ESI) is that higher concentrations of corticosteroid are delivered to the inflamed nerve root(s) than with oral, intravenous or intramuscular routes, resulting in enhanced pain relief and reduced side effects. ESI have been studied predominantly in patients with radicular pain, which is most commonly caused by a disk herniation. Disk herniations can produce radicular symptoms both by mechanical compression of a nerve root as well as chemical inflammation, as described by Olmarker *et al.* using a porcine model [2]. Inflammatory cytokines have been shown to mediate pain, promote intraneural edema, and reduce nerve conduction velocity in affected spinal nerves, all of which can be reversed by cytokine inhibition [3].

There are three ways to access the epidural space: the caudal, interlaminar, and transforaminal approaches. The interlaminar and transforaminal techniques can be used in the cervical, thoracic and lumbar spine. The caudal epidural space is accessed via the sacral hiatus, and hence is reserved for lumbosacral symptomatology.

The interlaminar approach is the most common way to access the epidural space. However, medication injected by this approach may fail to reach the ventral epidural space, which is closest to the site of pathology (i.e. the ventral aspect of the lumbar nerve root sleeve and the dorsal aspect of the disk herniation). In a multicenter analysis by Stojanovic *et al.* [4] evaluating contrast dispersal patterns for cervical ESI, the authors found that spread into the ventral epidural space occurred only 28% of the time using 2 ml of injectate. This obstacle can usually be overcome by using the transforaminal approach, which in one study resulted in ventral epidural spread in all cases [5].

A key methodologic flaw is that many studies evaluating the efficacy of interlaminar ESI were done without fluoroscopic guidance. Previous studies have demonstrated high rates (8.8–70%) of false loss of resistance for blinded (without fluoroscopic guidance) ESI [4, 6, 7]. Even when the epidural space is successfully accessed, blinded injections may not deliver the medication to the area of pathology. In a study conducted in 50 patients with failed back surgery syndrome, Fredman et al. found that 5 ml of blindly administered injectate reached the targeted area only 26% of the time [6].

Many reviews have been written on the efficacy of ESI [8–20]. These reviews are limited by reviewer bias (reviews conducted by people who perform epidural injections tend to be more favorable than those done by people who do not), the inclusion of studies with small sample sizes, serious methodologic flaws, inadequate outcome measures, and heterogeneity with respect to route of injection and use of fluoroscopy. In one of the earliest reviews, Koes et al. [8] illustrated the difficulty of properly evaluating the literature in a systematic review of 12 randomized clinical trials with disparate methodologic qualities, six of which were deemed positive and six negative. The primary care physicians who conducted this review concluded that the benefits of epidural steroids, if any, seem to be of short duration only. A similar review conducted 4 years later by a French task force of rheumatologists determined that eight of 13 randomized studies demonstrated no measurable benefit [13]. The authors of this analysis concluded that no determination could be made regarding the efficacy of epidural steroids for sciatica. The main weaknesses in the studies analyzed in these reviews were that none utilized fluoroscopic guidance, and all used an interlaminar approach which has been shown to be clinically inferior to fluoroscopically guided transforaminal ESI [21].

In the recent European guidelines for the management of chronic low back pain, Airaksinen et al. [22] concluded that epidural corticosteroid injections should be considered only for radicular pain, if a contained disk prolapse is the cause of the pain, and if the corticosteroid is injected close to the site of pathology. They further noted that injections should be fluoroscopically guided towards the ventral epidural space. These recommendations are in direct contrast with those outlined in a recent report by a subcommittee of the American Academy of Neurology which concluded that lumbosacral ESI for radicular pain do not improve function, provide long-term pain relief (>3 months) or obviate the need for surgery [20] For cervical ESI, the authors found insufficient data to draw a conclusion. This review contained six high-quality randomized controlled trials, but there was marked heterogeneity among the studies with respect to outcomes, method of injection, and use of fluoroscopy.

Recent systematic reviews by Abdi et al. [19] and Boswell et al. [23] evaluating ESI based on route of administration reached a different conclusion. The consensus from these reviews is that the evidence supporting lumbar transforaminal, cervical interlaminar and caudal epidural injections is strong for short-term pain relief and functional improvement, and moderate for long-term pain relief. The evidence for lumbar interlaminar injections is strong for short-term improvement but limited for long-term benefit.

Tables 28.1–28.3 summarize the randomized controlled trials that evaluate caudal, interlaminar and transforaminal epidural steroid injections (TFESI), respectively. Of note, fluoroscopic guidance was not used in any study in Table 28.1 or 28.2. Also noteworthy is that five studies in Table 28.2 were conducted in patients hospitalized for their pain. One prospective, randomized, double-blind study by Thomas et al. [21] compared the efficacy of transforaminal and interlaminar ESI in patients with sciatica. At 30 days post procedure, pain relief was significantly better in the transforaminal group. At 6 months, significant benefit continued to be observed with respect to pain relief, daily activities, work activity, anxiety and depression in the transforaminal group. This study demonstrated a difference in clinical outcome based on the method of injection. In a randomized controlled study conducted by an orthopedic surgery group, Riew et al. [24, 25] found that a majority of patients who underwent lumbar TFESI elected not to undergo decompression surgery.

Table 28.1 Randomized controlled trials evaluating caudal epidural steroid injections

Author, method	Patients	Interventions	Results	Comments
Bush & Hillier [54] Double-blind randomized controlled trial	23 patients with lumbosacral radiculopathy	2 injections performed at 2-week intervals. 12 pts received 25 ml steroid, saline and LA and 11 pts received saline	At 4 weeks the RX group had statistically significant improvements in pain, lifestyle, and SLR compared to controls	Both groups improved at 1 year, with no statistical difference between groups. 25 ml saline may be therapeutic
Mathews et al. [55] Double-blind randomized controlled trial	57 patients with single-level radiculopathy	Maximum of 3 injections at 2-week intervals. 23 pts received up to 3 injections of 20 ml of LA with steroid vs trigger point injections with 2 ml of LA	At 1 month 67% of treated patients improved compared to 56% of controls. At 3 months, treatment group had larger decrease in pain score	3-month pain score was the only statistically significant difference
Breivik et al. [56] Double-blind randomized controlled trial	35 patients with radiculopathy	16 pts received 20 ml of LA and steroid and 19 pts received 20 ml of LA followed by 100 ml of saline. Up to 3 injections at weekly intervals	63% of pts who received steroid reported good short-term pain relief vs 25% in control group. At 6 months, 50% reported pain relief in the RX group vs 20% in the control group	50% of pts treated with steroids returned to work vs 20% of the pts treated with LA and saline

*None of the studies were conducted with fluoroscopic guidance.
LA, local anesthetic; SLR, straight leg raising.

Table 28.2 Randomized controlled trials evaluating interlaminar epidural steroid injections

Author, method	Patients	Intervention	Results	Comments
Wilson-McDonald et al. [57] Single-blind randomized controlled trial	93 patients with lumbosacral radiculopathy secondary to herniated disk or spinal stenosis	Pts received either a 10 ml injection of LA and steroid injected epidurally or intra-muscularly. Control group could cross-over to ESI if no benefit	Treatment group had better pain relief at 35 days. No difference between groups at 1 year or difference in rate of surgical intervention	Significant difference was noted 10 days after the treatment. Fluoroscopy was not used
Arden et al. [58] Multicenter double-blind randomized controlled trial	228 patients with unilateral lumbosacral radiculopathy	3 injections at weeks 0, 3, and 6. Treatment group received 10 ml of LA and steroid epidurally vs 2 ml of saline in interspinous ligament	Improvement in treatment group at 3 weeks. No differences noted after 6 weeks. NNT was 11.4	At study conclusion 55% of patients in the active group and 45% in control group believed they had received an epidural injection. Fluoroscopy not used
Valat et al. [59] Multicenter double-blind randomized controlled trial	85 hospitalized patients with lumbosacral radiculopathy	3 injections at 2-day intervals. Treatment group received prednisolone vs 2 ml of epidural saline in control group	At 20 and 35 days no difference in any primary or secondary outcome. NNT to achieve one more success with steroids than saline was 6.5	51% in the treatment group and 36% in the control group were considered a success. Fluoroscopy not used
Buchner et al. [60] Single-blind randomized controlled trial	36 hospitalized patients with lumbosacral radiculopathy from a herniated disk	3 injections within 14 days. Treatment group received 10 ml of LA and steroid vs standard rehabilitation in control group	Statistically significant improvement of straight leg raise test at 2 weeks. Treatment group had nonstatistically significant improvements in pain relief and mobility	Final results at the 6-month follow-up not statistically significant. Treatment group: 88% return-to-work rate, 12% surgery rate. Control group: 74% return-to-work rate, 24% surgery rate. Fluoroscopy not used
Carette et al. [26] Double-blind placebo-controlled trial	158 patients with lumbosacral radiculopathy due to a herniated disk	Injections at 0, 3 and 6 weeks only if no improvement. Treatment group received steroid mixed with 8 ml saline. Control group received 1 ml of epidural saline	No difference in the primary outcome (Oswestry Disability Index score). No difference in rate of back surgery between groups over 1 year	Epidural steroid injections did afford mild-to-moderate improvement in leg pain and sensory deficits at 6 weeks and reduced the need for analgesics. Fluoroscopy not used

Study	Population	Intervention	Results	Comments
Kraemer et al. [61] Randomized controlled trial	133 hospitalized patients with lumbosacral radiculopathy	3 injections in 1 week. Pts randomized to receive 10 mg of transforaminal epidural triamcinolone with 1 ml of LA vs interlaminar epidural steroid or paravertebral local anesthetic. Dose not reported	68% in transforaminal group had good result vs 53% in interlaminar epidural group. 65% of control group did not improve	Follow-up period was 3 months. No major side effects were reported in either group. CT guidance used for perineural injections
Ridley et al. [62] Randomized controlled trial	35 patients with lumbosacral radiculopathy	Treatment group received 10 ml of saline and steroid. Control group received 2 ml interspinous saline	90% reported improvement at 2 weeks in treatment group vs 19% in control group	Significant difference in pain relief up to 12 weeks. Fluoroscopy not used
Cuckler et al. [63] Double-blind randomized controlled trial	73 patients hospitalized with lumbosacral radicular pain secondary to herniated disk or spinal stenosis	Single injection with 2nd nonblinded injection after 24 hours if no improvement. Treatment group received steroid with 5 ml LA vs 2 ml of saline and 5 ml LA in control group	No significant long- or short-term differences between groups. Average long-term follow-up was 20.2 months	61% of patients in the treatment group and 62.5% of patients in the control group reported improvement 24 hours post injection. Fluoroscopy not used
Dilke et al. [64] Double-blind randomized controlled trial	100 hospitalized patients with lumbosacral radiculopathy	Single injection, with 2nd injection after 1 week if no improvement. Treatment group received 80 mg of steroid in 10 ml of saline. Control group received interspinous ligament injection of 1 ml of saline	31% of treatment group had clear-cut pain relief vs 8.3% of controls at final 3-month follow-up.	Improvement in disability also noted. 92% return-to-work rate in RXgroup vs. 60% in control group. Fluoroscopy not used

ESI, epidural steroid injection; LA, local anesthetic; NNT, number needed to treat.

Table 28.3 Transforaminal epidural steroid injection randomized controlled trials

Author, method	Patients	Intervention	Results	Comments
Riew et al. [24, 25] Double-blind randomized controlled trial	55 patients with spinal stenosis or disk herniation referred for surgical evaluation	Pts received up to 4 injections with fluoroscopic guidance. Treatment group received 1 ml of LA plus steroid vs. 1 ml of LA in control group	8/28 in the treatment group and 18/27 in the control group chose surgery (P<0.04)	At 5 years, 17 of the 21 patients who avoided surgery at initial analysis (13–28 mos) had not had surgery. No difference between groups. All patients who avoided surgery had improvements in neurologic symptoms and back pain
Ng et al. [65] Double-blind randomized controlled trial	88 patients with unilateral leg pain > back pain > 6 weeks duration. 2 patients terminated for blinding failure	Single injection with fluoroscopic guidance with contrast. Treatment group received 2 ml of LA with steroid vs 2 ml of LA in control group	No significant difference noted between groups. Prolonged pain duration associated with less favorable outcomes at 3 months	Clinical improvement noted in both groups at 3-month follow-up
Vad et al. [66] Randomized (by patient choice) controlled trial	50 patients with lumbosacral radiculopathy	Treatment group received 1–3 fluoroscopically guided transforaminal ESI with 1.5 ml of LA and steroid vs 1–2 paraspinal trigger point injections in control group	84% successful outcomes in treatment group versus 48% in control at 1-year follow-up	Patients in the treatment group with symptoms lasting over 1 year had a 50% success rate. Mean follow-up 16 months
Karppinen et al. [67, 68] Double-blind placebo-controlled trial	160 patients with lumbosacral radiculopathy <6 months duration	Single injection with fluoroscopic guidance. Treatment group 2–3 ml of steroid and LA vs. transforaminal saline in the control group	Treatment was superior to control at 2 weeks for leg pain, straight leg raise test and range of motion. Control was superior at 3 and 6 months for back pain and at 6 months for leg pain	Subgroup analysis found treatment superior to control for contained herniations, resulting in prevention of surgery and reduced medical cost
Kraemer et al. [61] Prospective double-blind trial	49 hospitalized patients with intractable sciatica	Treatment group received epidural/ perineural injection of corticosteroid and saline vs saline alone in control group. Saline volume not specified	At 3 months perineural injections had a significantly better outcome than control group (55% good results vs 40% good results)	Surgery rates were under 5% in both groups without significant differences. CT guidance used for perineural technique

ESI, epidural steroid injection; LA, local anesthetic.

Fluoroscopic guidance and method of injection (interlaminar versus transforaminal) appear to account for most of the heterogeneity among the systematic reviews. The reviews with heterogeneity among methods of injection did not find a clinical benefit for the procedure [8, 20] while those which stratified trials based on the method of injection did find evidence to support a clinical benefit for transforaminal and caudal ESI performed with fluoroscopic guidance [19, 23]. Considering that transforaminal and caudal ESI more reliably deliver medication to the ventral epidural space, this finding is not surprising [4, 5]. Transforaminal ESI have also been found to decrease the rate of surgical interventions while interlaminar ESI have not [24, 26]. Additionally, transforaminal injections were found to be clinically superior in a head-to-head RCT [21].

Although fewer studies have evaluated cervical interlaminar and transforaminal injections, the ones that did are predominantly positive. In separate systematic reviews, Boswell et al. [23] and Abdi et al. [19] both concluded that there is moderate evidence to support interlaminar and transforaminal cervical ESI to treat cervical radiculopathy. In a Cochrane review assessing conservative treatment for mechanical neck disorders, Peloso et al. [18] also found cervical interlaminar ESI to be beneficial, although the conclusion was limited by the inclusion of only a single controlled trial. In a randomized, controlled study, Stav et al. [27] compared cervical epidural injections of methylprednisolone and lidocaine to intramuscular methylprednisolone and lidocaine in patients with cervical radicular symptoms. One year after their injection(s), 68% of patients in the epidural group continued to experience improved pain and function, compared to only 12% in the intramuscular group. Finally, Castagnera et al. [28] randomized 42 patients with cervical radicular symptoms to receive either a single cervical epidural injection with local anesthetic plus corticosteroid, or local anesthetic with steroid and low-dose morphine. One year after injection, 80% of patients in both groups reported good to excellent pain relief. There are presently no published controlled trials on cervical TFESI. The four prospective case series showed good short- and long-term results [29–32].

These results, however, must be weighed against the increased risk of cervical TFESI compared to all other types of epidural injection. There are numerous reports of death and paraplegia following cervical and thoracic TFESI [33–35] and several reports of paraplegia after lumbar TFESI [36]. In a cross-sectional study that surveyed members of the American Pain Society about complications of cervical TFESI, 287 respondents out of 1340 physicians reported 78 serious complications that included 30 cases of brain or spinal cord infarcts, and 13 fatalities. However, the complication rate cannot be determined from these data since the denominator remains unknown. In a 2003 Medicare claims study, 37,651 cervical and thoracic TFESI were performed [37]. Scanlon et al. reported 12 serious complications for 2003 [38].

Proposed mechanisms of injury include spinal cord infarct from particulate injection into radicular arteries, vertebral artery perforation, and needle-induced vasospasm. In contrast, serious complications resulting from lumbar transforaminal, cervical interlaminar and caudal ESI are exceedingly rare (see Table 28.4 for common complications) [39–42].

In summary, the preponderance of evidence supports the use of ESI for carefully selected candidates with a predominance of radicular symptomatology. There is strong evidence for short-term pain relief, and limited evidence for benefits lasting longer than 6 weeks. The best candidates for ESI are patients with acute, mostly extremity pain secondary to a herniated disk. Transforaminal ESI appear to afford better and longer lasting relief than interlaminar and caudal ESI, but the added benefit must be balanced against the higher risk associated with the procedure. For cervical radiculopathy, the evidence supporting cervical ESI is positive but limited by the paucity of data.

The practice of limiting injections to three in 6 months is not based on sound, scientific evidence in the form of prospective randomized studies [43]. Rather, the law of diminishing returns both anecdotally and theoretically dictates an inverse relationship between the number of injections and the added benefit for each successive injection, since the inflammatory component of chronic pain is limited. Moreover, the risk of complications and steroid-induced adverse effects is a direct function of the number of injections. Thus, it would appear to be prudent to limit the number of injections, though the exact number and timing of injections need to be defined in clinical trials.

Table 28.4 Common epidural steroid injection complication rates

	Headache	Axial Pain	Flushing	Vasovagal reaction	Other	Other	Other	Minor complication rate
Cervical interlaminar 345 injections/157 patients [41]	4.6%	6.7%	1.5%	1.7%	Fever 0.3%	Dural Puncture 0.3%	NR	16.8%
Thoracic interlaminar 39 injections/21 patients [42]	2.6%	7.7%	5.1%	NR	Fever 2.6%	Insomnia 2.6%	NR	20.5%
Lumbar transforaminal 322 injections/207 patients [39]	3.1%	2.4%	1.2%	0.3%	HTN 0.3%	Increased blood sugar 0.3%	NR	9.6%
Caudal 257 injections/139 patients [40]	3.5%	3.1%	2.3%	0.8%	N 0.8%	Insomnia 4.7%	Leg Pain 0.4%	15.6%

HTN, hypertension; Insomnia, night of procedure only; N, nausea; NR, not reported.

Epidural adhesiolysis

Percutaneous epidural adhesiolysis and spinal endoscopic adhesiolysis are interventional pain management techniques used to treat patients with refractory low back pain presumably due to epidural scarring. These techniques trace their foundation back to the 1930 s when Evans [44] described the caudal epidural injection of 100 ml of fluid. Evans reasoned that physical displacement of neural elements by injected fluid might lead to lysis of adhesions and possibly even anesthesia. He reported a 60% "cure" rate in 40 patients with chronic sciatica.

Whether epidural scar formation is a chief component of postlaminectomy pain or an innocuous byproduct of surgery remains a subject of intense debate. A recent preclinical postlaminectomy rat model demonstrated evidence of prominent nerve root scarring and adherence to the adjacent disk and pedicle after laminectomy, with subsequent behavioral evidence of tactile allodynia [45]. Formation of scar and entrapment of peripheral nerves have been found to result in neuropathic pain processes at peripheral sites [46–49] but radiologic evidence of scar formation has not been found to be predictive of postlaminectomy pain [50]. Clearly, further research into the etiology of postlaminectomy pain is needed to shed light on this common clinical condition.

Trescot *et al.* [51] recently performed a systematic review of the effectiveness and complications of adhesiolysis. The authors concluded there was strong evidence for short-term and moderate evidence for long-term effectiveness of percutaneous adhesiolysis and spinal endoscopy to relieve chronic low back and extremity pain. Percutaneous adhesiolysis and spinal endoscopy randomized controlled trials are presented in Table 28.5. Definitive conclusions based on clinical trials evaluating these interventions are difficult to reach due to the many procedural variables present in these complex procedures. Perhaps the best study evaluating epidural adhesiolysis is that of Dashfield *et al.* [52], who randomized 60 patients with lumbosacral radiculopathy to receive either a caudal ESI or ESI plus lysis of adhesions via epiduroscopy and infusion of large volumes of saline. Whereas both groups demonstrated improvements up to 6 months post procedure, no differences were noted between groups in any outcome variable at any follow-up period. Shortcomings in this study included not

selecting patients with demonstrated epidural fibrosis (those with prior back surgery were excluded), and not injecting medications that may enhance adhesiolysis such as hypertonic saline and hyaluronidase.

In summary, there is conflicting evidence supporting any advantage of epidural adhesiolysis over conventional ESI for low back pain with radicular symptoms. This view is consistent with that of the UK National Institute of Health and Clinical Excellence (NICE)[53], which declared that current evidence does not support the routine use of epidural lysis of adhesions for low back or leg pain.

Facet interventions

Since Goldthwaite [74] first noted in 1911 that zygapophysial (aka facet) joints could be a source of back pain, thousands of scientific papers have been published on the subject. Today, facet interventions represent the second most common type of procedure performed in pain management centers throughout the United States [37].

The two most commonly used methods to treat facet-mediated pain are intra-articular corticosteroid injections and medial branch radiofrequency (RF) denervation, which destroys the afferent nerve supply to the joint(s). Since the facet articulation is a true synovial joint, many physicians have advocated treating zygapophysial joint (z-joint) pain with intra-articular corticosteroid injections, as is done with varying degrees of success in most other joints in the body. The use of fluoroscopically guided RF facet denervation to treat facet pain was pioneered by Shealy [75] in the mid 1970s. Each facet joint receives dual innervation from the medial branch arising from the posterior primary rami at the same level and one level above the joint [76]. The randomized controlled trials evaluating RF denervation are reviewed in Tables 28.6 and 28.7.

The efficacy of intra-articular injections is a subject of controversy. In five recent reviews, the authors were split as to whether intra-articular steroids constituted an effective treatment for facet joint pain, with three concluding they did not [77–81]. In the most recent comprehensive review, Cohen & Raja [82] concluded that intra-articular steroid injections may provide intermediate-term relief to a small subset of patients with facet pain associated with

Table 28.5 Randomized controlled trials evaluating percutaneous adhesiolysis and spinal endoscopy

Author, Method	Patients	Intervention	Results	Comments
Viehelmann et al. [69] Randomized controlled trial	99 patients with chronic low back pain and lumbosacral radiculopathy (13 with prior back surgery)	Treatment group: catheter inserted through sacral hiatus to level of pathology. 9 ml of LA and 1 ml steroid injected, followed 30 minutes later by 10 ml of hypertonic saline. Control group received standard physiotherapy	Through 1-year follow-up, leg and back pain was significantly reduced and functional improvement noted in the treatment group. Pain medication usage was reduced in both groups	No major complications. 15 patients had transient sensory deficits
Manchikanti et al. [70] Double-blind randomized controlled trial	75 patients with epidural fibrosis, spinal stenosis, and/ or disk degeneration	Group I: control group with catheter placement followed by injection of 14 ml of LA, steroid and saline. Group II: adhesiolysis with 14 ml of LA, steroid and saline after epidurography. Group III: adhesiolysis with same solution except hypertonic saline used instead of normal saline	Group II and group III had statistically significant reductions in pain scores compared to group I at 3, 6, and 12 months	Only difference between adhesiolysis and nonadhesiolysis groups was catheter placement guided by contrast. Significant improvement noted for depression, anxiety, and somatization scores as well as decreased opioid use
Manchikanti et al. [71] Randomized controlled trial	45 patients with chronic low back and leg pain	Treatment group (n = 30): adhesiolysis with 11 ml of hypertonic saline and LA plus steroid (1–10 injections over 1.5–3 year period). Control group (n = 15): standard physical therapy program and medications	93% of pts in RX group improved at 6 months. 47% at 1 year. Improvement noted for anxiety, pain and function	Patients received up to 10 procedures. No complications noted. Control group consisted of pts who refused or insurance would not pay for injections
Heavner et al. [72] Double-blind randomized trial	83 patients with chronic low back pain due to epidural fibrosis	Group I: hypertonic saline plus hyaluronidase. Group II: hypertonic saline. Group III: isotonic saline. Group IV: isotonic saline plus hyaluronidase. All patient received epidural local anesthetic and steroid	Percentage of patients with improved pain scores did not differ between groups. 49% of the patients reported pain relief at 12 months	Only 59 completed study. Infused volumes not noted. No additional benefit with hyaluronidase
Manchikanti et al. [73] Double-blind randomized trial	83 patients with chronic low back and leg pain (84% with prior back surgery)	Group I: control group (n = 33) placement of endoscope with injection of 10 ml of LA and steroid. Group II: treatment group (n = 50) same as group I plus irrigation of up to 100 ml of saline and video-assisted adhesiolysis	Statistically significant decrease in VAS score compared to baseline and control group at 3 and 12 months. 48% of patients had over 50% pain relief at 1 year	Return-to-work rate and anxiety improved in RX group at 12 months
Dashfield et al. [52] Double-blind randomized controlled trial	60 patients with lumbosacral radiculopathy between 6 and 18 months duration	Treatment group received spinal epiduroscopy with LA and steroid injection as well as visualized adhesiolysis. Mean volume infused 132 ml. Control group received caudal epidural with 10 ml LA plus steroid	Both groups benefited from the treatment with no difference between groups	Postsurgical patients were excluded and few adhesions were found on epiduroscopy

LA, local anesthetic.

Table 28.6 Prospective clinical trials evaluating intra-articular steroid injections for lumbar and cervical facet joint pain

Author, method	Patients	Intervention	Results	Comments
Lynch & Taylor [106] Prospective trial	50 pts with chronic LBP accompanied by paraspinal tenderness and pain worsened by hyperextension	Underwent attempted intra-articular steroid injections at 2 most caudal l-z joints. Failed "extra-articular" injections designated as "control" group	Relief of pain at 2 weeks and 6 months was better in pts who had 2 intra-articular injections than the other groups. Pts who had 1 intra-articular injection had better relief than those who had no successful injections	Flaws include lack of randomization, poor outcome assessment, failure to identify pts based on diagnostic injections, and failure to blind the examining physician
Lilius et al. [107] Prospective randomized controlled trial	109 pts with unilateral chronic LBP	Received 8 ml of LA & steroid injected into 2 l-z joints (n = 28), around 2 joints (n = 39) or 8 ml of NS into 2 joints (n = 42)	All 3 groups demonstrated significant improvement in pain scores (at 3 months), disability scores, clinical exam findings and return to work at 6 weeks post injection. No differences were noted on any variable between groups	Pts were not diagnosed with l-z joint pain before injection. Large volumes utilized rendered injections nonspecific. Large standards of deviation were found for variables measured. Other flaws include suboptimal outcomes measures & lack of a blinded observer. Pain scores measured at 3 months by questionnaire
Nash [108] Prospective randomized controlled trial	67 pts with chronic LBP	Randomized by pairs to receive either 1.5 ml of intra-articular LA & steroid or MBB with 2 ml of LA	At 1-month follow-up, 12 pairs reported MBB to be more beneficial, 11 reported intra-articular injection to be better and 3 reported no difference	11 pts lost to follow-up. Flaws include not using l-z joint blocks for diagnosis, lack of a blinded observer, poor outcome measures, and no true control group
Carette et al. [109] Double-blind randomized controlled trial	97 pts with chronic LBP who reported immediate relief after LA facet injections	Received either 2 ml of steroid & saline (n = 49) or saline (n = 48) into L4-5 and L5-S1 l-z joints	42% of pts who received steroid and 33% who received placebo reported marked improvement for up to 3 months (P = NS). At 6 months the steroid group reported less pain and disability. Only 22% of pts in steroid group and 10% in placebo group had sustained improvement thru 6 months	Differences between groups at 6 months reduced when co-interventions taken into account. Although this is the only study that identified study pts based on diagnostic injections, these injections were not "controlled." NS is known to provide pain relief > than expected from placebo
Marks et al. [110] Prospective randomized controlled trial	86 pts with chronic LBP	Randomized to receive either 1.5 ml of steroid and LA MBB or intra-articular injections (2 ml at lowest level)	Pts who had facet joint injections had better pain relief than those who had MBB at all follow-up visits up to 3 months, but this was only significant at 1-month review	Flaws include no true control group, failure to identify pts based on diagnostic injections, no monitoring of co-interventions, lack of a blinded observer and poor outcome assessment

Continued on p.380

Table 28.6 *Continued*

Author, method	Patients	Intervention	Results	Comments
Barnsley *et al.* [86] Double-blind randomized controlled trial	41 pts with chronic neck pain following MVA	Randomized to either 1 ml of 0.5% bupivacaine or 5.7 mg betametasone into painful cervical facet joints diagnosed by comparative LA MBB	Less than half the pts reported relief for more than 1 week, and less than 1 in 5 pts reported relief for more than 1 month, irrespective of treatment group. Median time to return of 50% of preprocedure pain was 3 days in steroid group and 3.5 in LA group (P = NS)	All pts with neck pain following whiplash injury. May be different fromchronic neck pain of other etiologies. Some pts with long-lasting benefit in both groups
Fuchs *et al.* [111] Prospective randomized comparative trial	60 pts with chronic LBP	Randomized to receive either 1 ml of hyaluronic acid or steroid into the 3 lowest facet joints at weekly intervals x 6	Pts who received HA injections experienced a 40% decrease in pain scores vs a 56% reduction in those who received steroid (P = NS). Greatest pain reduction observed 3 months post treatment in HA group and 1 week post treatment in steroid group	Inclusion criteria included at least moderate facet degeneration on radiologic imaging. Flaws include lack of a control group, failure to identify pts based on diagnostic injections, no monitoring of co-interventions and multiple injections
Pneumaticos *et al.* [84] Prospective randomized comparative trial	47 pts with chronic LBP worse with lumbar extension and radiologic evidence of l-z joint abnormalities	Randomized in a 2:1 ratio to undergo intra-articular LA & steroid injections (3 ml) based on SPECT scans or physical examination	1-month post injection, 87% of pts with (+)SPECT had significant pain improvement vs 12.5% of pts with (−)SPECT and 31% of pts who underwent injections based on physical exam	Differences remained significant at 3 months but not 6 months post injection. Pain scores obtained by mailed questionnaire. No functional assessment done. Use of SPECT was cost effective

HA, hyaluronic acid; LA, local anesthesia; LBP, low back pain; l-z, lumbar zygapophysial; MBB, medial branch block; MVA, motor vehicle accident; NS, normal saline; pts, patients; SPECT, single photon emission computed tomography.

Table 28.7 Outcomes for randomized, controlled studies assessing medial branch radiofrequency denervation for lumbar and cervical facet joint pain

Author, method	Type and number of patients	Interventions	Results	Comments
King & Lagger [112] Prospective randomized controlled trial	Subjects were 60 pts with chronic low back and leg pain plus paraspinal tenderness	Randomized to 3 groups. Group I had RF denervation of the primary posterior ramus, group II had RF performed using a 1.25 inch needle inserted within the area of maximum tenderness (assumed to be a myotomy) and group III received stimulation but no coagulation (control)	In group I, 27% had ≥50% relief at 6 months vs 53% in group II and 0% in group III	Did not use diagnostic blocks before randomization. Likely included many pts with sciatica. In some pts, 1.25 inches may be sufficient to reach medial branch. Used 120 s lesion; 3 lesions were empirically made without electrical stimulation
Gallagher et al. [97] Double-blind randomized controlled trial	Subjects were 41 pts with chronic LBP who obtained "clear-cut or equivocal" relief from single intra-articular facet joint injections with LA and steroid	18 pts with a good response and 6 pts with an equivocal response underwent RF denervation. 12 pts with a good response and 5 with an equivocal response underwent sham denervation	Significant differences in pain scores noted only between patients with a good response to LA blocks who underwent true RF denervation (n = 18) and those with a good response who underwent sham treatment (n = 12). Differences were noted 1 and 6 months after procedures	Did not define "good" or "equivocal" response to diagnostic injections. Anatomic landmarks not well described. Observer not blinded. Electrode not placed parallel to nerve. In "Methods" stated only LA used, but in abstract stated LA and steroid were used. Used 90 s lesions
van Kleef et al. [98] Double-blind randomized controlled trial	Subjects were 31 pts with chronic LBP who obtained ≥50% pain relief after a single MBB (1 drop-out)	Compared true denervation to sham. Treatment: 60 s RF lesion after electrode placement with multifidus stimulation to identify the medial branch. Control: needle placement with sham denervation	After 3 mos, 9 of 15 pts in lesion group vs 4 of 16 in sham group had ≥50% pain relief. At 1-yr follow-up, 7/15 in lesion group & 2/16 in sham group had ≥50% relief	Used 0.75 ml of injectate for diagnostic blocks. Electrode not placed perpendicular to target nerve. Used multifidus rather than sensory stimulation to identify medial branch. Used 60 s lesions
Saunders & Zuurmond [113] Double-blind randomized controlled trial	Subjects were 34 pts with chronic LBP who obtained ≥50% relief after single intra-articular injection with lidocaine	Half the pts received medial branch RF denervation and half intra-articular denervation. 3 month follow-up	Both groups improved at 3 months, but intra-articular denervation group improved more than medial branch RF group	Used 1 ml for diagnostic blocks. Medial branch lesions done at inferolateral aspect of facet capsule & upper border of transverse process. 3 intra-articular facet lesions done. Used 60 s lesions

Continued on p.382

Table 28.7 *Continued*

Author, method	Type and number of patients	Interventions	Results	Comments
Leclaire et al. [90] Double-blind randomized controlled trial	Subjects were 70 pts with chronic LBP who obtained "significant" pain relief lasting >24 h after single intra-articular facet injection with lidocaine & steroid (4 drop-outs)	Compared true denervation to sham. Treatment: 2 lesions of 90 s duration with localization of the medial branch with sensory stimulation. Control: needle placement with sham denervation. 12-week follow-up	At 4 wks there were modest improvements in Roland-Morris ($P = 0.05$) and VAS pain scores ($P = NS$), but not Oswestry score. No difference in any outcome measure at 12 wks	Did not define "significant pain relief" with diagnostic injection. Inclusion criteria of >24 hr pain relief is inconsistent with pharmacology of lidocaine. Performed 2 lesions, each for 90 s. Anatomical landmarks not noted. Electrode not placed parallel to nerve
van Wijk et al. [102] Double-blind randomized controlled trial	81 pts with chronic LBP who obtained ≥50% pain relief after 2-level intra-articular facet injection with LA (no drop-outs)	Compared true denervation to sham. Treatment: 60 s lesions with localization of the medial branch with sensory stimulation. Control: needle placement with sham denervation. 3 month follow-up	Combined outcome measure (pain score, physical activity and analgesic intake) showed no differences between groups at 3 months. VAS pain score improved in both groups at 3 months. Global perceived effect was greater in treatment than sham group at 3 months	Blinding ended at 3 months in >70% of pts. Improvement in pain scores persisted throughout 12-month follow-up. Used 60 s lesions
Lord et al. [91] Double-blind randomized controlled trial	24 pts (12 per group) with neck pain lasting more than 3 months after MVA and failed conservative therapy. Included pts with positive response to placebo-controlled, diagnostic blocks	Treatment: medial branch RF lesion 90 s at 80°C. Control: electrode insertion with sham treatment. Follow-up 3 months (12 months in pts with persistent relief)	Mean time to return of 50% of preoperative pain was 263 days in RF group and 8 days in placebo group ($P = 0.04$); At 27 weeks, 7 pts in RF group and 1 in control group remained pain free	Excluded pts with solely C2–3 facet pain. Five pts in RF group with numbness in territory of treated nerves
Stovner et al. [96] Double-blind randomized controlled trial	12 pts with unilateral cervicogenic HA received comparative LA blocks and a greater occipital nerve block	Randomized to cervical facet RF or sham procedure. Follow-up 24 months	At 3 months, 4 of 6 RF pts had meaningful clinical response (≥30% improvement) vs 2 of the 6 in the sham group. 6 months post procedure, no differences noted between groups. Concluded cervical facet denervation is not effective for cervicogenic HA	RF group had better response to diagnostic blocks. Only able to recruit 12 pts in 2.9 years. Excluded pts with ongoing litigation

HA, headache; LA, local anesthetic; LBP, low back pain; MBB, medial branch block; MVA, motor vehicle accident; pts, patients; RF, radiofrequency; VAS, visual analog scale.

an active inflammatory process. Inflammation of the facet joint cannot be detected clinically, though radionuclide bone scintigraphy is capable of depicting synovial changes caused by inflammation, degenerative changes associated with bone remodeling, and increased metabolic function. Radionuclide bone scintigraphy may be a useful screening test prior to invasive facet injections since it is a sensitive indicator of active inflammation. Several prospective and observational studies evaluating low to intermediate volume (1–3 ml) local anesthetic (LA) and steroid intra-articular l-z joint injections performed in over 160 patients with axial low back pain (LBP) [83–85] support this assertion. In these studies, patients with positive single photon emission computed tomography experienced dramatically better pain relief (>75% success rate) for up to 3 months compared to those with negative or no single photon emission computed tomography (<40% success rate). With respect to cervical z-joint pain, the sole RCT conducted following whiplash injury [86] provided strong evidence for the ineffectiveness of intra-articular corticosteroids.

The evidence for benefit from RF neurolysis is more supportive, though still mixed. The correct diagnosis of facet-mediated pain continues to be a confounding factor in the study of facet interventions since neurolysis would not be expected to relieve nonfacet-mediated pain. False-positive rates of diagnostic z-joint blocks range from 25% to 40% [77, 87, 88] due to a number of factors including the placebo response, use of sedation, liberal use of superficial local anesthetic, and spread of local anesthetic to adjacent potential pain generators [89]. For example, the study by Leclarie et al. [90] was seriously compromised by the diagnostic criteria (i.e. "significant pain relief lasting over 24 hours after intra-articular z-joint block with lidocaine and steroid"). A local anesthetic block lasting over 24 hours is not consistent with local anesthetic pharmacology, and the efficacy of corticosteroids is questionable; even if they do work in some patients, the beneficial effect is not immediate. Consequently, they may have included many patients with nonfacetogenic (e.g. disk, myofascial, ligament) sources of pain. In contrast, the study evaluating cervical RF neurolysis by Lord et al. [91] conducted in patients with chronic cervical facet joint pain after whiplash injury instituted a rigorous regimen of controlled, comparative diagnostic blocks (0.5 ml of lidocaine, bupivacaine or saline) performed in random order (a positive comparative block requires the duration of pain relief to be concordant with the duration of action of the LA, and absence of pain relief with the saline control). Among 12 patients randomized to RF neurolysis, seven were pain free at 27 weeks versus only one of 12 in the sham group.

The evidence for cervical medial branch RF denervation provides moderate support. The randomized, controlled trial by Lord et al., detailed in Table 28.7, was positive for long-term relief, with the main criticism being trial size. There are four additional prospective studies that support long-term relief in patients with facet pain diagnosed by comparative, controlled LA blocks [92–95]. However, not all studies have been positive. In a more recent study, Stovner et al. randomized 12 patients diagnosed with cervicogenic headaches based on clinical symptoms and a positive response to comparative LA blocks to receive either cervical facet RF denervation or a sham procedure [96]. At their 3-month follow-up, four of six patients in the RF denervation group obtained a meaningful clinical response versus two of six patients in the sham group. At 6 months, no differences were noted between groups.

The evidence for lumbar medial branch RF denervation is similarly mixed, but none of the randomized controlled trials used diagnostic criteria comparable with those employed by Lord et al. [91] Two randomized controlled trials conducted by Gallagher et al. [97] and van Kleef et al. [98] in patients with chronic low back pain who experienced greater than 50% pain relief after uncontrolled medial branch blocks were positive, with the study by van Kleef et al. widely regarded as the most methodologically sound RCT to date. Five positive prospective trials lend support to the efficacy of lumbar facet denervation [99–101]. Of note, the prospective trial by Dreyfus et al. used comparative local anesthetic blocks, a larger 16 gauge electrode, and EMG of the multifidus muscle to confirm the accuracy of neurotomy. In this study 87% of the patients had at least 60% pain relief at 12 months. To date, only two studies [98, 100] used multifidus stimulation to determine electrode placement, with both yielding positive results.

Although the results of these studies are encouraging, the two most recent randomized controlled trials evaluating lumbar medial branch denervation have been negative. In addition to suboptimal selection criteria, reviewed earlier in this section, the study by Leclarie *et al.* [90] contained several other methodologic flaws including the use of small gauge electrodes (22 gauge) placed perpendicular rather than parallel to the nerve, which resulted in a smaller lesion size. Although the study by van Wijk *et al.* [102] was large and methodologically sound, many experts feel it was technically flawed. Specifically, the needle tips were positioned perpendicular to the nerve and too far lateral to reliably ensure denervation [103]. Another valid criticism is that the study suffered from an overly optimistic primary endpoint that combined VAS pain score, functional capacity, and analgesic intake. Additionally, 75% of patients in both groups had pain for over 2 years, which makes it less likely that any single treatment will decrease analgesic intake or significantly improve functional capacity. The global perceived effect at 3 months was statistically significant in favor of RF lesioning, with 61.5% of treatment and 39% of control patients reporting over 50% pain relief. They also found an overall cost saving per point VAS pain reduction in the RF versus the control group for the first 3 months after the procedure.

Serious complications and side effects are rare after facet interventions. The most common complication after facet joint RF denervation is neuritis, with a reported incidence of less than 5% per level [104]. Other rare events include septic arthritis, epidural abscess, meningitis, spinal anesthesia, postdural puncture headache and transient numbness and or dysesthesias [82].

There is currently little evidence evaluating the risk:benefit ratio of repeating lumbar facet RF denervation. Schofferman *et al.* published a small retrospective review in 20 patients that found similar efficacy and duration of relief between primary and repeat procedures [105]. Although positive, this study was not powered to detect the small but clinically significant risk of worsening pain following neurotomy. Although the practice of performing multiple RF denervation seems clinically valid, larger, prospective studies with longer follow-up are needed to better weigh the risks and benefits of repeat denervation.

In summary, intra-articular facet steroid injections do not appear to provide reliable short- or intermediate-term relief, except in those patients with an active inflammatory process confirmed by radiologic imaging. For both lumbar and cervical facet RF denervation,

the evidence for intermediate-term (<12 months) efficacy is mixed. However, a review of the existing literature does support RF lesioning in appropriately selected candidates, provided stringent selection and technical criteria are applied. Given the mixed nature of the evidence, large well-designed randomized controlled trials are needed. Future studies should pay careful attention to the diagnosis of facet pain with the use of comparative blocks, consider multifidus stimulation for needle localization, place electrodes parallel to the targeted nerves, and use bigger electrodes to create larger lesions. Study designs should also take into account secondary outcome measures such as functional improvement, medication reduction and work status. Additionally, since l-z joints are seldom the sole contributor to the pain, these procedures should be supported by a comprehensive rehabilitation program.

Sacroiliac joint interventions

The sacroiliac (SI) joint is the largest axial joint in the body, averaging 17 cm² in adults. The SI articulation is a true synovial joint only inferiorly, with the rest of the junction composed of an intricate set of ligamentous connections. The prevalence of pain generated from this joint in carefully screened patients with axial LBP appears to be in the 15–25% range [114].

The treatment of SI joint pain is widely acknowledged to be challenging, although new interventional techniques offer promise. Similar to facet-mediated pain, the two main interventional treatment options are intra-articular steroid injections and RF denervation of the joint.

There are only four randomized controlled trials evaluating SI joint corticosteroid injections (see Table 28.8). Two concluded that periarticular corticosteroid injections were beneficial in the short term in patients with and without spondyloarthropathy [115]. One study concluded that CT-guided SI joint injections provided long-term pain relief in children with spondyloarthropathy who were resistant to NSAID. In the only placebo-controlled study evaluating intra-articular steroid injections, Maugars *et al.* [116] injected 13 joints in 10 patients with spondyloarthropathy with either corticosteroid without local anesthetic or normal saline. At 1 month, only one patient in the control group reported good pain relief versus five of six in the steroid group. Six of

Table 28.8 Randomized controlled trials evaluating sacroiliac (SI) steroid injections

Author, method	Patients	Interventions	Results	Comments
Maugars *et al.* [116] Double-blind randomized controlled trial	10 patients with spondyloarthropathy, 13 joints. Pts with degenerative SI joints and complete ankylosis excluded	13 total joints injected. 6 were injected with corticosteroid without LA and 7 with normal saline. 6 of 7 placebo pts were reinjected with steroid at 1 month	5 steroid joints had good or very good pain relief at 1 month vs 1 in placebo group. Overall, 12/14 SI joints had good or very good results at 1 month, 8/13 at 3 months and 7/12 at 6 months	Dx made by PE and radiologic studies. Fluoroscopy used to guide injections. One pt developed radicular pain that lasted 3 weeks
Luukkainen *et al.* [124] Randomized controlled trial	20 pts with seronegative spondyloarthropathy received steroid and LA; 10 pts received saline and LA. All pts had unilateral blocks	All pts underwent unilateral, periarticular injections. 10 received corticosteroid without LA; 10 received normal saline with LA	At 2-month follow-up, VAS pain scores decreased significantly in the steroid but not saline group	Injections were periarticular, not intra-articular. Dx made by PE and radiologic studies. Fluoroscopy used to guide injections
Luukkainen *et al.* [115] Randomized controlled trial	24 pts with spondyloarthropathy	All pts underwent unilateral, periarticular injections. 13 pts received corticosteroid and LA, with 11 pts receiving normal saline and LA	At 1-month follow-up, VAS pain scores decreased significantly more in the steroid group than in the saline group	Injections were periarticular, not intra-articular. Dx made by PE. No pt had radiologic evidence of sacroiliitis. Fluoroscopy used to guide injections
Fischer *et al.* [125] Randomized controlled trial	89 children with juvenile spondyloarthropathy. 56 were responders to NSAIDs (control group) and 33 were nonresponders (treatment group)	Treatment group received corticosteroid without LA injections plus NSAID (27 bilateral injections). The control group was continued on NSAID without injections	87.5% of children who received injections reported significant decrease in their pain complaints over the 20-month follow-up period (mean VAS pain score decreased from 6.9 to 1.8). The control group showed similar improvement in pain scores, with no difference between groups	Dx made clinically and by MRI evidence of sacroiliitis. CT used to guide injections. One-third of patients who received injections demonstrated continued joint destruction despite absence of subjective complaints

CT, computed tomography; Dx, diagnosis; LA, local anesthetic; MRI, magnetic resonance imaging; PE, physical exam; SI, sacroiliac; VAS, visual analog scale.

the patients in the control group were then reinjected with steroid. Good pain relief was reported in seven of the 12 injected joints at 6 months. To summarize the existing data, Cohen [114] reported that most but not all investigators have found radiologically guided SI joint injections to provide good to excellent inter-mediate-term (3–6 months) pain relief.

There have been several uncontrolled studies evaluating SI joint RF denervation. In a retrospective study, Ferrante et al. [117] attempted to perform SI joint denervation by performing serial strip lesions with an RF electrode at <1 cm intervals in the pos-teroinferior aspect of the joint. At 6-month follow-up, 36% of patients reported ≥50% pain relief. Gervargez et al. [118] created three lesions in the posterior interosseous SI ligament and a lesion of the L5 dor-sal ramus in a prospective observational study con-ducted in 38 patients. At 3-month follow-up, 65.6% of patients reported either no pain or a substantial decrease in symptoms. Neither of these studies speci-fied the degree of pain relief during the diagnostic SI joint block required for study inclusion.

Four uncontrolled studies have evaluated dorsal rami and lateral branch RF denervation for injection-confirmed SI joint pain [119–122]. All used slightly different techniques and inclusion criteria. Yin et al. [122] selected patients based on two high-volume SI joint ligamentous (rather than intra-articular) injections, and chose the dorsal rami branches for lesioning based on concordant electrical stimula-tion. Burnham & Yasui [119] strategically placed four electrodes around each sacral foramen to create con-tinuous strip lesions to maximize the lesion volume. Cohen [119] & Burnham [120] used both SI joint and lateral branch blocks as inclusion criteria. Employing prognostic lateral branch blocks before RF lesion-ing apparently increased the success rate. Whereas Yin et al., Gervargez et al. and Buijs et al. all reported good outcomes in around 66% of patients, Cohen & Burnham reported identical 89% success rates.

Cohen et al. [123] recently conducted a bi-center placebo-controlled study evaluating L4–5 primary dor-sal rami and S1–3 lateral branch RF denervation. At 1 and 6 months postprocedure, 79% and 57% of patients in the treatment group experienced ≥50% pain relief and significant functional improvement, which favo-rably compared to the 14% success rate in the sham group at 1-month follow-up. Three months after the

procedure, no patient in the control group experienced significant benefit. In summary, there is moderate to strong evidence that carefully selected patients who obtain good but short-lasting pain relief with SI joint blocks will obtain intermediate-term (6–12 months) pain relief after SI joint RF denervation.

Spinal cord stimulation

Spinal cord stimulation (SCS) is an interventional technique used to treat a variety of chronic pain conditions. In 1967 Shealy et al. [126] described the use of dorsal column stimulation to treat chronic pain as a clinical application of the gate control theory [127]. The procedure involves placement of an electrode with metal contacts in the dorsal epi-dural space in order to produce an electric field that stimulates the dorsal column of the spinal cord. Despite its widespread use, the exact mechanisms of SCS have not been fully elucidated. Based on exist-ing data, it appears that SCS best attenuates contin-uous and evoked pain (in particular tactile/thermal allodynia), while acute nociceptive pain (e.g. wound pain or arthritis) remains relatively unaffected [128]. In neuropathic pain, SCS may have an inhibi-tory effect on A-β fiber-mediated hyperexcitability of dorsal horn neurones via a γ-aminobutyric acid (GABA)-mediated mechanism. Research is under way to evaluate the neuromodulatory effects of SCS in the dorsal horn [128]. Currently, SCS is most commonly used to treat pain of neuropathic and ischemic origin.

Evidence does exist to support SCS in the treat-ment of pain of ischemic origin. A recent Cochrane review by Ubbink et al. concluded that there is suf-ficient evidence favoring SCS over standard con-servative treatment to improve limb salvage and clinical signs and symptoms in patients with non-reconstructible chronic critical leg ischemia [129]. A placebo-controlled randomized study by Eddicks et al. also found that SCS improved functional sta-tus and angina-related symptoms in patients with refractory angina [130]. Although SCS shows prom-ise for ischemic pain, this section will focus on SCS evidence to treat complex regional pain syndrome (CRPS) and failed back surgery syndrome (FBSS) since these are the two most frequent indications for the therapy.

A review of the evidence to evaluate the efficacy of SCS to treat CRPS found one randomized controlled study and seven recent reviews. The seven reviews all concluded that SCS is effective in the management of pain in patients with CRPS [131–137] but differed in their evaluations of the level of evidence and recommendation grades [138] A Cochrane review by Mailis-Gagnon et al. [133], a review by Grabow et al. [132], and a review by Cameron et al. [134] found the existing literature limited in quality and quantity, but concluded that the available evidence suggests that SCS is effective for CRPS (grade B/C evidence). Reviews by Taylor et al. [131, 136] and de Andres et al. [135, 137] based their recommendations primarily on evidence from systematic reviews. They both concluded that grade A evidence based on the Harbour & Miller scale [138] existed to support the efficacy of SCS to treat CRPS type I. There is also evidence that SCS is a cost-effective treatment for CRPS type I [131].

The evidence used in the first three reviews consisted of case reports, case series, retrospective data and one RCT (reviewed in Table 28.9), with only one negative case study reported [139]. Both prospective trials reported positive results for SCS treatment. Calvillo et al. [140] reported a 45.3% overall success rate with a 41% return-to-work rate 36 months after implantation. Oakley et al. [141] reported an 80% success rate with an 8-month average follow-up. A more recent prospective study by Harke et al. [142] not included in the first three reviews also found positive results for SCS treatment in 29 patients with CRPS type I responsive to sympathetic blockade. After a mean follow-up period of 35.6 months, significant improvements in function were reported in a majority of patients. Twelve of 16 patients with an affected upper limb showed a significant increase in grip strength and eight of 10 patients with affected lower extremities resumed walking without crutches. Significant decreases in pain and analgesic usage were also reported. The randomized study by Kemler et al. [143] detailed in Table 28.9 found positive results for SCS compared to physical therapy when evaluated on an intention-to-treat basis, with additional benefits noted in the SCS treated group when the results were evaluated "as treated" (i.e. SCS trial failures were not included in the calculations). The mean VAS score decrease was 2.4 cm in the intention-to-treat analysis and 3.6 cm in the "as treated" analysis. However, the 5-year follow-up data revealed a significant diminution in the analgesic benefit occurring 3 years after implantation [144]. A subgroup analysis of patients actually implanted in the SCS group was not provided in this letter to the editor.

In summary, there is moderate evidence, including one RCT, three prospective trials, and many other positive studies summarized in systematic reviews, to support the use of SCS in the treatment of CRPS type I. However, most of the studies are of low methodologic quality and/or have small sample sizes. Further well-designed studies are needed to provide clinically useful information to guide clinicians in the rational use of SCS (i.e. how best to identify candidates for SCS), and to enhance the technical aspects of the procedure.

The literature to evaluate the efficacy of SCS to treat FBSS includes six recent reviews and one RCT. All the reviews concur that there is evidence to support the use of SCS to treat FBSS [133–137, 145]. However, they are also agreed on the recommendation that more well-designed, robust studies are needed.

A meta-analysis of pooled outcomes showed that 62% of SCS patients with FBSS achieved greater than 50% pain relief, and 53% of patients no longer required analgesics. Furthermore, 70% of SCS patients expressed satisfaction with their treatment [135]. The only well-designed RCT, conducted by North et al. [146] comparing SCS versus reoperation for the treatment of FBSS, provided direct evidence to support the conclusions of the meta-analysis. The study, detailed in Table 28.9, found SCS to be more effective than reoperation in patients with FBSS who had greater leg than back pain with the presence of a surgically correctable diagnosis. Several other key benefits for early SCS were also found. There was a statistically significant increase (P = 0.025) in opioid use among those patients randomized to reoperation. In addition, patients randomized to reoperation reported more loss of function than improvement with respect to motor strength, bladder control, and sleep. There were no categories in which loss of function was reported more frequently than benefit in the SCS patients. The authors concluded that SCS is not only cost-effective, but that it obviates the need for repeat surgery in the majority of patients treated.

Similar to CRPS, there is moderate evidence consisting of one RCT [146] and two meta-analyses [135, 136] to support SCS for FBSS provided the

Table 28.9 Efficacy of randomized controlled trials evaluating SCS, IDET and IDDS

Author, method	Patients	Intervention	Results	Comments
North et al. [146] Randomized controlled trial with crossover **SCS**	50 patients with FBSS and a surgically correctable diagnosis	24 SCS trials, 17 successful* with subsequent implant, 5 cross-overs to surgery, 2 lost to follow-up. 26 lumbosacral reoperations, 14 post-op cross-overs to SCS	SCS was more successful than reoperation (47% vs 12%) (P < 0.01) at 2-year follow-up. Patients initially randomized to SCS were also less likely to cross over (5/24 SCS vs 14/26 reoperation) (P = 0.02)	Concluded SCS is more effective than reoperation as a treatment for persistent radicular pain after lumbosacral spine surgery
Kemler et al. [143] Randomized controlled trial **SCS**	54 patients with CRPS involving one hand or foot. 2:1 randomization	36 SCS trials, 24 successful** trials with subsequent implant. All 36 patients continued with physical therapy. 18 pts randomized to physical therapy alone	Mean VAS pain reduction 2.4 cm SCS vs +0.6 cm in PT group (P<0.01). 39% of SCS pts had (+) global perceived effect vs 6% in PT group (P = 0.01)	Health-related quality of life also significantly improved in favor of SCS
Pauza et al. [148] Double-blind randomized controlled trial **IDET**	64 patients with axial back pain >6 months and a single positive diskogram	37 patients were treated with IDET-36 per protocol and 1 with unacceptable catheter placement. 27 treated with needle placement to annulus only	NNT to obtain 75% relief pain was 5. At 6 months the IDET group had a significant reduction in mean VAS compared to control (2.3 vs 1.1) (P = 0.45). Improvement in disability was also significant (P = 0.05) at 6 months	Subgroup analysis found IDET to be statistically superior to control in patients with pre-treatment pain scores below 7, ODI disability >40, and SF-36 physical function <55
Freeman et al. [149] Double-blind randomized controlled trial **IDET**	57 patients with axial low back pain >3 months and 1 or 2 positive diskograms	38 patients were treated with IDET. 19 were treated with intradiskal needle placement and sham heating	No subject in either treatment arm met the joint criteria for "success" at 6 months = no neurologic deficit, improvement in LBOS > 7 and improvement on SF-36 subscales of bodily pain and physical functioning of >1 SD from the mean	At 6 months neither group had any mean intragroup improvement in LBOS or ODI and the placebo group worsened in both parameters

Table 28.9 *Continued*

Author, method	Patients	Intervention	Results	Comments
Smith *et al.* [150] Multicenter randomized controlled trial with cross-over **IDDS**	202 patients with advanced cancer and refractory pain despite >200 mg/d oral morphine equivalents	IDDS started with morphine, other analgesics added as needed per algorithm by Staats [151]. Comprehensive medical management performed per guidelines	At 4 weeks 84.5% IDDS vs 70.8% CMM were clinical successes (P = 0.05). Significant (50%) toxicity reduction in IDDS group compared to CMM (P = 0.004). Clinical success = ≥20% reduction in VAS or equal VAS score with ≥20% reduction in toxicity	IDDS group had improved pain control, significantly decreased side effects and a trend toward increased survival at 6 months (53.9% vs 37.2%)

*Successful trial criteria: >50% pain relief, stable or improved analgesic intake, and improved physical activity. ** Successful trial criteria: >50% pain relief or a score of "much improved." CMM, comprehensive medical management; CRPS, complex regional pain syndrome; FBSS, failed back surgery syndrome; IDDS, intrathecal drug delivery systems; IDET,intradiskal electrothermal therapy; LBOS, low back pain outcome score; ODI, Oswestry Disability Index; QOL, quality of life; SCS, spinal cord stimulation; SD, standard deviation.

patients present with leg greater than back pain. The justification for SCS is further supported by its relative safety compared to reoperation. More robust randomized controlled trials are needed to confirm these results, and determine which patients are most likely to succeed with treatment. Evidence is especially needed to evaluate SCS in FBSS patients who present with a predominantly axial pain component.

Complications of permanent implantation of SCS are fairly common. The proportion of patients with at least one complication ranges from 9% to 50%, with the reoperation rate ranging between 11.1% to 50% [132]. The most common reported complication is lead migration (27%), followed by infection (6%) and battery failure (6%) [145]. Although rare, cases of epidural hematoma and paralysis have been reported [147].

Intradiskal electrothermal therapy (IDET)

The treatment of chronic diskogenic low back pain (CDLBP) remains a challenge for patients, physicians, and society as a whole. Failed conservative treatment has traditionally been followed by spinal fusion. However, little evidence exists to support the long-term benefit of spinal fusion over a comprehensive

rehabilitation program [152–154]. Since ethical concerns preclude conducting well-designed controlled studies evaluating spine surgery, the proportion of surgical success that is attributable to the placebo effect remains unknown. In part motivated by the questionable cost:benefit ratio of spinal fusion, Saal & Saal [155] introduced the use of intradiskal electrothermal therapy (IDET) in 2000 as a safer and less invasive alternative to treat diskogenic pain. The IDET procedure involves the placement of a navigable intradiskal catheter with a 6 cm electrothermal tip around the posterolateral border of the inner annulus, which is subsequently heated to a peak temperature of 90°C. Mechanisms of action for IDET remain a subject of debate, but may include nociceptor denervation, collagen denaturation and the sealing of annular tears [156]. Over the past few years, several variations of IDET have emerged including intradiskal radiofrequency intradiskal thermocoagulation, intradiskal biacuplasty and discTRODE, in which the RF electrode is directly inserted into the posterolateral mid-annulus. However, the evidence supporting or refuting any of these techniques is severely limited.

Four systematic reviews have recently been conducted to evaluate the efficacy of IDET and similar techniques in the treatment of CDLBP [157–160]. Two reviews concluded that there was no evidence to support IDET [158, 159] while the other two concluded that there was evidence of safety and efficacy [157, 160].

Urrutia *et al.* [159] reviewed the two RCT that compared IDET to placebo, which are reviewed in Table 28.9, and concluded that the available evidence does not support the efficacy of IDET. Among the two controlled studies comparing IDET with sham heating, one demonstrated modest benefit for IDET [148], while the other, more methodologically robust study conducted by a group of orthopedic surgeons found no benefit in either group [149]. In the one placebo-controlled study evaluating intradiskal RF thermocoagulation, no significant differences were noted between the control and treatment groups [161]. No differences were also noted in a randomized study assessing different methods for percutaneous intradiskal RF thermocoagulation, with both groups demonstrating only short-term relief [162]. In two prospective comparative studies, both groups of authors found IDET to be beneficial [163, 164]. In the earlier study, Bogduk & Karasek found that patients who received IDET were more likely to obtain significant pain reduction up to 2 years post procedure than those who participated in a comprehensive rehabilitation program. In a study comparing IDET to intradiskal RF thermocoagulation, Kapural *et al.* found IDET to be superior for both pain reduction and functional improvement up to 1 year post procedure.

In concordance with Urrutia, an orthopedic group led by Freeman *et al.* [158] conducted a systematic review evaluating five retrospective and 11 prospective trials as well as the two RCT. The 11 prospective trials included a total of 256 patients with a mean follow-up of 17.1 months. The mean improvement in VAS for back pain was 3.4 points and the mean improvement in Oswestry Disability Index (ODI) was 5.2 points (<10 minimal disability, maximum score 50). They concluded that the evidence for the efficacy of IDET remains weak and has not passed the standard of scientific proof. In contrast [157], a group associated with the manufacturers of IDET performed a meta-analysis of 17 studies evaluating the treatment. They found the overall mean VAS improvement to be 2.9 points, the mean improvement in SF-36 physical function to be 21.1 points (normal >84.2, maximum score 100), a mean improvement in SF-36 bodily pain of 18.0 points (normal >75.2, maximum score 100),

and a mean improvement in ODI of 7.0 points. They also reported a 0.8% complication rate. They concluded that the published studies provide compelling evidence of the relative efficacy and safety of IDET.

Andersson *et al.* [160] performed a systematic review that compared IDET with spinal fusion outcomes. The results of the two therapies were similar with respect to pain relief (50–51%) and quality of life improvement (43–46%). However, spinal surgery resulted in greater improvements than IDET with regard to back function (42% versus 14%). This improvement did come at the expense of a greater incidence of complications, which ranged between 2–54% in the 31 studies evaluating fusion and 0–15% in the 14 studies evaluating IDET. The authors concluded that IDET offers similar symptomatic relief with a lower risk for complications.

Perhaps more than any other procedure, the four mentioned reviews appeared to be at least somewhat influenced by the reviewer's perspective, with those conducted by practitioners who perform or who have a vested interest in the procedure tending to report more positive results. This is clearly illustrated by the fact that Appleby and Freeman evaluated very similar data but came up with contradictory conclusions. This specialty bias also pervades the cadaveric literature on IDET. Whereas Bono *et al.* reported that IDET heating achieved sufficient temperatures to alter collagen architecture and coagulate nociceptors, Kleinstueck *et al.* (an orthopedic group) concluded the opposite [165, 166]. The same contradictory conclusions based on specialty bias were also reported for spinal stability after IDET [167, 168].

Given that only two RCT have been performed and divergent results were reported, it is not surprising that different reviews arrived at contradictory conclusions. The studies by Pauza *et al.* [148] and Freeman *et al.* [149] are markedly different. The one by Pauza *et al.* was a highly selective study involving only 64 subjects among over 1300 screened. This study also had a sham group success rate of 38%, suggesting a profound placebo effect associated with either the procedure itself or the conduct of the trial in general. In contrast, the study by Freeman *et al.* used liberal inclusion criteria more consistent with the majority of patients treated in specialty clinics for chronic diskogenic LBP, and very strict success criteria (no patient in either group experienced a "successful outcome"). Six months post-IDET, whereas the control group worsened, clinically insignificant improvement occurred across all parameters in the IDET group. Since patients in this study were not asked what their expectations were, it is impossible to determine if there was a systemic issue that contributed to the absence of any beneficial effect (i.e. a nocebo effect) [169, 170].

Intradiskal electrothermal therapy is widely considered to be safer than open surgery, with a reported complication rate of around 1%. However, serious complications have been reported including catheter breakage [171], vertebral osteonecrosis [172], herniated disk [173], and cauda equina syndrome [174].

In summary, the clinical utility of IDET is dependent on the perspective of the reviewer. Prospective and retrospective evidence provide mixed support for its efficacy as summarized in the reviews detailed above. The study by Pauza et al. [148] provides support for its efficacy in carefully selected patients, whereas the study by Freeman et al. [149] provides evidence against its use as a "cure" for diskogenic LBP. Given that there is not a current gold standard in the treatment of diskogenic LBP, IDET should remain a viable interventional technique for patients who meet strict inclusion criteria [148]. Future studies should focus on further identifying prognostic factors for success and complications, and should include comparative groups treated with comprehensive rehabilitation, surgery and sham controls.

Continuous neuraxial infusions

Since the discovery of specific opioid receptors in the CNS in the 1970s, attempts have been made to optimize medical therapy by delivering medications centrally rather than parenterally [175–178]. Wang et al. [179] reported the first case of intrathecal morphine administration to relieve pain in humans. Since that time, neuraxial drug delivery has been increasingly used to treat both malignant and nonmalignant pain. Although this section focuses on the treatment of malignant pain, there are many experts advocating its use in nonmalignant pain (see Erdine & de Andres [180] for a contemporary review).

The current literature consists predominantly of uncontrolled trials comprising a mix of retrospective case series and prospective cohort studies. One prospective, randomized trial was found which is detailed in Table 28.9. In a recent Cochrane systematic review comparing the efficacy of epidural, subarachnoid, and intracerebroventricular opioids in patients with cancer pain, Ballantyne & Carwood [181] found that neuraxial opioid therapy is often effective for treating cancer pain that is not adequately controlled by systemic treatment. A pooled analysis of data from uncontrolled studies reported excellent pain relief among 72% of patients treated with epidural opioids and 62% of those treated with subarachnoid opioids. The incidence of unsatisfactory relief was low in all three groups.

A large, well-designed multicenter randomized trial by Smith et al. [150] lends further support to the efficacy of intrathecal drug delivery systems (IDDS) to manage refractory cancer pain. In addition to improved pain control, a key finding in the study was the reduction in composite drug toxicity score. The authors found that a reduction in drug toxicity score was associated with improved survival, which suggests that the improved 6-month survival found in the IDDS group might be a function of reduced drug toxicity. Specifically, statistically significant reductions in fatigue and depressed level of consciousness were reported. However, the finding of improved survival should be interpreted cautiously since it was not designated as a primary endpoint. The authors concluded that IDDS improved pain control, significantly reduced common drug toxicities, and enhanced survival in patients with refractory cancer pain.

Epidural administration might be expected to have similar efficacy but similar RCT have not been performed. One key difference between the two therapies is the cost of an external epidural system versus an implanted subarachnoid system. Hassenbusch et al. [182] developed an economic model that predicted that the break-even point at which it becomes less expensive to administer opioids with an implanted intrathecal pump than via an external epidural pump is between 3 and 6 months. A similar point was found to be between 1.5 and 2.5 years with respect to IDDS versus systemic treatment.

Complications are fairly common with neuraxial infusions. They are due to pharmacologic side effects, surgical complications, and device-related complications. All opioid-related side effects also occur when the medication is given neuraxially, but many are reduced compared to systemic administration, as reported by Smith *et al.* [150]. The incidence of major infection reported by Ballantyne & Carwood [181] was 1.44% for epidural and 2.54% for subarachnoid systems. Overall, the combined surgical and device complication rates are typically in line with the 25% rate reported by Smith *et al.*

In conclusion, there is moderate evidence that neuraxial infusion techniques are effective in treating cancer pain when parenteral treatment has failed. However, there is little evidence present to guide clinical use with respect to the timing of implantation. Robust studies with cost analysis and length of survival as primary endpoints are still needed.

The evidence supporting IDDS in chronic nonmalignant pain is not as robust as the evidence in cancer pain. To some extent, this may be due to the different mechanisms characterizing pain in the two conditions. In patients with cancer, between 75% and 90% of pain is either nociceptive or mixed nociceptive-neuropathic in origin [183, 184]. In chronic nonmalignant pain, the etiology is more variable. In the chronic pain conditions most amenable to spinal analgesia such as CRPS and FBSS, neuropathic pain plays the most prominent role. Numerous preclinical [185] and clinical studies [186, 187] have shown that neuropathic pain is less responsive to opioids than nociceptive pain.

Thimineur *et al.* [188] performed a prospective study to investigate long-term outcomes of intrathecal (IT) opioid therapy in patients with severe, refractory chronic nonmalignant pain. The authors compared treatment outcomes between 31 patients who received IT opioid therapy, 38 patients who either failed their trial or refused pump implantation, and 41 newly referred patients who were not offered IT therapy. During the 3-year study, pain scores, functional capacity and mood scores significantly improved in the recipients, while they either declined or stayed the same in nonpump recipients. However, most IT patients continued to suffer from moderate to severe pain. The authors concluded that "when patients with extremely severe pain are selected as pump candidates, they will likely improve with therapy, but their overall severity of pain and symptoms will remain

high." Multiple prospective studies support the notion that IDDS can be a safe and effective therapy in the management of severe refractory nonmalignant pain in carefully selected patients [189–192] although this conclusion is by no means universal [193].

Conclusion

As is readily apparent from this review evaluating interventional techniques for pain management, more research is needed to guide clinical decision making. One area in which this is especially true is the documentation of complication rates. Currently, complication rates are based on extrapolation from controlled trials, insurance registries and retrospective chart reviews. In the present system, common complication rates vary widely among sources and rare complications often go unreported altogether, as evidenced in the case of cervical transforaminal epidural steroid injections. The recent survey by Scanlon *et al.* [38] provides some perspective as to the scope of adverse events, but fails to provide any insight into the incidence since a denominator cannot be determined from the survey. Other flaws included the low response rate (21%) and database used to query respondents, which contains relatively few interventionalists. Surveys in the future would benefit from a design similar to that of Auroy *et al.* [194] who conducted a prospective survey of French anesthesiologists regarding regional anesthetic complications. The study resulted in data involving 103,730 regional anesthetics, with useful information garnered for each complication.

The future also offers a great deal of promise. Surveillance systems similar to the regional anesthesia surveillance system (RASS) [195] can be designed and implemented across practices, institutions, states or countries through the use of shared information technologies. However, financial support and political will are required at each level. Open reporting of complications without fear of litigation is crucial to the future of medicine, especially with regard to pain management, which is a specialty field still in its infancy. The cost of therapy will continue to be a factor, but "do no harm" must remain one of the primary tenets of medicine. If the true incidence of complications is known, then more informed decisions could be made with regard to therapy.

Some interventional procedures can be difficult or impossible to study with RCT due to ethical concerns (IDDS), cost (IDDS/SCS) or the fact that the nature of the treatment unavoidably entails unblinding (SCS). These same issues also apply to surgical interventions for similar conditions. A Cochrane systematic review by Gibson & Waddell [153] reported no surgical trials which compared surgery to sham surgery. The surgical literature, much like the IDDS and SCS literature, is full of positive retrospective and prospective trials, as well as positive randomized trials comparing the relevant intervention to a standard suboptimal conservative treatment that in many cases had already failed. In contrast, epidural, facet joint, SI joint and intradiskal treatments are more amenable to double-blind studies, and have all been compared to placebo interventions, albeit with somewhat mixed results. Given the current push toward evidence-based medicine as currently defined [138, 196], IDDS, SCS and open surgery, as well as other interventions, will require methods other than true RCT to assess efficacy.

Pain and, more to the point, pain treatment is a complex, multifactorial endeavor that involves treating both the organic pathology as well as the patient as a whole. Toward this end, more research needs to be performed to not only provide better evidence for interventions that cannot be studied by RCT, but for pain procedures in general. Interventional studies should be evaluated by comparison to comprehensive noninterventional treatment which may include cognitive behavioral therapy, physical therapy and functional restoration, and pharmacologic treatment, similar to those described by Brox et al. [152]. Comparison to these types of programs ensures that patients are provided with the best conservative treatment available, which then allows patients and clinicians to make informed decisions based on the degree and likelihood of pain relief as well as the relative risk. Any significant treatment benefit reported in the intervention group compared to the conservative treatment group can then be attributed to the efficacy of the procedure with the expectation that it can be reproduced in clinical practice. With this knowledge, patients and doctors could make personalized, informed decisions regarding medical care.

References

1. Sicard MA. Les injections medicamenteuse extraduraqles per voie saracoccygiene. *Comptes Renues des Senances de la Societe de Biolgie et de ses Filliales* 1901; **53**: 452–453.
2. Olmarker K, Rydevik B, Nordborg C. Autologous nucleus pulposus induces neurophysiologic and histologic changes in porcine cauda equina nerve roots. *Spine* 1993; **18**: 1425–1432.
3. Olmarker K, Rydevik B. Selective inhibition of tumor necrosis factor-alpha prevents nucleus pulposus-induced thrombus formation, intraneural edema, and reduction of nerve conduction velocity: possible implications for future pharmacologic treatment strategies of sciatica. *Spine* 2001; **26**: 863–869.
4. Stojanovic MP, Vu T, Caneris O, Slezak J, Cohen SP, Sang CN. The role of fluoroscopy in cervical epidural steroid injections. *Spine* 2002; **27**(5): 509–514.
5. Botwin K, Natalicchio J, Brown LA. Epidurography contrast patterns with fluoroscopic guided lumbar transforaminal epidural injections: a prospective evaluation. *Pain Physician* 2004; **7**(2): 211–215.
6. Fredman B, Nun MB, Zohar E, Iraqi G, Shapiro M, Gepstein R, *et al.* Epidural steroid for treating "Failed back surgery syndrome": is fluoroscopy really necessary? *Reg Anesth Pain Med* 1999; **88**: 367–372.
7. White AH, Derby R, Wynne G. Epidural injections for the diagnosis and treatment of low back pain. *Spine* 1980; **5**: 78–86.
8. Koes B, Scholten R, Mens J, Bouter L. Efficacy of epidural steroid injections for low back pain and sciatica: a systematic review of randomized clinical trials. *Pain* 1995; **63**: 279–288.
9. Koes B, Scholten R, Mens J, Bouter L. Epidural steroid and sciatica: an updated systematic review of randomized clinical trials. *Pain Digest* 1999; **9**: 241–247.
10. Watts R, Silagy C. A meta-analysis on the efficacy of epidural corticosteroids in the treatment of sciatica. *Anaesth Intens Care* 1995; **23**: 564–569.
11. Weinstein S, Herring S, Derby R. Contemporary concept in spine care. Epidural steroid injections. *Spine* 1995; **20**: 1842–1846.
12. McQuay H, Moore R, Eccleston C, Morley S, Williams A. Systematic review of outpatient services for chronic pain control. *Health Technol Assess* 1997; **1**: 1–135.
13. Rozenberg S, Dubourg G, Khalifa P, Paolozzi L, Maheu E, Ravaud P. Efficacy of epidural steroids in low back pain and sciatica. *Revue Rhumatisme* 1999; **66**: 79–85.
14. Tonkovich-Quaranta L, Winkler S. Use of epidural corticosteroids in low back pain. *Ann Pharmacother* 2000; **34**: 1165–1172.
15. Vroomen P, de Krom M, Slofstra P, Knottnerus J. Conservative treatment of sciatica: a systematic review. *J Spinal Disord* 2000; **13**(6): 463–469.
16. Nelemans P, de Bie R, de Vet H, Sturmans F. Injection therapy for subacute and chronic benign low back pain. *Spine* 2001; **26**: 501–515.

17. Singh V, Manchikanti L. Role of caudal epidural injections in the management of chronic low back pain. *Pain Physician* 2002; **5**(2): 133–148.

18. Peloso PMJ, Gross A, Haines T, Trinh K, Goldsmith CH, Burnie SJ, Cervical Overview Group. Medicinal and injection therapies for mechanical neck disorders. Cochrane Database of Systematic Reviews 2007, Issue 3. Art. No.: CD000319. DOI: 10.1002/14651858.CD000319.pub4.

19. Abdi S, Datta S, Trescot A, Schultz D, Adlaka R, Atluri S, *et al*. Epidural steroids in the management of chronic spinal pain: a systematic review. *Pain Physician* 2007; **10**: 185–212.

20. Armon C, Argoff C, Samuels J, Backonja M. Assessment: use of epidural steroid injections to treat radicular lumbosacral pain. *Neurology* 2007; **68**: 723–729.

21. Thomas E, Cyteval C, Abiad L, Picot MC, Taourel P, Blotman F. Efficacy of transforaminal versus interspinous corticosteroid injection in discal radiculalgia-a prospective, randomised, double-blind study. *Clin Rheumatol* 2003; **22**: 299–304.

22. Airaksinen O, Brox J, Cedraschi C, Hildebrandt J, Klaber-Moffett J, Kovacs F, *et al*. European guidelines for the management of chronic nonspecific low back pain. *Eur Spine J* 2006; **15**: S192–S300.

23. Boswell MV, Colson JD, Sehgal N, Dunbar EE, Epter R. A systematic review of therapeutic facet joint interventions in chronic spinal pain. *Pain Physician* 2007; **10**: 229–253.

24. Riew KD, Yuming Y, Gilula L, Bridwell K, Lenke L, Lauryssen C, *et al*. The effect of nerve-root injections on the need for operative treatment of lumbar radicular pain: A prospective, randomized, controlled, double-blind study. *J Bone Joint Surg (Am)* 2000; **82**-A(11): 1589–1593.

25. Riew KD, Park JB, Cho YS, Gilula L, Patel A, Lenke L, *et al*. Nerve root blocks in the treatment of lumbar radicular pain. *J Bone Joint Surg (Am)* 2006; **88**-A(8): 1722–1725.

26. Carette S, Leclaire R, Marcoux S, Morin F, Blaise G. Epidural corticosteroid injections for sciatica due to herniated nucleus pulposus. *N Engl J Med* 1997; **336**: 1634–1640.

27. Stav A, Ovadia L, Sternberg A, Kaadan M, Weksler N. Cervical epidural steroid injection for cervicobrachialgia. *Acta Anaesth Scand* 1993; **37**: 562–566.

28. Castagnera L, Maurette P, Pointillart V, Vital J, Erny P, Senegas J. Long-term results of cervical epidural steroid injection with and without morphine in chronic cervical radicular pain. *Pain* 1994; **58**: 239–243.

29. Bush K, Hillier H. Outcome of cervical radiculopathy treated with periradicular/epidural corticosteroid injections: a prospective study with independent clinical review. *Eur Spine J* 1996; **5**: 319–325.

30. Lin EL, Lieu V, Halevi L, Shamie AN, Wang JC. Cervical epidural steroid injections for symptomatic disc herniations. *J Spinal Disord Tech* 2006; **19**: 183–186.

31. Kolstad F, Leivseth G, Nygaard O. Transforaminal steroid injections in the treatment of cervical radiculopathy. A prospective outcome study. *Acta Neurochir (Wein)* 2005; **147**: 1065–1070.

32. Cyteval C, Thomas E, Decoux E, Sarrabere MP, Cottin A, Blotman F, *et al*. Cervical radiculopathy: open study on percutaneous periradicular foraminal steroid infiltration performed under CT control in 30 patients. *Am J Neuroradiol* 2004; **25**: 441–445.

33. Rosin L, Rozin R, Koehler SA, Shakir A, Ladham S, Barmada M, *et al*. Death during transforaminal epidural steroid nerve root block (C7) due to perforation of the left vertebral artery. *Am J Forensic Med Pathol* 2003; **24**: 351–355.

34. Glaser SE, Falco F. Paraplegia following a thoracolumbar transforaminal epidural steroid injection. *Pain Physician* 2005; **8**: 309–314.

35. Baker R, Dreyfuss P, Mercer S, Bogduk N. Cervical transforaminal injection of corticosteroids into a radicular artery: a possible mechanism for spinal cord injury. *Pain* 2004; **103**: 211–215.

36. Houten JK, Errico TJ. Paraplegia after lumbosacral nerve root block: report of three cases. *Spine J* 2002; **2**: 70–75.

37. Manchikanti L. The growth of interventional pain management in the new millennium: a critical analysis of utilization in the Medicare population. *Pain Physician* 2004; **7**: 465–482.

38. Scanlon G, Moeller-Bertram T, Romanowsky S, Wallace M. Cervical transforaminal epidural steroid injections. *Spine* 2007; **32**(11): 1249–1256.

39. Botwin KP, Gruber RD, Bouchlas CG, Torres-Ramos FM, Freeman TL, Slaten Wk. Complications of fluoroscopically guided transforaminal lumbar epidural injections. *Arch Phys Med Rehabil* 2000; **81**: 1045–1050.

40. Botwin KP, Gruber RD, Bouchlas CG, Torres-Ramos FM, Hanna A, Rittenberg J, *et al*. Complications of fluoroscopically guided caudal epidural injections. *Arch Phys Med Rehabil* 2001; **80**: 416–424.

41. Botwin KP, Castellanos R, Rao S, Hanna AF, Torres-Ramos FM, Gruber RD, *et al*. Complications of fluoroscopically guided interlaminar cervical epidural injections. *Arch Phys Med Rehabil* 2003; **84**: 627–633.

42. Botwin KP, Baskin M, Rao S. Adverse effects of fluoroscopically guided interlaminar thoracic epidural steroid injections. *Am J Phys Med Rehabil* 2006; **85**: 14–23.

43. Cluff R, Mehio A, Cohen S, Chang Y, Sang C, Stojanovic MP. The technical aspects of epidural steroid injections: a national survey. *Anesthes Analges* 2002; **95**: 403–408.

44. Evans W. Intrasacral epidural injection in the treatment of sciatica. *Lancet* 1930; **2**: 1225–1229.

45. Massie J, Huang B, Malkmus S, Yaksh T, Kim C, Garfin S, *et al*. A preclinical laminectomy rat model mimics the human post laminectomy syndrome. *J Neurosci Methods* 2004; **137**: 283–289.

46. Burchiel KJ, Johan T, Ochoa J. Painful nerve injuries: bridges the gap between basic neuroscience and neurosurgical treatment. *Acta Neurochir* 1993; **58**(suppl): 131–135.

47. Campbell J. Nerve lesions and the generation of pain. *Muscle Nerve* 2001; **24**: 1261–1273.

48. Carlton S, Lekan H, Kim S, Chung J. Behavioral manifestations of an experimental model for peripheral neuropathy produced by spinal nerve ligation in the primate. *Pain* 1994; **56**: 155–166.

49. Millesi H. Forty-two years of peripheral nerve surgery. *Microsurgery* 1993; **14**: 228–233.

50. Vogelsang J, Finkenstaedt M, Vogelsang M, Markakis E. Recurrent pain after lumbar discectomy: the diagnostic value of peridural scar on MRI. *Eur Spine J* 1999; **8**: 475–479.

51. Trescot A, Chopra P, Abdi S, Datta S, Schultz D. Systematic review of effectiveness and complications of adhesiolysis in the management of chronic spinal pain: an update. *Pain Physician* 2007; **10**: 129–146.

52. Dashfield A, Taylor M, Cleaver J, Farrow D. Comparison of caudal steriod epidural with targeted steroid placement during spinal endoscopy for chronic sciatica: a prospective, randomized, double-blind trial. *Br J Anaesth* 2005; **94**(4): 514–519.

53. Interventional procedures overview of endoscopic division of epidural adhesions. National Institute for Clinical Excellence. 2004. www.nice.org.uk/IPG088guidance.

54. Bush K, Hillier S. A controlled study of caudal epidural injections of triamcinolone plus procaine for the management of intractable sciatica. *Spine* 1991; **16**(5): 572–575.

55. Mathews J, Mills S, Jenkins V, Grimes S, Morkel M, Mathews W, *et al.* Back pain and sciatica: controlled trials of manipulation, traction, sclerosant and epidural injections. *Br J Rheumatol* 1987; **26**: 416–423.

56. Breivik H, Helsa PE, Molnar I, Lind B. Treatment of chronic low back pain and sciatica. Comparison of caudal epidural injections of bupivacaine and methylprednisolone with bupivacaine followed by saline. In: Bonica JJ, AlbeFesard D (eds) *Advances in Pain Research and Therapy*, vol 1. Raven Press, New York, 1976: 927–932.

57. Wilson-MacDonald J, Burt G, Griffin D, Glynn C. Epidural steroid injection for nerve root compression. *J Bone Joint Surg* 2005; **87–B**(3): 352–355.

58. Arden NK, Price C, Reading I, Stubbing J, Hazelgrove J, Dunne C, *et al.* A multicentre randomized controlled trial of epidural corticosteroid injections for sciatica: the WEST study. *Rheumatology* 2005; **44**(11): 1399–1406.

59. Valat J-P, Giraudeau B, Rozenberg S, Goupille P, Bourgeois P, Micheau-Beaugendre V, *et al.* Epidural corticosteroid injections for sciatica: a randomised, double blind, controlled clinical trial. *Ann Rheum Dis* 2003; **62**: 639–643.

60. Buchner M, Zeifang F, Brocai DRC, Schiltenwolf M. Epidural corticosteroid injection in the conservative management of sciatica. *Clin Orthop Relat Res* 2000; **375**: 149–156.

61. Kraemer J, Ludwig J, Bickert U, Owczarek V, Traupe M. Lumbar epidural perineural injection: a new technique. *Eur Spine J* 1997; **6**: 357–361.

62. Ridley MG, Kingsley GH, Gibson T, Grahame R. Outpatient lumbar epidural corticosteroid injection in the management of sciatica. *Br J Rheumatol* 1988; **27**: 295–299.

63. Cuckler JM, Bernini PA, Wiesel SW, Booth REJ, Rothman RH, Pickens GT. The use of epidural steroids in the treatment of lumbar radicular pain. A prospective, randomized, double-blind study. *J Bone Joint Surg (Am)* 1985; **67**(1): 63–66.

64. Dilke TFW, Burry HC, Grahame R. Extradural corticosteroid injection in management of lumbar nerve root compression. *BMJ* 1973; **2**: 635–637.

65. Ng L, Chaudhary N, Sell P. The efficacy of corticosteroids in periradicular infiltration for chronic radicular pain. *Spine* 2005; **30**(8): 857–862.

66. Vad VB, Bhat AL, MD, Lutz GE, Cammisa F. Transforaminal epidural steroid injections in lumbosacral radiculopathy. *Spine* 2002; **27**(1): 11–16.

67. Karppinen J, Malmivaara A, Kurunlahti M, Kyllönen E, Pienimäki T, Nieminen P, *et al.* Periradicular infiltration for sciatica: a randomized controlled trial. *Spine* 2001; **26**(9): 1059–1067.

68. Karppinen J, Ohinmaa A, Malmivaara A, Kurunlahti M, Kyllonen E, Pienimaki T. Cost effectiveness of periradicular infiltration for sciatica *Spine* 2001; **26**(23): 2587–2595.

69. Veihelmann A, Devens C, Trouiller H, Birkenmaier C, Gerdesmeyer L, Refior H. Epidural neuroplasty versus physiotherapy to relieve pain in patients with sciatica: a prospective randomized blinded clinical trial. *J Orthop Sci* 2006; **11**: 365–369.

70. Manchikanti L, Rivera J, Pampati V, Damron KS, McManus CD, Brandon DE, *et al.* One day lumbar epidural adhesiolysis and hypertonic saline neurolysis in treatment of chronic low back pain. *Pain Physician* 2004; **7**: 177–186.

71. Manchikanti L, Pampati V, Fellows B, Rivera J, Beyer C, Damron K. Role of one day epidural adhesiolysis in management of chronic low back pain: a randomized clinical trial. *Pain Physician* 2001; **4**(2): 153–166.

72. Heavner J, Racz G, Raj P. Percutaneous epidural neuroplasty. Prospective evaluation of 0.9% NaCl versus 10% NaCl with or without hyaluronidase. *Reg Anesth Pain Med* 1999; **24**: 202–207.

73. Manchikanti L, Boswell M, Rivera J, Pampati V, Damron K, McManus C, *et al.* A randomized, controlled trial of spinal endoscopic adhesiolysis in chronic refractory low back and lower extremity pain. *BMC Anesthesiol* 2005; **5**(10).

74. Goldthwaite J. The lumbosacral articulation: an explanation of many cases of lumbago, sciatica, and paraplegia. *Boston Med Surg J* 1911; **164**: 365–372.

75. Shealy C. Percutaneous radiofrequency denervation of spinal facets: treatment for chronic back pain and sciatica. *J Neurosurg* 1975; **43**: 448–451.

76. Pedersen H, Blunck C, Gardner E. The anatomy of the lumbosacral posterior rami and meningeal brances of spinal nerves (sinuvertebral nerves) – with an experimental study of their function. *J Bone Joint Surg* 1956; **38**: 377–391.

77. Dreyfus P, Dreyer S. Lumbar zygapophysial joint (facet) injections. *Spine J* 2003; **3**: 50S–9S.

78. Berven S, Tay B, Colman W, Hu S. The lumbar zygapophyseal (facet) joints: a role in the pathogenesis of spinal pina syndromes and degenerative spondylolisthesis. *Semin Neurol* 2002; **22**: 187–195.

79. Resnick D, Choudhri T, Dailey A, Groff M, Khoo L, Matz P, *et al.* American Association of Neurological Surgeons/ Congress of Neurological Surgeons. Guidelines for the performance of fusion procedures for degenerative disease of the lumbar spine Part 13: Injection therapies, low-back pain, and lumbar fusion. *J Neurosurg Spine* 2005; **2**: 707–715.

80. Bogduk N. A narrative review of intra-articular corticosteroid injections for low back pain. *Pain Med* 2005; **6**: 287–296.

81. Slipman C, Bhat A, Gilchrist R, Isaac Z, Chou L, Lenrow D. A critical review of the evidence for the use of zygapophysial injections and radiofrequency denervation in the treatment of low back pain. *Spine J* 2003; **3**: 310–316.

82. Cohen SP, Raja SN. Pathogenesis, diagnosis, and treatment of lumbar zygapophysial (facet) joint pain. *Anesthesiology* 2007; **106**: 591–614.

83. Dolan AL, Ryan PJ, Arden NK, Statton R, Wedley JR, Hamann W, *et al.* The value of SPECT scans in identifying back pain likely to benefit from facet joint injection. *Br J Rheumatol* 1996; **35**: 1269–1273.

84. Pneumaticos SG, Chatziioannou SN, Hipp JA, Moore WH, I ES. Low back pain: prediction of short-term outcome of facet joint injection with bone scintigraphy. *Radiology* 2006; **238**: 693–698.

85. Holder LE, Machin JL, Asdourian PL, Links JM, Sexton CC. Planar and high-resolution SPECT bone imaging in the diagnosis of facet syndrome. *J Nucl Med* 1995; **36**(1): 37–44.

86. Barnsley L, Lord S, Wallis B, Bogduk N. Lack of effect of intraarticular corticosteroids for chronic pain in the cervical zygapophyseal joints. *N Engl J Med* 1994; **330**: 1047–1050.

87. Manchikanti L, Pampati V, Fellows B, Bakhit C. The diagnostic validity and therapeutic value of lumbar facet joint nerve blocks with or without adjuvant age nts. *Curr Rev Pain* 2000; **4**: 337–344.

88. Schwarzer AC, Aprill CN, Derby R, Fortin L, Kine G, Bogduk N. The false-positive rate of uncontrolled diagnostic blocks of the lumbar zygapophysial joints. *Pain* 1994; **58**: 195–200.

89. Hogan QH, Abram SE. Neural blockade for diagnosis and prognosis: a review. *Anesthesiology* 1997; **86**: 216–241.

90. Leclaire R, Fortin L, Lambert R, Bergeron YM, Rossignol M. Radiofrequency facet joint denervation in the treatment of low back pain. *Spine* 2001; **26**: 1411–1417.

91. Lord S, Barnsley L, Wallis B, McDonald G, Bogduk N. Percutaneous radiofrequency neurotomy for chronic cervical zygapophyseal joint pain. *N Engl J Med* 1996; **335**: 1721–1726.

92. Barnsley L. Percutaneous radiofrequency neurotomy for chronic neck pain: outcomes in a series of consecutive patients. *Pain Med* 2005; **6**: 282–286.

93. Shin WR, Kim HI, Shin DG, Shin DA. Radiofrequency neurotomy of cervical medial branches for chronic cervicobrachialgia. *J Korean Med Sci* 2006; **21**: 119–125.

94. Sapir D, Gorup JM. Radiofrequency medial branch neurotomy in litigant and non-litigant patients with cervical whiplash. *Spine* 2001; **26**: E268–E273.

95. McDonald GJ, Lord SM, Bogduk N. Long-term follow-up of patients treated with cervical radiofrequency neurotomy for chronic neck pain. *Neurosurgery* 1999; **45**: 61–68.

96. Stovner LJ, Kolstad F, Helde G. Radiofrequency denervation of facet joints C2–C6 in cervicogenic headache: a randomized, double-blind, sham-controlled study. *Cephalalgia* 2004; **24**: 821–830.

97. Gallagher J, Petriccione DVP, Wedley J, Hamann W, Ryan P, Chikanza I, *et al.* Radiofrequency facet joint denervation in the treatment of low back pain: a prospective controlled double-blind study to assess its efficacy. *Pain Clin* 1994; **7**: 193–198.

98. van Kleef M, Barendse G, Kessels A, Voets H, Weber W, de Lange S. Randomized trial of radiofrequency lumbar facet denervation for chronic low back pain. *Spine* 1999; **24**: 1937–1942.

99. Staender M, Maerz U, Tonn JC, Steude U. Computerized tomography-guided kryorhizotomy in 76 patients with lumbar facet joint syndrome. *J Neurosurg* 2005; **3**: 444–449.

100. Dreyfuss P, Halbrook B, Pauza K, Joshi A, McLarty J, Bogduk N. Efficacy and validity of radiofrequency neurotomy for chronic lumbar zygapophysial joint pain. *Spine* 2000; **25**: 1270–1277.

101. Vad VB, Cano WG, Basrai D, Lutz GE, Bhat AL. Role of radiofrequency denervation in lumbar zygapophyseal joint synovitis in baseball pitchers: a clinical experience. *Pain Physician* 2003; **6**: 307–312.

102. van Wijk RM, Geurts JW, Wynne HJ, Hammink E, Buskens E, Lousberg R, *et al.* Radiofrequency denervation of lumbar facet joints in the treatment of chronic low back pain: a randomized, double-blind, sham lesion-controlled trial. *Clin J Pain* 2005; **21**: 335–344.

103. Bogduk N. Lumbar radiofrequency neurotomy (commentary). *Clin J Pain* 2005; **21**: 335–344.

104. Kornick C, Kramarich S, Lamer T, Sitzman B. Complications of lumbar facet radiofrequency denervation. *Spine* 2004; **29**: 1352–1354.

105. Schofferman J, Kine G. Effectiveness of repeated radiofrequency neurotomy for lumbar facet pain. *Spine* 2004; **29**: 2471–2473.

106. Lynch MC, Taylor JF. Facet joint injection for low back pain: a clinical study. *J Bone Joint Surg (Br)* 1986; **1**: 138–141.

107. Lilius G, Laasonen EM, Harilainen A, Gronlund G. Lumbar facet joint syndrome: a randomised clinical trial. *J Bone Joint Surg (Br)* 1989; **71**: 746–750.

108. Nash TP. Facet joints: intra-articular steroids or nerve block? *Pain Clin* 1990; **3**: 77–82.

109. Carette S, Marcoux S, Truch on R, Grondin C, Gagnon J, Allard Y, *et al.* A controlled trial of corticosteroid injections into facet joints for chronic low back pain. *N Engl J Med* 1991; **325**: 1002–1007.

110. Marks RC, Houston T, Thulbourne T. Facet joint injection and facet nerve block: a randomized comparison in 86 patients with chronic low back pain. *Pain* 1992; **49**: 325–328.

111. Fuchs S, Erbe T, Fischer HL, Tibesku CO. Intraarticular hyaluronic acid versus glucocorticoid injections for nonradicular pain in the lumbar spine. *J Vasc Interv Radiol* 2005; **16**: 1493–1498.

112. King J, Lagger R. Sciatica viewed as a referred pain syndrome. *Surg Neurol* 1976; **5**: 46–50.

113. Sanders M, Zuurmond WW. Percutaneous intra-articular lumbar facet joint denervation in the treatment of low back pain. A comparison with percutaneous extra-araticular lumbar facet denervation. *Pain Clin* 1999; **11**: 329–335.

114. Cohen SP. Sacroiliac joint pain: a comprehensive review of anatomy, diagnosis, and treatment. *Anesthes Analges* 2005; **101**: 1440–1453.

115. Luukkainen R, Wennerstrand PV, Kautiainen HH. Efficacy of periarticular corticosteroid treatment of the sacroiliac joint in non-spondyloarthropathic patients with chronic low back pain in the region of the sacroiliac joint. *Clin Exp Rheumatol* 2002; **20**: 52–54.

116. Maugars Y, Mathis C, Berthelot JM, Charlier C, Prost A. Assessment of the efficacy of sacroiliac corticosteroid injections in spondyloarthropathies: a double-blind study. *Br J Rheumatol* 1996; **35**: 767–770.

117. Ferrante FM, King LF, Roche EA, Kim PS, Aranda M, Delaney LR, et al. Radiofrequency sacroiliac joint denervation for sacroiliac syndrome. *Reg Anesth Pain Med* 2001; **26**: 137–142.

118. Gervargez A, Groenemeyer D, Schirp S, Braun M. CT-guided percutaneous radiofrequency denervation of the sacroiliac joint. *Eur Radiol* 2002; **12**: 1360–1365.

119. Burnham RS, Yasui Y. An alternate method of radiofrequency neurotomy of the sacroiliac joint: a pilot study of the effect on pain, function, and satisfaction. *Reg Anesth Pain Med* 2007; **32**(1): 12–19.

120. Cohen SP, Abdi S. Lateral branch blocks as a treatment for sacroiliac joint pain: a pilot study. *Reg Anesth Pain Med* 2003; **28**: 113–119.

121. Buijs EJ, Kamphuis ET, Groen GJ. Radiofrequency treatment of sacroiliac joint-related pain aimed at the first three sacral dorsal rami: a minimal approach. *Pain Clin* 2004; **16**: 139–146.

122. Yin W, Willard F, Carreiro J, Dreyfus P. Sensory stimulation guided sacroiliac joint radiofrequency neurotomy: technique based on neuroanatomy of the dorsal sacral plexus. *Spine* 2003; **28**: 2419–2425.

123. Cohen SP, Hurley RW, Buckenmaier CC 3rd, Kurihara C, Morlando B, Dragovich A. Randomized placebo-controlled study evaluating lateral branch radiofrequency denervation for sacroiliac joint pain. *Anesthesiology* 200; **109**(2): 167–8.

124. Luukkainen R, Wennerstrand PV, Kautiainen HH. Periarticular corticosteroid treatment of the sacroiliac joint in patients with seronegative spondyloarthropathy. *Clin Exp Rheumatol* 1999; **17**: 88–90.

125. Fischer T, Biedermann T, Hermann KG. Sacroiliitis in children with spondyloarthropathy: therapeutic effect of CT-guided intra-articular corticosteroid injection (in German). *Rofo* 2003; **175**: 814–821.

126. Shealy CN, Mortimer JT, Reswick JB. Electrical inhibition of pain by stimulation of the dorsal columns: preliminary clinical report. *Anesthes Analges* 1967; **46**: 489–491.

127. Melzack R, Wall PD. Pain mechanisms: a new theory. *Science* 1965; **150**: 971–979.

128. Meyerson BA, Linderoth B. Mechanisms of spinal cord stimulation in neuropathic pain. *Neurol Res* 2000; **22**(3): 285–292.

129. Ubbink DT, Vermeulen H. Spinal cord stimulation for non-reconstructable chronic critical leg ischaemia. Cochrane Database of Systematic Reviews 2005, Issue 3. Art. No.: CD004001. DOI: 10.1002/14651858.CD004001.pub2.

130. Eddicks S, Maier-Hauff K, Schenk M, Muller A, Baumann G, Theres H. Thoracic spinal cord stimulation improves functional status and relieves symptoms in patients with refractory angina pectoris: the first placebo-controlled randomised study. *Heart* 2007; **93**: 585–590.

131. Taylor RS, van Buyten JP, Buchser E. Spinal cord stimulation for complex regional pain syndrome: a systematic review of the clinical and cost-effectiveness literature and assessment of prognostic factors. *Eur J Pain* 2006; **10**: 91–101.

132. Grabow TS, T PK, Srinivasa N. Raja M. Spinal cord stimulation for complex regional pain syndrome: an evidence-based medicine review of the literature. *Clin J Pain* 2003; **19**: 371–383.

133. Mailis-Gagnon A, Furlan MD, Sandoval JA, Taylor RS. Spinal cord stimulation for chronic pain. Cochrane Database of Systematic Reviews 2004, Issue 3. Art. No.: CD003783. DOI: 10.1002/14651858.CD003783.pub2.

134. Cameron T. Safety and efficacy of spinal cord stimulation for the treatment of chronic pain: a 20-year literature review. *J Neurosurg* 2004; **100**(3 suppl): 254–267.

135. de Andres J, van Buyten JP. Neural modulation by stimulation. *Pain Pract* 2006; **6**(1): 39–45.

136. Taylor RS. Spinal cord stimulation in complex regional pain syndrome and refractory neuropathic back and leg pain/failed back surgery syndrome: results of a systematic review and meta-analysis. *J Pain Symptom Manage* 2006; **31**(4S): S13–S19.

137. Turner JA, Loeser JD, Deyo RA, Sanders SB. Spinal cord stimulation for patients with failed back surgery syndrome or complex regional pain syndrome: a systematic review of effectiveness and complications. *Pain* 2004; **108**: 137–147.

138. Harbour R, Miller J. A new system for grading recommendations in evidence based guidelines. *BMJ* 2001; **323**: 334–336.

139. Miles J, Lipton S, Hayward M. Pain relief by implanted electrical stimulators. *Lancet* 1974; **1**: 777–779.

140. Calvillo O, Racz GB, Didie J. Neuroaugmentation in the treatment of complex regional pain syndrome of the upper extremity. *Acta Orthop Belg* 1998; **64**: 57–63.

141. Oakley J, Weiner R. Spinal cord stimulation for complex regional pain syndrome: a prospective study of 19 patients at two centers. *Neuromodulation* 1999; **2**: 47–50.

142. Harke H, Gretenkort P, Ladleif HU, Rahman S. Spinal cord stimulation in sympathetically maintained complex regional pain syndrome type I with severe disability. A prospective clinical study. *Eur J Pain* 2005; **9**: 363–373.

143. Kemler MA, Barendse GA, van Kleef M, de Vet H, Rijks C, Furnee CA, et al. Spinal cord stimulation in patients with chronic reflex sympathetic dystrophy. *N Engl J Med* 2000; **343**: 618–624.

144. Kemler MA, de Vet H, Barendse GA, van den Wildenberg F, van Kleef M. Spinal cord stimulation for chronic reflex sympathetic dystrophy: five-year follow-up. *N Engl J Med* 2006; **354**: 2394–2396.

145. Taylor RS, van Buyten JP, Buchser E. Spinal cord stimulation for chronic back and leg pain and failed back surgery

syndrome: a systematic review and analysis of prognostic factors. *Spine* 2005; **30**: 152–160.

146. North RB, Kidd DH, Farrokhi F, Piantadosi SA. Spinal cord stimulation versus repeated lumbosacral spine surgery for chronic pain: a randomized, controlled trial. *Neurosurgery* 2005; **56**(1): 98–107.

147. Markman JD, Philip A. Interventional approaches to pain management. *Med Clin North Am* 2007; **91**: 271–286.

148. Pauza KJ, Howell S, Dreyfus P, Peloza JH, Dawson K, Bogduk N. A randomized, placebo-controlled trial of intradiscal electrothermal therapy for the treatment of discogenic low back pain. *Spine J* 2004; **4**: 27–35.

149. Freeman BJ, Fraser RD, Cain CMJ, Hall DJ, Chappe DCL. A randomized, double-blind, controlled trial. Intradiscal electrothermal therapy versus placebo for the treatment of chronic discogenic low back pain. *Spine* 2005; **30**(21): 2369–2377.

150. Smith TJ, Staats PS, Deer T, Stearns LJ, Rauck RL, Boortz-Marx RL, *et al.* Randomized clinical trial of an implantable drug delivery system compared with comprehensive medical management for refractory cancer pain: impact on pain, drug-related toxicity, and survival. *J Clin Oncol* 2002; **20**: 4040–4049.

151. Staats PS. Neuraxial infusion for pain control: when, why, and what to do after the implant. *Oncology* 1999; **13**: 58–62.

152. Brox JI, Sorensen R, Friis A, Nygaard O, Indahl A, Keller A, *et al.* Randomized clinical trial of lumbar instrumented fusion and cognitive intervention and exercises in patients with chronic low back pain and disc degeneration. *Spine* 2003; **28**(17): 1913–1921.

153. Gibson JNA, Waddell G. Surgery for degenerative lumbar spondylosis. Cochrane Database of Systematic Reviews 2005, Issue 4. Art. No.: CD001352. DOI: 10.1002/14651858.CD001352.pub3.

154. Fairbank J, Frost H, Wilson-MacDonald J, Yu L, Barker K, Collins R. Randomised controlled trial to compare surgical stabilisation of the lumbar spine with an intense rehabilitation programme for patients with chronic low back pain: the MRC spine stabilisation trial. *BMJ* 2005; **330**(7502): 1233.

155. Saal JS, Saal JA. Management of chronic discogenic low back pain with a thermal intradiscal catheter: a preliminary report. *Spine* 2000; **25**: 382–388.

156. Cohen SP, Larkin T, Abdi S, Chang A, Stojanovic MP. Risk factors for failure and complications of intradiscal electrothermal therapy: a pilot study. *Spine* 2003; **28**(11): 1142–1147.

157. Appleby D, Andersson G, Totta M. Meta-analysis of the efficacy and safety of intradiscal electrodthermal therapy (IDET). *Pain Med* 2006; **7**(4): 308–316.

158. Freeman BJ. IDET: a critical appraisal of the evidence. *Eur Spine J* 2006; **15**: S448–457.

159. Urrutia G, Kovacs F, Nishishinya MB, Olabe J. Percutaneous thermocoagulation intradiscal techniques for discogenic low back pain. *Spine* 2007; **32**(10): 1146–1154.

160. Andersson GBJ, Mekhail NA, Block JE. Treatment of intractable discogenic low back pain. A systematic review

161. Barendse GA, van den Berg SG, Kessels AH, Weber WE, van Kleef M. Randomized controlled trial of percutaneous intradiscal radiofrequency thermocoagulation for chronic discogenic back pain: lack of effect from a 90-second 70 C lesion. *Spine* 2001; **26**(3): 287–292.

162. Ercelen O, Bulutcu E, Oktenoglu T, Sasani M, Bozkus H, Cetin Saryoglu A, *et al.* Radiofrequency lesioning using two different time modalities for the treatment of lumbar discogenic pain: a randomized trial. *Spine* 2003; **28**(17): 1922–1927.

163. Bogduk N, Karasek M. Two-year follow-up of a controlled trial of intradiscal electrothermal anuloplasty for chronic low back pain resulting from internal disc disruption. *Spine J* 2002; **2**(5): 343–350.

164. Kapural L, Hayek S, Malak O, Arrigain S, Mekhail N. Intradiscal thermal annuloplasty versus intradiscal radiofrequency ablation for the treatment of discogenic pain: a prospective matched control trial. *Pain Med* 2005; **6**(6): 425–431.

165. Bono CM, Iki K, Jalota A, Dawson K, Garfin SR. Temperatures within the lumbar disc and endplates during intradiscal electrothermal therapy: formulation of a predictive temperature map in relation to distance from the catheter. *Spine* 2004; **29**: 1124–1129.

166. Kleinstueck FS, Diederich CJ, Nau WH, Puttlitz CM, Smith JA, Bradford DS, *et al.* Temperature and thermal dose distributions during intradiscal electrothermal therapy in the cadaveric lumbar spine. *Spine* 2003; **28**: 1700–1708.

167. Lee J, Lutz GE, Campbell D, Rodeo SA, Wright T. Stability of the lumbar spine after intradiscal electrothermal therapy. *Arch Phys Med Rehabil* 2001; **82**: 120–122.

168. Kleinstueck FS, Diederich CJ, Nau WH, Puttlitz CM, Smith JA, Bradford DS, *et al.* Acute biomechanical and histological effects of intradiscal electrothermal therapy on human lumbar discs. *Spine* 2001; **26**: 2198–2207.

169. Wagner TD, Rilling JK, Smith EE, Sokolik A, Casey KL, Davidson RJ, *et al.* Placebo-induced changes in fMRI in the anticipation and experience of pain. *Science* 2004; **303**: 1162–1167.

170. Goffaux P, Redmond WJ, Rainville P, Marchand S. Descending analgesia. When the spine echoes what the brain expects. *Pain* 2007; **130**(1–2): 137–143.

171. Biyani A, Andersson G, Chaudhary H. Intradiscal electrothermal therapy: a treatment option in patients with internal disc disruption. *Spine* 2003; **28**: 8–14.

172. Djurasovic M, Galassman SD, Dimar JR. Vertebral osteonecrosis associated with the use of intradiscal electrothermal therapy: a case report. *Spine* 2002; **27**: E325–328.

173. Cohen SP, Larkin T, Polly DWJ. A giant herniated disc following intradiscal electrothermal therapy. *J Spinal Disord Tech* 2002; **15**: 537–541.

174. Wetzel FT. Cauda equina syndrome from intradiscal electrothermal therapy. *Neurology* 2001; **56**: 1607.

175. Goldstein A, Lowney LI, Pal BK. Stereospecific and non-stereospecific interactions of the morphine congener

levorphanol in the subcelluar fractions of mouse brain. *Proc Natl Acad Sci USA* 1971; **68**: 1742–1747.

176. Pert CB, Snyder SH. Opiate receptor: demonstration in nervous tissue. *Science* 1973; **179**: 1011–1014.

177. Lamotte C, Pert CB, Snyder SH. Opiate receptor binding in primate spinal cord: distribution and changes after dorsal root section. *Brain Res* 1976; **112**: 407–412.

178. Yaksh TL, Rudy TA. Analgesia mediated by a direct spinal action of narcotic. *Science* 1976; **192**: 1357–1358.

179. Wang JK, Nauss LA, Thomas JE. Pain relief by intrathecally applied morphine in man. *Anesthesiology* 1979; **50**: 149–151.

180. Erdine S, de Andres J. Drug delivery systems. *Pain Pract* 2006; **6**(1): 51–57.

181. Ballantyne JC, Carwood C. Comparative efficacy of epidural, subarachnoid, and intracerebroventricular opioids in patients with pain due to cancer. Cochrane Database of Systematic Reviews 2005, Issue 2. Art. No.: CD005178. DOI: 10.1002/14651858.CD005178.

182. Haaenbusch SJ. Cost modeling for alternate routes of administration of opioids for cancer pain. *Oncology* 1999; **13**(5): 63–67.

183. Zeppetella G, O'Doherty CA, Collins S. Prevalence and characteristics of breakthrough pain in patients with non-malignant terminal disease admitted to a hospice. *Palliat Med* 2001; **15**: 243–246.

184. Portenoy RK, Hagen NA. Breakthrough pain: definition, prevalence and characteristics. *Pain* 1990; **41**: 273–281.

185. Idanpaan-Heikkila JJ, Guilbaud G. Pharmacological studies on a rat model of trigeminal neuropathic pain: baclofen, but not carbamazepine, morphine or tricyclic antidepresants, attenuates the allodynia-like behavior. *Pain* 1999; **79**: 281–290.

186. Hanks GW, Forbes K. Opioid responsiveness. *Acta Anaesth Scand* 1997; **41**: 154–158.

187. Benedetti F, Vighetti S, Amanzio M. Dose-response relationship of opioids in nociceptive and neuropathic post operative pain. *Pain* 1998; **74**: 205–211.

188. Thimineur MA, Kravitz E, Vodapally MS. Intrathecal opioid treatment for chronic non-malignant pain: a 3-year prospective study. *Pain* 2004; **109**: 242–249.

189. Anderson VC, Burchiel KJ. A prospective study of long-term intrathecal morphine in the management of chronic nonmalignant pain. *Neurosurgery* 1999; **44**: 289–300.

190. Kumar K, Kelly M, Pirlot T. Continuous intrathecal morphine treatment for chronic pain of nonmalignant etiology: long-term benefits and efficacy. *Surg Neurol* 2001; **55**: 79–86.

191. Angel IF, Gould HJ, Carey ME. Intrathecal morphine pump as a treatment option in chronic pain of nonmalignant origin. *Surg Neurol* 1998; **49**: 92–98.

192. Hassenbusch SJ, Portenoy RK, Cousins M. Polyanalgesic consensus conference 2003: an update on the management of pain by intraspinal drug delivery – report of an expert panel. *J Pain Symptom Manage* 2004; **276**: 540–563.

193. Yoshida GM, Nelson RW, Capen DA, Nagelberg S, Thomas JC, Rimodi RL, *et al.* Evaluation of continuous intraspinal narcotic analgesia for chronic pain from benign causes. *Am J Orthop* 1996; **25**: 693–694.

194. Auroy Y, Narchi P, Messiah A, Litt L, Rouvier B, Samii K. Serious complications related to regional anesthesia: results of a prospective survey in France. *Anesthesiology* 1997; **87**: 479–486.

195. Schulz-Stuber S, Kelly J. Regional anesthesia surveillance system: first experiences with a quality assessment tool for regional anesthesia and analgesia. *Acta Anaesthesiol Scand* 2007; **51**: 305–315.

196. Moher D, Schulz KF, Altman D. The CONSORT Statement: revised recommendations for improving the quality of reports of parallel-group randomized trials. *JAMA* 2001; **285**: 1987–1991.

CHAPTER 29

Spinal cord stimulation for refractory angina

Mats Börjesson[1], *Clas Mannheimer*[1], *Paulin Andréll*[1] *and Bengt Linderoth*[2]

[1] Pain Centre, Department of Medicine, Sahlgrenska University Hospital/Östra, Göteborg University, Göteborg, Sweden
[2] Department of Neurosurgery, Karolinska University Hospital, Stockholm, Sweden

Introduction

Patients with severe symptomatic angina pectoris, despite optimum conventional pharmacologic and invasive therapy, i.e. refractory angina, constitute a major problem in the clinical setting [1]. Several additional treatment methods, such as enhanced external counterpulsation (EECP) and stem cell therapy, have been developed and have also been found to provide symptom relief in several studies of varying quality. Neurostimulation in the form of spinal cord stimulation (SCS) is the best studied alternative method and has been shown in randomized controlled trials (RCT) to have positive effects on symptom relief, improved functional status and improved quality of life.

Treatment of refractory angina

Today, patients with refractory angina pectoris are mainly treated by cardiologists and internal medicine specialists, often in an emergency setting. These patients are only occasionally assessed by an algologist for consideration of additional treatment methods. Several different therapies have been introduced [1], including transcutaneous electrical nerve stimulation (TENS), SCS, thoracoscopic sympathectomy (ETS), thoracic epidural analgesia (EDA), transmyocardial and percutaneous myocardial laser revascularization

(TMR and PMR), stem cell therapy and, most recently, EECP, in addition to new pharmacologic therapies [2].

It has been possible to demonstrate symptom-relieving effects of most additional treatment methods in long-term studies, of varying quality [1]. However, several of these studies suffer from limitations, such as no control group, too short treatment period, and too few patients. Furthermore, it has been difficult to evaluate the methods, due to the absence of comparative studies.

The first systematic survey of available treatment methods, resulting in international treatment recommendations, was published in 2002 by the European Society of Cardiology [1]. The recommended first-line therapy alternatives are TENS and SCS, which are considered to be adequately documented, are used by several different centers and have been shown to have an effect on symptoms and coronary ischemia in addition to a favorable side effect profile.

Neurostimulation in ischemic pain

Spinal cord stimulation and TENS have been directly developed on the basis of experimental findings and are based on Melzack and Wall's famous gate control theory [3] and its general principles of segmental pain inhibition.

Electrical stimulation of the dorsal columns of the spinal cord was the first form of electrical stimulation that was used clinically. The first spinal cord stimulator was implanted in 1967 [4]. Towards the end of the 1970s, the method was brought into use for

Evidence-Based Chronic Pain Management. Edited by C. Stannard, E. Kalso and J. Ballantyne. © 2010 Blackwell Publishing.

patients with severe peripheral arterial circulatory insufficiency of the lower extremities, with favorable effects on both circulation and pain [5]. At about the same time, TENS was first used in patients with therapy-resistant angina pectoris, with good clinical results [6, 7]. As 10–20% of patients using TENS developed discomforting skin irritation after a period of use, treatment with SCS was tried instead for patients with severe angina pectoris [8].

Mechanisms of action

Results from human and animal studies

Early experimental studies in the monkey [9] showed that SCS produced inhibition of the influx of nociceptive signals from the heart, suggesting a primary pain-blocking effect of SCS. Later studies and clinical experience have shown that this is not the case. Instead, a reduction in cardiac ischemia appears to be the primary effect and in its absence, no symptom relief will be achieved [10, 11].

Increased/changed coronary blood flow

Angina pectoris typically occurs as a consequence of an imbalance between oxygen supply and oxygen demand in the myocardium [12]. Therefore, it was natural that the first hypotheses concerning the mechanisms behind the favorable effects of SCS in angina pectoris focused on a possible increase in the blood flow to ischemic regions, in particular as SCS had been found to increase the circulation in peripheral vascular beds [13]. However, so far, there is no stable experimental support for this redistributing effect of SCS ("the Robin Hood effect") on coronary flow [14], despite the findings in an early Dutch PET study in humans, indicating such a redistribution of the blood flow as a result of SCS therapy [15]. The study by Kingma et al. [14] was, however, performed on healthy animals which were subjected to an acute LAD occlusion, which does not replicate the clinical course adequately.

To simulate these conditions experimentally, a chronic animal model has been developed in which a coronary artery is slowly occluded [16], resulting in collateral-dependent myocardial ischemia. In subsequent experiments, the basal heart rate was kept at 150 beats/minute using a pacemaker. To provoke critical ischemia, angiotensin II was injected.

Resulting ST elevations over the left ventricle were markedly attenuated by SCS. This indicates that SCS may mitigate the effect of stressors on a heart with diminished reserve capacity.

Reduced oxygen consumption in the myocardium

The other main hypothesis concerning the mechanism of action of SCS focuses instead on an SCS-induced reduction in myocardial oxygen demand [11].

Several experimental and clinical studies from different centers have shown that symptom relief by TENS and SCS in angina in humans is secondary to an anti-ischemic effect, associated with a reduction in the oxygen consumption of the myocardium at comparable workload. Specifically, a favorable change in the metabolism of lactate in the heart has been demonstrated, as well as reduced ST segment depression on ECG during stress and concomitant stimulation [6, 7, 11, 12]. Evidence supporting the anti-ischemic effect is also provided by infarction studies in the rabbit [17, 18], where application of SCS produced a reduction in infarction size after controlled occlusion of a large coronary vessel. However, this protective effect was only seen if the SCS was initiated before the ischemic episode.

Spinal cord stimulation may give rise to reduced oxygen consumption via a number of putative mechanisms. It has been shown in animal experimental studies that β-endorphin reduces oxygen consumption, via antagonistic effects on local opioid receptors (μ receptors) in the myocardium. In a study on humans, SCS stimulation caused release of β-endorphin in the myocardium, which could lead to reduced oxygen consumption [19]. There are also indications that the anti-ischemic effect could be secondary to a lowered sympathetic tone in the heart [20].

Other possible mechanisms

More recent studies also show that SCS gives rise to catecholamine release in the myocardium, which may contribute to the development of protective changes similar to those occurring in "ischemic preconditioning"; however, in this case, without any signs of ischemia. SCS also appears to have the potential to induce other types of changes that may be observed in connection with ischemic preconditioning, such as activation of protein kinase C [17].

The intrinsic cardiac nervous system is forcefully activated in coronary ischemia. The system consists of several ganglia (with autonomous and somato-sensory nerve cells), embedded in the epicardial fat across the surface of the heart. Interestingly, it has been observed that SCS appears to be able to stabilize the activity in these nerve ganglia, especially in connection with ischemic stress [21, 22].

Clinical effects

Many studies have been published on the sympto-matic effects of SCS in angina pectoris. Most are of limited scientific value. Initially, only case reports were published, later followed by case–control studies of limited follow-up time. Due to the short follow-up periods, the small number of patients and/or lack of control group, these studies offered interesting clinical information but limited scientific evidence for the efficacy of SCS.

Beginning in the 1990s, RCT of high quality started to be published in this field. However, today most reports still do not have all the requirements of a high-quality study (i.e. proper randomization, concealed allocation, control group, proper blinding (difficult) and description of withdrawals, for example). Most commonly, noncontrolled follow-up case–control studies are reported, making scientific statements regarding efficacy difficult. However, eight RCT (and two additional substudies) of medium-high to high scientific value have been published in recent years [23–30]. The results of these RCTs are presented in the systematic review on SCS in severe angina [31].

In summary, there is strong scientific evidence that SCS reduces symptoms in patients with severe angina pectoris. Four available studies of high quality [27–30] show a reduction in the number of anginal attacks, comsumption of short-acting nitrates and/or an improvement of anginal classification (Canadian Classification Score, CCS). Clinically, this allows the patient to be more physically active, before experiencing anginal symptoms, which will also influence the functional status of the patient. Indeed, there is strong scientific evidence that SCS improves functional status in patients with severe angina pectoris, as measured by increased walking time on 6-minute walk test [27] or improved working capacity on treadmill/exercise test [28–30].

In addition, there is strong scientific evidence that SCS improves quality of life in patients with angina pectoris, as shown in three studies of high quality [27, 28, 30]. One of these studies [27] showed improvement in the Seattle Angina Questionnaire (SAQ), which includes five parts: physical limitation, angina stability, angina frequency, treatment satisfaction and disease perception. Eddicks' study also showed improvement in global quality of life as measured by the EuroQol visual analog scale [27].

There is limited scientific evidence that SCS is clinically safe in patients with severe angina pectoris. One RCT suggests that SCS is associated with reduction in mortality compared to CABG at 6 months, which is attributed to the periprocedureal mortality of CABG [29]. A Dutch study found the mortality of SCS retrospectively to be similar to an external matched control group with angina pectoris [32].

Overall, SCS has a low complication rate in patients with angina pectoris, of 0–12% [27–30]. Specifically, no severe complications such as severe deep infection were reported. In the ESBY study [29], one patient had a subcutaneous infection, while the other most common complications are electrode dislocations and generator dislocation [28].

In the selection of patients who are suitable for implantation, it is important to identify whether the patient's current chest pain really is related to reversible myocardial ischemia, is of nonischemic origin or is even noncardiac [33]. The presence of current myocardial ischemia must therefore be confirmed using conventional methods such as exercise tests, myocardial scintigraphy or stress echocardiography.

Conclusion

Angina pectoris is a growing clinical problem and a large number of patients with coronary disease remain symptomatic, despite conventional pharmacologic treatment, and are left without (further) surgical treatment options, i.e. refractory angina pectoris. Results from available high-quality studies show that SCS has positive long-term effects on quality of life and symptoms (anginal pain) as well as functional status, compared with untreated controls or standard treatment. Hence, SCS is the first-line treatment recommended by the ESC in refractory angina pectoris [1].

Table 29.1 Medium-to-high quality studies on SCS and angina pectoris, $n = 10$. Reproduced from Börjesson *et al.* [31] with permission.

Study	Design	Patients	Lost to follow-up	Intervention	Follow-up	Results	Complications
de Jongste *et al.* [23]	RCT	24	1	SCS vs placebo	2 months + 1 year	1 year: • QoL ↑ • Ischemia ↓ (n.s)	Six electrode dislocations
de Jongste *et al.* [30]	RCT	17	3	SCS vs waiting list (8 weeks) and then all SCS	8 weeks + 1 year	8 weeks: • Working capacity ↑ • Ischemia ↓ • Symptoms ↓ • QoL ↑ 1 year: • Working capacity ↑ • QoL ↑	Two electrode dislocations
Mannheimer *et al.* [29]	RCT (ESBY study)	104 (21 women/ 83 men)	8 deaths (1 SCS 7 CABG)	SCS vs CAB (51/53)	6 months	• Symptoms ↓ (same both groups) • Working capacity ↑ (more in CABG) • Mortality (1.9% SCS vs 13.7% CABG)	0
Hautvast *et al.* [24]	RCT	25	0	SCS + standard treatment vs standard treatment	6 weeks	SCS + standard treatment: • Working capacity ↑ • Symptoms ↓ • QoL ↑	?
Ekre *et al.* [26]	RCT (ESBY follow-up)	104	29 deaths (13 SCS/ 16 CABG)	SCS vs CABG	5 years	6 months: • QoL ↑ in both groups (n.s) 5 years: • QoL ↑ in both (n.s) • Mortality 28% (n.s)	SCS: 1 sc infection and 3 electrode dislocations
Andrell *et al.* [25]	RCT (ESBY follow-up)	104	17 deaths (5 SCS/ 10 CABG, other: 0/2)	SCS vs CABG	2 years	SCS group: • Hospitalisation ↓ • Cardiac morbidity ↓ • Total costs ↓	SCS: 1 sc infection and 3 electrode dislocations

Continued on p. 404

Table 29.1 *Continued*

McNab et al. [28]	RCT	68	7(3 SCS/4 PMR) deaths: 1/10	SCS vs PMR (34/34)	12 months	• Exercise time ↑ • Symptoms ↓ • QoL↓ (no difference between groups) • Time to angina ↑ in SCS	0 infections, electrode dislocation 1, generator dislocation 2 (SCS)
Eddicks et al. [27]	RCT (cross-over design)	12		SCS at 3 stimulation regimes vs placebo stimulation	4 months (4 weeks × 4)	• Symptoms ↓ • Walking distance ↑ with all regimes vs placebo stimulation	0
Jessurun et al. [32]	CT (retrospective)	57	?	SCS vs external control group	?	SCS: mortality 6.5% (similar to external control group)	Unipolar electrode: 83% rep.; Quadripolar electrodes: 33% reop.
Jessurum et al. [34]	CT	24	?	SCS vs controls	4 weeks	Symptoms similar after 4 weeks of non-stimulation	?

CABG, coronary artery bypass graft; CT, controlled trial; ESBY, electrical stimulation versus bypass surgery in severe angina pectoris; PMR, percutaneous myocardial laser revascularization; RCT, randomized controlled trial; SCS, spinal cord stimulation; QoL, quality of life.

All cardiology units treating a large number of patients with symptomatic coronary disease should have a clear strategy for the handling of patients with refractory angina. This requires development of local expert knowledge, together with the cardiologists in charge, preferably in collaboration with algologists. From this perspective, SCS is an effective treatment method that has the potential for considerably greater use.

References

1. Mannheimer C, Camici P, Chester MR, Collins A, de Jongste M, Eliasson T, *et al.* The problem of chronic refractory angina: report from the ESC Joint Study Group on the Treatment of Refractory Angina. *Eur Heart J* 2002; **23**: 355–370.
2. Gowda R, Khan IA, Punukollu G, Vasavada BC, Nair CK. Treatment of refractory angina pectoris. *Int J Cardiol* 2005; **101**: 1–7.
3. Melzack R, Wall PD. Pain mechanisms: a new theory. *Science* 1965; **150**: 971–979.
4. Shealy CN, Mortimer JT, Reswick JB. Electrical inhibition of pain by stimulation of the dorsal columns: preliminary clinical report. *Anesth Analg* 1967; **46**: 489–491.
5. Ubbink DT, Vermeulen H. Spinal cord stimulation for non-reconstructible chronic critical leg ischaemia. Cochrane Database of Systematic Reviews, 2003(3).
6. Mannheimer C, Carlsson CA, Emanuelsson H, Vedin A, Waagstein F, Wilhelmsson C. The effects of transcutaneous electrical nerve stimulation in patients with severe angina pectoris. *Circulation* 1985; **71**: 308–316.
7. Mannheimer C, Carlsson CA, Ericsson K, Vedin A, Wilhelmsson C. Transcutaneous electrical nerve stimulation in severe angina pectoris. *Eur Heart J* 1982; **3**: 297–302.
8. Murphy D, Gibs K. Dorsal column stimulation for pain relief from intractable angina pectoris. *Pain* 1987; **28**: 365–368.
9. Chandler MJ, Brennan TJ, Garrison DW, Kim KS, Schwartz PJ, Foreman RD. A mechanism of cardiac pain suppression by spinal cord stimulation: implications for patients with angina pectoris. *Eur Heart J* 1993; **14**: 96–105.
10. Eliasson T, Augustinsson LE, Mannheimer C. Spinal cord stimulation in severe angina pectoris – presentation of current studies, indications, and clinical experience. *Pain* 1996; **65**: 169–179.
11. Mannheimer C, Eliasson T, Andersson B, Berg CH, Augustinsson LE, Emanuelsson H, *et al.* Effects of spinal cord stimulation in angina pectoris induced by pacing and possible mechanisms of action. *BMJ* 1993; **307**: 477–480.
12. de Jongste M, Haaksma J, Hautvast RW, Hillege HL, Meyler PW, Staal MJ, *et al.* Effects of spinal cord stimulation on myocardial ischaemia during daily life in patients with severe coronary artery disease. A prospective ambulatory electrocardiographic study. *Br Heart J* 1994; **71**: 413–418.
13. Wu M, Linderoth B, Foreman RD. Putative mechanisms behind effects of spinal cord stimulation on vascular diseases: a review of experimental studies. *Auton Neurosci* 2008: **138**(1–2): 9–23.
14. Kingma J, Linderoth B, Ardell JL, *et al.* Neuromodulation therapy does not influence blood flow distribution or left-ventricular dymanics during acute myocardial ischemia. *Auton Neurosci Basic Clin* 2001; **91**: 47–54.
15. Hautvast R, Blanksma PK, de Jongste MJ, *et al.* Effect of spinal cord stimulation on myocardial blood flow assessed by positron emission tomography in patients with refractory angina pectoris. *Am J Cardiol* 1996; **77**: 462–467.
16. Cardinal R, Ardell J, Linderoth B, Vermeulen M, Foreman RD, Armour JA. Spinal cord activation differently modulates ischemic electrical responses to different stressors in canine ventricels. *Auton Neurosci Basic Clin* 2004; **111**: 34–47.
17. Southerland EM, Milhorn D, Foreman RD, Linderoth B, de Jongste MJ, Armour JA, *et al.* Pre-emptive, but not reactive, spinal cord stimulation mitigates transient ischemia-induced myocardial infarction via cardiac adrenergic neurons. *Am J Physiol Heart Circ Physiol* 2007; **292**: H311–317.
18. Ardell JL, Dellitallia LJ, Millhorn DM, Linderoth B, de Jongste MJ, Foreman RD, *et al.* Spinal cord stimulation modulates catecholamine release into interstitial fluid in the canine myocardium. *FASEB J* 2002; **16**: A118.
19. Eliasson T, Mannheimer C, Waagstein F, Andersson B, Bergh CH, Augustinsson LE, *et al.* Myocardial turnover of endogenous opioids and calcitonin-gene-related peptide in the human heart and the effects of spinal cord stimulation on pacing-induced angina pectoris. *Cardiology* 1998; **89**: 170–177.
20. Norrsell H, Eliasson T, Mannheimer C, Augustinsson LE, Bergh CH, Andersson B, *et al.* Effects of pacing-induced myocardial stress and spinal cord stimulation on whole body and cardiac norepinephrine spillover. *Eur Heart J* 1997; **18**: 1890–1896.
21. Issa ZF, Zhou X, Ujhelyi MR, Rosenberger J, Bhakta D, Groh WJ, *et al.* Thoracic spinal cord stimulation reduces the risk of ischemic ventricular arrhythmias in postinfarction heart failure canine model. *Circulation* 2005; **111**: 3217–3220.
22. Foreman RD, Linderoth B, Ardell JL, Barron KW, Chandler MJ, Hull Jr SS, *et al.* Modulation of intrinsic cardiac neurons by spinal cord stimulation: implications for therapeutic use in angina pectoris. *Cardiovasc Res* 2000; **47**: 367–375.
23. de Jongste MJ, Staal MJ. Preliminary results of a randomized study on the clinical efficacy of spinal cord stimulation for refractory angina pectoris. *Acta Neurochir* 1993; **58**(suppl): 161–164.
24. Hautvast R, de Jongste MJ, Staal MJ, van Gilst WH, Lie KI. Spinal cord stimulation in chronic intractable angina pectoris: a randomized controlled efficacy study. *Am Heart J* 1998; **136**: 1114–1120.
25. Andrell P, Ekre O, Eliasson T, Blomstrand C, Börjesson M, Nilsson M, *et al.* Cost-effectiveness of spinal cord stimulation versus coronary artery bypass grafting in patients with severe angina pectoris – long-term results from the ESBY study. *Cardiology* 2003; **99**: 20–24.
26. Ekre O, Eliasson T, Norrsell H, Währborg P, Mannheimer C. Long-term effects of spinal cord stimulation and coronary

artery bypass grafting on quality of life and survival in the ESBY study. *Eur Heart J* 2002; **23**: 1938–1945.

27. Eddicks S, Maier-Hauff K, Schenk M, Muller A, Baumann G, Theres H. Thoracic spinal cord stimulation imporves functional status and relieves symptoms in patients with refractory angina pectoris: the first placebo-controlled randomised study. *Heart* 2007; **93**: 585–590.

28. McNab D, Khan SN, Sharples LD, Ryan JY, Freeman C, Caine N, *et al.* An open label, single-centre, randomized trial of spinal cord stimulation vs. percutaneous myocardial laser revascularization in patients with refractory angina pectoris: the SPiRiT trial. *Eur Heart J* 2006; **27**: 1048–1053.

29. Mannheimer C, Eliasson T, Augustinsson LE, Blomstrand C, Emanuelsson H, Larsson S, *et al.* Electrical stimulation versus coronary artery bypass surgery in severe angina pectoris: the ESBY study. *Circulation* 1998; **97**: 1157–1163.

30. de Jongste M, Hautvast RW, Hillege HL, Lie KI. Efficacy of spinal cord stimulation as adjuvant therapy for intractable angina pectoris: a prospective, randomized clinical study.

Working Group on Neurocardiology. *J Am Coll Cardiol* 1994; **23**: 1592–1597.

31. Börjesson M, Andrell P, Lundberg D, Mannheimer C. Spinal cord stimulation in severe angina pectoris – a systematic review based on the Swedish Council on Technology Assessment in Health Care report on long-standing pain. *Pain* 2008; **140**: 501–508.

32. Jessurun GA, ten Vaarwerk IA, de Jongste MJ, Tio RA, Staal MJ. Sequelae of spinal cord stimulation for refractory angina pectoris. Reliability and safety profile of long-term clinical application. *Cor Art Dis* 1997; **8**: 33–38.

33. Borjesson M, Dellborg M. Before intervention – is the pain really cardiac? *Scand Cardiovasc J* 2003; **37**(3): 124–127.

34. Jessurun GA, DeJongste MJ, Hautvast RW, Tio RA, Brouwer J, van Lelievaid S, *et al.* Clinical follow-up after cessation of chronic electrical neuromodulation in patients with severe coronary artery disease: a prospective randomized controlled study on putative involvement of sympathetic activity. *Pacing Clin Electrophysiol* 1999; **22**: 1432–9.

CHAPTER 30

Rehabilitative treatment for chronic pain

James P. Robinson[1], Raphael Leo[2], Joseph Wallach[2], Ellen McGough[3] and Michael Schatman[4]

[1] Department of Rehabilitation Medicine, University of Washington, Washington, DC, USA
[2] Department of Psychiatry, School of Medicine and Biomedical Sciences, State University of New York at Buffalo, Buffalo, NY, USA
[3] Biobehavioral Nursing and Health Systems, University of Washington, Washington, DC, USA
[4] Pacific Northwest University of Health Sciences, College of Osteopathic Medicine, Yakima, WA, USA

Introduction

In an ideal world, therapies for chronic pain would be so effective that most patients could be cured. Unfortunately, this goal is often unrealistic, for the simple reason that reliable cures for chronic pain syndromes are generally not available. This somber conclusion comes from an examination of the tenacity of chronic pain syndromes such as fibromyalgia [1], and from a wealth of data about the natural history of disabling painful conditions treated in the workers' compensation system [2].

In the absence of definitive cures for many chronic pain disorders, physicians rely on a number of strategies to manage the conditions. For the most part, these strategies can be divided into two large groups: palliative and rehabilitative. Palliative strategies focus directly on symptom relief, and generally do not require any special effort by patients. Opioid therapy is a good example of palliative treatment. Rehabilitation has been defined as: "the restoration of the ill or injured patient to optimal functional level in the home and community in relation to physical, psychosocial, vocational, and recreational activity" [3, p. 1443]. Rehabilitation involves patients taking an active role in optimizing recovery from their medical condition via learning and practice. For example,

a patient who has sustained a cerebrovascular accident (CVA) can practice walking with a cane, and can learn one-handed techniques for donning and doffing clothes.

Rehabilitative approaches for patients with chronic musculoskeletal pain typically focus on physical conditioning and on strategies that patients can use to manage pain and associated emotional distress. The most comprehensive pain rehabilitation programs are those provided in multidisciplinary pain centers and functional restoration programs. These often involve a wide range of therapeutic interventions – including vocational counseling, medication management and various interventional pain therapies such as epidural injections. However, two therapeutic approaches are used in all multidisciplinary pain rehabilitation programs – exercise therapy and psychologic treatment.

In this chapter, we conceptualize exercise therapy and psychologic treatment as core elements of rehabilitative treatment for chronic musculoskeletal pain. We first examine evidence regarding their efficacy as stand-alone treatments. We then evaluate the efficacy of combinations of exercise therapy and psychologic treatment, and finally evaluate multidisciplinary pain rehabilitation programs. The chapter will focus on low back pain (LBP), rather than attempting an evidence-based review of a wide range of disorders.

Psychologic therapy

Psychologic therapies have emerged as relatively noninvasive approaches to the management of LBP. Various considerations rationalize their use. One is that

Evidence-Based Chronic Pain Management. Edited by C. Stannard, E. Kalso and J. Ballantyne. © 2010 Blackwell Publishing.

extensive research has demonstrated the importance of psychologic factors in the onset and maintenance of LBP [4, 5]. This assertion does not negate the role of biomechanical derangements in LBP, but does assert that the experiences and behaviors of LBP patients are influenced by factors in addition to strictly mechanical ones. Secondly, like patients with many chronic disorders, such as diabetes or breast cancer, LBP patients can benefit from the disease management skills that psychologists teach.

Psychologic therapies focus on modifying the behavioral, cognitive and physiologic responses to pain [6, 7]. A variety of psychologic techniques have been advocated, including cognitive behavioral therapy (CBT), self-regulatory treatment interventions, and behavioral (operant) therapy. These therapies differ with regard to their approach, perspectives, and goals, described below.

Cognitive behavioral therapy

Cognitive behavioral therapy (CBT) focuses on belief systems and coping strategies that contribute to problematic behaviors of patients with LBP [7a]. Cognitive restructuring, an interactive process involving the socratic method, is used to teach patients to identify and modify maladaptive, negatively distorted thoughts that may lead them to avoid activities and to experience negative feelings, such as depression, anxiety and anger. Patients are encouraged to reappraise irrational, self-defeating thoughts and discriminate between these and more rational alternatives. Faulty appraisals and misattributions are reframed and replaced with those that are less irrational. The presumption is that as a result of cognitive restructuring, patients will demonstrate less avoidance of physical activity, and will experience less physiologic arousal and less intense pain. Coping skills training is aimed at assisting patients to develop a repertoire of skills for managing pain as well as problem-solving strategies that may be useful in a wide range of situations that induce pain. Using homework completed by the patient and issues discussed in sessions, the therapist assists the patient in identifying currently employed strategies, assessing the utility of the existing strategies, e.g. whether they facilitate the patient's relief, and developing/refining alternatives.

The efficacy of CBT is related to the modification of distorted cognitions that may interfere with rehabilitative efforts. Previous investigations have supported the notion that cognitive misinterpretations, e.g. catastrophizing, i.e. the tendency to expect the worst, are predictive of subsequent disability, and that the association is often mediated by fear avoidance [8–10]. Other research indicates that patients' expectations regarding their treatment and their ability to work influence adherence to treatment [11] and return to work [12].

Meta-analyses reveal that in comparison to no treatment or to standard treatment, CBT leads to improvements in perceived pain intensity, life interference from pain, health-related quality of life, and depression severity [13]. However, controversy attends the effectiveness of CBT when such treatment is compared to alternative active treatments [14–16]. Studies relying predominantly on multiple self-report outcome measures suggest that CBT is effective in facilitating psychologic adjustment and reducing reported pain levels as compared with standard medical treatment conditions [14, 17, 18] or wait-list control conditions [15, 19]. By contrast, when observational outcome measures were employed, e.g. pain behaviors and functional status, no significant benefits were demonstrated with CBT post treatment [15, 19] and differential effects of CBT as compared with other psychologic treatment modalities were not always apparent [7, 20, 21]. For example, when return to work was assessed among LBP patients, CBT was not any more effective than control situations [22]. Additionally, while back pain patients administered physical therapy and CBT versus being in a conventional treatment program fared better with regard to subjective assessments of performance, leisure activity, pain and disability perception, there were no significant differences between the two groups with regard to sick leave in the follow-up period 1 year later [23].

There are several factors that can undermine the effectiveness of CBT. These include patients' failure to complete homework assignments [24] or failure to implement the strategies acquired during therapy (cognitive structuring and coping skills) at home when they are no longer in session [21].

Self-regulatory (respondent) treatments

Self-regulatory treatments (SRT) are intended to teach patients techniques to mitigate the experience of pain by reducing the physiologic responses that pain tends to elicit. SRT therefore serve to facilitate the patient's abilities to reduce muscle tension, sympathetic arousal or mental distress (e.g. anxiety) by inducing a state of relaxation. In so doing, an internal state that is incompatible with tension and distress is created. In addition to the general effects of producing a relaxed state, such measures foster in patients a sense of mastery over their pain experiences. Customarily, SRT approaches include biofeedback, relaxation training, guided imagery and hypnosis.

A major problem in determining the effectiveness of SRT is that they are often provided in combination with behavioral and CBT therapies. In such cases, it is difficult to ascertain the independent contribution that SRT approaches make. Meta-analyses of RCT in which SRT were combined with CBT in the treatment of chronic LBP have shown that such combinations produced short-term reductions in pain severity compared with patients in wait-list control conditions [15, 16]. However, the added contributory role of SRT could not be confirmed [25, 26].

The nature of SRT suggests that they would influence perceptions of pain intensity severity, but would have less influence on functional restoration. This has largely been borne out in available research. There are limited data available from RCT suggesting that relaxation and imagery techniques moderately reduce perceived pain severity, and, as expected, poor evidence to support that such interventions influence patients' general functional status [15, 16].

Behavior (operant) therapy

The goal of behavior therapy is to mitigate excessive problematic pain-associated behaviors, e.g. over-reliance on medication and inactivity, and increase the frequency of adaptive behaviors that at baseline occur infrequently or not at all, e.g. walking, exercise, self-care, work [27]. Behavior therapy is predicated on the principles of operant conditioning, i.e. the patient engages in behavior(s) maintained by social and environmental contingencies. Simply put, behaviors that are followed by pleasant or desirable consequences (reinforcements) are likely to be repeated in the future, whereas those followed by negative consequences are not likely to recur [28]. To influence behavior, the therapist actively modifies the consequences that follow the patient's behavior;

therefore, behavioral approaches rely on adapting reinforcement contingencies to increase the patient's activity levels and to increase health behaviors, while withholding reinforcements for maladaptive behaviors.

When originally described, operant therapy was conducted with chronic pain patients undergoing multidisciplinary pain rehabilitation on an inpatient basis [29, 30]. Although operant conditioning principles guided various aspects of the rehabilitation program (e.g. tapers of opioid medications), their most obvious application was to exercise therapy.

Operant therapy differs in critical respects from other kinds of psychologic treatment [16, 28]. Instead of direct patient treatment, the role of the psychologist is to teach the principles and procedures of operant conditioning to other team members. Thus, psychologists instruct physical therapists who construct and co-ordinate the regimen of a patient's exercise therapy program such that reinforcements are consistently applied to optimize adherence. Ultimately, the professional who provides the treatment is a physical therapist. The psychologist contributes expertise only with respect to specific issues related to the exercise program, e.g. the reinforcement schedule that should be followed as demands are increased, and the way in which the physical therapist should behave when the patient succeeds or fails on established quotas. Choices regarding the specific exercises to be given to patients are made by the physical therapist or the supervising physician.

One potential weakness of operant programs as envisaged by Fordyce [28] is that they require a great deal of control over the environment of patients. This could be achieved during inpatient pain rehabilitation programs but in outpatient settings, such environmental control can generally not be achieved. A related problem is that the changes produced during a treatment program can dissipate at home or work, where reinforcement patterns are less systematic or consistent. Ideally, effective behavioral programs also include training for partners/significant others with whom the patient resides or is closely connected. The partners/significant others are taught to recognize the difference between healthy and unhealthy behaviors, and to reinforce healthy adaptive behaviors while withholding attention from unhealthy behaviors exhibited by the patient. The goal of such training is to bolster treatment programs by the implementation of comparable reinforcement programs in the home [21].

Several studies on the efficacy of physical therapy based on operant principles have shown that such therapy produces better outcomes than various other treatment programs [25, 31–33] or than participation in a wait list control group [21, 34, 35]. However, some studies have found no difference between operant treatment and various other kinds of treatment [36–38]. It is reasonable to conclude from the above research that operant treatment probably has a positive effect on LBP patients, but that the efficacy of the approach has not been conclusively demonstrated.

One possible reason for inconsistencies in the results of research on operant activity programs is that experienced physical therapists (PT) may already have developed effective strategies for addressing behavioral issues that come up during exercise therapy. For example, Fordyce and other behavior therapists have argued that an exercise program should be progressed on the basis of a prearranged schedule rather than on the basis of the pain behaviors of a patient. It is quite possible that experienced PT have intuitively learned this strategy or equally effective behavioral strategies as a result of their interactions with large numbers of patients. To the extent that PT have developed effective behavioral strategies without the help of psychologists, comparisons between operant programs and usual exercise programs are likely to be inconclusive.

Also, it is possible that operant treatment rests on a conceptualization of human behavior that is too narrow. By focusing exclusively on outcome contingencies, the behavioral approach fails to address subjective experiences that influence behavior. For example, expectation, anticipation, thinking, planning, and remembering can also influence behavior and mediate pain-related behavior and perception [6]. As an illustration, passivity and inactivity can be particularly problematic in LBP, resulting in generalized deconditioning, muscle weakness, and reduced endurance – all of which can exacerbate pain once an effort is undertaken. From a behavioral perspective, such passivity might be reinforced by others, e.g. the solicitous spouse who tends to the patient's needs every time the inactivity is noticed. An alternative explanation might attribute the inactivity to the patient's expectations that activity will exacerbate pain, i.e. fear avoidance.

Thus, the patient is avoiding the prospect of pain, a factor that may be more pivotal in determining the inactivity. Yet another explanation suggests that passivity arises from learned helplessness. For example, a patient might conclude that his/her pain will inevitably cause permanent disablement, and that it is pointless to try to change this fate by exercising.

The broad point is that many psychologists believe that an exclusive emphasis on the overt behavior of a LBP patient is inadequate. Instead, they emphasize that both the overt behavior and the subjective experiences of patients must be considered in psychologic theories that purport to understand them, and in psychologic treatments to modify the behavior. This is the perspective taken by supporters of CBT.

Summary

The aim of various psychotherapeutic approaches is to modify the behavior, cognitions, and physiologic reactivity associated with pain [7, 10]. In the aggregate, there is evidence that psychologic interventions benefit LBP patients with respect to clinical outcomes such as pain relief, improved mood, and improved functional capacities. However, the efficacy of psychologic intervention remains unclear with regard to influence on vocational outcomes.

It is important to note that these general conclusions obscure several issues that have not been resolved in the studies cited above. One problem in evaluating psychologic therapies is that they are often embedded in broad-based rehabilitation programs that include several other types of treatment. As a result, it is difficult to determine the independent effect of the psychologic treatments.

Another problem is that research to date has not determined the relative efficacy of different psychologic approaches. Generally, comparisons of the relative efficacy of varied psychotherapeutic approaches have demonstrated few differential findings. In some cases, behavioral approaches were reported to be more effective than cognitively based approaches [25, 35] whereas in other studies, a combined operant-cognitive approach was superior to a unimodal operant approach [7, 39]. Furthermore, in studies comparing the efficacies of psychotherapeutic approaches, any differences in effects noted at the conclusion of time-limited treatment programs was generally found to disappear at follow-up some time later [7].

A related issue is that it may be pointless to attempt to assess the effectiveness of any specific psychologic approach in the abstract. The key challenge may be one of matching the psychologic treatment that is provided to the specific psychologic needs of an individual patient. A study by George et al. [40] exemplifies this point. They found that a graded activity (i.e. operant) exercise program facilitated improvement among LBP patients with high levels of fear of reinjury, but impeded the progress of patients with low fear levels.

Finally, several recurring methodologic issues cloud the interpretation of research on psychologic therapies. For example, factors obscuring determination of differential treatment effects across psychotherapeutic approaches include the heterogeneity of definitions and content of treatments described as cognitive behavioral or behavioral, varying outcome measures, varying use of co-interventions, e.g. medication, and different sample characteristics, e.g. mild versus moderately to severely disabled individuals [41]. Combined, these methodologic issues impede efforts to ascertain which psychologic treatments, or combinations of treatments, are essential in optimizing rehabilitation efforts.

Physical therapy

Physical therapy exercise interventions for LBP patients range from specific exercises, aimed at symptom reduction and movement control, to general exercises for improving strength, flexibility and aerobic conditioning. Evidence is stronger for the effectiveness of exercise therapy than for the effectiveness of other PT interventions such as heat modalities [42, 43]. However, many questions regarding the effectiveness of specific elements of exercise therapy remain.

Multiple systematic reviews have shown that therapeutic exercise in PT reduces pain and improves activity in patients with chronic LBP [44]. In a systematic review of exercise therapy for nonspecific LBP involving 61 trials (43 of which included chronic LBP), Hayden et al. [45–47] reported that exercise therapy decreased pain and improved function by modest amounts. When considering work disability, Kool et al. [48] reported significantly reduced sick leave within the first year, in a meta-analysis of 14 RCT of exercise for nonacute, nonspecific LBP. This

effect was strongest in the most severely disabled patients (>90 days of sick leave). While the strength of this effect has been questioned [49], there is clearly support for prescribing therapeutic exercise for patients with chronic low back pain.

Program design, exercise intensity, delivery type, and individualization of exercise interventions all impact the effectiveness of exercise interventions [45–47]. Exercise programs that have a higher exercise dosage (>20 h intervention) and are delivered in a supervised format (which may include home-based exercises with regular practitioner follow-up) are associated with greater improvements in patients with chronic LBP [45–47]. Also, better results are obtained when programs are individualized based on the patient's pretreatment level of physical function, severity of pain and tolerance to exercise-induced pain [50].

Specific approaches to therapeutic exercise for chronic LBP

The reviews cited above [44–47] included studies of a variety of exercise programs. In combining exercise programs that are quite different from each other, the authors may have obscured important differences in effectiveness among various programs. In addressing this issue, it is helpful to distinguish between: (1) general conditioning programs which emphasize flexibility, aerobic fitness and strengthening of major muscle groups throughout the body, and (2) specific exercise programs based on hypotheses about the pathophysiology underlying patients' symptoms.

One such specific exercise approach is called spinal stabilization. Spinal stabilization programs include specific exercises designed to enhance the control of spinal orientation and control of intervertebral translation and rotation via training of deep trunk muscles, specifically the lumbar multifidus and transversus abdominis [51], and sometimes also the rectus abdominis, quadratus lumborus, internal oblique abdominals, and erector spinae [52].

Hides et al. [53] reported reduced LBP recurrence in 20 first-episode LBP patients who received spinal stabilization training for multifidus and transversus abdominis muscles, compared to control patients (n = 19) receiving advice and medication only. However, spinal stabilization programs have generally not been shown to be superior to general exercise programs or usual PT [54–56]. For example, Critchley *et al.* [55] reported no significant difference in physical performance or self-rated disability between groups of randomized patients in three intervention groups: (1) usual outpatient PT (n = 71), (2) spinal stabilization (n = 69), and (3) PT-led pain management classes (n = 72). The only significant difference between groups was that patients in the PT-led pain management group had lower levels of healthcare consumption and costs following treatment than patients in the other two groups.

Another form of specific exercise is the Mckenzie approach to low back pain. Directional preference (DP) is at the foundation of this approach and is identified when posture or repeated end-range movements in a single direction (flexion, extension or side-glide/rotation) decrease lumbar midline pain or reduce the extent of peripheralization of symptoms [57]. Long *et al.* [57] demonstrated better outcomes after 2 weeks in patients who received treatment based on directional matching, compared to those matched with the opposite direction or given multidirectional exercises. Since 46% of patients were considered chronic, using the patient's directional preference as a guide may benefit patients with chronic LBP during initial phases of the exercise programs.

Pooled results of four trials comparing passive therapy with McKenzie exercises for acute LBP showed a statistically significant decrease in pain and disability favoring the Mckenzie approach at 1-week follow-up. However, no difference in disability was found between the groups at 4 weeks [58]. Peterson [59] found that in comparison to an intensive strengthening program, a McKenzie approach showed a greater reduction in pain at 2 months (P = 0.01) but no significant difference at 8 months in pain, function, and disability levels. Thus, while there may be short-term benefits of McKenzie exercises for LBP, they do not appear to enhance function and disability at later stages of rehabilitation.

Matching treatments to patients

Subgroups or classifications that match patient baseline characteristics and examination factors with a specific treatment approach have been studied for physical therapy interventions [60].

A preliminary clinical prediction rule for determining which patients are likely to respond to segmental stabilization exercises was developed by Hicks [61]. For patients completing a spinal stabilization program, a higher likelihood for improvement at 8 weeks (>50% on the Oswestry Disability Questionnaire) was associated with four variables: age <40 years, straight leg raise >91°, positive prone instability test, and aberrant movement patterns. Using segmental spine mobility assessment, Fritz *et al.* [62] reported a higher success rate among patients receiving stabilization exercises who were categorized with segmental hypermobility than those categorized with segmental hypomobility. Selecting specific exercises based on subgroups, based on physical examination findings, may be most beneficial during the acute and subacute stages [63]. However, there are likely to be a different set of characteristics or classifications that are more appropriate for chronic LBP. Although much research is needed, it appears that classification systems for chronic LBP may assist in the selection of therapeutic exercise approaches.

Physical versus psychologic changes during exercise therapy

The rationale for exercise therapy in LBP patients seems obvious. If patients can increase their strength, flexibility and co-ordination through such therapy, these improvements should translate into increases in their ability to engage in the physical activities required for normal participation in work, family life, and recreation. This analysis suggests that exercise therapy helps LBP patients via a fairly straightforward transfer of physical capacities developed in the gym to activities of daily living.

It is possible, though, that the connection between participation in an exercise program in the gym and improvement in activities of daily living is indirect, and is mediated primarily by psychologic processes. For example, it is possible that participation helps patients not so much by increasing their physical capacities as by increasing their confidence that they can use their bodies safely or their ability to maintain emotional equanimity in the face of pain increases.

These alternative explanations for the benefits from exercise therapy can be tested empirically by examining the extent to which changes in physical capacities versus changes in psychologic measures of coping during rehabilitation programs predict important outcome variables such as self-reported disability and return to work. Wessels *et al.* [64] reviewed 13 studies of rehabilitative care that permitted such comparisons to be made, and concluded: "The results show that functional coping mechanisms and pain reduction seem associated with a decrease in disability and return to work, but not physical performance factors" (p. 1640). Thus, it appears that changes in patients' perceptions and coping strategies are at least as important as changes in physical capacity in the functional improvements that occur as a result of exercise therapy.

Support for the importance of psychologic factors in exercise therapy also comes from intensive multidisciplinary pain rehabilitation programs (see below). These programs typically produce substantial changes in patients' physical performance in only a few weeks. This time interval provides ample opportunity for patients to change their attitudes and coping mechanisms, but is too short to produce major changes in patients' physical capabilities [65]. A plausible hypothesis to account for the rapid changes is that prior to starting rehabilitation programs, patients perform well below their physiologic limits because of concern that they might injure themselves. As their fears subside, their performance improves so that it approximates their physiologic limits by the time the rehabilitation program ends. Thus, the improvements in physical performance that occur during the programs are mediated primarily by psychologic changes rather than physical ones.

Summary

- In general, exercise is effective for reducing pain and improving function in individuals with chronic LBP.
- Higher dosage, individualized programs and supervised programs are associated with better outcomes.
- Specific stabilization exercises have shown some effect in reducing recurrence when applied to acute LBP, when compared to no treatment. However,

stabilization exercises compared to general exercise or usual physical therapy have not shown better outcomes.
- Specific exercises based on directional preferences may benefit patients with acute LBP, but there is limited evidence supporting this approach for chronic LBP.
- The benefits that accrue from exercise therapy appear to depend at least as much on psychologic changes such as improved coping mechanisms as on changes in physical capacity.

Combination therapy – physical and psychologic

As has been discussed above, there is empirical support for both psychologic therapy and exercise therapy in the treatment of chronic LBP. These findings beg the question of whether the combination of these therapies produces better results than either one given in isolation. Unfortunately, the body of literature examining the efficacy of the combination of psychologic therapies and exercise is somewhat limited, and most of the relevant studies do not address the issue of combination therapy in an unambiguous way.

As one example of the ambiguity of PT/psychologic combination therapy, treatment programs based on operant principles involve an integration of behavioral principles and exercise therapy (see above). However, in typical operant programs or graded activity programs, patients receive both exercise and instruction in a conceptual model regarding factors that underlie persistent LBP. Thus, it is difficult to determine whether benefits from such programs should be attributed to the exercises in which patients engage or the psychoeducational inputs they receive.

Hints about the benefits of combined PT and psychologic therapy come from studies examining the use of these treatments within the context of multidisciplinary/interdisciplinary treatment programs. The efficacy of multidisciplinary chronic pain management is well established (see below), and programs essentially always include psychologic and exercise components. However, since the programs also include various other therapies (e.g. medications, interventional approaches, the therapeutic milieu), it is difficult, if not impossible, to draw conclusions specifically regarding the combination of psychologic and exercise therapies.

The same interpretive problem applies to a Cochrane review by Schonstein *et al.* [66] on the effectiveness of work conditioning, work hardening, and functional restoration programs for disabled workers with neck or back pain. The authors concluded that exercise programs foster return to work among these patients only if they are accompanied by CBT. But inspection of the 18 studies included in the review indicates that many of them evaluated multidisciplinary rehabilitation programs which included several treatment elements other than just PT and CBT.

We are aware of only one study that nominally attempted to assess the effects of exercise therapy, CBT, and the combination of the two. Jensen *et al.* [67] randomly assigned work-disabled individuals with nonspecific spinal pain to one of four treatment conditions: PT; CBT; a behavioral medicine program (BM) that combined PT and CBT; and a treatment as usual control group. They found modest support for the efficacy of combined treatment, in that female patients given the BM treatment had better outcomes with respect to self-reported well-being and return to work than ones in the control group. Outcomes for the PT and CBT participants fell between those of the BM participants and the control participants.

Unfortunately, the study was designed in a way that precluded any clear interpretation about effects of PT, CBT, and combined therapy. One complicating design issue is that there was substantial blurring between PT and psychologic therapy. Participants in the PT group received relaxation training and lectures on psychologic aspects of chronic pain in addition to exercise therapy. Also, the exercise therapy they received was described as a "behavior-oriented" exercise program. Although the program was not described in detail, it appears to have followed the graded activity approach originally outlined by Fordyce [28]. Thus, participants in the PT group could best be described as receiving integrated CBT/PT, rather than PT alone. Another complicating issue is that participants in the BM group received more total hours of treatment than did participants in the PT or CBT groups.

In summary, common sense and clinical experience support the combination of psychologic therapies and exercise programs for the treatment of chronic low back pain, and there is ample evidence for the effectiveness of multidisciplinary pain rehabilitation programs, which include the two types of treatment along with various other therapies. However, there is a paucity of research on treatment programs that include combinations of only psychologic therapy and exercise therapy. Thus, no conclusions can be reached about the efficacy of combining these two treatment approaches.

Multidisciplinary pain rehabilitation

Multidisciplinary chronic pain treatment is distinguished by integrative and co-ordinated interventions from different disciplines with common goals [68]. The approach includes a thorough evaluation, establishment of a treatment plan, and cohesive team treatment [69]. Treatment provides training in various tools to create a sense of control over pain and life, through changing emotional, behavioral, cognitive, and sensory experiences [70]. Multidisciplinary pain management/treatment/rehabilitation programs (PMP) frequently include physicians, nurses, physical therapists, psychologists or social workers, biofeedback therapists, occupational therapists, recreational therapists, and vocational counselors [69, 71]. The treatment provided by PMP is typically intensive. Early programs were carried out in an inpatient setting. In recent years, most PMP have used a day treatment model, in which patients come to a center approximately 40 hours per week for 3 weeks or more.

Pain management programs differ substantially from each other in a number of ways. Some of the differences among them are shown in Table 30.1. The differences complicate research on PMP effectiveness and render the definition of a PMP somewhat ambiguous. In the present discussion, we define a PMP as a chronic pain treatment program that: adheres to a rehabilitative model; includes at least medical monitoring, active physical therapy, and psychologic treatment; and provides at least 100 hours of treatment.

Table 30.1 Factors on which multidisciplinary pain centers vary

Patient variables at start of treatment

Social context of treatment – injured workers versus other patient groups

Pain condition being treated – low back pain versus other specific pain condition versus mixture of patients with different painful conditions

Chronicity

Level of function required of patients at start of program, e.g. bedbound versus ambulatory and able to stay up all day

Treatment variables – general

Intensity – inpatient versus outpatient; hours per week; number of weeks

Setting in which treatment is carried out:
  Medical setting – hospital or outpatient clinic
  Home
  At job site

Strict rehabilitative model versus mixture of rehabilitation and palliative treatment

Tone of program:
  Strict, "tough love" approach versus permissive approach
  Alliance with patients versus alliance with workers' compensation carrier or employer

Specialists comprising treatment team

Physician
Psychologist
Physical therapist
Occupational therapist
Vocational rehabilitation counselor
Nurse

Treatment inputs

Medical monitoring
Medication management:
  Discontinuation of opioids and sedatives
  Addition of medications, e.g. antidepressants
  Other treatments – injections; indwelling epidural catheter
Physical therapy:
  Exercise – graded activity versus other
  PT modalities – heat, myofascial release
Psychologic treatment – many types
Vocational rehabilitation
Education
Team meetings; co-ordination

Outcome variables

Pain
Self-reported functional status, e.g. SF-36, Oswestry
Observed functional capacity
Use of medical resources, e.g. more surgeries
Patient satisfaction
Psychologic improvement – self-efficacy; reduced fear; reduced depression
Vocational – return to work; declared employable; claim resolution

Outcome evaluation – overview

More than 100 outcome studies on PMP have been published. The earliest studies were case series [29]. During the 1980s investigators published results of prospective or retrospective cohort studies in which patients receiving PMP were compared to those receiving other kinds of treatment [72]. During the 1990s several large RCT were conducted in which PMP treatment was compared to a variety of alternatives [73, 74]. For the most part, published studies have supported the efficacy of PMP. They have demonstrated that following PMP treatment, patients show reductions in pain, emotional distress, and perceived disability [26, 75–79]. PMP graduates have also demonstrated reduced use of medical services and increased return to work [76, 80, 81]. Even without significant changes in pain, significant improvements in mood, coping skills, physical disability, and medication consumption have been reported following PMP treatment [78].

Reviews and meta-analytic reviews of PMP

Because of the multitude of studies on PMP, several literature reviews on the effectiveness of the programs have been undertaken. Flor et al. [82] evaluated 65 studies of multidisciplinary pain treatment using meta-analytic methodology. In contrast to the previous meta-analytic research by Malone & Strube [83] which provided evidence that nonmedical treatments of chronic pain were effective, Flor et al. evaluated *only* multidisciplinary programs. The results of both within- and between-group effect sizes demonstrated greater improvements following PMP relative to no treatment, wait list, and single discipline interventions. These positive results were obtained for a variety of outcome measures, including subjective ones (pain and mood) and objective ones (return to work and healthcare utilization). Results supported the superiority of PMP over standard care and continued stability over 12 months.

Cutler et al. [84] performed a review and meta-analysis of work outcomes among LBP patients who received PMP. They evaluated 164 publications for inclusion that focused on nonsurgical interventions for pain management, including physical therapy, occupational therapy, TENS, behavioral techniques (individual and group psychotherapy, cognitive retraining, relaxation training, hypnosis, biofeedback, education, etc.), nerve blocks, medication management, and combinations of these treatments. They systematically evaluated 37 studies that used return to work as an outcome variable. Most of these studies reported treatment in PMP. Results indicated that nonsurgical interventions (primarily PMP treatment) more than doubled the rate of return to work post treatment.

Guzmán et al. [85] performed a systematic review that was limited to RCT of PMP. The review included 10 such trials. The authors concluded: "There was strong evidence that intensive multidisciplinary biopsychosocial rehabilitation with functional restoration improves function when compared with inpatient or outpatient nonmultidisciplinary treatments. There was moderate evidence that intensive multidisciplinary biopsychosocial rehabilitation with functional restoration reduces pain when compared with outpatient nonmultidisciplinary rehabilitation or usual care. There was contradictory evidence regarding vocational outcomes of intensive multidisciplinary biopsychosocial intervention" (p. 1511).

The systematic reviews by Flor et al., Cutler et al., and Guzman et al. are not strictly comparable, because they included different studies. The reviews agreed that PMP promote improvement in important clinical measures such as pain, mood and functional capacity. They disagreed with respect to the effectiveness of PMP in promoting return to work.

Recent research

No additional systematic reviews of PMP have been published since 2001. In fact, there has been a dearth of research on PMP during the past several years. This may reflect the fact that PMP have been on the decline for many years [86], largely because of lack of support from the insurance industry.

In one recent RCT [87], 86 disabled LBP patients were randomly assigned to a functional restoration program (30 hours per week for 5 weeks) or individual PT (3 hours per week for 5 weeks). After statistical adjustments were made, patients in the functional restoration group demonstrated better outcomes at 6 months than those in the PT with respect to sick leave days, satisfaction with treatment, and physical capacities. Two other RCT dealt with treatment programs that included elements of traditional PMP but were less intensive. Kaapa et al. [88] compared the effects of a 70-hour multidisciplinary rehabilitation

program to those of an individual PT program lasting 10 hours. The treatment groups did not differ significantly with respect to pain intensity, sick leave or healthcare consumption at 24-month follow-up. Haldorsen et al. [89] identified injured workers as low, medium or high risk for continued work disability, and randomly assigned patients within each group to one of three treatments: ordinary treatment, light multidisciplinary treatment (approximately 6 hours of treatment), and extensive multidisciplinary treatment (120 hours). They found that the three treatments promoted return to work equally well for low-risk patients, that light and extensive multidisciplinary treatment promoted return to work more effectively than ordinary treatment for medium-risk patients, and that only extensive multidisciplinary treatment facilitated return to work for high-risk patients.

Both Kaapa et al. and Haldorsen et al. investigated the efficacy of less intensive PMP that were less expensive than traditional ones. These studies can be viewed as a first step in addressing the broad issue of how to streamline PMP so that they are both clinically effective and cost-effective. Cost-effectiveness for a "light" PMP was specifically addressed by Skouen et al. [90] in a follow-up of the study by Haldorsen et al. They concluded that when both medical and disability costs were considered, a light PMP program was cost-effective for males with disabling back pain. In contrast, light PMP was not cost-effective in the treatment of disabled women, and an extensive PMP was not cost-effective for either gender.

Several studies published during the past 7 years have looked at predictors of positive response to PMP rather than at the overall effectiveness of such programs. Studies on gender differences have produced mixed results, with men being more responsive to PMP in some studies [90–92], women being more responsive in at least one [93], and no gender difference being obtained in three studies [94–96]. These findings leave open the question of whether men or women respond better to PMP.

Other studies have looked at a variety of other potential predictors of outcome of PMP treatment, including scores on the SF-36 [97] and the Pain Disability Questionnaire [98], patient beliefs and coping patterns [99], readiness to self-manage pain [100], obesity [101], opioid use or dependence [102, 103], healthcare utilization prior to enrollment in a PMP [94], various DSM-IV psychiatric diagnoses [103], and miscellaneous other psychosocial variables [104, 105]. In the aggregate, these studies suggest that several different demographic and psychosocial characteristics of patients influence the likelihood that they will respond to PMP. But it is extremely difficult to integrate findings from the above studies into a coherent profile of the type of individual who is likely to respond well to PMP treatment. One recent review attempted to do this [106], but the authors concluded that it was "impossible to define a generic set of predictors of outcome of multidisciplinary rehabilitation" (p. 813). The main problem they encountered was that the studies they reviewed were so disparate that it was essentially impossible to identify consistent, replicable results.

Summary

Overall, the above research demonstrates the efficacy of PMP. Chronic pain patients demonstrate improvements on multiple measurements after treatment, at both short-term and long-term follow-up. The positive treatment outcomes from PMP are higher than those achieved with standard medical intervention and unimodal treatments.

It is important to note, though, that there are significant gaps in the evidence regarding PMP. One important issue that has not been adequately studied is the optimal mixture of specific treatment modalities offered in PMP. As noted above and documented in Table 30.1, PMP differ greatly with respect to treatment modalities and several other factors that may influence the effectiveness of their treatment. This variation can be traced to the historical fact that PMP have been established not on the basis of empirical evidence but rather on the basis of the intuitions of clinicians about the combinations of treatments that would produce optimal results. Although individual studies and systematic reviews provide empirical support for many of the PMP that have been developed, the significance of most of the factors in Table 30.1 has not been systematically explored. As an example of the kind of research that is needed, a few recent studies have evaluated "light" PMP and have thus addressed one important

dimension on which PMP vary – the intensity of treatment.

Similarly, although there is a growing body of research on predictors of success from PMP treatment, the research has not yet progressed to a point where practical strategies can be developed for deciding which chronic pain patients should be referred to PMP. In the current environment of skepticism about the effectiveness and cost-effectiveness of PMP, it is exceedingly important for clinicians to refer only those patients with a good chance of profiting from PMP treatment.

Conclusion

The literature cited above supports the conclusion that two of the core ingredients of rehabilitative treatment for chronic LBP are effective – exercise therapy and psychologic therapy. Indirect evidence supports the conclusion that combinations of exercise therapy and psychologic therapy produce better outcomes than either approach provided in isolation. Finally, there is evidence for the effectiveness of intensive multidisciplinary pain rehabilitation programs, which include exercise therapy and psychologic therapy in combination with various other inputs such as medication management.

As is often the case, significant methodologic issues limit the strength of the conclusions that can be reached from this review. As noted in virtually every relevant systematic review [16, 45, 66, 85], the research literature on rehabilitative therapies is plagued by a host of methodologic problems related to subject selection, randomization, definition of treatments, subject attrition leading to missing data, blinding of subjects and examiners, definition of outcome variables, and statistical methods. These issues have been addressed in detail in the above reviews, and will not be repeated here.

Another problem that complicates interpretation of the literature is the enormous variation across studies that superficially address the same treatment modality. For example, Table 30.1 describes the numerous factors that differentiate various PMP. Similar variation exists across studies of exercise therapy and psychologic therapy. This variation makes it difficult to combine studies, even when the component studies are methodologically rigorous.

Of the many unresolved issues related to rehabilitative treatment for chronic pain, we believe that the following deserve special attention.

Specific issues regarding exercise therapy

The aggregation of studies on exercise therapy for the purposes of systematic review embodies the assumption that exercise therapy represents a well-defined, homogeneous form of treatment. Most physical therapists bristle at this idea and emphasize the substantial differences among different approaches to exercise therapy for LBP. A related issue is that it may be pointless to evaluate the effectiveness of a specific exercise program in the abstract, because its effectiveness may depend primarily on whether it matches the biomechanical deficits and psychosocial make-up of an individual patient. Also, legitimate questions can be raised about the extent to which the effectiveness of physical therapy depends on "art" versus "science." It is certainly possible that the successes of PT depend more on their unique combinations of communication skills and knowledge of biomechanics than on the specific "schools" of physical therapy to which they subscribe, or the names they give to the treatments that they provide.

Specific issues regarding psychologic therapies

Research on psychologic therapies runs into problems very similar to those outlined above for exercise therapy. Specifically, there are multiple treatment approaches that are loosely included under the "psychologic therapy" rubric. The fact that psychologic therapies in the aggregate are effective in treating LBP leaves multiple questions unanswered about the specific therapies that are likely to be most helpful for specific patient groups. Moreover, it is quite possible that the benefit from psychologic therapies depends as much on the interpersonal skill of the individual psychologist as on the specific "school" to which the psychologist adheres.

The optimal setting for multidisciplinary rehabilitative treatment

For many years after PMP were started in the 1960s, programs were established in medical facilities such as hospitals or outpatient rehabilitation centers. Implicitly, programs run in such settings conveyed the message that pain rehabilitation is a medical process that needs to be treated in a medical facility. This message may be inappropriate for injured workers with chronic LBP. As Fordyce [107] has argued, workers with persistent LBP might better be construed as having activity intolerance than as having a medical condition that is amenable to medical therapy. From this perspective, it might be more appropriate for rehabilitation of injured workers to occur in a work-like setting than in a medical setting [108–110].

Complementary and alternative treatments

Another historical legacy from the 1960s is that PMP have generally been run by physicians and have focused on allopathic therapies. Very little attention has been given to the role of complementary and alternative medicine (CAM) therapies such as chiropractic treatment or acupuncture in PMP. Given the heavy reliance on such therapies by patients with musculoskeletal disorders, it will be important in the future to consider ways to integrate them into rehabilitation programs, and to evaluate PMP that include CAM therapies.

Patient populations – medical conditions

This chapter has focused on LBP for the practical reason that research on rehabilitative therapies is much more extensive for disorders of the lumbar spine than for any other kind of chronic pain disorder. Obviously, though, questions can be raised about the generalizability of the conclusions summarized above. In the absence of conclusive evidence, we speculate that the rehabilitative approaches that have shown efficacy in the treatment of LBP are also likely to be efficacious for most chronically painful musculoskeletal conditions. But their relevance to painful disorders that involve other organ systems (e.g. endometriosis or diabetic neuropathy) is unclear.

Patient populations – injured workers

It is important to distinguish between injured workers and other patient groups when discussing rehabilitative therapies for LBP. One reason for this distinction is that different outcome variables are needed for workers versus nonworkers. A related point is that PMP have been less successful in achieving outcomes of special relevance to injured workers – return to work and resolution of disability claim – than in achieving clinical outcomes such as pain reduction and improvements in physical functioning [85]. Our understanding of all rehabilitative therapies will be enhanced if researchers pay consistent attention to whether the patients being treated are injured workers versus others, and whether the benefits that accrue from treatment are primarily subjective ones (e.g. pain relief or improved mood) versus objective ones (especially return to work).

A final word

Finally, it is important to note an important paradox regarding rehabilitative therapies for LBP. Given that: (1) research supports the effectiveness of individual rehabilitative treatments and their combination in the form of PMP, and (2) experts routinely support the importance of combinations of therapies [111], one would expect enthusiastic support for PMP. In fact, the trend in the United States has been in the direction of fewer PMP [86]. The reasons for this are not entirely clear. It is quite possible that too much was expected from PMP when they were started, and that insurers and some physicians are now experiencing a wave of disappointment. In any case, we believe that it will be important to reverse the current downward spiral in PMP. To do this, research will be needed to identify the most effective combinations of rehabilitative therapies, so that the cost-effectiveness of combination treatment programs can be maximized. At the same time, it will be important for specialists in pain medicine and rehabilitation medicine to communicate to their colleagues and to the insurance community regarding the effectiveness of rehabilitative treatment for chronic LBP.

References

1. Forseth KO, Forre O, Gran JT. A 5.5 year prospective study of self-reported musculoskeletal pain and of fibromyalgia in a female population: significance and natural history. *Clin Rheumatol* 1999; **18**(2): 114–121.
2. Hashemi L, Webster BS, Clancy EA. Trends in disability duration and cost of workers' compensation low back pain claims (1988–1996). *J Occup Environ Med* 1998; **40**(12): 1110–1119.
3. *Dorland's Illustrated Medical Dictionary*, 28th edn. Saunders, Philadelphia, 1994.
4. Manek NJ, MacGregor AJ. Epidemiology of back disorders: prevalence, risk factors, and prognosis. *Curr Opin Rheumatol* 2005; **17**(2): 134–140.
5. Carragee E, Alamin T, Cheng I, Franklin T, Hurwitz E. Does minor trauma cause serious low back illness? *Spine* 2006; **31**(25): 2942–2049.
6. Leo RJ. *Clinical Manual of Pain Management in Psychiatry*. American Psychiatric Press, Washington, DC, 2007.
7. Vlaeyen JWS, Haazen IW, Schuerman JA, Kole-Snijders AM, van Eek H. Behavioural rehabilitation of chronic low back pain: comparison of an operant treatment, an operant-cognitive treatment and an operant-respondent treatment. *Br J Clin Psychol* 1995; **34** (Pt 1): 95–118.
7a. Waddell G. The biopsychosocial model. In: Waddell G (ed) *The Back Pain Revolution*. Churchill Livingstone, Edinburgh, 2004.
8. Vlaeyen JWS, Kole-Snijders AMJ, Boeren RGB, van Eek H. Fear of movement/(re)injury in chronic low back pain and its relation to behavioral performance. *Pain* 1995; **62**: 363–372.
9. Vlaeyen JW, Linton SJ. Fear-avoidance and its consequences in chronic musculoskeletal pain: a state of the art. *Pain* 2000; **85**(3): 317–332.
10. Leeuw M, Goossens ME, Linton SJ, Crombez G, Boersma K, Vlaeyen JW. The fear-avoidance model of musculoskeletal pain: current state of scientific evidence. *J Behav Med* 2007; **30**(1): 77–94.
11. Mondloch MV, Cole DC, Frank JW. Does how you do depend on how you think you'll do? A systematic review of the evidence for a relation between patients' recovery expectations and health outcomes. *Can Med Assoc J* 2001; **165**(2): 174–179.
12. Cole DC, Mondloch MV, Hogg-Johnson S. Listening to injured workers: how recovery expectations predict outcomes – a prospective study. *Can Med Assoc J* 2002; **166**(6): 749–754.
13. Hoffman BM, Papas RK, Chatkoff DK, Kerns RD. Meta-analysis of psychological interventions for chronic low back pain. *Health Psychol* 2007; **26**(1): 1–9.
14. Morley S, Eccleston C, Williams A. Systematic review and meta-analysis of randomized controlled trials of cognitive behaviour therapy and behaviour therapy for chronic pain in adults, excluding headache. *Pain* 1999; **80**: 1–13.
15. van Tulder M, Malmivaara A, Esmail R, Koes B. Exercise therapy for low back pain: a systematic review within the framework of the cochrane collaboration back review group. *Spine* 2000; **25**(21): 2784–2796.
16. Ostelo RWJG, van Tulder MW, Vlaeyen JWS, Linton SJ, Morley S, Assendelft WJJ. Behavioural treatment for chronic low-back pain. Cochrane Database of Systematic Reviews 2005, Issue 1. Art. No.: CD002014. DOI: 10.1002/14651858.CD002014.pub2.
17. Compas BE, Haaga DA, Keefe FJ, Leitenberg H, Williams DA. Sampling of empirically supported psychological treatments from health psychology: smoking, chronic pain, cancer, and bulimia nervosa. *J Consult Clin Psychol* 1998; **66**(1): 89–112.
18. Keefe FJ, Dunsmore J, Burnett R. Behavioral and cognitive-behavioral approaches to chronic pain: recent advances and future directions. *J Consult Clin Psychol* 1992; **60**(4): 528–536.

19. Newton-John TR, Spence SH, Schotte D. Cognitive behavioural therapy versus EMG biofeedback in the treatment of chronic low back pain. *Behav Res Ther* 1995; **33**: 691–697.

20. Smeets RJEM, Vlaeyen JWS, Hidding A, *et al.* Active rehabilitation for chronic low back pain: cognitive-behavioral, physical or both? First direct post-treatment results from a randomized controlled trial. *BMC Musculoskelet Disord* 2006; 7: 5.

21. Kole-Snijders AMJ, Vlaeyen JWS, Goossens MEJB, *et al.* Chronic low-back pain: what does cognitive coping skills training add to operant behavioral treatment? Results of a randomized clinical trial. *J Consult Clin Psychol* 1999; **67**(6): 931–944.

22. Scheer SJ, Watanabe TK, Radack KL. Randomized controlled trials in industrial low back pain. Part 3. Subacute/chronic pain interventions. *Arch Phys Med Rehabil* 1997; **78**(4): 414–423.

23. Alaranta H, Rytokoski U, Rissanen A, *et al.* Intensive physical and psychosocial training program for patients with chronic low back pain. A controlled clinical trial. *Spine* 1994; **19**(12): 1339–1349.

24. Goossens ME, Rutten-van Molken MP, Kole-Snijders AM, *et al.* Health economic assessment of behavioural rehabilitation in chronic low back pain: a randomised clinical trial. *Health Econ* 1998; **7**(1): 39–51.

25. Nicholas MK, Wilson PH, Goyen J. Operant-behavioural and cognitive-behavioural treatment for chronic low back pain. *Behav Res Ther* 1991; **29**; 225–238.

26. Turner JA, Jensen MP. Efficacy of cognitive therapy for chronic low back pain. *Pain* 1993; **52**(2): 169–177.

27. Sanders SH. Operant therapy with pain patients: evidence for its effectiveness. In: Lebovits AH (ed) *Seminars in Pain Medicine. 1.* W.B. Saunders, Philadelphia, 2003: 90–98.

28. Fordyce WE. *Behavioral Methods for Chronic Pain and Illness.* Mosby, St Louis, 1976.

29. Fordyce WE, Fowler RS Jr, Lehmann JF, Delateur BJ, Sand PL, Trieschmann RB. Operant conditioning in the treatment of chronic pain. *Arch Phys Med Rehabil* 1973; **54**(9): 399–408.

30. Fordyce WE, Shelton JL, Dundore DE. The modification of avoidance learning pain behaviors. *J Behav Med* 1982; **5**(4): 405–414.

31. Turner JA, Clancy S, McQuade KJ, Cardenas DD. Effectiveness of behavioral therapy for chronic low back pain: a component analysis. *J Consult Clin Psychol* 1990; **58**: 573–579.

32. Lindstrom I, Ohlund C, Eek C, *et al.* The effect of graded activity on patients with subacute low back pain: a randomized prospective clinical study with an operant-conditioning behavioral approach. *Phys Ther* 1992; **72**: 279–293.

33. Staal JB, Hlobil H, Twisk JW, Smid T, Koke AJ, van Mechelen W. Graded activity for low back pain in occupational health care: a randomized, controlled trial. *Ann Intern Med* 2004; **140**(2): 77–84.

34. Linton SJ, Bradley LA, Jensen I, *et al.* The secondary prevention of low back pain: a controlled study with follow-up. *Pain* 1989; **36**: 197–207.

35. Turner JA, Clancy S. Comparison of operant behavioral and cognitive-behavioral group treatment for chronic low back pain. *J Consult Clin Psychol* 1988; **56**: 261–266.

36. van der Hout JHC, Vlaeyen JWS, Heuts PH, *et al.* Secondary prevention of work-related disability in non-specific low back pain: does problem solving therapy help? *Clin J Pain* 2003; **19**(2): 87–96.

37. Ostelo RW, de Vet HC, Vlaeyen JW, *et al.* Behavioral graded activity following first-time lumbar disc surgery: 1-year results of a randomized clinical trial. *Spine* 2003; **28**(16): 1757–1765.

38. Steenstra IA, Anema JR, Bongers PM, de Vet HC, Knol DL, van Mechelen W. The effectiveness of graded activity for low back pain in occupational healthcare. *Occup Environ Med* 2006; **63**(11): 718–725.

39. Vlaeyen JWS. *Chronic Low Back Pain. Assessment and Treatment from a Behavioral Rehabilitation Perspective.* Swets and Zeitlinger, Lisse, 1991.

40. George SZ, Fritz JM, Bialosky JE, Donald DA. The effect of a fear-avoidance-based physical therapy intervention for patients with acute low back pain: results of a randomized clinical trial. *Spine* 2003; **28**(23): 2551–2560.

41. Nielson WR, Weir R. Biopsychosocial approaches to the treatment of chronic pain. *Clin J Pain* 2001; **17**(4 suppl): 114–127.

42. Airaksinen O, Brox JI, Cedraschi C, *et al.*, COST B13 Working Group on Guidelines for Chronic Low Back Pain. European guidelines for the management of chronic nonspecific low back pain. *Eur Spine J* 2006; 15(msuppl 2): S192–S300.

43. Albright J, Allman R, Bonfiglio RP, *et al.* Philadelphia Panel evidence-based clinical practice guidelines on selected rehabilitation interventions for low back pain. *Phys Ther* 2001; **81**(10): 1641–1674.

44. Taylor NF, Dodd KJ, Shields N, Bruder A. Therapeutic exercise in physiotherapy practice is beneficial: a summary of systematic reviews 2002–2005. *Aust J Physiother* 2007; **53**: 7–16.

45. Hayden JA, van Tulder MW, Malmivaara A, Koes BW. Exercise therapy for treatment of non-specific low back pain. Cochrane Database of Systematic Reviews 2005, Issue 3. Art. No.: CD000335.pub2. DOI: 10.1002/14651858. CD000335.pub2.

46. Hayden JA, van Tulde MW, Malmivaara AV, Koes BW. Meta-analysis: exercise therapy for nonspecific low back pain. *Ann Intern Med* 2005; **142**(9): 767–775.

47. Hayden JA, van Tulde MW, Tomlinson G. Systematic review: strategies for using exercise therapy to improve outcomes in chronic low back pain. *Ann Intern Med* 2005; **142**(9): 776–785.

48. Kool J, de Bie R, Oesch P, Knusel O, van den Brandt P, Bachman S. Exercise reduces sick leave in patients with non-acute non-specific low back pain: a meta-analysis. *J Rehab Med* 2004; **36**: 49–62.

49. van Tulder M, Malmivaara A, Hayden J, Koes B. Statistical significance versus clinical importance: trials on exercise therapy for chronic low back pain as example. *Spine* 2007; **32**(16): 1785–1790.

50. Mannerkorpi K, Henriksson C. Non-pharmacological treatment of chronic widespread musculoskeletal pain. *Best Pract Res Clin Rheumatol* 2007; **21**(3): 513–534.

51. Hodges P. Spinal segmental stabilization training. In: Liebenson C (ed) *Rehabilitation of the Spine*. Lippincott Williams and Wilkins, Philadelphia, 2007: 585–611.

52. McGill S. Lumbar spine stability: mechanisms of injury and restabilization. In: Liebenson C (ed) *Rehabilitation of the Spine*. Lippincott Williams and Wilkins, Philadelphia, 2007: 93–111.

53. Hides JA, Jull GA, Richardson CA. Long-term effects of specific stabilizing exercises for first-episode low back pain. *Spine* 2001; **26**(11): E243–E248.

54. Cairns MC, Foster N E, Wright C. Randomized controlled trial of specific spinal stabilization exercises and conventional physiotherapy for recurrent low back pain. *Spine* 2006; **31**(19): E670–E681.

55. Critchley DJ, Ratcliffe J, Noonan S, Jones RH, Hurley MV. Effectiveness and cost-effectiveness of three types of physiotherapy used to reduce chronic low back pain disability: a pragmatic randomized trial with economic evaluation. *Spine* 2007; **32**(14): 1474–1481.

56. Koumantakis GA, Watson PJ, Oldham JA. Trunk muscle stabilization training plus general exercise versus general exercise only: randomized controlled trial of patients with recurrent low back pain. *Phys Ther* 2005; **85**(3): 209–225.

57. Long A, Donelson R, Fung T. Does it matter which exercise? A randomized control trial of exercise for low back pain. *Spine* 2004; **29**(23): 2593–2602.

58. Machado LA, de Souza MS, Ferreira PH, Ferreira ML. The Mckenzie method for low back pain: a systematic review of the literature with a meta-analysis approach. *Spine* 2006; **31**: E254–E262.

59. Peterson T, Kryger P, Ekdahl C, Olsen S, Jacobsen S. The effect of Mckenzie therapy as compared with that of intensive strengthening training for treatment of patients with subacute or chronic low back pain: a randomized controlled trial. *Spine* 2002; **27**(16): 1702–1709.

60. Fritz JM, Cleland JA, Childs JD. Subgrouping patients with low back pain: evolution of a classification approach to physical therapy. *J Orthop Sports Phys Ther* 2007; **37** (6): 290–302.

61. Hicks GE, Fritiz JM, Delitto A, Mcgill SM. Preliminary development of a clinical prediction rule for determining which patients with low back pain will respond to a stabilization exercise program. *Arch Phys Med Rehabil* 2005; **86**: 1753–1762.

62. Fritz JM, Whitman JM, Childs JD. Lumbar spine segmental mobility assessment: an examination of validity for determining intervention strategies in patients with low back pain. *Arch Phys Med Rehabil* 2005; **86**: 1745–1752.

63. Brennan GP, Fritz JM, Hunter SJ, Thackeray A, Delitto A, Erhard RE. Identifying subgroups of patients with acute/subacute "nonspecific" low back pain: results of randomized clinical trial. *Spine* 2006; **31**(6): 623–631.

64. Wessels T, van Tulder M, Sigl T, Ewert T, Limm H, Stucki G. What predicts outcome in non-operative treatments of chronic low back pain? A systematic review. *Eur Spine J* 2006; **15**(11): 1633–1644.

65. Astrand, P, Rodahl K, Dahl, HA, Stromme SB. *Textbook of Work Physiology*, 4th edn. Human Kinetics, Champaign, IL, 2003.

66. Schonstein E, Kenny DT, Keating J, Boes BW. Work conditioning, work hardening and functional restoration for workers with back and neck pain. Cochrane Database of Systematic Reviews 2003, Issue 3, Art. No.: CD001822. DOI: 10.1002/14651858.CD001822.

67. Jensen IB, Bergstrom G, Ljungquist T, Bodin L. A 3-year follow-up of a multidisciplinary rehabilitation programme for back and neck pain. *Pain* 2005; **115**: 273–283.

68. Jacobson L, Mariano AJ. General considerations of chronic pain. In: Loeser JD, Butler SH, Chapman CR, Turk DC (eds) *Bonica's Management of Pain*. Lippincott, Williams, and Wilkins, Philadelphia, 2001.

69. Aronoff GM. Pain centers: treatment for intractable suffering and disability resulting from chronic pain. In: Aronoff GM (ed) *Evaluation and Treatment of Chronic Pain*, 3rd edn. Williams and Wilkins, Baltimore, MD, 1989.

70. Gatchel RJ, Turk DC. *Psychological Approaches to Pain Management: A Practitioner's Handbook*. Guilford Press, New York, 1996.

71. Hardin KN. Chronic pain management. In: Camic P Knight S (eds) *Clinical Handbook of Health Psychology*. Hogrefe and Huber Publishers, Seattle, WA, 1998: 123–165.

72. Mayer TG, Gatchel RJ, Mayer H, Kishino ND, Keeley J, Mooney V. A prospective two-year study of functional restoration in industrial low back injury. An objective assessment procedure. *JAMA* 1987; **258**(13): 1763–1767.

73. Bendix AF, Bendix T, Labriola M, Bœgaard P. Functional restoration for chronic low back pain: two-year follow-up of two randomized clinical trials. *Spine* 1998; **23**(6): 717–725.

74. Bendix T, Bendix AF, Labriola M, Haestrup C, Ebbehoj N. Functional restoration versus outpatient physical training in chronic low back pain: a randomized comparative study. *Spine* 2000; **25**(19): 2494–2500.

75. Keller S, Ehrhardt-Schmelzer S, Herda C, Schmid S, Basler HD. Multidisciplinary rehabilitation for chronic back pain in an outpatient setting: a controlled randomized trial. *Eur J Pain* 1997; **1**(4): 279–292.

76. Lofland KR, Burns JW, Tsoutsouris J, Laird MM, Blonsky ER, Hejna WF. Predictors of outcome following multidisciplinary treatment of chronic pain: effects of change in perceived disability and depression. *Int J Rehabil Health* 1997; **3**(4): 221–232.

77. Nicholas MK, Wilson PH, Goyen J. Comparison of cognitive-behavioral group treatment and an alternative non-psychological treatment for chronic low back pain. *Pain* 1992; **48**: 339–347.

78. Skinner JB, Erskine A, Pearce SA, Rubenstein I, Taylor M, Foster C. The evaluation of a cognitive behavioural treatment programme in outpatients with chronic pain. *J Psychosom Res* 1990; **34**: 13–19.

79. Turner JA, Jensen MP. Efficacy of cognitive therapy for chronic low back pain. *Pain* 1993; **52**: 169–177.

80. Cassisi JE, Sypert GW, Salamon A, Kapel L. Independent evaluation of a multidisciplinary rehabilitation program for chronic low back pain. *Neurosurgery* 1989; **25**: 877–883.

81. Jensen MP, Turner JA, Romano JM. Correlates of improvement in multidisciplinary treatment of chronic pain. *J Consult Clin Psychol* 1994; **62**: 172–179.

82. Flor H, Fydrich T, Turk DC. Efficacy of multidisciplinary pain treatment centers: a meta-analytic review. *Pain* 1992; **49**: 221–230.

83. Malone MD, Strube MJ. Meta-analysis of non-medical treatments for chronic pain. *Pain* 1988; **34**(3): 231–244.

84. Cutler RB, Fishbain DA, Rosomoff HL, Abdel-Motsy E, Khalil TM, Rosomoff RS. Does nonsurgical pain center treatment of chronic pain return patients to work? A review and meta-analysis of the literature. *Spine* 1994; **19**(6): 643–652.

85. Guzmán J, Esmail R, Karjalainen K, Malmivaara A, Irvin E, Bombardier C. Multidisciplinary rehabilitation for chronic low back pain: systematic review. *BMJ* 2001; **322**: 1511–1516.

86. Schatman ME. The demise of multidisciplinary pain management clinics? *Pract Pain Manage* 2006; **6**: 30–41.

87. Jousset N, Fanello S, Bontoux L, *et al.* Effects of functional restoration versus 3 hours per week physical therapy: a randomized controlled study. *Spine* 2004; **29**(5): 487–493.

88. Kaapa EH, Frantsi K, Sarna S, Malmivaara A. Multidisciplinary group rehabilitation versus individual physiotherapy for chronic nonspecific low back pain: a randomized trial. *Spine* 2006; **31**(4): 371–376.

89. Haldorsen EM, Grasdal AL, Skouen JS, Risa AE, Kronholm K, Ursin H. Is there a right treatment for a particular patient group? Comparison of ordinary treatment, light multidisciplinary treatment, and extensive multidisciplinary treatment for long-term sick-listed employees with musculoskeletal pain. *Pain* 2002; **95**(1–2): 49–63.

90. Skouen JS, Grasdal AL, Haldorsen EM, Ursin H. Relative cost-effectiveness of extensive and light multidisciplinary treatment programs versus treatment as usual for patients with chronic low back pain on long-term sick leave: randomized controlled study. *Spine* 2002; **27**(9): 901–909.

91. Keogh E, McCracken LM, Eccleston C. Do men and women differ in their response to interdisciplinary chronic pain management? *Pain* 2005; **114**(1-2): 37–46.

92. McGeary DD, Mayer TG, Gatchel RJ, Anagnostis C, Proctor TJ. Gender-related differences in treatment outcomes for patients with musculoskeletal disorders. *Spine J* 2003; **3**(3): 197–203.

93. Jensen IB, Bergstrom G, Ljungquist T, Bodin L. A 3-year follow-up of a multidisciplinary rehabilitation programme for back and neck pain. *Pain* 2005; **115**(3): 273–283.

94. Gross DP, Battie MC. Predicting timely recovery and recurrence following multidisciplinary rehabilitation in patients with compensated low back pain. *Spine* 2005; **30**(2): 235–240.

95. Edwards RR, Doleys DM, Lowery D, Fillingim RB. Pain tolerance as a predictor of outcome following multidisciplinary treatment for chronic pain: differential effects as a function of sex. *Pain* 2003; **106**(3): 419–426.

96. Gatchel RJ, Mayer TG, Kidner CL, McGeary DD. Are gender, marital status or parenthood risk factors for outcome of treatment for chronic disabling spinal disorders? *J Occup Rehabil* 2005; **15**(2): 191–201.

97. Loyd R, Fanciullo GJ, Hanscom B, Baird JC. Cluster analysis of SF-36 scales as a predictor of spinal pain patients response to a multidisciplinary pain management approach beginning with epidural steroid injection. *Pain Med* 2006; **7**(3): 229–236.

98. Gatchel RJ, Mayer TG, Theodore BR. The pain disability questionnaire: relationship to one-year functional and psychosocial rehabilitation outcomes. *J Occup Rehabil* 2006; **16**(1): 75–94.

99. Jensen MP, Turner JA, Romano JM. Changes after multidisciplinary pain treatment in patient pain beliefs and coping are associated with concurrent changes in patient functioning. *Pain* 2007; **131**(1-2): 38–47.

100. Jensen MP, Nielson WR, Turner JA, Romano JM, Hill ML. Changes in readiness to self-manage pain are associated with improvement in multidisciplinary pain treatment and pain coping. *Pain* 2004; **111**(1-2): 84–95.

101. Mayer T, Aceska A, Gatchel RJ. Is obesity overrated as a "risk factor" for poor outcomes in chronic occupational spinal disorders? *Spine* 2006; **31**(25): 2967–2972.

102. Maclaren JE, Gross RT, Sperry JA, Boggess JT. Impact of opioid use on outcomes of functional restoration. *Clin J Pain* 2006; **22**(4): 392–398.

103. Dersh J, Mayer T, Gatchel RJ, Towns B, Theodore B, Polatin P. Psychiatric comorbidity in chronic disabling occupational spinal disorders has minimal impact on functional restoration socioeconomic outcomes. *Spine* 2007; **32**(17): 1917–1925.

104. Lillefjell M, Krokstad S, Espnes GA. Prediction of function in daily life following multidisciplinary rehabilitation for individuals with chronic musculoskeletal pain; a prospective study. *BMC Musculoskelet Disord* 2007; **8**: 65.

105. Talo S, Forssell H, Heikkonen S, Puukka P. Integrative group therapy outcome related to psychosocial characteristics in patients with chronic pain. *Int J Rehabil Res* 2001; **24**(1): 25–33.

106. van der Hulst M, Vollenbroek-Hutten MMR, Ijzerman MJ. A systematic review of sociodemographic, physical, and psychological predictdors of multidisciplinary rehabilitation – or, back school treatment outcome in patients with chronic low back pain. *Spine* 2005; **30**: 813–825.

107. Fordyce WE. *Back Pain in the Workplace*. IASP Press, Seattle, WA, 1995.

108. Lemstra M, Olszynski WP. The effectiveness of standard care, early intervention, and occupational management in Workers' Compensation claims: part 2. *Spine* 2004; **29**(14): 1573–1579.

109. Anema JR, Steenstra IA, Bongers PM, *et al.* Multidisciplinary rehabilitation for subacute low back pain: graded activ-

ity or workplace intervention or both? A randomized controlled trial. *Spine* 2007; **32**(3): 291–298; discussion 299–300.

110. Loisel P, Durand MJ, Diallo B, Vachon B, Charpentier N, Labelle J. From evidence to community practice in work

rehabilitation: the Quebec experience. *Clin J Pain* 2003; **19**(2): 105–113.

111. Bergman S. Strategies for prevention and management of musculoskeletal conditions. *Best Pract Res Clin Rheumatol* 2007; **21**(1): 153–166.

CHAPTER 31

Drug treatment of chronic pain

Henry McQuay

Nuffield Department of Anaesthetics, John Radcliffe Hospital, Oxford, UK

Introduction

The lessons learned from systematic reviews of analgesic drug interventions fall into three main groups:

- the guidance we can glean about relative efficacy and safety in populations
- the principle of add rather than replace
- the trial designs and outcome measures which we could adopt to make things better.

The issue of the appropriateness of the relative efficacy and safety advice is an important one. There is controversy about whether we should be thinking of relative efficacy and safety in the context of a particular procedure (e.g. type of operation in the acute context) rather than across all procedures or, in the chronic pain context, thinking of a particular pain syndrome rather than across syndromes. In an ideal world we would of course have sufficient data to enable precision when giving clear advice about medication for a particular procedure or pain syndrome. In the absence of that adequacy of data, the argument becomes whether it is legitimate or illegitimate to lump data from all procedures or pain conditions (lumping allowing us to achieve an adequate amount of data). To date, in acute pain the lumped efficacy estimates have proved robust across procedures and have extrapolated credibly to nociceptive chronic pain, and similarly pharmacologic remedies effective in one peripheral neuropathic

pain syndrome have shown efficacy in others. We would argue that thus far, lumping across procedure or across condition or syndrome has been necessary because we do not have sufficient data within procedure or condition, but that lumping has produced credible and robust estimates which have extrapolated well. These arguments are put in more detail elsewhere [1].

Figure 31.1 shows the relative efficacy league table derived from postoperative placebo-controlled studies. The number needed to treat (NNT) for at least 50% relief over the 6 hours post dose on the horizontal axis show better performance to the left; the NNT point estimate is at the center of the bar with the 95% confidence intervals extending laterally. Oral nonsteroidal anti-inflammatory drugs (NSAIDs) perform at least as well as intramuscular morphine 10 mg, and single-dose oral opioids do relatively poorly. The internal validity of the league table shows in the better performance of a bigger dose, as with paracetamol. The better the analgesic, the fewer patients we need to study to have convincing efficacy estimates, but 500 is a rule of thumb minimum. This minimum is important when we come to chronic neuropathic pain analyses. The nub of the argument from this figure is that these relative efficacy estimates are the best we have at present, and that they extrapolate well to other nociceptive pain contexts such as chronic arthritis. One enigma is that oral opioids may perform better on multiple dosing than they do in these single-dose studies.

What the relative efficacy league table gives us is a feel for the relative efficacy in the population – relative efficacy on average. This is different from performance

Evidence-Based Chronic Pain Management. Edited by
C. Stannard, E. Kalso and J. Ballantyne. © 2010 Blackwell
Publishing.

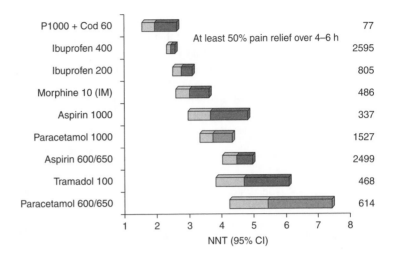

Figure 31.1 Relative efficacy analgesic league table (postoperative pain).

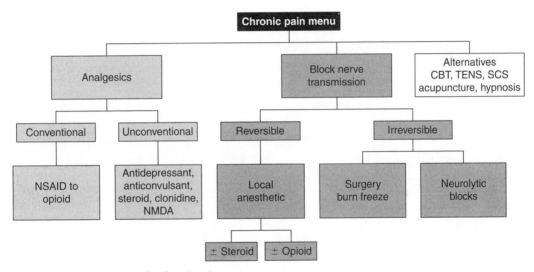

Figure 31.2 A treatment menu for chronic pain.

in the individual. It is a guide, a prediction, but we all vary. Didactic application of these performance estimates, using them as rules rather than tools, should be avoided.

Menus and ladders

Figure 31.2 shows the major ways in which we can treat chronic pain – the "menu." The important split in the analgesic choice is between the conventional analgesics, drugs used throughout medicine to treat nociceptive pain, and the unconventional analgesics, primarily drawn from the antidepressants and antiepileptics. The downside of picturing the choices as

a menu like this is the impression it gives of a static pain – find the right remedy and you are home and dry. For most patients, life is more complicated than that, with pain intensity that varies, either for a reason such as increased activity or for no good reason. The row headings in Figure 31.3 are an attempt to map this acute, acute on chronic or more chronic timing onto the variety of chronic pain syndromes.

Perhaps the most effective way to give patients a strategy to deal with pain intensity that varies is time spent explaining a stepped approach to the drug management of their pain. This applies to management of both nociceptive and neuropathic pain, although the exemplar given is for nociceptive pain alone. The start point is the WHO pain "ladder." Turning it on its head, because that reduces the likelihood that patients and carers will omit the step 1 drug when treating severe pain, we end up with a picture like Figure 31.4. Detailed explanation of the reasoning behind this "DOAS" ladder may be found elsewhere [2]. Increasing pain severity moves from left to right, and to deal with severe pain we have three remedies rather than just the one we need for mild pain. Precisely what goes in each of the three pots should (hopefully) be guided by data such as shown in Figure 31.1, tempered by the patient's experience. Perhaps the crucial point is to

	1. Nociceptive	2. Neuropathic		3. Visceral	Combined
		a. Peripheral	b. Central		
Acute	Post-op Burns "Sprains & strains"			"Stone" pain ulcer	
Intermittent/ incidental	Headache Migraine Osteo-arthritis	Trigeminal neuralgia		Dysmenorrhea Endometriosis Pelvic IBS Dyspepsia	Cancer (1,2,3)
Chronic	Rheumatoid arthritis Osteo-arthritis FM Myofascial (e.g. neck-shoulder) Low back pain	Postherpetic neuralgia (PHN) Diabetic mono/poly neuropathy Nerve trauma	Spinal cord injury Central post stroke Multiple sclerosis Parkinson's disease	Pelvic	Cancer (1,2,3) LBP with radiculo- pathy (1, 2a) Whiplash (1, 2a)

Figure 31.3 Pain conditions, by timing and by mechanism.

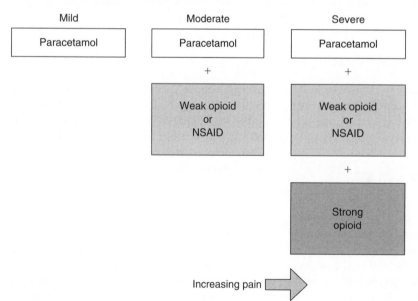

Figure 31.4 The DOAS (Do Once And Share) basic pain care pathway.

appreciate the concept of "add rather than replace" as pain intensity increases, and then come back down to just the step 1 drug as pain intensity decreases.

Choosing drugs to treat nociceptive pain

Choosing between the various drugs which treat nociceptive pain is governed by the three pot principle, one pot for each of the three ladder stages shown in Figure 31.4, with the extra thought that we should be minimizing NSAID or COXIB exposure, in terms of both drug and duration of prescribing. This is particularly important in chronic pain, where doses may be prescribed over long periods of time and where our patients are often older. The risk of gastrointestinal bleeding increases with age, with increased dose and with longer duration prescribing, so it makes good sense to teach the patient to boost their paracetamol with NSAID if the paracetamol alone is inadequate to deal with a flare of pain, and then to reduce the NSAID and go back to paracetamol alone as soon as that is possible. The standard therapeutic doses of NSAID differ little on the league table of relative efficacy (see Fig. 31.1). Increasing the dose increases the duration of analgesia more than the peak pain relief. The dose–response curves for efficacy are relatively flat, and indeed dose–response curves for adverse effects may be steeper, so that increased dose may increase duration of analgesia (rather than peak pain relief) at the price of increased adverse effect incidence.

Part of the tactic of minimizing NSAID or COXIB exposure is to consider the alternatives in the second ladder stage pot if NSAID are absolutely or relatively contraindicated. Figure 31.5 shows the meta-analytic evidence to support the use of paracetamol opioid combinations, supporting the good performance of a small number of patients given paracetamol 1000 mg with codeine 60 mg (see Fig. 30.1). Fixed-dose combinations are frowned on by the purists because the drugs have disparate kinetics, but by using them either as single tablets or capsules or indeed giving the paracetamol and codeine or other opioid separately, patients can achieve a good balance between efficacy and adverse effects.

We can use the relative efficacy to make these "global" statements about which drug should be in which pot but we are still bedevilled by the fact that these are averages, and everybody is different. Figure 31.6 makes this point powerfully. The percentage of patients achieving different extent of pain relief (percentage of maximum pain relief) is shown for rofecoxib 50 mg, ibuprofen 400 mg and placebo. Lots of patients achieved little relief. A few achieved substantial relief. The average, however, is just over 40% relief. Choice based on the average will be inadequate for many patients.

Another area in which the evidence can be misleading is when attempts are made to compare very different treatment approaches for the same condition. Figure 31.7 shows the efficacy estimates Bjordal et al. calculated for a range of different interventions for osteo-arthritic knee pain [3]. The paper by Bjordal and colleagues examines clinical trials in

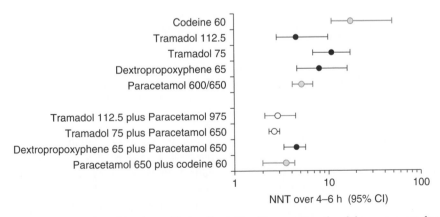

Figure 31.5 Relative efficacy of combinations of "minor" opioids with paracetamol and the component drugs alone. NNT to obtain at least 50% pain relief over 4–6 h: comparison of single-dose oral tramadol and tramadol plus paracetamol with other combination drugs and their components.

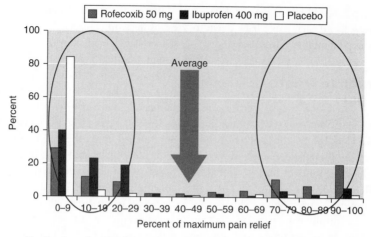

Figure 31.6 Frequency distribution of analgesic response to rofecoxib 50 mg, ibuprofen 400 mg and placebo in postoperative pain.

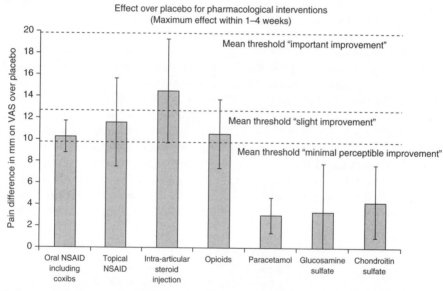

Figure 31.7 Comparison of treatment efficacy for painful osteo-arthritis of the knee. Reprinted from Jan Magnus Bjordal, Atle Klovning, Anne Elisabeth Ljunggren and Lars Slørdal. Short-term efficacy of pharmacotherapeutic interventions in osteoarthritic knee pain: a meta-analysis of randomised placebo-controlled trials. *European Journal of Pain*, **11**, 125-138 Copyright ©2007, with permission from Elsevier.

osteo-arthritic knee pain, and the difference in VAS pain intensity between intervention and placebo after 4 weeks. In 14,000 patients (63 trials) the analysis showed that four treatments (intra-articular steroid injections, oral NSAID including COXIBs, opioids (presumably oral), and topical NSAID) were similar at producing 10–14 mm difference, while others, including paracetamol and glucosamine, produced only 3 mm improvement. Pooling all NSAID and COX-IBs at all doses above specified minima makes it very difficult to say anything about a particular drug or dose. Oral opioids can be different, particularly with regard to dose. Intra-articular injections may or may not contain local anesthetic or agents other than steroid. Some topical NSAIDs are known to work, others not. We are also limited because we have no real

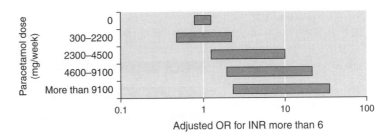

Figure 31.8 Paracetamol and warfarin interaction.

knowledge from this analysis of the sensitivity of these trials, no dose–response for low and high doses of any particular NSAID, for instance, which would give a clear signal that the analysis was capable of showing differences in relative efficacy. We have no such index of internal sensitivity here. The clinical pitfall is that relative efficacy of drugs or other interventions crosses clinical conditions that are too broad, for instance, all postoperative pain or all neuropathic pain, rather than focusing in on a particular situation, context or condition. The clinician may be glad to have the overall relative efficacy but would prefer the information specific to the individual patient in front of them.

There are also additional clinical legitimacy questions of an analysis like this, producing relative efficacy data for a condition which changes over time, whether patients in the trials used in the analysis are like our patients, and whether clinical trials can directly affect clinical practice. For example, a patient who is "satisfied" on paracetamol is unlikely to enrol in a trial, which will therefore recruit paracetamol nonresponders, people for whom paracetamol does not provide sufficient analgesia; paracetamol will then do badly in the trial. Again, efficacy of different treatment approaches will vary according to the point in the disease process when the treatment is tested. Patients may be satisfied with paracetamol at an early phase of their knee arthritis but not later, so testing paracetamol in people with a more advanced condition could produce a negative result. Topical NSAID would be an inappropriate sole treatment for most patients late in the disease when surgery is needed, or in more widespread conditions, but can be very helpful early on when single joints are affected. Therein lies the problem. Neither this nor any other analysis can help us tease out clinically important subtleties. Instead, the authors make the sweeping conclusion "that it is time to reconsider the place of these drug therapies in osteoarthritis of the knee management."

The issue of "lumping" all NSAID doses together crops up too in the adverse effect reviews, for instance with celecoxib [4]. Just like the Bjordal efficacy analysis, which lacks face validity, the adverse effect analysis which lumps doses together deprives us of anything more than phenomenologic data.

Two examples, then, of why we need to think about averaging and its legitimacy. The first is the interaction between paracetamol and warfarin (Fig. 31.8). The analysis by Hylek *et al.* shows a relationship between higher paracetamol doses and greater anti-clotting efficacy of warfarin [5]. The catch is that this relationship was found in those who had higher INR values, so the moral of the story is that the sensitive should avoid high-dose paracetamol if they take warfarin. Once again, we are not all average.

The second example is codeine metabolism. It has been known for many years that roughly 10% of the Caucasian population are "slow" metabolizers of codeine, with demonstrated lower efficacy in experimental pain models. Now there is evidence of ultra-rapid CYP2D6 metabolism. These patients get greater efficacy from a given dose of codeine, with potentially dire consequences [6]. We can glean average values for codeine efficacy from published trials, but at the individual patient level all may not be average.

The choice of which opioid to prescribe is determined more by adverse effects (and custom and practice) than by proven differences in efficacy. Logic would predict that at equi-analgesic doses one opioid is much like another, unless there are quirks in metabolism as in the codeine example above. Between different pain conditions, however, it is worth remembering that opioid efficacy may also be different. Kalso *et al.* drew together trials of opioids in nonmalignant chronic pain [7]. Figure 31.9 shows that on average, the opioid doses required in neuropathic pain syndromes, phantom limb pain, painful diabetic neuropathy and postherpetic neuralgia

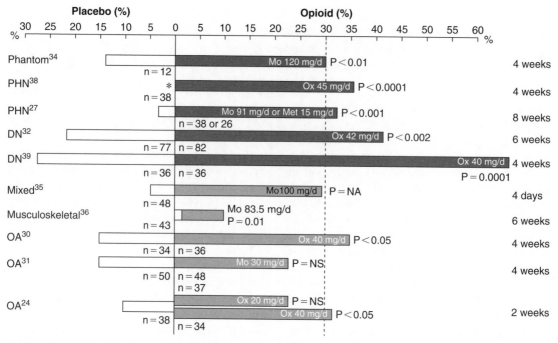

Figure 31.9 Opioid efficacy in nonmalignant pain.

were greater than those needed in musculoskeletal and osteo-arthritic pain. This links back to the old controversy about opioid efficacy in neuropathic pain. The need for quite substantial opioid doses to achieve pain relief in neuropathic pain, doses likely to engender higher adverse effect incidence, is perhaps reflected in the reluctance of some patients to continue on opioids long term.

While the prevalence of opioid adverse effects may be well known, the relative incidence with different opioids at equi-analgesic dose is not. Figure 31.10 shows the adverse effects reported in randomized trials of opioids in nonmalignant pain (34 trials, 5600 patients) [8]. These were mostly 4-week trials with tramadol, paracetamol plus tramadol, codeine or dextropropoxyphene. Few were titrated dosing regimens. What the data do give us is an overall prevalence with step 2 opioids, with little indication of substantial difference between different pain conditions to support the views expressed above. This may reflect the largely fixed-dose nature of the studies. What we lack, then, are data to compare different opioids at equi-analgesic dose in the various pain conditions to see if there are indeed differences in relative adverse

effect incidence. This lack of evidence about differential adverse effect incidence is very relevant to the opioid switching debate. Switching between opioids to improve efficacy with fewer adverse effects is common and empirical. We need better evidence.

Evidence and neuropathic pain numbers

Our focus in testing putative remedies for neuropathic pain has been the two "classic" neuropathic pain conditions, postherpetic neuralgia (PHN) and painful diabetic neuropathy (PDN). The reasoning has probably been that these two conditions present little diagnostic difficulty and trials in PHN and PDN are acceptable to the regulatory authorities.

However, PDN and PHN are not that common. Using the general practice research database (GPRD) for records between January 1992 and April 2002, the incidence per 100,000 person-years observation for PHN was 40 (95% confidence interval (CI) 39–41), for PDN 15 (15–16), for trigeminal neuralgia 27 (26–27), and for phantom limb pain 1 (1–2). Rates decreased over time for PHN and phantom limb pain but were increasing for PDN [9].

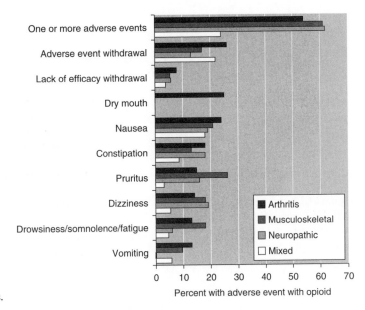

Figure 31.10 Opioids and adverse effects.

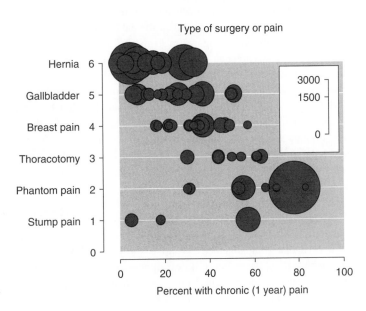

Figure 31.11 Chronic pain after surgery.

One major cause of neuropathic pain is of course back pain, but that is so notoriously diagnostically difficult or heterogeneous that few trials of neuropathic pain remedies are done in back pain. Perhaps the biggest change over recent years has been the recognition that chronic pain after surgery is one of the major causes of neuropathic pain. Figure 31.11 is redrawn from the seminal publication by Perkins & Kehlet [10]. It shows the percentage of people

reporting pain at 1 year after various different types of surgery.

Choosing drugs to treat neuropathic pain

There is perhaps a false sense of security when it comes to talking about the evidence for drug treatments for neuropathic pain. We've all been talking about the

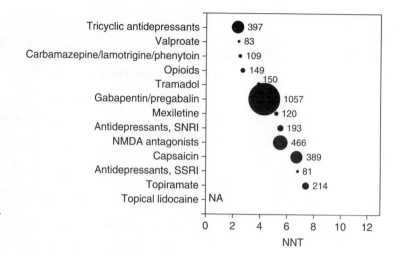

Figure 31.12 Numbers needed to treat (NNT) for different drug treatments for peripheral neuropathic pain.

relative efficacy for a decade now, which is excellent, but sometimes it feels as though we are making too much out of an evidence base which is really not that robust.

This is easy to illustrate by looking at the data used to assemble the treatment algorithm in the influential review by Finnerup *et al.* [11]. Figure 31.12 shows the NNT for different drug treatments for peripheral neuropathic pain. These were derived by taking all the randomized trials which met specified quality standards, and which compared the drug with placebo, and then pooling the data for that particular drug and producing an NNT for at least 50% pain relief compared with placebo. The best performing drugs have the lower NNT values.

The first point to notice in the figure is the absence of any dose information, which leaves the data open to the criticisms made above about lumping all doses for a particular drug together. Second is the lumping together of all drugs (at all doses) in a particular drug class, such as tricyclic antidepressants. Is it really legitimate to combine the data from all the different tricyclic antidepressants, particularly when we know there are differences in responsiveness with the different drugs?

The third point to notice is the numbers just beside each of the dark circles. These numbers tell us how many patients were studied with that drug (or drug class) to derive the NNT. You will notice that some of the numbers are really quite small, for instance 81 for the selective serotonin reuptake inhibitors (SSRI). Within the pain world, there is a dogma that SSRI are

ineffective in the management of neuropathic pain. Many people are surprised when they learn that the dogma is based on just 81 patients studied, and that in one of the trials paroxetine performed as well as imipramine. One trial in which fluoxetine performed badly, and which was widely known, is, I think, the basis of the dogma. It really is not safe to base our conclusions on data from just 81 patients. One small trial in which the drug performs worse than average, or better for that matter, and just by random chance can shift the efficacy estimate, the NNT, disproportionately. The robustness of the efficacy estimate needs data based on many more patients than 81, and ideally 500 or more.

Conclusion

So I am cautious about putting too much emphasis on data which I think are not robust. I question the legitimacy of lumping all doses of a particular drug together, and I question the legitimacy of lumping all drugs (and all doses of all drugs) in a particular drug class together. There comes a point where in the desire to make our work, our guideline or our treatment algorithm look evidence based, we overstretch. As an example, I do not disagree with the conclusion of the Finnerup paper, it is the process that I question.

It seems to me far healthier that we ask for evidence to support our decisions rather than make decisions without evidence. It also seems healthier if we debate the legitimacy of our methodology, and that we acknowledge the shortcomings.

References

1. McQuay HJ. What we have learned about trials from systematic reviews. In: McQuay HJ, Kalso E, Moore RA (eds) *Systematic Reviews in Pain Research: Methodology Refined.* IASP Press, Seattle, WA, 2008.

2. McQuay HJ. Pain ladders, systematic reviews and trials. In: McQuay HJ, Kalso E, Moore RA (eds) *Systematic Reviews in Pain Research: Methodology Refined.* IASP Press, Seattle, WA, 2008.

3. Bjordal JM, Klovning A, Ljunggren AE, Slørdal L. Short-term efficacy of pharmacotherapeutic interventions in osteoarthritic knee pain: a meta-analysis of randomised placebo-controlled trials. *Eur J Pain* 2007; **11**: 125–138.

4. Deeks JJ, Smith LA, Bradley MD. Efficacy, tolerability, and upper gastrointestinal safety of celecoxib for treatment of osteoarthritis and rheumatoid arthritis: systematic review of randomised controlled trials. *BMJ* 2002; **325**: 1–8.

5. Hylek EM, Heiman H, Skates SJ. Acetaminophen and other risk factors for excessive warfarin anticoagulation. *JAMA* 1998; **279**(9): 657–662.

6. Gasche Y, Daali Y, Fathi M, Chiappe A, Cottini S, Dayer P, *et al.* Codeine intoxication associated with ultrarapid CYP2D6 metabolism. *N Engl J Med* 2004; **351**(27): 2827–2831.

7. Kalso E, Edwards JE, Moore RA, McQuay HJ. Opioids in chronic non-cancer pain: systematic review of efficacy and safety. *Pain* 2004; **112**: 372–380.

8. Moore RA, McQuay HJ. Prevalence of opioid adverse events in chronic non-malignant pain: systematic review of randomised trials of oral opioids. *Arthritis Res Ther* 2005; **7**: R1046–R1051.

9. Hall GC, Carroll D, Parry D, McQuay HJ. Epidemiology and treatment of neuropathic pain: The UK primary care perspective. *Pain* 2006; **122**: 156–162.

10. Perkins FM, Kehlet H. Chronic pain as an outcome of surgery. *Anesthesiology* 2000; **93**: 1123–1133.

11. Finnerup N, Otto M, McQuay H, Jensen T, Sindrup S. Algorithm for neuropathic pain treatment: An evidence based proposal. *Pain* 2005; **118**: 289–305.

CHAPTER 32

Complementary therapies for pain relief

Edzard Ernst

Department of Complementary Medicine, Peninsula Medical School, Universities of Exeter and Plymouth, Exeter, UK

Introduction

Complementary/alternative medicine (CAM) can be defined as "diagnosis, treatment and/or prevention which complements mainstream medicine by contributing to a common whole, by satisfying a demand not met by orthodoxy or by diversifying the conceptual frameworks of medicine" [1]. It comprises a wide range of heterogeneous modalities (Table 32.1) which have in common mainly that they are outside conventional medicine and emphasize a holistic approach to healthcare. Surveys from different parts of the world have shown repeatedly that CAM is popular and that pain is one of the most common complaints for which it is employed [2]. This applies in particular for those types of pain which conventional medicine is unable to treat successfully without significant risks.

Effectiveness

This popularity of CAM for pain management begs the question of which CAM modalities are of proven effectiveness for which type of pain [2]. The most reliable answer comes from randomized clinical trials (RCT) or systematic reviews of such studies. We have recently reviewed this evidence for (or against) CAM related to a wide range of pain syndromes [3]. The following is a brief summary of this extensive review. It focuses on conditions for which CAM is used frequently and on those CAM modalities for which

Evidence-Based Chronic Pain Management. Edited by
C. Stannard, E. Kalso and J. Ballantyne. © 2010 Blackwell
Publishing.

the evidence is positive. Sadly, for many therapies the evidence is unconvincing or even negative; for the sake of brevity, these treatments are omitted in the following text and the reader is referred to our original overview [3].

Back pain

Many surveys imply that back pain is the most frequent reason for patients to try CAM [4]. Many therapies have been tested for back problems but frequently the results have been less than convincing. Some of the most encouraging evidence exists for acupuncture [5], the herbal medicine devil's claw (*Hapargophytum procumbens*) [6], massage [7] and spinal manipulation [8]. Unfortunately, there are caveats for all of these: the primary studies are frequently flawed and their results are often contradictory. The bottom line therefore is that no CAM modality has been unequivally shown to be effective for back pain [3].

Cancer pain

The situation is similar for cancer pain. Again, numerous CAM modalities have been submitted to RCT but the findings have not been compelling. The most promising results relate to exercise [9] (which arguably is a conventional form of healthcare) and hypnotherapy [10]. It follows that no CAM modality has been demonstrated to be effective in the management of cancer pain [3].

Complex regional pain syndrome

This condition is often difficult to treat and several CAM options are supported by the results of positive RCT: acupuncture, imagery, massage and qigong [3].

Table 32.1 Some of the most important modalities in CAM

Therapy	Description
Acupuncture	Insertion of a needle into the skin and underlying tissues in special sites, known as points, for therapeutic or preventive purposes
Biofeedback	The use of apparatus to monitor, amplify and feed back information on physiological responses so that a patient can learn to regulate these responses. It is a form of psychophysiologic self-regulation
Chiropractic	A system of healthcare which is based on the belief that the nervous system is the most important determinant of health and that most diseases are caused by spinal subluxations which respond to spinal manipulation
Herbal medicine	The medical use of preparations that contain exclusively plant material
Hypnotherapy	The induction of a trance-like state to facilitate the relaxation of the conscious mind and make use of enhanced suggestibility to treat psychologic and medical conditions and effect behavioral changes
Massage	A method of manipulating the soft tissue of whole body areas using pressure and traction
Osteopathy	Form of manual therapy involving massage, mobilization and spinal manipulation
Relaxation therapy	Techniques for eliciting the "relaxation response" of the autonomic nervous system

Unfortunately, this evidence invariably relies on single, small studies. Therefore independent replication of these results would be required before positive recommendations can be issued.

Fibromyalgia

Survey data suggest that practically all fibromyalgia patients try some form of CAM [11]. A plethora of CAM modalities are being recommended and many have been submitted to RCT [3]. The only treatment for which the evidence is strongly positive is exercise (arguably not a CAM) [12]. For some other therapies the results are encouraging: biofeedback and massage [3]. Due to methodologic weaknesses of the primary studies and the paucity of such data, the evidence is, however, not fully convincing.

Migraine

Biofeedback and relaxation are both supported by strong, positive evidence of effectiveness [13]. Several other CAM modalities have generated promising results. For acupuncture, a sizable number of RCT are available, yet their findings are somewhat contradictory [14]. Feverfew (*Tanacetum parthenium*) may be a herbal preventive of migraine attacks but some RCT fail to support this view [15]. Encouraging results also were reported for co-enzyme Q10 [16] but they require independent confirmation.

Neck pain

Spinal manipulation, massage and acupuncture are commonly used for this condition. The best evidence, however, fails to show that spinal manipulation is effective as a sole intervention [17]. For acupuncture, the evidence is encouraging but not fully convincing [18]. For massage therapy, both positive and negative findings have been reported [3]. Thus no CAM intervention has been proven to be effective for neck pain.

Osteo-arthritis pain

Most patients suffering from this chronic condition try some form of CAM. The RCT evidence is strongly positive for acupuncture [19], for Phytodolor™, a herbal mixture containing *Populus tremula, Fraxinus excelsior* and *Solidago virgaurea* [20], and for S-adenosylmethionine [21]. For many other CAM modalities, the evidence is encouraging but not fully convincing, e.g. balneotherapy, avocado/soybean unsaponifables, devil's claw (*Hapargophytum procumbens*), ginger (*Zingiber officinalis*), topical capsaicin, chondroitin, glucosamine and tai chi [3].

Postoperative pain

The only treatment for which the evidence is strongly positive is TENS [22] (which may not be considered a CAM by many experts) and hypnotherapy [23].

Several other CAM modalities are supported by encouraging evidence which, however, fails to be totally convincing: acupuncture, massage, music therapy and relaxation [3].

Procedural pain

Pain caused by diagnostic or nonsurgical procedures, such as injections, change of dressings, etc., can be effectively alleviated by distraction therapy and hypnotherapy according to unanimous findings from multiple RCT [3]. Other CAM modalities that may be effective but are not supported by equally strong evidence are music therapy and acupuncture [3].

Rheumatoid arthritis

Many CAM interventions have been tested for the management of pain caused by rheumatoid arthritis. Fasting and strict vegetarian diets have been shown to reduce inflammation and thus pain [24]. Other CAM modalities are supported by less conclusive yet encouraging evidence: fish oils supplements [25] and tai chi [26]. Many other CAM interventions have been tested but mostly with less than convincing results [3].

Tennis elbow

This common condition can be difficult to treat with conventional therapies; many patients thus turn to CAM, particularly as most CAM practitioners are confident of being able to treat this condition

effectively. The RCT evidence is, however, not convincing. Only three treatments (acupuncture, joint manipulation and massage) have been submitted to rigorous tests. For none of these is the evidence convincingly positive.

Risks

The popular media frequently portray CAM as natural and therefore free of adverse effects. The reality shows that this is a potentially dangerous misunderstanding. Table 32.2 gives examples of known adverse effects of some popular forms of CAM. Most types of CAM can cause adverse effects which sometimes can be serious [27]. As there is no equivalent of a postmarketing surveillance system for any CAM (with the exception of herbal medicines which are covered by the "yellow card scheme" in the UK), the incidence of serious adverse effects is usually unknown.

In addition to such direct adverse effects, indirect safety issues must be considered. These mostly relate to the behavior of CAM practitioners. For instance, UK nonmedically trained acupuncturists regularly interfere with their patient's drug prescriptions [28] and chiropractors often fail to inform their patients about serious risks of spinal manipulation [29]. The message which seems to emerge here is that a given CAM intervention might be safe but the CAM practitioner administering it might not in all cases be low risk.

Table 32.2 Adverse effects of some popular forms of CAM. Examples of potentially serious, direct adverse effects associated with CAM

Therapy	Adverse effects (example)	Comment
Acupuncture	Puncture of vital organs, infections	Rare with adequately trained therapists, deaths are on record
Chiropractic	50% of patients experience minor adverse effects. Serious complications e.g. vertebral arterial dissections, occur in unknown number of cases	Numerous cases are described. Deaths are on record
Herbalism traditional (e.g. TCM*, Ayurveda)	Intrinsic toxicity (e.g. liver damage), drug interactions, contamination with heavy metals	Nature of adverse effect caused by contaminants depends on contaminant
Herbalism/phytotherapy	Intrinsic toxicity, e.g. liver damage, drug interactions	Frequency of adverse effect depends on remedy, deaths are on record

* TCM = Traditional Chinese Medicine.

Conclusion

Many CAM modalities are currently being promoted and used for pain management. Relatively few have been rigorously tested for effectiveness or safety. Even fewer have been shown beyond reasonable doubt to generate more good than harm. Considering the popularity of CAM and the huge gap in our knowledge about this subject, the inescapable conclusion is that rigorous research is needed with some urgency.

References

1. Ernst E, Resch KL, Mills S, Hill R, Mitchell A, Willoughby M, *et al.* Complementary medicine – a definition. *Br J Gen Pract* 1995; **45**: 506.

2. Ernst E, Pittler MH, Wider B, Boddy K. *The Desktop Guide to Complementary and Alternative Medicine*, 2nd edn. Elsevier Mosby, Edinburgh, 2006.

3. Ernst E, Pittler MH, Wider B, Boddy K. *Complementary Therapies for Pain Management. An Evidence-Based Approach.* Elsevier, London, 2007.

4. Eisenberg D, David RB, Ettner SL, Appel S, Wilkey S, van Rompay M, *et al.* Trends in alternative medicine use in the United States; 1990–1997. *JAMA* 1998; **280**: 1569–1575.

5. Manheimer E, White A, Berman B, Ernst E. Meta-analysis: acupuncture for low back pain. *Ann Intern Med* 2005; **142**: 651–663.

6. Gagnier JJ, Chrubasik S, Manheimer E. Harpagophytum procumbens for osteoarthritis and low back pain: a systematic review. *BMC Compl Alt Med* 2004; **4** : 13.

7. Furlan AD, Brosseau L, Imamura M, Irvin E. Massage for low-back pain: a systematic review within the framework of the Cochrane Collaboration Back Review Group. *Spine* 2002; **27**: 1896–1910.

8. Assendelft WJJ, Morton SC, Yu EI, Suttorp MJ, Shekelle PG. Spinal manipulative therapy for low-backpain. Cochrane Database of Systematic Reviews 2004, Issue 1. Art No.: CD000447.pub2. DOI: 10.1002/14651858.CD000447. pub2. 2004.

9. Dimeo F. Welche Rolle spielt körperliche Aktivität in der Prävention, Therapie und Rehabilitation von neoplastischen Erkrankungen? *Deutsche Zeitschr Sportmed* 2004; **55**: 177–182.

10. Rajasekaran M, Edmonds PM, Higginson IL. Systematic review of hypnotherapy for treating symptoms in terminally ill adult cancer patients. *Palliat Med* 2005; **19**:418–426.

11. Pioro-Boisset M, Esdaile JM, Fitzcharles M-A. Alternative medicine use in fibromyalgia syndrome. *Arthritis Care Res* 1996; **9**: 13–17.

12. Busch AJ, Barber KA, Overend TJ, Peloso PMJ, Schachter CL. Exercise for treating fibromyalgia syndrome. Cochrane Database of Systematic Reviews 2007, Issue 4. Art. No.: CD003786. DOI: 10.1002/14651858.CD003786.pub2.

13. Holroyd KA, Penzien DB. Pharmacological versus non-pharmacological prophylaxis of recurrent migraine headache: a meta-analytic review of clinical trials. *Pain* 1990; **42**: 1–13.

14. Melchart D, Linde K, Fischer P, Berman B, White A, Vickers A, *et al.* Acupuncture for idiopathic headache. Cochrane Database of Systematic Reviews 2001, Issue 1, Art No: CD001218. 2001.

15. Pittler MH, Ernst E. Feverfew for preventing migraine. Cochrane Database of Systematic Reviews 2004, Issue 1. Art. No.: CD002286. DOI: 10.1002/14651858.CD002286.pub2.

16. Sándor PS, di Clemente L, Coppola G, Saenger U, Magis D, Seidel L, *et al.* Efficacy of coenzyme Q10 in migraine prophylaxis: a randomised controlled trial. *Neurology* 2005; **64**: 713–715.

17. Gross AR, Hoving JL, Haines TA, Goldsmith CH, Kay T, Aker P, *et al.* A Cochrane review of manipulation and mobilization for mechanical neck disorders. *Spine* 2004; **29**: 1541–1548.

18. White AR, Ernst E. A systematic review of randomized controlled trials of acupuncture for neck pain. *Rheumatology* 1999; **38**:143–147.

19. Kwon YD, Pittler MH, Ernst E. Acupuncture for peripheral joint osteoarthritis: a systematic review and meta-analysis. *Rheumatology (Oxford)* 2006; **45**(11): 1331–1337.

20. Long L. Herbal medicines for the treatment of osteoarthritis a systematic review. *Rheumatology* 2001; **40**: 779–793.

21. Soeken KL, Lee WL, Bausell RB, Agelli M, Berman BM. Safety and efficacy of S-adenosylmethionine (SAMe) for osteoarthritis. *J Fam Pract* 2002; **51**(5): 425–430.

22. Bjordal JM, Johnson MI, Ljunggreen AE. Transcutaneous electrical nerve stimulation (TENS) can reduce postoperative analgesic consumption. A meta-analysis with assessment of optimal treatment parameters for postoperative pain. *Eur J Pain* 2003; **7**(2): 181–188.

23. Mongomery GH, David D, Winkel G, Silverstein JH, Bovbjerg DH. The effectiveness of adjunctive hypnosis with surgical patients: a meta-analysis. *Anesth Analg* 2002; **94**:1639–1645.

24. Müller H, de Toledo FW, Resch KL. Fasting followed by vegetarian diet in patients with rheumatoid arthritis: a systematic review. *Scand J Rheumatol* 2001; **30**: 1–10.

25. Fortin PR, Lew RA, Liang MH, Wright EA, Beckett LA, Chalmers TC, *et al.* Validation of a meta-analysis: the effects of fish oil in rheumatoid arthritis. *J Clin Epidemiol* 1995; **48**: 1379–1390.

26. Han A, Judd M, Welch V, Wu T, Tugwell P, Wells GA. Tai chi for treating rheumatoid arthritis. Cochrane Database of Systematic Reviews 2004, Issue 3. Art. No.: CD004849. DOI: 10.1002/14651858.CD004849.

27. Ernst E. Complementary and alternative medicine. In: Dukes MNG (ed) *Meyler's Side Effects of Drugs,* vols 2 and 3. Elsevier, Edinburgh, 2006.

28. MacPherson H, Scullion A, Thomas KJ, Walters S. Patient reports of adverse events associated with acupuncture treatment: a prospective national survey. *Qual Saf Health Care* 2004; **13**: 348–355.

29. Langworthy JM, Le Fleming C. Consent or submission? The practice of consent within UK chiropractic. *J Manipul Physiol Ther* 2005; **28**: 15–24.

Index